Chronic Fatigue Syndrome/Myalgic Encephalomyelitis: Diagnosis and Treatment

Chronic Fatigue Syndrome/Myalgic Encephalomyelitis: Diagnosis and Treatment

Editors

Giovanni Ricevuti
Lorenzo Lorusso

MDPI • Basel • Beijing • Wuhan • Barcelona • Belgrade • Manchester • Tokyo • Cluj • Tianjin

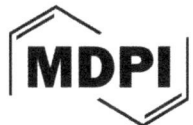

Editors
Giovanni Ricevuti
University of Pavia
Italy

Lorenzo Lorusso
ASST Lecco
Italy

Editorial Office
MDPI
St. Alban-Anlage 66
4052 Basel, Switzerland

This is a reprint of articles from the Special Issue published online in the open access journal *Journal of Clinical Medicine* (ISSN 2077-0383) (available at: https://www.mdpi.com/journal/jcm/special_issues/Chronic_Fatigue).

For citation purposes, cite each article independently as indicated on the article page online and as indicated below:

LastName, A.A.; LastName, B.B.; LastName, C.C. Article Title. *Journal Name* **Year**, *Volume Number*, Page Range.

ISBN 978-3-0365-5969-8 (Hbk)
ISBN 978-3-0365-5970-4 (PDF)

© 2023 by the authors. Articles in this book are Open Access and distributed under the Creative Commons Attribution (CC BY) license, which allows users to download, copy and build upon published articles, as long as the author and publisher are properly credited, which ensures maximum dissemination and a wider impact of our publications.

The book as a whole is distributed by MDPI under the terms and conditions of the Creative Commons license CC BY-NC-ND.

Contents

Lorenzo Lorusso and Giovanni Ricevuti
Special Issue "Chronic Fatigue Syndrome/Myalgic Encephalomyelitis: Diagnosis and Treatment"
Reprinted from: *J. Clin. Med.* 2022, 11, 4563, doi:10.3390/jcm11154563 1

Jessica Van Oosterwijck, Uros Marusic, Inge De Wandele, Mira Meeus, Lorna Paul, Luc Lambrecht, et al.
Reduced Parasympathetic Reactivation during Recovery from Exercise in Myalgic Encephalomyelitis/Chronic Fatigue Syndrome
Reprinted from: *J. Clin. Med.* 2021, 10, 4527, doi:10.3390/jcm10194527 5

Jesús Castro-Marrero, Mario Zacares, Eloy Almenar-Pérez, José Alegre-Martín and Elisa Oltra
Complement Component C1q as a Potential Diagnostic Tool for Myalgic Encephalomyelitis/Chronic Fatigue Syndrome Subtyping
Reprinted from: *J. Clin. Med.* 2021, 10, 4171, doi:10.3390/jcm10184171 25

Juan Rodríguez-Mansilla, Abel Mejías-Gil, Elisa María Garrido-Ardila, María Jiménez-Palomares, Jesús Montanero-Fernández and María Victoria González-López-Arza
Effects of Non-Pharmacological Treatment on Pain, Flexibility, Balance and Quality of Life in Women with Fibromyalgia: A Randomised Clinical Trial
Reprinted from: *J. Clin. Med.* 2021, 10, 3826, doi:10.3390/jcm10173826 39

Helma Freitag, Marvin Szklarski, Sebastian Lorenz, Franziska Sotzny, Sandra Bauer, Aurélie Philippe, et al.
Autoantibodies to Vasoregulative G-Protein-Coupled Receptors Correlate with Symptom Severity, Autonomic Dysfunction and Disability in Myalgic Encephalomyelitis/Chronic Fatigue Syndrome
Reprinted from: *J. Clin. Med.* 2021, 10, 3675, doi:10.3390/jcm10163675 55

Elisha K. Josev, Rebecca C. Cole, Adam Scheinberg, Katherine Rowe, Lionel Lubitz and Sarah J. Knight
Health, Wellbeing, and Prognosis of Australian Adolescents with Myalgic Encephalomyelitis/Chronic Fatigue Syndrome (ME/CFS): A Case-Controlled Follow-Up Study
Reprinted from: *J. Clin. Med.* 2021, 10, 3603, doi:10.3390/jcm10163603 69

Ramón Martín-Brufau, Manuel Nombela Gómez, Leyre Sanchez-Sanchez-Rojas and Cristina Nombela
Fibromyalgia Detection Based on EEG Connectivity Patterns
Reprinted from: *J. Clin. Med.* 2021, 10, 3277, doi:10.3390/jcm10153277 87

Ingrid H. Baklund, Toril Dammen, Torbjørn Åge Moum, Wenche Kristiansen, Daysi Sosa Duarte, Jesus Castro-Marrero, et al.
Evaluating Routine Blood Tests According to Clinical Symptoms and Diagnostic Criteria in Individuals with Myalgic Encephalomyelitis/Chronic Fatigue Syndrome
Reprinted from: *J. Clin. Med.* 2021, 10, 3105, doi:10.3390/jcm10143105 101

Diana Araja, Uldis Berkis, Asja Lunga and Modra Murovska
Shadow Burden of Undiagnosed Myalgic Encephalomyelitis/Chronic Fatigue Syndrome (ME/CFS) on Society: Retrospective and Prospective—In Light of COVID-19
Reprinted from: *J. Clin. Med.* 2021, 10, 3017, doi:10.3390/jcm10143017 115

Carmen Scheibenbogen, Franziska Sotzny, Jelka Hartwig, Sandra Bauer, Helma Freitag, Kirsten Wittke, et al.
Tolerability and Efficacy of s.c. IgG Self-Treatment in ME/CFS Patients with IgG/IgG Subclass Deficiency: A Proof-of-Concept Study
Reprinted from: *J. Clin. Med.* **2021**, *10*, 2420, doi:10.3390/jcm10112420 133

Sławomir Kujawski, Joanna Słomko, Lynette Hodges, Derek F. H. Pheby, Modra Murovska, Julia L. Newton and Paweł Zalewski
Post-Exertional Malaise May Be Related to Central Blood Pressure, Sympathetic Activity and Mental Fatigue in Chronic Fatigue Syndrome Patients
Reprinted from: *J. Clin. Med.* **2021**, *10*, 2327, doi:10.3390/jcm10112327 147

Sławomir Kujawski, Jo Cossington, Joanna Słomko, Monika Zawadka-Kunikowska, Małgorzata Tafil-Klawe, Jacek J. Klawe, et al.
Relationship between Cardiopulmonary, Mitochondrial and Autonomic Nervous System Function Improvement after an Individualised Activity Programme upon Chronic Fatigue Syndrome Patients
Reprinted from: *J. Clin. Med.* **2021**, *10*, 1542, doi:10.3390/jcm10071542 159

Alvaro Murillo-Garcia, Juan Luis Leon-Llamas, Santos Villafaina, Paloma Rohlfs-Dominguez and Narcis Gusi
MoCA vs. MMSE of Fibromyalgia Patients: The Possible Role of Dual-Task Tests in Detecting Cognitive Impairment
Reprinted from: *J. Clin. Med.* **2021**, *10*, 125, doi:10.3390/jcm10010125 177

Angelica Varesi, Undine-Sophie Deumer, Sanjana Ananth and Giovanni Ricevuti
The Emerging Role of Gut Microbiota in Myalgic Encephalomyelitis/Chronic Fatigue Syndrome (ME/CFS): Current Evidence and Potential Therapeutic Applications
Reprinted from: *J. Clin. Med.* **2021**, *10*, 5077, doi:10.3390/jcm10215077 187

Undine-Sophie Deumer, Angelica Varesi, Valentina Floris, Gabriele Savioli, Elisa Mantovani, Paulina López-Carrasco, et al.
Myalgic Encephalomyelitis/Chronic Fatigue Syndrome (ME/CFS): An Overview
Reprinted from: *J. Clin. Med.* **2021**, *10*, 4786, doi:10.3390/jcm10204786 205

Eun-Jin Lim and Chang-Gue Son
Prevalence of Chronic Fatigue Syndrome (CFS) in Korea and Japan: A Meta-Analysis
Reprinted from: *J. Clin. Med.* **2021**, *10*, 3204, doi:10.3390/jcm10153204 227

Eun-Jin Lim, Eun-Bum Kang, Eun-Su Jang and Chang-Gue Son
The Prospects of the Two-Day Cardiopulmonary Exercise Test (CPET) in ME/CFS Patients: A Meta-Analysis
Reprinted from: *J. Clin. Med.* **2020**, *9*, 4040, doi:10.3390/jcm9124040 235

Do-Young Kim, Jin-Seok Lee and Chang-Gue Son
Systematic Review of Primary Outcome Measurements for Chronic Fatigue Syndrome/Myalgic Encephalomyelitis (CFS/ME) in Randomized Controlled Trials
Reprinted from: *J. Clin. Med.* **2020**, *9*, 3463, doi:10.3390/jcm9113463 249

Salvatore Chirumbolo, Luigi Valdenassi, Marianno Franzini, Sergio Pandolfi, Giovanni Ricevuti and Umberto Tirelli
Male vs. Female Differences in Responding to Oxygen–Ozone Autohemotherapy (O_2-O_3-AHT) in Patients with Myalgic Encephalomyelitis/Chronic Fatigue Syndrome (ME/CFS)
Reprinted from: *J. Clin. Med.* **2022**, *11*, 173, doi:10.3390/jcm11010173 261

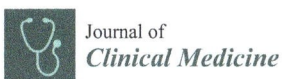

Editorial

Special Issue "Chronic Fatigue Syndrome/Myalgic Encephalomyelitis: Diagnosis and Treatment"

Lorenzo Lorusso [1,*] and Giovanni Ricevuti [2,*]

1. Neuroloy and Stroke Unit, Neuroscience Department, A.S.S.T.-Lecco, 23807 Merate, Italy
2. Department of Drug Sciences, School of Pharmacy, University of Pavia, 27100 Pavia, Italy
* Correspondence: l.lorusso@asst-lecco.it (L.L.); giovanni.ricevuti@unipv.it (G.R.)

Chronic fatigue syndrome, or myalgic encephalomyelitis (CFS/ME), is a debilitating disease with unknown causes that is more common in women and tends to develop between patients' mid-20s and mid-40s. From the perspectives on the etiology and pathophysiology, CFS/ME has been labeled differently, which has influenced changes in case definitions and terminologies. CFS/ME is characterized by persistent asthenia with associated musculoskeletal pain, cognitive disturbance (including attention, memory, and concentration), psychological troubles (depression, anxiety), sleep disorders, and a variety of neurovegetative symptoms. The best appropriate therapeutic is an integrative approach, based on a personalized medical plane that includes distinct groups of procedures: educational, cognitive-behavioral, pharmacological and non-pharmacological such as occupational therapy and rehabilitation. CFS/ME has some common clinical features with fibromyalgia, and a differential diagnosis is difficult for General Practitioners (GPs) [1,2].

The recent opinion is that CFS/ME pathogenesis is dependent on several factors or causes. Different studies have shown evidence for an alteration in immunity system in patients with CFS/ME. A modification in cytokine subsets, a diminished activity of natural killer (NK) lymphocytes, the detection of autoantibodies and a decreased response of T cells to mitogens and specific antigens have been observed. An increased level of pro-inflammatory cytokines may explain some of the clinical features, such as fatigue and flulike symptoms, with an effect on NK activity. Anomalous activation of the T lymphocyte profile and a reduction in antibody-dependent cell-mediated cytotoxicity have been reported. An increased number of CD8+ cytotoxic T lymphocytes and CD38 and HLA-DR activation markers have been demonstrated, and a reduced CD11b expression associated with an increased expression of CD28+ T subsets has been described [3]. An interest towards CFS/ME is increased with the recent pandemic by SARS-CoV-2 because, after the acute phase of disease, some patients have clinical features similar to CFS/ME called Long-COVID, characterized by tiredness, brain fog and headache. There is debate on common aspect between these pathologies but in especially a possible effect of COVID-19 on CFS/ME and the consequences [4].

This Special Issue on CFS/ME collects 18 papers with an interdisciplinary view on the current demographic and epidemiological data and immunological characteristics of CFS/ME and examines the different pathogenic hypotheses, as well as giving information about the latest knowledge on diagnostic investigations, pharmacological, integrative, physical, cognitive-behavioral and psychological curative approaches.

It is known that CFS/ME affects young adults, but there are little studies in pediatric and adolescent age. Australian colleagues Elisha K. Josev and colleagues have carried out a case-controlled follow-up study on the health, wellbeing and prognosis of Australian adolescents with CFS/ME on the comprehension of the important relation between physical and psychological health factors to adolescent' long-term outcome for approaching future prevention, management and treatment [5]. Concerning epidemiological data, there

Citation: Lorusso, L.; Ricevuti, G. Special Issue "Chronic Fatigue Syndrome/Myalgic Encephalomyelitis: Diagnosis and Treatment". *J. Clin. Med.* 2022, 11, 4563. https://doi.org/10.3390/jcm11154563

Received: 19 April 2022
Accepted: 2 August 2022
Published: 4 August 2022

Publisher's Note: MDPI stays neutral with regard to jurisdictional claims in published maps and institutional affiliations.

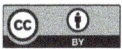

Copyright: © 2022 by the authors. Licensee MDPI, Basel, Switzerland. This article is an open access article distributed under the terms and conditions of the Creative Commons Attribution (CC BY) license (https://creativecommons.org/licenses/by/4.0/).

is little information for Asian countries such Korea and Japan. Eun-Jn Lim and Chang-Gue Son evaluate and match the prevalence of CFS/ME in Korea and Japan, performing a meta-analysis analyzing the main characteristics of these nations [6]. The emerging data of the involvement of immune system confirmed the hypothesis that CFS/ME is an autoimmune disease; recent studies have shown the role of autoantibodies towards the vegetative nervous system. Freitag H. and colleagues reported the reactivity of autoantibodies to vasoregulative G-Protein-Coupled Receptor correlates with autonomic dysfunction, clinical gravity and disability in CFS/ME patients [7]. Another paper, by Kujawski S. and collaborators, studies the differences in CFS patients applying post-exertional malaise (PEM) as indicators of aortic stiffness, autonomic nervous system function and severity of fatigue [8]. Always on the role of the autonomic nervous system dysfunction, Jessica Van Oosterwijck et al. published a paper showing decreased parasympathetic reactivation from physical exercise that could be correlated with a bad prognosis or high risk for adverse cardiac event [8]. Varesi A. and colleagues investigated the emerging role of the modified composition of gut microbiota in relationship with genetic, infection, immunological and other influences that have seen in CFS/ME individuals [9]. The authors discuss the change and the potential therapeutic application of treating the gut in CFS/ME patients [10].

A collection of papers investigates the importance of the diagnostic tools in clinical practice. We start with Baklund H. I. et al., who evaluated the blood test in relationship with clinical features and diagnostic classification, suggesting muscle damage and metabolic abnormalities [11].

A potential blood diagnostic tool, by Castro-Marrero J. and his Spanish collaborators, could be the complement C1 examining in CFS/ME three-symptom clusters, identified as severe, moderate and mild, presenting important differences in five blood parameters [12]. Another objective measurement for PEM, which is a hallmark of CFS/ME, is the application of the two-days cardiopulmonary exercise test (CPET) to assess functional impairment: Eun-Jin Lim and Korean collaborators, in their paper, published the results of a meta-analysis on this diagnostic tool [13]. Moreover, Do-Young Kim and his Korean colleagues examined a systematic review to provide an overview of the adoption of the main measurements in RCTs for CFS/ME. Around 40% of RCTs utilized multiple primary measurements. This information could be helpful in clinical practice in the design of medical studies for CFS/ME-linked therapeutic development [14].

The therapy of CFS/ME is problematic due to lack of knowledge on the etiopathogenesis of this disease, with application of the unconventional and conventional treatments: Tirelli and colleagues compared the application of oxygen–ozone autohemotherapy (O_2-O_3-AHT) in male vs. female patients, evaluating the differences in their responses to this approach [15]. The effects of exercise from a structured activity program have been disputed; Kujawski S. et al., with a multidisciplinary study, examined the impact of a personalized program of activities associated with cardiovascular, mitochondrial and fatigue parameters, showing a reduction in fatigue and an improving functional performance [16]. An important conventional therapeutic approach is the effect of s.c. IgG self-treatment in ME/CFS patients with IgG/IgG subgroup deficiency. The aim of Scheibenbogen C. and her German collaborators was to study the IgG administration for its immunomodulatory effects. [17].

There are few studies relationship CFS/ME patients and COVID-19 patients [18]. Araja D. and Latvian collaborators researched undiagnosed CFS/ME patients, hypothesizing the expansion of post-viral CFS as an effect of COVID-19 and its social impact. The Latvian research results show that patients with CFS/ME are not a risk group for COVID-19; however, COVID-19 causes symptoms similar to CFS/ME. They concluded that CFS/ME creates a significant social consequence, considering the direct medical costs of undiagnosed patients. At the same time, COVID-19 is responsible for long-lasting complications and a chronic course, such as post-viral CFS [19].

Deumer U-S et al. discuss the role of the gut microbiota on disease progression, highlighting a potential biomarker in non-coding RNA (ncRNA) as a probable diagnostic tool and suggesting the possibility that SARS-CoV-2 infection may result in symptoms similar to CFS [20].

CFS/ME has an overlap with Fibromyalgia, and differential diagnosis is difficult for some clinicians because the diagnosis of fibromyalgia is based only on clinical features that are characterized by widespread pain, fatigue, stiffness and troubles in cognitive functions, such as attention, executive function and verbal memory deficits [21]. It is important to add more tests beyond the Mini-Mental State Examination (MMSE) and the Montreal Cognitive Assessment (MoCA) test in fibromyalgia patients to assess the relationship between physical and cognitive performance, as reported by Murillo-Garcia A. and colleagues [22]. Another potential diagnostic tool is studied by Martin-Brufau R. and collaborators using electroencephalography for patients with fibromyalgia that present lower levels of brain activity with reduced connectivity than controls. The Spanish group identified a possible neurophysiological pattern that could adapt to the clinical features of the disease [23]. The therapeutic approach to this disease is a difficult choice. Rodriguez-Mansilla J. and Spanish collaborators studied the effects of non-pharmacological treatment in terms of the effectiveness of an exercise program compared to wellness activities by improving pain, flexibility, static balance, perceived effort and quality of life in patients with fibromyalgia. Participants in the active exercise program performed better than exercise for well-being [24]. This proposal in fibromyalgia is associated with other conventional treatments based on a multidisciplinary approach.

In conclusion, the papers published within this research topic, with the major contribution of the members of the European Network on Myalgic Encephalomyelitis/Chronic Fatigue Syndrome (EUROMENE), give us the recent highlight perspective and opportunities for the discovery and development of possible specific biomarkers, diagnostic and therapeutic approaches for these immunological disorders.

Funding: This research received no external funding.

Conflicts of Interest: The authors declare no conflict of interest.

References

1. Nacul, L.; Authier, F.J.; Scheibenbogen, C.; Lorusso, L.; Helland, I.B.; Martin, J.A.; Sirbu, C.A.; Mengshoel, A.M.; Polo, O.; Behrends, U.; et al. European Network on Myalgic Encephalomyelitis/Chronic Fatigue Syndrome (EUROMENE): Expert Consensus on the Diagnosis, Service Provision, and Care of People with ME/CFS in Europe. *Medicina* **2021**, *57*, 510. [CrossRef] [PubMed]
2. Pheby, D.F.H.; Araja, D.; Berkis, U.; Brenna, E.; Cullinan, J.; de Korwin, J.-D.; Gitto, L.; Hughes, D.A.; Hunter, R.M.; Trepel, D.; et al. A Literature Review of GP Knowledge and Understanding of ME/CFS: A Report from the Socioeconomic Working Group of the European Network on ME/CFS (EUROMENE). *Medicina* **2020**, *57*, 7. [CrossRef] [PubMed]
3. Sotzny, F.; Blanco, J.; Capelli, E.; Castro-Marrero, J.; Steiner, S.; Murovska, M.; Scheibenbogen, C.; European Network on ME/CFS (EUROMENE). Myalgic Encephalomyelitis/Chronic Fatigue Syndrome—Evidence for an autoimmune disease. *Autoimmun. Rev.* **2018**, *17*, 601–609. [CrossRef]
4. White, P. Long COVID: Don't consign ME/CFS to history. *Nature* **2020**, *587*, 197. [CrossRef]
5. Josev, E.K.; Cole, R.C.; Scheinberg, A.; Rowe, K.; Lubitz, L.; Knight, S.J. Health, Wellbeing, and Prognosis of Australian Adolescents with Myalgic Encephalomyelitis/Chronic Fatigue Syndrome (ME/CFS): A Case-Controlled Follow-Up Study. *J. Clin. Med.* **2021**, *10*, 3603. [CrossRef] [PubMed]
6. Lim, E.-J.; Son, C.-G. Prevalence of Chronic Fatigue Syndrome (CFS) in Korea and Japan: A Meta-Analysis. *J. Clin. Med.* **2021**, *10*, 3204. [CrossRef]
7. Freitag, H.; Szklarski, M.; Lorenz, S.; Sotzny, F.; Bauer, S.; Philippe, A.; Kedor, C.; Grabowski, P.; Lange, T.; Riemekasten, G.; et al. Autoantibodies to Vasoregulative G-Protein-Coupled Receptors Correlate with Symptom Severity, Autonomic Dysfunction and Disability in Myalgic Encephalomyelitis/Chronic Fatigue Syndrome. *J. Clin. Med.* **2021**, *10*, 3675. [CrossRef]
8. Kujawski, S.; Słomko, J.; Hodges, L.; Pheby, D.F.H.; Murovska, M.; Newton, J.L.; Zalewski, P. Post-Exertional Malaise May Be Related to Central Blood Pressure, Sympathetic Activity and Mental Fatigue in Chronic Fatigue Syndrome Patients. *J. Clin. Med.* **2021**, *10*, 2327. [CrossRef]
9. Lupo, G.F.D.; Rocchetti, G.; Lucini, L.; Lorusso, L.; Manara, E.; Bertelli, M.; Puglisi, E.; Capelli, E. Potential role of microbiome in Chronic Fatigue Syndrome/Myalgic Encephalomyelits (CFS/ME). *Sci. Rep.* **2021**, *11*, 7043. [CrossRef]
10. Varesi, A.; Deumer, U.-S.; Ananth, S.; Ricevuti, G. The Emerging Role of Gut Microbiota in Myalgic Encephalomyelitis/Chronic Fatigue Syndrome (ME/CFS): Current Evidence and Potential Therapeutic Applications. *J. Clin. Med.* **2021**, *10*, 5077. [CrossRef]

11. Baklund, I.H.; Dammen, T.; Moum, T.Å.; Kristiansen, W.; Duarte, D.S.; Castro-Marrero, J.; Helland, I.B.; Strand, E.B. Evaluating routine blood tests according to clinical symptoms and diagnostic criteria in individuals with Myalgic Encephalomyelitis/Chronic Fatigue Syndrome. *J. Clin. Med.* **2021**, *10*, 3105. [CrossRef] [PubMed]
12. Castro-Marrero, J.; Zacares, M.; Almenar-Pérez, E.; Alegre-Martín, J.; Oltra, E. Complement Component C1q as a Potential Diagnostic Tool for Myalgic Encephalomyelitis/Chronic Fatigue Syndrome Subtyping. *J. Clin. Med.* **2021**, *10*, 4171. [CrossRef] [PubMed]
13. Lim, E.-J.; Kang, E.-B.; Jang, E.-S.; Son, C.-G. The Prospects of the Two-Day Cardiopulmonary Exercise Test (CPET) in ME/CFS Patients: A Meta-Analysis. *J. Clin. Med.* **2020**, *9*, 4040. [CrossRef] [PubMed]
14. Kim, D.-Y.; Lee, J.-S.; Son, C.-G. Systematic Review of Primary Outcome Measurements for Chronic Fatigue Syndrome/Myalgic Encephalomyelitis (CFS/ME) in Randomized Controlled Trials. *J. Clin. Med.* **2020**, *9*, 3463. [CrossRef]
15. Chirumbolo, S.; Valdenassi, L.; Franzini, M.; Pandolfi, S.; Ricevuti, G.; Tirelli, U. Male vs. Female Differences in Responding to Oxygen–Ozone Autohemotherapy (O_2-O_3-AHT) in Patients with Myalgic Encephalomyelitis/Chronic Fatigue Syndrome (ME/CFS). *J. Clin. Med.* **2021**, *11*, 173. [CrossRef]
16. Kujawski, S.; Cossington, J.; Słomko, J.; Zawadka-Kunikowska, M.; Tafil-Klawe, M.; Klawe, J.J.; Buszko, K.; Jakovljevic, D.G.; Kozakiewicz, M.; Morten, K.J.; et al. Relationship between Cardiopulmonary, Mitochondrial and Autonomic Nervous System Function Improvement after an Individualised Activity Programme upon Chronic Fatigue Syndrome Patients. *J. Clin. Med.* **2021**, *10*, 1542. [CrossRef]
17. Scheibenbogen, C.; Sotzny, F.; Hartwig, J.; Bauer, S.; Freitag, H.; Wittke, K.; Doehner, W.; Scherbakov, N.; Loebel, M.; Grabowski, P. Tolerability and Efficacy of s.c. IgG Self-Treatment in ME/CFS Patients with IgG/IgG Subclass Deficiency: A Proof-of-Concept Study. *J. Clin. Med.* **2021**, *10*, 2420. [CrossRef]
18. Jason, L.A.; Islam, M.F.; Conroy, K.; Cotler, J.; Torres, C.; Johnson, M.; Mabie, B. COVID-19 symptoms over time: Comparing long-haulers to ME/CFS. *Fatigue* **2021**, *9*, 59–68. [CrossRef]
19. Araja, D.; Berkis, U.; Lunga, A.; Murovska, M. Shadow Burden of Undiagnosed Myalgic Encephalomyelitis/Chronic Fatigue Syndrome (ME/CFS) on Society: Retrospective and Prospective—In Light of COVID-19. *J. Clin. Med.* **2021**, *10*, 3017. [CrossRef]
20. Deumer, U.-S.; Varesi, A.; Floris, V.; Savioli, G.; Mantovani, E.; López-Carrasco, P.; Rosati, G.M.; Prasad, S.; Ricevuti, G. Myalgic Encephalomyelitis/Chronic Fatigue Syndrome (ME/CFS): An Overview. *J. Clin. Med.* **2021**, *10*, 4786. [CrossRef]
21. Mckay, P.G.; Walker, H.; Martin, C.R.; Fleming, M. Exploratory study into the relationship between the symptoms of chronic fatigue syndrome (CFS)/myalgic encephalomyelitis (ME) and fibromyalgia (FM) using a quasiexperimental design. *BMJ Open* **2021**, *11*, e041947. [CrossRef] [PubMed]
22. Murillo-Garcia, A.; Leon-Llamas, J.L.; Villafaina, S.; Rohlfs-Dominguez, P.; Gusi, N. MoCA vs. MMSE of Fibromyalgia Patients: The Possible Role of Dual-Task Tests in Detecting Cognitive Impairment. *J. Clin. Med.* **2021**, *10*, 125. [CrossRef] [PubMed]
23. Martín-Brufau, R.; Gómez, M.N.; Sanchez-Sanchez-Rojas, L.; Nombela, C. Fibromyalgia Detection Based on EEG Connectivity Patterns. *J. Clin. Med.* **2021**, *10*, 3277. [CrossRef] [PubMed]
24. Rodríguez-Mansilla, J.; Mejías-Gil, A.; Garrido-Ardila, E.M.; Jiménez-Palomares, M.; Montanero-Fernández, J.; González-López-Arza, M.V. Effects of Non-Pharmacological Treatment on Pain, Flexibility, Balance and Quality of Life in Women with Fibromyalgia: A Randomised Clinical Trial. *J. Clin. Med.* **2021**, *10*, 3826. [CrossRef]

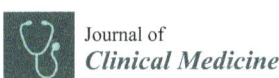

Article

Reduced Parasympathetic Reactivation during Recovery from Exercise in Myalgic Encephalomyelitis/Chronic Fatigue Syndrome

Jessica Van Oosterwijck [1,2,*,†], Uros Marusic [3,4], Inge De Wandele [2], Mira Meeus [2,5,†], Lorna Paul [6], Luc Lambrecht [7], Greta Moorkens [8], Lieven Danneels [2] and Jo Nijs [1,9,†]

1. Departments of Physiotherapy, Human Physiology and Anatomy, Vrije Universiteit Brussel, 1090 Brussels, Belgium; jo.nijs@vub.ac.be
2. Spine, Head and Pain Research Unit Ghent, Department of Rehabilitation Sciences, Faculty of Medicine and Health Sciences, Ghent University, Campus UZ Ghent, Corneel Heymanslaan 10, B3, 9000 Ghent, Belgium; Inge.DeWandele@UGent.be (I.D.W.); mira.meeus@ugent.be (M.M.); lieven.danneels@ugent.be (L.D.)
3. Institute for Kinesiology Research, Science and Research Centre Koper, 6000 Koper, Slovenia; uros.marusic@zrs-kp.si
4. Department of Health Sciences, Alma Mater Europaea—ECM, 2000 Maribor, Slovenia
5. Department of Rehabilitation Sciences and Physiotherapy, Faculty of Medicine and Health Sciences, University of Antwerp, 2610 Antwerp, Belgium
6. Nursing and Health Care, School of Medicine, University of Glasgow, Glasgow G12 8LL, UK; Lorna.Paul@glasgow.ac.uk
7. Medical Private Practice for Internal Medicine, 9000 Ghent, Belgium; Lambrechtlj@skynet.be
8. Department of Internal Medicine, University Hospital Antwerp (UZA), 2650 Antwerp, Belgium; Greta.Moorkens@uza.be
9. Department of Physical Medicine and Physiotherapy, University Hospital Brussels, 1090 Brussels, Belgium
* Correspondence: Jessica.VanOosterwijck@UGent.be; Tel.: +32-9-332-69-19; Fax: +32-9-332-38-11
† Member of Pain in Motion International Research Group.

Citation: Van Oosterwijck, J.; Marusic, U.; De Wandele, I.; Meeus, M.; Paul, L.; Lambrecht, L.; Moorkens, G.; Danneels, L.; Nijs, J. Reduced Parasympathetic Reactivation during Recovery from Exercise in Myalgic Encephalomyelitis/Chronic Fatigue Syndrome. *J. Clin. Med.* **2021**, *10*, 4527. https://doi.org/10.3390/jcm10194527

Academic Editors: Giovanni Ricevuti and Lorenzo Lorusso

Received: 30 June 2021
Accepted: 22 September 2021
Published: 30 September 2021

Publisher's Note: MDPI stays neutral with regard to jurisdictional claims in published maps and institutional affiliations.

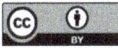

Copyright: © 2021 by the authors. Licensee MDPI, Basel, Switzerland. This article is an open access article distributed under the terms and conditions of the Creative Commons Attribution (CC BY) license (https:// creativecommons.org/licenses/by/ 4.0/).

Abstract: Although autonomic nervous system (ANS) dysfunction in Myalgic Encephalomyelitis/Chronic Fatigue Syndrome (ME/CFS) has been proposed, conflicting evidence makes it difficult to draw firm conclusions regarding ANS activity at rest in ME/CFS patients. Although severe exercise intolerance is one of the core features of ME/CFS, little attempts have been made to study ANS responses to physical exercise. Therefore, impairments in ANS activation at rest and following exercise were examined using a case-control study in 20 ME/CFS patients and 20 healthy people. Different autonomous variables, including cardiac, respiratory, and electrodermal responses were assessed at rest and following an acute exercise bout. At rest, parameters in the time-domain represented normal autonomic function in ME/CFS, while frequency-domain parameters indicated the possible presence of diminished (para)sympathetic activation. Reduced parasympathetic reactivation during recovery from exercise was observed in ME/CFS. This is the first study showing reduced parasympathetic reactivation during recovery from physical exercise in ME/CFS. Delayed HR recovery and/or a reduced HRV as seen in ME/CFS have been associated with poor disease prognosis, high risk for adverse cardiac events, and morbidity in other pathologies, implying that future studies should examine whether this is also the case in ME/CFS and how to safely improve HR recovery in this population.

Keywords: autonomic nervous system; autonomic function; electrodermal activity; electrocardiogram; heart rate

1. Introduction

Myalgic Encephalomyelitis/Chronic Fatigue Syndrome (ME/CFS) is a debilitating complex disorder characterized by extreme fatigue and pain complaints [1]. As fatigue and pain are often correlated to symptoms of autonomic dysfunction, involvement of the autonomic nervous system (ANS) has been proposed [2,3]. Two recent systematic reviews examining the existing evidence in ME/CFS have emphasized that controversial findings have been reported and that not all parameters of autonomic function have been studied extensively in this disorder [4,5]. As a consequence, it has been difficult to draw firm conclusions regarding ANS activity at rest in ME/CFS.

Furthermore, little attempts have been made to study ANS activation in response to physical exercise, which is remarkable, as severe exercise intolerance is one of the core features of ME/CFS. More specifically, these patients show decreased cerebral oxygen and blood volume/flow, decreased pain thresholds, impaired oxygen delivery to muscles, elevated levels of oxidative stress and complement proteins, delayed recovery of peripheral muscle fatigue, and symptom exacerbations in response to/during exercise [6]. The impaired cardiodynamic responses to exercise that have been reported in ME/CFS include a slow acceleration of heart rate (HR) and decreased maximum HR during incremental exercise and diminished HR and blood pressure (BP) responses during isometric handgrip exercise [7–12]. While heart rate variability (HRV) analysis is the most commonly used measure for the evaluation of cardiac autonomic function at rest and during exercise, studies in ME/CFS have been limited to HR (in beats/minute) and BP responses to physical acute exercise.

Moreover, to date, no studies have examined whether ME/CFS patients have normal autonomic activation during exercise recovery. Yet the ANS does not only play a crucial role in the cardiovascular response to acute exercise, it is also implicated in the recovery from exercise when the balance between the sympathetic and parasympathetic activity needs to be restored [13]. Furthermore, HR recovery after exercise has recently been shown to predict all-cause and cardiovascular mortality as well as sudden death [14–17].

Therefore, the objective of this study was to assess autonomic function in patients with ME/CFS at rest, during an acute exercise bout, and during recovery from this exercise bout. During these conditions, different autonomous variables, including cardiac, respiratory, and electrodermal responses, were studied concomitantly and were compared to the responses of a healthy control group.

2. Materials and Methods

2.1. Ethical Approval

This study was designed as a blinded case-control study in line with the STROBE Statement (http://www.strobe-statement.org/) and conducted in accordance with the Declaration of Helsinki with the protocol being approved by the Ethics Committee of the University Hospital Brussels/Vrije Universiteit Brussel (BUN 143201316368). The study was conducted at the department of human physiology from the Vrije Universiteit Brussel, and all participants provided written informed consent prior to study initiation. The abstract of conference presentation of this study has been published [18].

2.2. Subjects

Twenty ME/CFS patients and 20 healthy sedentary controls participated in this study. Patients were diagnosed according to the CDCP criteria for ME/CFS [19]. Healthy subjects with a medical history of endocrine abnormalities or diseases known to affect the function of the cardiovascular, immune, or autonomic system were excluded. Sedentary was defined as having a seated occupation and performing ≤3 h of moderate physical activity/week [20]. Moderate activities correspond to activities demanding at least threefold the energy spent passively [20].

All subjects were between 18 and 65 years of age and female as pooling of gender data forms an important source of bias in studies examining exercise physiology and as ME/CFS is predominant in females [21,22]. In order to preclude other confounding factors, subjects were excluded when pregnant, lactating, or <1 year postnatal.

ME/CFS patients were recruited from the department of internal medicine at a university hospital and from a private practice for internal medicine, where co-authors GM and LL respectively checked which patients fulfilled the inclusion criteria and informed them of the study and the possibility of participating in the study. Patients were voluntarily able to decide whether they were willing to participate, without this choice having any effect on their health care. The healthy subjects were recruited amongst healthy friends and relatives from the ME/CFS patients and volunteers who replied to advertisements.

2.3. Procedure

During the 1st visit study, one of the researchers (JVO) examined whether the included ME/CFS patients also fulfilled the more recent Canadian criteria for ME/CFS [1], which was the case for all patients. Sociodemographic and disease-related information was collected via a self-composed questionnaire. In order to prevent stress on the day of the assessment each subject was guided through the lab, the different assessment methods and materials were shown, and the full test procedure was explained. The 2nd visit took place within 7–21 days following the 1st visit.

During the 2nd visit, participants performed a submaximal bicycle exercise test with continuous cardiorespiratory monitoring. The Aerobic Power Index test [23–25] was performed as described in our previous study [26]. In summary, the exercise protocol commenced at 25 W, and the workload (W) was linearly increased by 25 W/minute, maintaining a cycling rate of 70 rotations/minute until 75% of the age-predicted target HR was reached. The exercise test was concluded by a short cooling down of 30 s, during which the subject kept cycling against a resistance of 25 W, to prevent venous pooling.

A portable cardiopulmonary indirect breath-by-breath calorimetry system (MetaMax 3B, Cortex Biophysik GmbH, Leipzig, Germany) was used to analyze the expired air for ventilatory and metabolic variables. HR during exercise was recorded using ECG electrodes allowing real-time determination of achieved target HR and post-determination of the mean and peak HR during exercise. Immediately following the exercise, subjects were asked to assess their perceived exertion using the Ratings of Perceived Exertion (RPE) Borg scale. The set-up of the exercise test is shown in Figure 1. Before the exercise test (at rest), during the exercise test, and during the subsequent passive recovery period, physiological measures of autonomic function were performed.

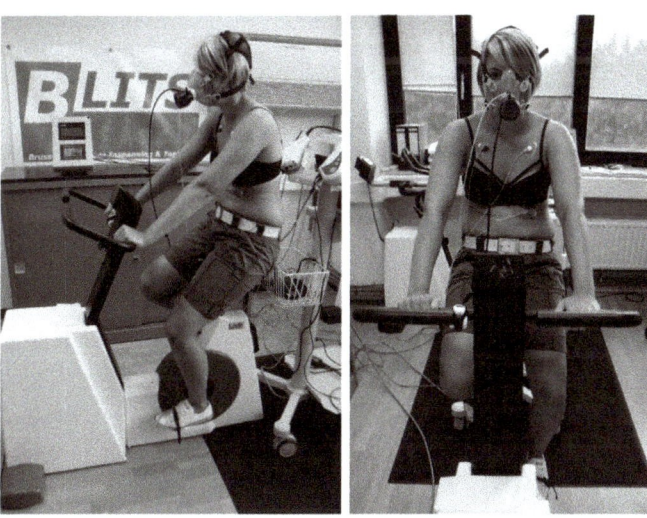

Figure 1. Set-up of the standardized submaximal bicycle exercise test.

All assessments took place in a quiet room with constant ambient temperature (21–23 °C). Subjects were asked to refrain from consuming caffeine, alcohol, nicotine, and physical exertion on the day of the experiment. If medically permissible, medication acting on (1) the cardiovascular system was withheld on the day of the examinations, as this type of medication can prevent achievement of the target HR during the exercise test; and (2) the central nervous or hormonal systems was withheld for at least 48 h before the examinations took place, as these types of medications can influence autonomic function. Subjects were asked to report whether they complied with these instructions.

2.4. Physiological Measures of Autonomic Function

The Nexus-10 wireless and portable telemetry data acquisition system (Mind Media BV, Roermond-Herten, The Netherlands) was used to physiologically assess autonomic responses such as skin conductance (SC), skin temperature (ST), electrocardiogram (ECG), and respiration rate (RR). Blood pressure (BP) was measured using an electronic blood pressure monitor. Placement of the sensors is presented in Figure 2. Measures were taken continuously during 10 min of rest before and following the bicycle exercise; the latter was considered as the recovery period. During the measurements at rest and recovery, the subject lay supine with the forearms in supination beside the body and was asked not to talk, move, or close the eyes. Measures during exercise were limited to ECG. Signals were analyzed offline with the BioSig toolbox in MATLAB software (MathWorks, Natick, MA, USA). For each measurement, the overall mean across the recording periods was calculated (mean PRE, mean DURING, mean POST) (Guideline on heart rate variability, 1996).

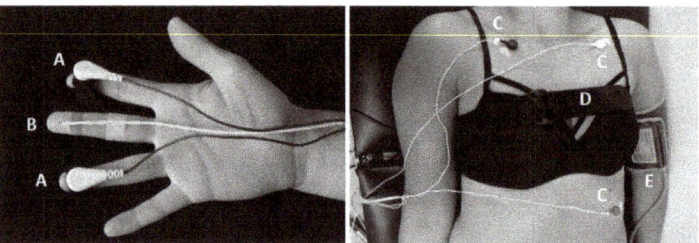

Figure 2. Electrode placement. Legends: A: skin conductance sensors, B: skin temperature sensor, C: ECG electrodes standard lead II placement, D: elastic belt with piezoelectric sensor to measure respiration rate, E: inflatable cuff placement of the electronic blood pressure monitor.

HRV was assessed through calculation of the root mean square of successive differences between NN intervals (RMSSD) and frequency analysis performed using the quotient (LF/HFratio) of low-frequency components (i.e., the power in the low-frequency (LF) range between 0.04 and 0.15 Hz) over high-frequency components (i.e., the power in the high-frequency (HF) range between 0.15 and 0.40 Hz) after fast Fourier transformation [27,28]. RMSSD reflects the integrity of vagus nerve-mediated autonomic control of the heart [29]. The LF/HF ratio is an indicator of cardiac sympathetic modulation and sympatho/vagal balance [28]. The efferent vagal activity is a major contributor to the HF component, while LF is mediated by both sympathetic and parasympathetic modulations. SC, a parameter of peripheral sympathetic activity, was assessed by extracting a measurement of the (tonic) background level i.e., skin conductance level (SCL), and of the time-varying (phasic) responses i.e., skin conductance responses (SCR) [30]. Changes in ST as small as 0.001 °C in a range of 10–40 °C were recorded. Peak detection was applied on the respiration data, and the number of peaks/minute reflected the RR. BP was measured at the start and at the end of the 10-min periods preceding and following the bicycle exercise.

2.5. Statistics

Data analysis was performed using SPSS 20.0. Descriptives were calculated, and the normality of the data was evaluated using the Shapiro–Wilk test and visual assessment of histograms, QQ-plots, and boxplots. When possible outliers were identified during this assessment, it was examined whether these were in the normal range of the according measures or whether they were considered as outliers using the outlier labeling rule [31].

Comparability of the groups at baseline and regarding exercise related outcome was evaluated using the Independent Samples *t*-test or Mann–Whitney U test depending on the distribution of the data. The Fisher exact test or the Pearson Chi-Square test were used to analyze binary and categorical data.

Not all outcome measures of autonomic function were normally distributed, and as logarithmically transformation did not resolve this issue for all parameters, further analysis was performed using univariate analyses. For each group (ME/CFS and CON), possible differences in the response of the outcome measures to exercise (PRE vs. DURING vs. POST) was examined using either the Paired Samples *t*-test or the Wilcoxon Signed Rank test. In case a significant difference was found regarding the recovery (PRE vs. POST), the 10-min baseline and recovery periods were additionally divided into five equal 2-min long periods to examine the course of the autonomic responses over time. The difference in exercise response between the two groups regarding autonomic function was examined using the Mann–Whitney U or Independent Samples *t*-testing.

The significance level was set at $p < 0.05$.

Since no studies had examined autonomic nervous function during/following physical exercise in ME/CFS before, no data were available to provide a basis for the a priori power analysis. Therefore, the sample size was based on a similar study [32] which evaluated autonomic dysfunction based on HRV parameters in time and frequency domains and HR recovery in response to a submaximal bicycle exercise test in females with chronic stroke on the one hand, and on a study [26] that used a submaximal bicycle exercise test to evaluate exercise intolerance in females with ME/CFS on the other hand. The calculations revealed that 16 to 21 subjects/group were required to obtain a power of 0.80 with $\alpha = 0.05$.

3. Results

3.1. Subjects

The sociodemographic data are shown in Table 1, and no significant group differences were found. Even though subjects were asked to refrain from central acting medication on the day of exercise testing, six ME/CFS and one control subject reported using medication (between-group $p = 0.091$). Only two ME/CFS patients took central acting selective serotonin reuptake inhibitors, while all other subjects took peripheral acting drugs including paracetamol, diclofenac, and non-steroid anti-inflammatory drugs.

Table 1. Demographic baseline characteristics.

	ME/CFS Group (n = 20)	Healthy Group (n = 20)	Between-Group Comparison (p-Value)
Age, years			
Mean (SD)	41.6 (9.8)	34.6 (15.2)	0.155
Length, cm			
Mean (SD)	168 (5)	168 (8)	0.935
Weight, kg			
Mean (SD)	68.1 (14.9)	73.9 (15.6)	0.168
Handedness			
Right (n)	17	16	1.000
Left (n)	3	4	
Employment status			
Student (n)	1	6	
Retired (n)	0	1	
Full-time (n)	4	2	0.208
Part-time (n)	6	4	
Non-employed (n)	9	7	
Years of education			
Mean (SD)	14.4 (2.8)	15.6 (2.7)	0.177
Highest degree of education			
Primary school (n)			
Secondary education (n)	9	12	
Higher education—university or college (n)	2	1	0.054
Higher education—adult education social	8	7	
advancement course (n)	1	0	
Marital status			
Single (n)	9	12	
Living together (n)	2	1	0.609
Married (n)	8	7	
Widow (n)	1	0	
Children			
Yes	7	12	0.205
No	13	8	
Mean number (SD)	1 (1.0)	1 (1.3)	0.640
Time from diagnosis, months			
Mean (SD)	70.3 (56.8)	NA	NA

Abbreviations: SD: standard deviation, n: number of, NA: not applicable.

3.2. Exercise-Related Outcomes

All subjects were able to complete the exercise test. There were no significant between-group differences regarding theoretical target HR, actual achieved peak HR and mean HR, cycling time, maximum workload achieved, and exercise capacity, as can been seen in Table 2. Although both groups performed a similar exercise test and showed similar exercise capacity, the exercise was perceived as heavier and more strenuous by the ME/CFS patients ($p < 0.001$).

Table 2. Exercise-related outcomes.

	ME/CFS Group (n = 20)	Healthy Group (n = 20)	Between-Group Comparison (p-Value)
HR, bpm			
Theoretical target HR peak *	134 (7)	140 (12)	0.149
Actual achieved HR peak	140 (9)	142 (10)	0.453
Mean HR	114 (10)	119 (10)	0.092
Cycling time, min	3.86 (1.00)	4.15 (1.15)	0.401
Peak Workload	109 (25)	118 (25)	0.327
VO2 peak, mL/min/kg	16.98 (4.25)	19.96 (6.80)	0.112
VE peak, L/min	31.81 (9.67)	31.61 (11.30)	0.758
RER peak	0.76 (0.89)	72 (0.08)	0.101
RPE	16 (0.3)	12 (2)	<0.001

Abbreviations: HR: heart rate, VO2 peak: peak oxygen uptake, VE peak: peak ventilation, RER peak: respiratory exchange ratio, RPE: rate of perceived exertion, * corresponds with 75% of the age-predicted target HR.

3.3. Autonomic Function

The mean PRE, DURING, and POST values for each group are presented in Figure 3; values of the 2-min intervals are presented in the supporting information (S1).

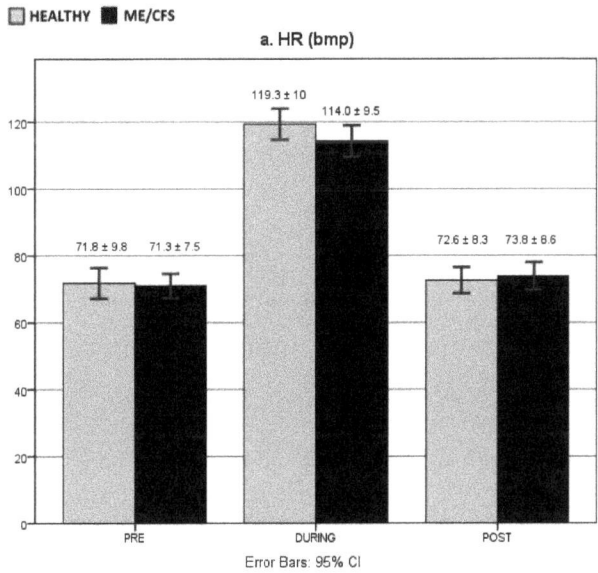

Figure 3. *Cont.*

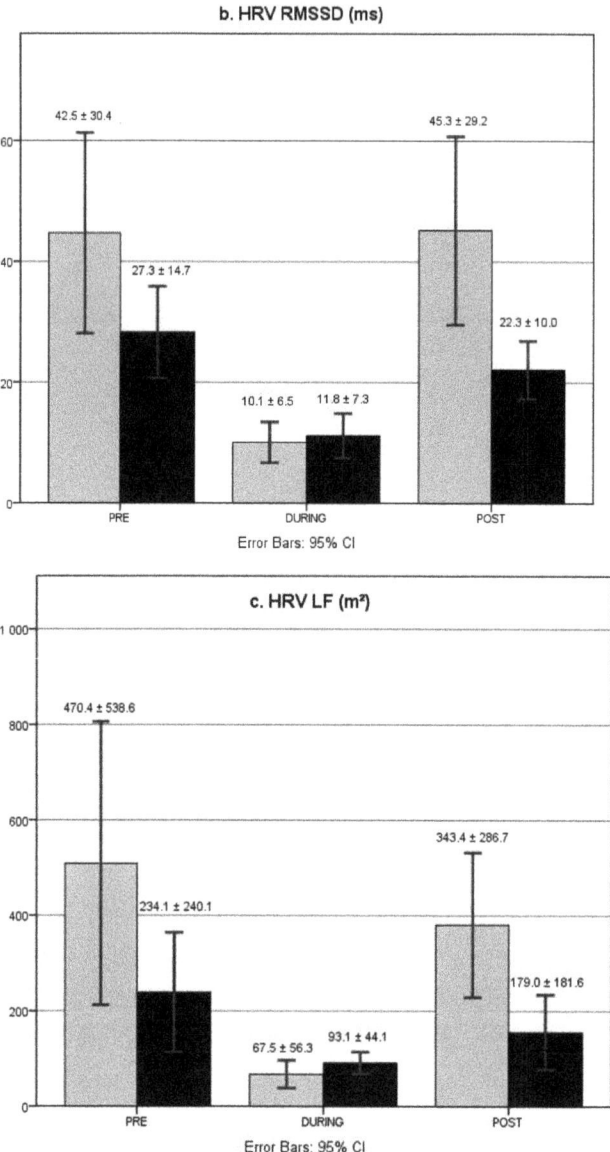

Figure 3. *Cont.*

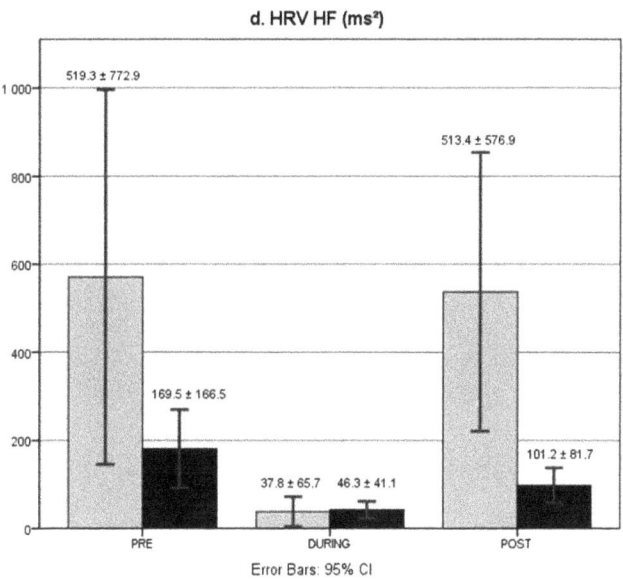

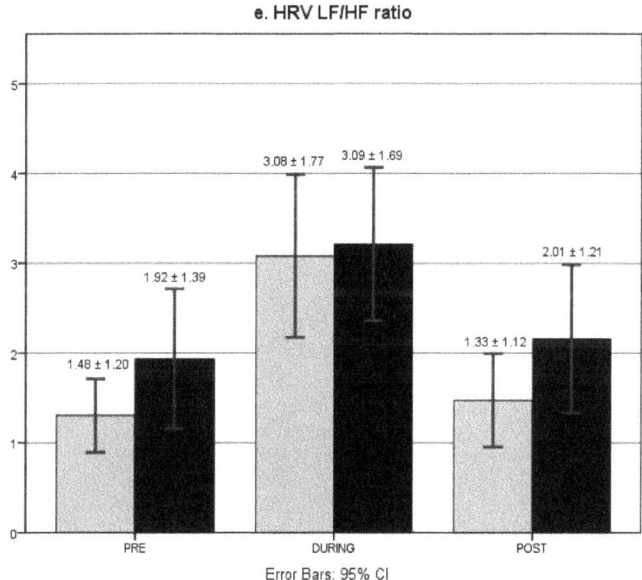

Figure 3. *Cont.*

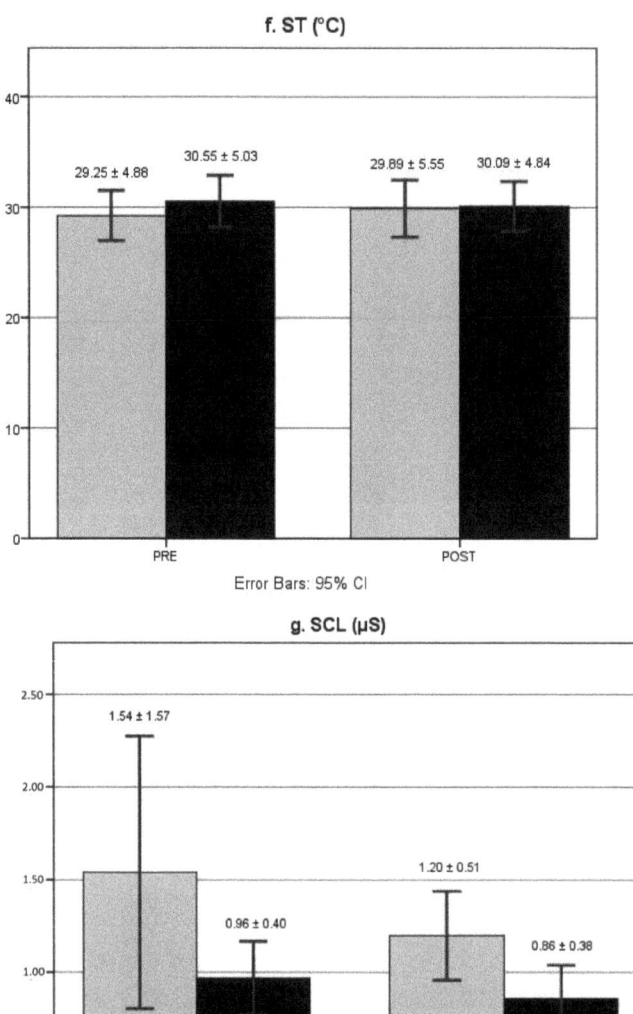

Figure 3. *Cont.*

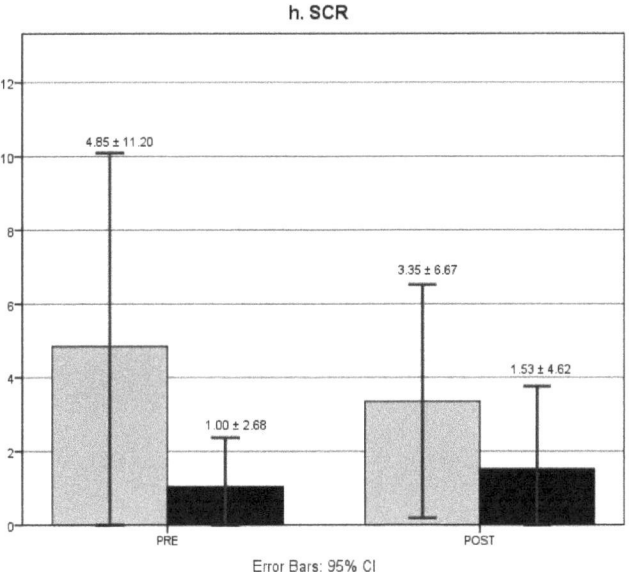

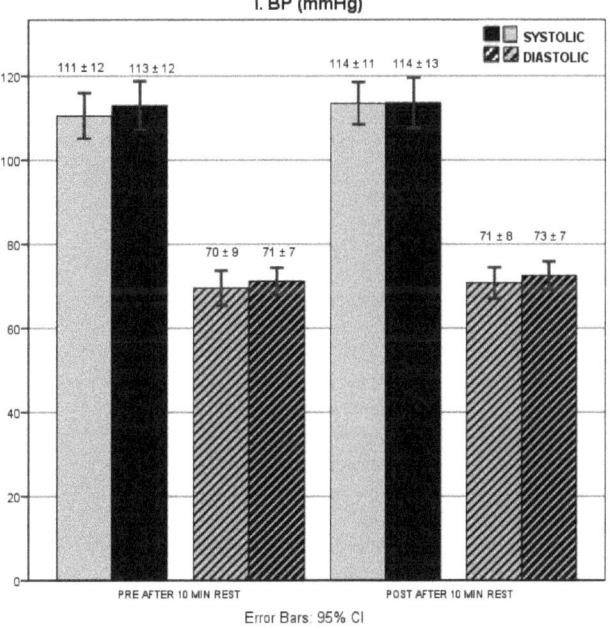

Figure 3. *Cont.*

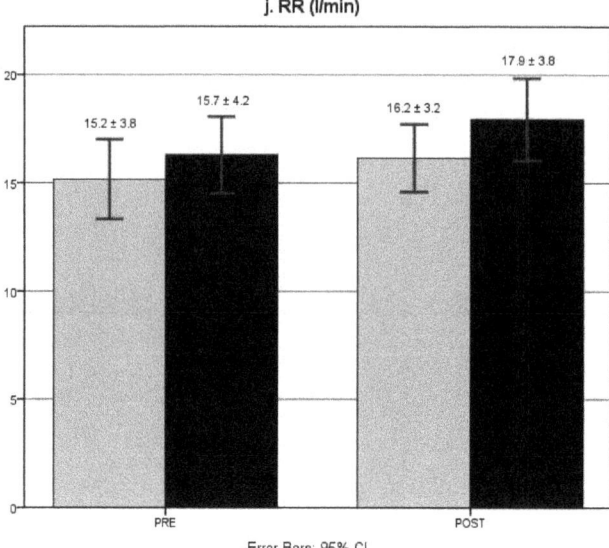

Figure 3. Means and standard deviations of autonomic outcome measures. The specific outcome measure each figure refers to is in depected in the figure itself. (**a**) HR (bpm); (**b**) HRV RMSSD (ms); (**c**) HRV LF (m^2); (**d**) HRV HF (ms^2); (**e**) The LF/HF ratio; (**f**) ST (°C); (**g**) SCL (µS); (**h**) SCR; (**i**) PB (mmHg); (**j**) RR (l/min). Legends: The y-axis represents the quantification of the measure, the x-axis represents the time point of the measure (PRE: measure taken prior to exercise, DURING: measure taken during exercise, POST: measure taken post-exercise). Gray bars: healthy controls, black bars: ME/CFS. Abbreviations: BP: blood pressure, bpm: beat per minute, CI: confidence interval, HR: high frequency, HR: heart rate, HRV: heart rate variability, LF: low frequency, ME/CFS: Myalgic Encephalomyelitis/Chronic Fatigue Syndrome, RMSSD: root mean square of successive differences between NN intervals, RR: respiration rate, SCL: skin conductance level, SCR: skin conductance response, ST: skin temperature.

3.4. HR

No between-group differences were found for mean HR at baseline (PRE $p = 0.870$), during exercise (DURING $p = 0.092$), and during recovery (POST $p = 0.655$) (Figure 3a). During exercise, the mean HR was higher than at rest in both groups (PRE vs. DURING $p < 0.001$). After the exercise, the mean HR declined in both groups (DURING vs. POST $p < 0.001$), but a differential response was seen regarding full recovery. The controls showed no significant differences between HR measured during recovery and HR at rest (PRE vs. POST $p = 0.578$), indicating a quick recovery to the original baseline levels following exercise. In ME/CFS, this was not the case, as a significantly higher HR was observed during recovery than at rest (PRE vs. POST $p = 0.031$), and at the end of the 10-min recovery, the HR remained above the baseline levels (PRE8-10 min vs. POST8-10 min $p = 0.020$), which was not the case for the controls.

3.5. HRV

No significant group differences were found regarding RMSSD at baseline (PRE $p = 0.060$) (Figure 3b). In both groups, a similar response to exercise was seen (DURING $p = 0.613$), with RMSSD decreasing (PRE vs. DURING ME/CFS $p = 0.003$, CON $p < 0.001$). After exercise, RMSSD values increased again (DURING vs. POST ME/CFS $p = 0.006$, CON $p < 0.001$), but RMSSD during recovery did differ significantly between groups. ME/CFS subjects showed lower values than the controls over the whole recovery period (POST $p = 0.010$) as well as at the different time intervals (p between 0.003 and 0.041). The overall RMSSD response during recovery was similar to baseline in both groups (PRE vs. POST ME/CFS $p = 0.059$, CON $p = 0.881$).

Both HF and LF were significantly lower in ME/CFS than in the controls at baseline (PRE HF $p = 0.024$, LF $p = 0.038$) and during recovery (POST HF $p = 0.001$, LF $p = 0.015$) (Figure 3c,d). During exercise, this difference between groups dissipated for HF ($p = 0.245$) but was sustained for LF ($p = 0.029$), and HF (PRE vs. DURING ME/CFS $p = 0.014$, CON $p < 0.001$) as well as LF (PRE vs. DURING ME/CFS = 0.022, CON $p < 0.001$) levels decreased in the two groups. In the controls, both HF and LF increased during recovery (DURING vs. POST respectively $p = 0.022$ and $p < 0.001$). While HF significantly increased during recovery in the ME/CFS patients, the increase in LF was not significant (DURING vs. POST respectively $p = 0.016$ and $p = 0.193$). The HF of the controls during exercise recovery was similar as in baseline (PRE vs. POST $p = 0.709$), while their LF was significantly lower during the recovery period (PRE vs. POST $p = 0.012$). In ME/CFS, the opposite effect was observed, where LF during recovery was similar to baseline (PRE vs. POST $p = 0.126$), and HF was significantly decreased during the whole recovery period (PRE vs. POST $p = 0.044$) and at the end of the 10-min recovery period (PRE8-10 min vs. POST8-10 min $p = 0.016$).

The LF/HF ratio was similar between groups at baseline (PRE $p = 0.314$) and during exercise (DURING $p = 0.961$) but higher in ME/CFS than in the controls during recovery (POST $p = 0.035$) (Figure 3e). At the end of the recovery period, the group difference was no longer present (POST8–10 min $p = 0.057$). While the LF/HF ratio increased significantly from rest to exercise in controls, this was not the case in the ME/CFS group (PRE vs. DURING ME/CFS $p = 0.078$, CON $p = 0.001$). However, values decreased in both groups during the post-exercise recovery period (DURING vs. POST ME/CFS $p = 0.009$, CON $p = 0.004$) until they were no longer significantly different from baseline (PRE vs. POST ME/CFS $p = 0.841$, CON $p = 0.502$).

3.6. Electrodermal Responses

SCL were lower in ME/CFS than in the controls, but only during recovery did this difference reach significance (PRE $p = 0.165$, POST $p = 0.016$) (Figure 3g). The group difference was observed throughout the whole recovery period (POST intervals between 0.018 and 0.044). Although SCL were lower during recovery than at baseline, the mean difference was not significant in either group (PRE vs. POST ME/CFS $p = 0.184$, CON $p = 0.351$). SCR at baseline and during recovery were not significantly different from each other (PRE vs. POST ME/CFS $p = 0.916$, CON $p = 0.575$) or between the two groups (PRE $p = 0.758$, POST $p = 0.569$, POST intervals p between 0.309 and 0.835) (Figure 3h and Figure S1).

ST during recovery did not significantly differ from the baseline value in neither group (PRE vs. POST ME/CFS $p = 0.135$, CON $p = 0.823$), and no group differences were observed (PRE $p = 0.383$, POST $p = 0.820$) (Figure 3f).

3.7. RR

RR was similar between groups at baseline (PRE $p = 0.656$) (Figure 3j). While RR was not measured during exercise, similar between-group ventilatory outcomes were shown from the ergospirometric measures (cfr. 3.2). At the start of the recovery period, the ME/CFS group had a higher RR than controls (POST1-2 min $p = 0.032$), their RR decreased in the following 8 min of recovery returning to similar values as in the control group (POST $p = 0.343$, POST3–4,5–6,7–8,8–10 min p between 0.155 and 0.851). However, throughout the recovery period, RR remained higher than at baseline for both groups (PRE vs. POST ME/CFS $p = 0.003$, CON $p = 0.005$).

3.8. BP

BP values at the start and at the end of 10 min of supine resting were similar (p between 0.094 and 0.617), and there were no group differences (p between 0.437 and 0.528) (Figure 3i). Both groups responded in the same way to the exercise test (systolic BP $p = 0.589$, diastolic

BP $p = 0.588$), with systolic BP increasing (ME/CFS $p = 0.001$, CON $p = 0.003$) while diastolic BP remained stable (ME/CFS $p = 0.262$, CON $p = 0.275$). After 10 min of supine recovery, both systolic and diastolic BP were similar to the values seen at rest (p between 0.063 and 0.767) and between groups (systolic BP $p = 0.979$, diastolic BP $p = 0.467$).

4. Discussion

This study assessed autonomic function in patients with ME/CFS at rest, during an acute bout of physical exercise, and during exercise recovery. HRV frequency-domain parameters indicated the possible presence of diminished cardiac (para)sympathetic activation at supine rest, while blood pressure, respiratory, electrodermal, and HRV parameters in the time-domain represented normal autonomic function at rest in ME/CFS. A similar (para)sympathetic modulation took place during exercise in ME/CFS as in healthy people; however, the magnitude of this modulation was impaired in those with ME/CFS. Reduced parasympathetic reactivation during recovery from exercise was observed in ME/CFS.

4.1. Autonomic Function at Rest in ME/CFS

In the present study HR, BP, RMSSD, RR, SCL, SCR, and ST suggest normal autonomic activity during supine lying in ME/CFS. A similar amount of studies exist that confirm or refute the presence of a differential HR and BP in ME/CFS at rest (reviewed in [4,5]). Our findings showed that ME/CFS patients have a similar resting HR and systolic/diastolic BP as healthy sedentary subjects. This was also the case for RMSSD, which is in line with previous observations (reviewed in [4,5]). Although LF and HF in ME/CFS were lower than in healthy subjects, the LF/HR ratio was similar in both groups. This observation could indicate reduced sympathetic and parasympathetic activity in ME/CFS at rest, while the sympatho/vagal balance is maintained. As LF is related to baroreflex function, a decreased LF could reflect baroreflex failure, which in turn is often observed in case of cardiac sympathetic denervation [33]. However, further research using beat-to-beat measures is necessary to confirm this assumption.

The current knowledge regarding electrodermal function in ME/CFS is very limited, as only one study [34] has examined this aspect of autonomic function before in this population. The findings from that study suggested that ME/CFS patients have normal SCR but reduced SCL and increased ST. Our findings could not confirm the latter observations. Although mean SCL were lower and mean ST was higher in ME/CFS than in the healthy group, the difference was not significant, and the mean values were lower than those reported by Pazderka-Robinson et al. [34].

4.2. Autonomic Function during an Acute Aerobic Exercise Bout in ME/CFS

Cardiac responses were studied during the performance of a submaximal, incremental aerobic exercise test on a cycle ergometer. Performance parameters such as the ability to complete the exercise protocol, exercise capacity, final power output, and cycled time were similar between ME/CFS and healthy subjects, which is in line with previous reports [26,35] and suggests equal demands were required from the ANS during exercise in both populations. In normal circumstances, exercise is accompanied with dynamic changes in cardiac responses, which results in an increased blood flow and redistribution of the blood to satisfy the energy demands of the working muscles. While systolic BP will increase during exercise, diastolic BP remains relatively constant. HR increases immediately at the onset of activity as a result of parasympathetic withdrawal [36]. As exercise continues, further increases in HR are due to the action of the sympathetic nervous system. The increased sympathetic nervous activity is reflected in an increased LF/HF ratio and has been described to occur when HR exceeds 100 bpm [37,38].

Our findings in ME/CFS are in line with these observations in healthy people. The BP responses during exercise were normal in ME/CFS, with systolic BP increasing while diastolic BP remained stable. The subjects' mean HR increased during exercise testing while the mean HF dropped, which can be interpreted as a decrease in parasympathetic modulation. As this was observed in both ME/CFS and healthy subjects, we can conclude that this autonomic mechanism functions normally in ME/CFS. Since sympathetic activity cannot be easily isolated from LF, the LF/HR ratio is a more adequate parameter to provide us with insights regarding sympathetic modulation and sympatho/vagal balance during the exercise test [28]. The LF/HF ratio increased in the controls, reflecting sympathetic dominance and parasympathetic inhibition during exercise. Although the mean LF/HF ratio also increased in ME/CFS in response to the exercise, the decrease was not large enough to reach significance. The latter observation might indicate that although a similar autonomic modulation seems to take place during exercise in ME/CFS as in healthy people, the magnitude of this modulation might be impaired in ME/CFS. Further research in larger sample sizes is warranted to confirm these assumptions.

4.3. Autonomic Function during Recovery from Exercise in ME/CFS

Autonomic activity was assessed during a 10-min passive recovery period following the aerobic exercise test. HR and BP responses during recovery were similar for both groups, although those with ME/CFS did not manage to fully restore their elevated HR to rest levels as healthy subjects did. It has been shown that a delayed HR recovery, which is the return of the HR during post-exercise recovery to the pre-exercise HR by parasympathetic reactivation, is an independent predictor of overall mortality and may be linked to adverse prognosis [14–17]. Therefore, the lack of HR recovery observed during the two first minutes of the passive recovery period and the delayed HR recovery observed over the full 10 min of the recovery period could have important implications, and this should be further examined. Specifically, future studies should attempt to evaluate HR recovery during the first or second minute after immediate cessations of the acute exercise bout (i.e., passive recovery) or during cooling down (i.e., active recovery) [39]. As aerobic endurance training has been shown to accelerate HR recovery after exercise in healthy people [40]), future studies are required to determine whether this type of training can also improve HR recovery in ME/CFS and if this can be performed without inducing symptom exacerbations [26].

Although RMSSD, LF, and HF evolved the same way in ME/CFS as in healthy subjects, again, the magnitude of these modulations was smaller in ME/CFS. More specifically, in ME/CFS, the increases of RMSSD and LF during recovery from exercise were reduced, and although a similar increase was seen for HF, HF did not manage to restore to pre-exercise levels. The latter observations indicate that ME/CFS patients manage to restore their HRV following exercise, but that the magnitude of their HRV following exercise is lower than in healthy people. The inability to restore HF to pre-exercise levels in ME/CFS suggest a reduced parasympathetic modulation during recovery from exercise in these patients.

It is generally agreed that there is parasympathetic withdrawal and sympathetic excitation during exercise and that these effects are reversed in recovery [36]). Hence, the LF/HF ratio will decrease during recovery. This was the case for both ME/CFS patients and healthy subjects, and the LF/HF reached similar values as at rest. Although the recovery of LF/HF took place in ME/CFS, the magnitude was smaller, and more time (8 min) was necessary to fully restore HF/LF as healthy people did. While both groups showed equal LF/HF ratios at baseline, during recovery, ME/CFS patients had higher LF/HF than healthy subjects, suggesting a dysfunctional balance between the parasympathetic and sympathetic nervous system following recovery. However, LF/HF was restored at the end of the 10-min recovery period, which possibly indicates a delayed recovery in ME/CFS.

It has been suggested that the HF or parasympathetic tone represents an individual's 'functional capacity' for exercise [41]. Our HRV results in ME/CFS demonstrate a reduced functional capacity for exercise (decreased HF power at rest). Since physical training has been shown to cause an increase in parasympathetic tone [42], it could be beneficial for ME/CFS. Nonetheless, the training intensity should be kept within the limits of the individual's capacity in order to not worsen the already present autonomic imbalance; yet, it needs to be high enough to invoke a training effect. The balance between accurate training stimuli and recovery is necessary to avoid post-exertional malaise. Since each training session causes an acute decrease in parasympathetic activity, enough rest is required to rebound back toward (and beyond) the original pre-training level. Hautala et al. [41] have suggested to use the HF power obtained by HRV analysis as guidance in determining the correct training volume. On days when decreased parasympathetic activity is observed in the morning, expressing insufficient recovery from the previous exercise, a lower training load or rest is prescribed; and conversely, on days with high parasympathetic activity, a higher training load is allowed. Unfortunately, there is currently little knowledge regarding the best exercise intensity for improving autonomic balance in individuals with a dysfunctional stress system.

Similar responses in RR were seen in both groups, with RR remaining above baseline levels during the 10 min of recovery. In the 2 first minutes of recovery, ME/CFS had higher RR than healthy people, but after 2 min, the RR of the patients had decreased to similar levels as the healthy group. Peripheral autonomic activity was studied by examining SC and ST during the recovery period. SCL, which were similar between groups at rest and showed an analogous evolution during recovery, were lower in the ME/CFS patients compared to the healthy subjects throughout the recovery period. While the difference in mean SCL did not seem to increase during the recovery period compared to baseline, this difference between the groups seems to be the consequence of the diminished SCL variability in the control group during the recovery period. SCR responses during recovery were similar as at rest, and ME/CFS patients showed the same reactions as healthy people. Currently, there is no literature available regarding electrodermal responses during exercise recovery in ME/CFS, but our findings indicate that overall, these responses are similar as in healthy people.

4.4. Strengths and Limitations

The results should be interpreted light of the following study limitations. As not all subjects were examined at the same time of the day, and not all subjects complied with instructions regarding the wash-out period of medication, we cannot exclude the possibility that this influenced the results. As only women were studied, care should be taken with the extrapolation of these results to the male ME/CFS population. As the study was performed at the Human Physiology lab and participants had to perform an exercise test, it is obvious that only patients with ME/CFS with mild to moderate disease severity participated in this study. When interpreting the study results, one should keep in mind that although post-exercise assessments were taken as quickly as possible, subjects needed to reposition themselves from the bicycle to supine position and finger sensors needed to be reattached before the assessments were started. In addition, using this protocol, it was not possible to evaluate respiratory measures during exercise in the same way as at rest or recovery, or to examine the electrodermal responses during exercise. Furthermore, the sample size was based on primary outcomes of interest, namely, HRV parameters in time and frequency domains and HR recovery, and thus, it cannot be excluded that for the other outcome variables that were studied, the sample size was too low in order to draw firm conclusions.

The study has several strengths by complying with previous recommendations regarding research in ME/CFS and preventing confounding factors. Patients fulfilled the diagnostic criteria for ME/CFS described by Fukuda et al. in 1994 [19] as well as the more recent Canadian criteria described by Carruthers et al. in 2011 [1]. As previously suggested, measures of cardiac, respiratory, and electrodermal activity were performed to study different aspects of the ANS [5]. Sedentary healthy subjects were included and showed similar exercise capacity levels and performance parameters as the ME/CFS group, which suggests that deconditioning was not primarily responsible for the observed group differences. A submaximal exercise protocol that is reliable and valid for testing these populations was used [23–25]. Finally, all measures were undertaken in a standardized way and in a temperature-controlled environment.

5. Conclusions

The findings of this study suggest reduced autonomic modulation during exercise/reactivation during exercise recovery in ME/CFS. As delayed HR recovery and/or a reduced HRV implicate a poor disease prognosis and have been associated with higher risk for cardiac events and morbidity, further studies on methods to improve HR recovery in ME/CFS are warranted. This mainly implies improving parasympathetic reactivation following physical exercise and providing sufficient long recovery periods following exercise.

Supplementary Materials: The following are available online at https://www.mdpi.com/article/10.3390/jcm10194527/s1, Figure S1: Means and standard deviations of autonomic outcome measures over 2-min intervals.

Author Contributions: Conception or design of the work: J.V.O., I.D.W., M.M., L.P., J.N. Subject recruitment: J.V.O., G.M., L.L. Acquisition, analysis, or interpretation of data for the work: J.V.O., U.M., L.L., G.M. Drafting the work or revising it critically for important intellectual content: J.V.O., U.M., I.D.W., M.M., L.P., L.L., G.M., L.D., J.N. Final approval of the version to be published: J.V.O., U.M., I.D.W., M.M., L.P., L.L., G.M., L.D., J.N. Agreement to be accountable for all aspects of the work: J.V.O., U.M., I.D.W., M.M., L.P., L.L., G.M., L.D., J.N. All persons designated as authors qualify for authorship, and all those who qualify for authorship are listed: J.V.O., U.M., I.D.W., M.M., L.P., L.L., G.M., L.D., J.N. All authors have read and agreed to the published version of the manuscript.

Funding: This study was funded by the Ramsay Research Fund of the ME Association (UK). Jessica Van Oosterwijck is a post-doctoral research fellow funded by the Special Research Fund of Ghent University and the ME Association's Ramsay Research Fund. Jo Nijs is holder of a Chair entitled 'Exercise immunology and chronic fatigue in health and disease' funded by the European College for Decongestive Lymphatic Therapy, The Netherlands.

Institutional Review Board Statement: The study was conducted according to the guidelines of the Declaration of Helsinki and approved by the Ethics Committee of the University Hospital Brussels/Vrije Universiteit Brussel (BUN 143201316368).

Informed Consent Statement: Informed consent was obtained from all subjects involved in the study.

Acknowledgments: The authors are grateful to Andrea Nees, Charissa Van Puymbroeck, Ellen Loots, and Heleen Van Cleynenbreugel for assisting during data collection.

Conflicts of Interest: None of the authors have potential conflict of interest to be disclosed.

Abbreviations

ANS	autonomic nervous system
ECG	electrocardiogram
CFS	chronic fatigue syndrome
HR	heart rate
HRV	heart rate variability
HF	high frequency
LF	low frequency
ME	myalgic encephalomyelitis
RMSSD	root mean square of successive differences between NN intervals
RPE	ratings of perceived exertion
RR	respiration rate
SC	skin conductance
SCL	skin conductance level
SCR	skin conductance responses
ST	skin temperature
W	workload

References

1. Carruthers, B.M.; van de Sande, M.I.; De Meirleir, K.L.; Klimas, N.G.; Broderick, G.; Mitchell, T.; Staines, D.; Powles, A.C.P.; Speight, N.; Vallings, R.; et al. Myalgic encephalomyelitis: International Consensus Criteria. *J. Int. Med.* **2011**, *270*, 327–338. [CrossRef]
2. Freeman, R.; Komaroff, A.L. Does the Chronic Fatigue Syndrome Involve the Autonomic Nervous System? *Am. J. Med.* **1997**, *102*, 357–364. [CrossRef]
3. Newton, J.; Okonkwo, O.; Sutcliffe, K.; Seth, A.; Shin, J.; Jones, D. Symptoms of autonomic dysfunction in chronic fatigue syndrome. *QJM Int. J. Med.* **2007**, *100*, 519–526. [CrossRef]
4. Meeus, M.; Goubert, D.; De Backer, F.; Struyf, F.; Hermans, L.; Coppieters, I.; De Wandele, I.; Da Silva, H.; Calders, P. Heart rate variability in patients with fibromyalgia and patients with chronic fatigue syndrome: A systematic review. *Semin. Arthrit. Rheum.* **2013**, *43*, 279–287. [CrossRef]
5. Van Cauwenbergh, D.; Nijs, J.; Kos, D.; Van Weijnen, L.; Struyf, F.; Meeus, M. Malfunctioning of the autonomic nervous system in patients with chronic fatigue syndrome: A systematic literature review. *Eur. J. Clin. Investig.* **2014**, *44*, 516–526. [CrossRef]
6. Nijs, J.; Nees, A.; Paul, L.; De Kooning, M.; Ickmans, K.; Meeus, M.; Van Oosterwijck, J. Altered immune response to exercise in patients with chronic fatigue syndrome/myalgic encephalomyelitis: A systematic literature review. *Exerc. Immunol. Rev.* **2014**, *20*, 94–116. [PubMed]
7. De Becker, P.; Roeykens, J.; Reynders, M.; McGregor, N.; De Meirleir, K. Exercise Capacity in Chronic Fatigue Syndrome. *Arch. Int. Med.* **2000**, *160*, 3270–3277. [CrossRef] [PubMed]
8. Gibson, H.; Carroll Clague, J.E.; Edwards, R.H. Exercise performance and fatiguability in patients with chronic fatigue syndrome. *J. Neurol. Neurosurg. Psychiatry* **1993**, *56*, 993–998. [CrossRef]
9. Montague, T.J.; Marrie, T.J.; Klassen, G.A.; Bewick, D.J.; Horacek, B.M. Cardiac Function at Rest and with Exercise in the Chronic Fatigue Syndrome. *Chest* **1989**, *95*, 779–784. [CrossRef] [PubMed]
10. Sisto, S.A.; LaManca, J.; Cordero, D.L.; Bergen, M.T.; Ellis, S.P.; Drastal, S.; Bodaad, W.L.; Tappac, W.N.; Natelsonac, B.H. Metabolic and cardiovascular effects of a progressive exercise test in patients with chronic fatigue syndrome. *Am. J. Med.* **1996**, *100*, 634–640. [CrossRef]
11. Soetekouw, P.M.; Lenders, J.W.; Bleijenberg, G.; Thien, T.; van der Meer, J.W. Autonomic function in patients with chronic fa-tigue syndrome. *Clin. Auton. Res.* **1999**, *9*, 334–340. [CrossRef] [PubMed]
12. Vanness, J.M.; Snell, C.R.; Strayer, D.R.; Dempsey, L., IV; Stevens, S.R. Subclassifying chronic fatigue syndrome through exer-cise testing. *Med. Sci. Sports Exerc.* **2003**, *35*, 908–913. [CrossRef] [PubMed]
13. Fink, G. *Stress Science: Neuroendocrinology*; Academic Press, Elsevier Ltd.: San Diego, CA, USA, 2009; p. 829.
14. Cole, C.R.; Blackstone, E.H.; Pashkow, F.J.; Snader, C.E.; Lauer, M.S. Heartrate recovery immediately after exercise as a preditor of mortality. *N. Engl. J. Med.* **1999**, *341*, 1351–1357. [CrossRef] [PubMed]
15. Jouven, X.; Empana, J.P.; Schwartz, P.J.; Desnos, M.; Courbon, D.; Ducimetière, P. Heart-Rate Profile during Exercise as a Predictor of Sudden Death. *N. Engl. J. Med.* **2005**, *352*, 1951–1958. [CrossRef] [PubMed]
16. Lauer, M.S. Autonomic function and prognosis. *Clevel. Clin. J. Med.* **2009**, *76*, S18–S22. [CrossRef]
17. Nishime, E.O.; Cole, C.R.; Blackstone, E.H.; Pashkow, F.J.; Lauer, M. Heart Rate Recovery and Treadmill Exercise Score as Predictors of Mortality in Patients Referred for Exercise ECG. *JAMA* **2000**, *284*, 1392–1398. [CrossRef]
18. Van Oosterwijck, J.; Uros, M.; De Wandele, I.; Meeus, M.; Paul, L.; Lambrecht, L.; Moorkens, G. Nijs Reduced Parasympathetic Reactivation During Recovery from Exercise in Myalgic Encephalomyelitis (ME)/chronic Fatigue Syndrome (CFS). *Physiothera-py* **2015**, *101*, e1091–e1092. [CrossRef]
19. Fukuda, K.; Straus, S.E.; Hickie, I.; Sharpe, M.C.; Dobbins, J.G.; Komaroff, A. The Chronic Fatigue Syndrome, a comprehensive approach to its definition and study. *Ann. Int. Med.* **1994**, *121*, 953–959. [CrossRef] [PubMed]
20. Bernstein, M.S.; Morabia, A.; Sloutskis, D. Definition and prevalence of sedentarism in an urban population. *Am. J. Public Health* **1999**, *89*, 862–867. [CrossRef] [PubMed]
21. Bleijenberg, G. Chronic fatigue and chronic fatigue syndrome in the general population. *Health Qual. Life Outcomes* **2003**, *1*, 52. [CrossRef] [PubMed]
22. Sheel, A.W.; Richards, J.C.; Foster, G.; Guenette, J.A. Sex Differences in Respiratory Exercise Physiology. *Sports Med.* **2004**, *34*, 567–579. [CrossRef]
23. Wallman, K.; Goodman, C.; Morton, A.; Grove, R.; Dawson, B. Test-Retest Reliability of the Aerobic Power Index Test in Patients with Chronic Fatigue Syndrome. *J. Chronic Fatigue Syndr.* **2003**, *11*, 19–32. [CrossRef]
24. Wallman, K.; Goodman, C.; Morton, A.; Grove, R.; Dawson, B. Test-retest reliability of the aerobic power index component of the tri-level fitness profile in a sedentary population. *J. Sci. Med. Sport* **2003**, *6*, 443–454. [CrossRef]
25. Wallman, K.E.; Morton, A.R.; Goodman, C.; Grove, R. Physiological Responses during a Submaximal Cycle Test in Chronic Fatigue Syndrome. *Med. Sci. Sports Exerc.* **2004**, *36*, 1682–1688. [CrossRef]
26. Van Oosterwijck, J.; Nijs, J.; Meeus, M.; Lefever, I.; Huybrechts, L.; Lambrecht, L.; Paul, L. Pain inhibition and postexertional malaise in myalgic encephalomyelitis/chronic fatigue syndrome: An experimental study. *J. Int. Med.* **2010**, *268*, 265–278. [CrossRef] [PubMed]
27. Koenig, A.; Omlin, X.; Zimmerli, L.; Sapa, M.; Krewer, C.; Bolliger, M.; Müller, F.; Riener, R. Psychological state estimation from physiological recordings during robot-assisted gait rehabilitation. *J. Rehabilit. Res. Dev.* **2011**, *48*, 367–385. [CrossRef] [PubMed]

28. Guideline: Standards of measurement, physiological interpretation and clinical use. Task Force of the European Society of Cardiology and the North American Society of Pacing and Electrophysiology. *Circulation* **1996**, *93*, 1043–1065. [CrossRef]
29. DeGiorgio, C.M.; Miller, P.; Meymandi, S.; Chin, A.; Epps, J.; Gordon, S.; Gornbein, J.; Harper, R.M. RMSSD, a measure of vagusmediated heart rate variability, is associated with risk factors for SUDEP: The SUDEP-7 Inventory. *Epilepsy Behav.* **2010**, *19*, 78–81. [CrossRef] [PubMed]
30. Novak, D.; Mihelj, M.; Munih, M. Psychophysiological responses to different levels of cognitive and physical workload in haptic interaction. *Robotica* **2010**, *29*, 367–374. [CrossRef]
31. Hoaglin, D.C.; Iglewicz, B. Fine tuning some resistant rules for outlier labelling. *J. Am. Statist. Assoc.* **1987**, *82*, 1147–1149. [CrossRef]
32. Francica, J.V.; Bigongiari, A.; Mochizuki, L.; Scapini, K.B.; Moraes, O.A.; Mostarda, C.; Caperuto, É.C.; Irigoyen, M.C.; De Angelis, K.; Rodrigues, B. Cardiac autonomic dysfunction in chronic stroke women is attenuated after submaximal exercise test, as evaluated by linear and nonlinear analysis. *BMC Cardiovasc. Disord.* **2015**, *15*, 105. [CrossRef] [PubMed]
33. Goldstein, D.S.; Bentho, O.; Park, M.Y.; Sharabi, Y. Low-frequency power of heart rate variability is not a measure of cardiac sympathetic tone but may be a measure of modulation of cardiac autonomic outflows by baroreflexes. *Exp. Physiol.* **2011**, *96*, 1255–1261. [CrossRef] [PubMed]
34. Pazderka-Robinson, H.; Morrison, J.W.; Flor-Henry, P. Electrodermal dissociation of chronic fatigue and depression: Evidence for distinct physiological mechanisms. *Int. J. Psychophysiol.* **2004**, *53*, 171–182. [CrossRef]
35. Nijs, J.; Van Oosterwijck, J.; Meeus, M.; Lambrecht, L.; Metzger, K.; Fremont, M.; Paul, L. Unravelling the nature of postexertional malaise in myalgic encephalomyelitis/chronic fatigue syndrome: The role of elastase, complement C4a and interleukin-1β. *J. Int. Med.* **2010**, *267*, 418–435. [CrossRef] [PubMed]
36. Rowell, L.B. *Human Circulation: Regulation During Physical Stress*; Oxford University Press: New York, NY, USA, 1986.
37. Billman, G.E.; Dujardin, J.P. Dynamic changes in cardiac vagal tone as measured by time-series analysis. *Am. J. Physiol. Content* **1990**, *258*, 896–902. [CrossRef] [PubMed]
38. Breuer, H.W.; Skyschally, A.; Schulz, R.; Martin, C.; Wehr, M.; Heusch, G. Heart rate variability and circulating catecholamine concentrations during steady state exercise in healthy volunteers. *Br. Heart J.* **1993**, *70*, 144–149. [CrossRef]
39. Tekin, G.; Tekin, A. Heart rate recovery and methodological issues. *Anadolu Kardiyol. Dergisi/The Anatol. J. Cardiol.* **2015**, *15*, 87–88. [CrossRef]
40. Sugawara, J.; Murakami, H.; Maeda, S.; Kuno, S.; Matsuda, M. Change in post-exercise vagal reactivation with exercise train-ing and detraining in young men. *Eur. J. Appl. Physiol.* **2001**, *85*, 259–263. [CrossRef]
41. Hautala, A.J.; Kiviniemi, A.; Tulppo, M. Individual responses to aerobic exercise: The role of the autonomic nervous system. *Neurosci. Biobehav. Rev.* **2009**, *33*, 107–115. [CrossRef]
42. Tulppo, M.P.; Hautala, A.J.; Makikallio, T.H.; Laukkanen, R.T.; Nissila, S.; Hughson, R.L.; Huikuri, H.V. Effects of aerobic training on heart rate dynamics in sedentary subjects. *J. Appl. Physiol.* **2003**, *95*, 364–372. [CrossRef]

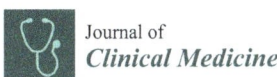

Article

Complement Component C1q as a Potential Diagnostic Tool for Myalgic Encephalomyelitis/Chronic Fatigue Syndrome Subtyping

Jesús Castro-Marrero [1,*], Mario Zacares [2], Eloy Almenar-Pérez [3], José Alegre-Martín [4] and Elisa Oltra [3,5,*]

1. ME/CFS Research Unit, Division of Rheumatology, Vall d'Hebron Research Institute, Universitat Autònoma de Barcelona, 08035 Barcelona, Spain
2. Departamento de Ciencias Básicas y Transversales, Facultad de Veterinaria y Ciencias Experimentales, Universidad Católica de Valencia San Vicente Mártir, 46001 Valencia, Spain; mario.zacares@ucv.es
3. Centro de Investigación Traslacional San Alberto Magno, Universidad Católica de Valencia San Vicente Mártir, 46001 Valencia, Spain; eloy.almenar@ucv.es
4. ME/CFS Clinical Unit, Division of Rheumatology, Vall d'Hebron University Hospital, Universitat Autònoma de Barcelona, 08035 Barcelona, Spain; jalegre@vhebron.net
5. Department of Pathology, School of Health Sciences, Universidad Católica de Valencia San Vicente Mártir, 46001 Valencia, Spain
* Correspondence: jesus.castro@vhir.org (J.C.-M.); elisa.oltra@ucv.es (E.O.)

Citation: Castro-Marrero, J.; Zacares, M.; Almenar-Pérez, E.; Alegre-Martín, J.; Oltra, E. Complement Component C1q as a Potential Diagnostic Tool for Myalgic Encephalomyelitis/Chronic Fatigue Syndrome Subtyping. *J. Clin. Med.* **2021**, *10*, 4171. https://doi.org/10.3390/jcm10184171

Academic Editors: Giovanni Ricevuti and Lorenzo Lorusso

Received: 27 August 2021
Accepted: 13 September 2021
Published: 15 September 2021

Publisher's Note: MDPI stays neutral with regard to jurisdictional claims in published maps and institutional affiliations.

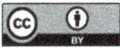

Copyright: © 2021 by the authors. Licensee MDPI, Basel, Switzerland. This article is an open access article distributed under the terms and conditions of the Creative Commons Attribution (CC BY) license (https://creativecommons.org/licenses/by/4.0/).

Abstract: Background: Routine blood analytics are systematically used in the clinic to diagnose disease or confirm individuals' healthy status. For myalgic encephalomyelitis/chronic fatigue syndrome (ME/CFS), a disease relying exclusively on clinical symptoms for its diagnosis, blood analytics only serve to rule out underlying conditions leading to exerting fatigue. However, studies evaluating complete and large blood datasets by combinatorial approaches to evidence ME/CFS condition or detect/identify case subgroups are still scarce. Methods: This study used unbiased hierarchical cluster analysis of a large cohort of 250 carefully phenotyped female ME/CFS cases toward exploring this possibility. Results: The results show three symptom-based clusters, classified as severe, moderate, and mild, presenting significant differences ($p < 0.05$) in five blood parameters. Unexpectedly the study also revealed high levels of circulating complement factor C1q in 107/250 (43%) of the participants, placing C1q as a key molecule to identify an ME/CFS subtype/subgroup with more apparent pain symptoms. Conclusions: The results obtained have important implications for the research of ME/CFS etiology and, most likely, for the implementation of future diagnosis methods and treatments of ME/CFS in the clinic.

Keywords: myalgic encephalomyelitis; chronic fatigue syndrome; C1q; complement system; blood analytics; diagnosis; symptoms; cluster analysis

1. Introduction

Myalgic encephalomyelitis/chronic fatigue syndrome (ME/CFS) constitutes a serious health problem that truncates the life of millions of people and their families around the world [1–3]. ME/CFS is a chronic condition characterized by profound fatigue which is exacerbated by physical/mental and emotional activity (also known as PEM; post-exertional malaise), lack of refreshing sleep and dysautonomia, and multiple additional comorbidities [4]; its diagnosis still solely relies on clinical symptom assessment [5–7] after ruling out potential subjacent illness that could explain patient's symptoms.

Despite a number of studies aimed at evidencing routine clinical parameters that may be useful, at least for the suspicion of an ME/CFS case, few are the differences that have been reported [8]. For example, Nacul et al. found significantly lower median values of serum creatine kinase (CK) in severely ill patients compared to healthy controls (HCs) and non-severe ME/CFS (median = 54, 101.5, and 84 U/L, respectively) [9], a finding confirmed by two additional studies [10,11]. While CK differences may be derived from patient sedentarism itself, some potential differences, including the levels of alkaline phosphatase, free T4 levels, or eosinophil counts, detected at lower significance ($p < 0.1$) in small cohorts ($n = 15$/group) [10] deserve further exploration in larger cohorts, individually or in combination with others.

Blood factors differentially altered in ME/CFS subgroups may constitute valuable tools in the clinic for achieving improved patient treatments, particularly for precision medicine purposes, while they may also serve to minimize patient heterogeneity in research studies. Unveiling the nature of ME/CFS, in fact, might well depend on homogeneous patient subset assessment, boosting the statistical robustness of data.

Therefore, in the current study we aimed at identifying clinical parameters that differentiate ME/CFS case subgroups by themselves or in relation to symptom severity, in a large cohort of female ME/CFS cases ($n = 250$), with potential therapeutic and/or research purposes.

2. Materials and Methods

2.1. Participants

In this observational, single-center, cross-sectional cohort study, a total of 250 females with ME/CFS were consecutively referred to a tertiary care referral center for clinical evaluation by a ME/CFS specialized clinician (Vall d'Hebron University Hospital, Barcelona, Spain) between March 2017 and December 2019. Participants were invited after eligibility was confirmed. Inclusion criteria consisted in adult female individuals fulfilling the 1994 CDC/Fukuda definition [5] and 2003 Canadian Consensus Criteria for ME/CFS [6]. Participants were excluded if they were previously diagnosed with any serious illnesses or comorbid diseases that could be associated with their symptoms. Participants donated a blood sample for routine blood testing, filled out validated standardized questionnaires, and provided demographic data and clinical characteristics at the time of their inclusion in the study.

The study procedures were reviewed and approved in accordance with the recommendations from the local Clinical Research Ethics Committee (Vall d'Hebron University Hospital, Barcelona, Spain; IRB protocol number: CEIC/PR-AG-VITAE-2015, approved in June 2015). All subjects voluntarily provided written signed informed consent prior to study participation, according to the guidelines of the Declaration of Helsinki and in compliance with current Spanish regulations on clinical research and the standards of EU good clinical practice.

2.2. Measures

Participants were asked to fill out validated self-reported outcome measures as symptom assessment tools. The measures described below were used to evaluate all participants under the supervision of two trained investigators (J.C.-M. and J.A.), who oversaw participant compliance.

2.2.1. Fatigue Impact Scale

The Fatigue Impact Scale (FIS-40) is a 40-item questionnaire designed to assess fatigue symptoms as part of an underlying chronic condition. It includes three domains reflecting the perceived feeling of fatigue: physical (10 items), cognitive (10 items), and psychosocial functions (20 items). Each item is scored from zero (no fatigue) to four (severe fatigue). The overall score is calculated by adding together the responses to the 40 questions (ranging from 0 to 160 points). Higher scores indicate more functional limitations due to fatigue [12].

2.2.2. Composite Autonomic Symptom Score

For measuring autonomic dysfunction, all participants were screened using the Composite Autonomic Symptom Score (COMPASS-31), a 31-item refined and abbreviated questionnaire designed to evaluate the frequency and severity of autonomic function symptoms, grouped in six domains: orthostatic intolerance (four items), vasomotor (three items), secretomotor (four items), gastrointestinal (12 items), bladder (three items), and pupillomotor symptoms (five items). Added together, the six domain scores provide a total COMPASS-31 score ranging from 0 to 100 points. Higher scores indicate more severe autonomic complaints [13].

2.2.3. Pittsburgh Sleep Quality Index

The Pittsburgh Sleep Quality Index (PSQI) is a 19-item self-administered questionnaire commonly used to assess sleep disturbances over a 1 month interval. Scores are acquired on each of the seven domains of sleep quality: subjective sleep quality, sleep latency, sleep duration, habitual sleep efficiency, sleep disturbances, use of sleeping medication, and daytime dysfunction. Each domain is scored from zero to three (zero = no problems and three = severe problems). The overall PSQI score ranges from 0 to 21 points, with scores ≥ 5 indicating poorer sleep quality [14].

2.2.4. Short-Form-36 Health Survey

The SF-36 Health Survey questionnaire, a generic scale that provides a health status profile, was used to assess quality of life. The SF-36 comprises 36 questions which explore eight dimensions of health status (physical function, role limitations due to physical health, bodily pain, general health, vitality, social functioning, emotional role, and mental health), as well as two general subscales covering the physical and mental health domains [15].

2.3. Blood Collection and Processing

Blood samples were collected via venipuncture after a 12 h overnight fasting for immediate routine lab tests by an experienced research nurse at the ME/CFS outpatient clinic (Vall d'Hebron University Hospital, Barcelona, Spain). Blood samples were delivered to the local core laboratory at the hospital within 2 h of collection and analyzed consecutively. Standard HUVH (Vall d'Hebron University Hospital Core Lab, Barcelona, Spain) laboratory protocols were used for the collection, transport and processing, and routine blood tests following standard operating procedures (SOPs).

2.4. Blood Analytics

Baseline laboratory tests were used primarily to exclude primary ME/CFS symptoms of other fatigue-related conditions. These fasting blood tests comprised full blood count, erythrocyte sedimentation rate (ESR), platelets, blood biochemistry parameters, creatinine, fasting glucose, urea, uric acid, bilirubin, electrolyte test (sodium, potassium, calcium), liver function tests (AST, ALT, ALP, GGT), lipid profile (cholesterol, triglycerides, LDL, HDL), thyroid function tests, vitamin D, immunoglobulin (IgA, IgM, IgG, and their isotypes), complement proteins (C1 inhibitor, C1q, C3, C4), and anti-phospholipid antibodies (cardiolipin, beta-2-glycoprotein I). Complement levels were measured by nephelometry using a BN II System (Siemens Healthcare Headquarters, Erlangen, Germany). Normal range reference levels provided by the Vall d'Hebron University Hospital, Barcelona, Spain for each studied variable are shown in Supplementary Table S1.

2.5. Cluster Analysis

Hierarchical cluster analysis was initially conducted using Ward's method [16] to identify the number of clusters chosen on the basis of interpretability and usefulness. A k-means cluster analysis was then carried out to assign participants to clusters. Welch's ANOVA was used on variables of interest to analyze differences among clusters, followed by pairwise comparisons between clusters when the univariate analyses were significant ($p < 0.05$).

2.6. Statistical Analysis and Plotting

Continuous data are shown as means ± SD (standard deviation). Statistical differences were determined using two-tailed unpaired Welch t-tests. Normal distribution was assessed by the Shapiro–Wilk normality test. Categorical variables are presented as n (%), normally distributed variables are presented as mean ± SD, and non-normally distributed variables are presented as median (interquartile range). Differences between groups were considered significant at $p \leq 0.05$. Variable correlations were evaluated by the simple linear regression method (least-squares approach). Statistical analyses were conducted with R 3.6.3 [17], and figures were produced using the package ggplot2 [18].

3. Results

3.1. Demographics and Clinical Characteristics of the Participants

This prospective observational study included 250 adult females diagnosed with ME/CFS by 1994 CDC/Fukuda and 2003 CCC [5,6], the analysis of 69 laboratory blood tests, demographic variables, and four validated self-reported questionnaires to assess disease severity and comorbidities [12–15]. In addition, cardiac variables and medication prescriptions were also recorded (Supplementary Table S1). Table 1 shows descriptive parameters of the study participants. The average age of participants was 45.9 ± 7.02 years, 11.6% (29/250) presented obesity (BMI ≥ 30), fitting with the 13% assessed for the general population [19], average heart rate was 78.5 ± 10.3 bpm, and systolic and diastolic blood pressure were 125.8 ± 2.5 and 76.3 ± 1.6, respectively, among participants. The overall FIS-40 score range reflected the presence of participants with different degrees of fatigue severity. The vast majority of participants had a severe fatigue score (98.8%) while only 1.2% had mild/moderate fatigue, as assessed by the FIS-40 questionnaire provided to the study participants. In addition, over 50% of subjects were taking at least more than one medication as usual/routine care treatment (Table 1).

Table 1. Demographics and clinical characteristics of participants at baseline. Data are expressed as the mean ± standard deviation (SD) for continuous variables and compared by Student t-test, whereas categorical variables are given as numbers with percentages (%) and compared by Fisher's exact test.

Variables	ME/CFS (n = 250)
Age, years	45.9 ± 7.02
BMI, kg/m² †	24.5 ± 4.72
SBP, mmHg	125.8 ± 2.5
DBP (mmHg)	76.3 ± 1.6
Medication, n (%)	
NSAIDs	9 (42.9)
Hypnotics	5 (23.8)
Antidepressants	6 (28.6)
Antipsychotics	4 (19.0)
Opioids	11 (52.4)
Measures	
FIS-40	
Global score (0–160)	
Physical	35.4 ± 2.4
Cognitive	34.0 ± 3.4
Psychosocial	63.9 ± 2.4
COMPASS-31	
Global score (0–100)	53.6 ± 3.5
Orthostatic intolerance	24.3 ± 2.1
Vasomotor	1.4 ± 2.7
Secretomotor	9.3 ± 3.4
Gastrointestinal	11.6 ± 2.9
Bladder	3.5 ± 4.1
Pupillomotor	3.7 ± 3.4

Table 1. *Cont.*

Variables	ME/CFS (*n* = 250)
PSQI	
Global score (0–21)	14.0 ± 0.7
Subjective sleep quality	1.9 ± 0.1
Sleep latency	2.2 ± 0.1
Sleep duration	1.5 ± 0.1
Habitual sleep efficiency	1.9 ± 0.2
Sleep disturbances	2.4 ± 0.1
Sleeping medication	1.9 ± 0.2
Daytime dysfunction	2.2 ± 0.1
SF-36	
Physical functioning	26.9 ± 0.6
Physical role	3.7 ± 0.81
Bodily pain	16.2 ± 1.55
General health perception	21.3 ± 2.18
Vitality	17.0 ± 1.58
Social role functioning	28.2 ± 1.87
Emotional role functioning	30.5 ± 2.78
Mental health	41.4 ± 3.12

Abbreviations: BMI, body mass index; DPB, diastolic blood pressure; SBP, systolic blood pressure; FIS-40, 40-item Fatigue Impact Scale; COMPASS-31, 31-item Composite Autonomic Symptom Score; PSQI, Pittsburgh Sleep Quality Index; SF-36, 36-item Short-Form Health Survey; NSAIDs, nonsteroidal anti-inflammatory drugs. [†] The body-mass index (BMI) is the weight in kilograms divided by the square of the height in meters.

3.2. Exploratory Case Cluster Analysis Based on Symptoms

After applying unbiased hierarchical clustering and optimal grouping based on k-means screenings to identify case clusters, as detailed in Section 2, a set of three clusters showing significant differences in their total FIS-40, total COMPASS-31, total PSQI, physical functioning, and bodily pain scores was obtained (Table 2). Plotting of the itemized standard score differences clearly illustrated the inverse distribution between scales of total FIS-40, total COMPASS-31, and total PSQI that attribute higher scores to more severe symptoms and SF-36 subscales that do the opposite. As a result, our cohort of 250 cases was subdivided into cluster 1, including cases showing more severe symptoms in all five selected parameters (*n* = 94), cluster 2 with cases presenting moderate affection (*n* = 107), and a smaller group of only 49 individuals with milder symptoms (cluster 3) (Figure 1). This shows that the cohort studied mostly contained severe to moderate cases, with <20% of mildly affected cases. The definition of severe in cluster 1 involve total FIS scores over 145 on average, scores over 65 for total COMPASS-31, scores over 15 on average for PSQI, and the lowest scores for physical functioning and bodily pain, which may translate into a more severe fatigue phenotype, accompanied by dysautonomia and sleep problems while experiencing higher levels of pain and compromised physical functioning than the other two clusters (Table 2, Figure 1).

Table 2. Clustering of ME/CFS cases according to symptom differences, as supported by k-means analysis. Data are presented as the mean ± SD for each item. Physical functioning and bodily pain were evaluated by two items of the 36-item Short-Form Health Survey (SF-36).

	Cluster 1	Cluster 2	Cluster 3	*p*-Value
Total FIS	147.93 (9.88)	131.79 (13.48)	108.1 (21.83)	<0.0001
Total COMPASS	66.82 (10.52)	50.9 (10.77)	34.26 (12.71)	<0.0001
Total PSQI	15.82 (3.4)	14.75 (2.94)	8.33 (2.78)	<0.0001
Physical functioning	12.82 (8.82)	31.27 (12.75)	44.39 (16.79)	<0.0001
Bodily pain	6.3 (7.77)	17.95 (11.79)	31.45 (11.83)	<0.0001
Size	94	107	49	

Standard deviation values are shown in parentheses.

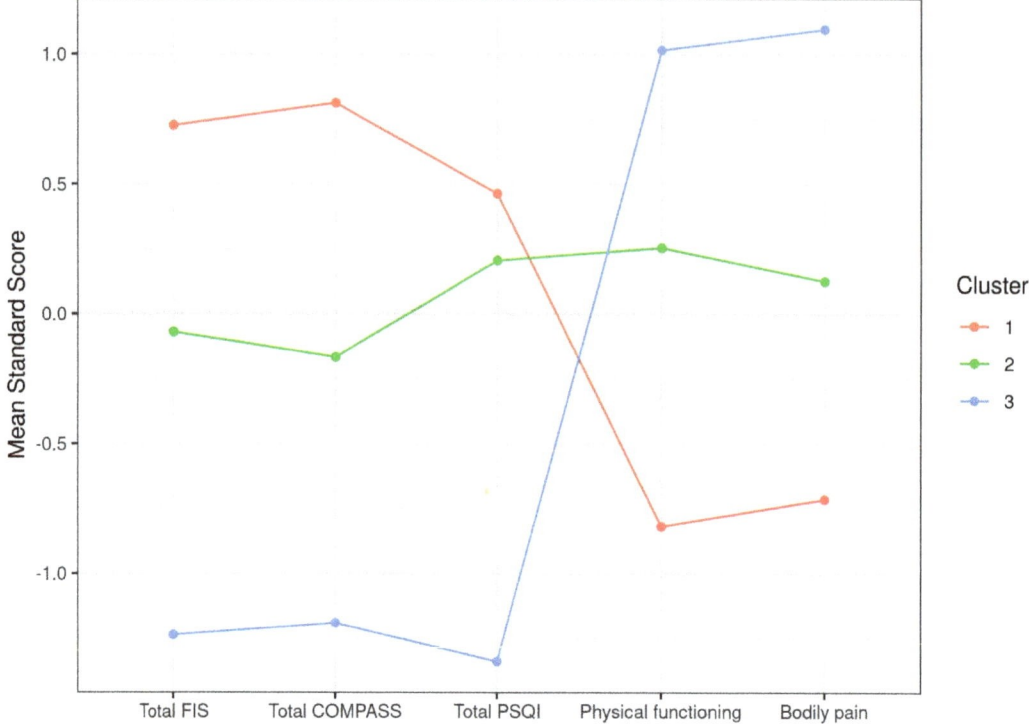

Figure 1. Graphic representation of ME/CFS clustering according to symptom standard mean scores.

3.3. Cluster-Based Differential Analysis of Blood Parameters

Next, we assessed potential differences in the blood analytical variables of these three clusters of cases (clusters 1, 2 and 3, as defined above) using univariate analyses (see Section 2 for details). The analyses intended to detect blood parameters within normal reference range values presented significant differences across case groups (clusters) and may, therefore, be associated with case symptoms. The statistical analysis detected five blood parameters fulfilling the requirements, with p-values < 0.05 (Table 3).

Table 3. Blood analytic differences between symptom-based case clusters. Data are presented as mean ± (SD) for each biochemical variable.

	Cluster 1	Cluster 2	Cluster 3	p-Value
Hb (g/dL)	13.16 (1.05)	13.57 (0.94)	13.07 (1.12)	0.0033
NT ($\times 10^9$/L)	3.99 (1.65)	3.58 (1.63)	3.3 (1.48)	0.0365
COL (mg/dL)	229.57 (36.69)	216.6 (37.42)	211.84 (33.73)	0.0077
HDL (mg/dL)	64.71 (14.44)	59.71 (12.48)	63.12 (12.65)	0.0292
C3 (mg/dL)	132.32 (24.65)	132.02 (29.96)	119.89 (28.09)	0.0246

Abbreviations: Hb, hemoglobin; NT, neutrophil counts; COL, cholesterol; HDL, high-density lipoprotein; C3 complement factor 3.

However, when looking at statistical differences between individual pair sets, we found that none of these five parameters could individually differentiate clusters 1, 2, and 3. For hemoglobin (Hb) levels, only the moderate group (cluster 2) differentiated from the other two, an observation with unclear physiologic interpretation. For neutrophil counts (NT), differences were found between severe (cluster 1) and mild (cluster 3) cases, but none were detected for the moderate group. For cholesterol levels (COL), severe cases (cluster 1) presented differences with moderate and mild (clusters 2 and 3), with no differences between the latter two, whereas high-density lipoproteins (HDL) differences appeared between clusters 1 and 2, but not with cluster 3. Lastly, the levels of complement factor 3 (C3) presented differences between the severe and mild clusters, as well as between the mild and the moderate, but no differences were detected between the severe and the moderate clusters, indicating potential value as a marker to differentiate mild cases from the rest (Figure 2).

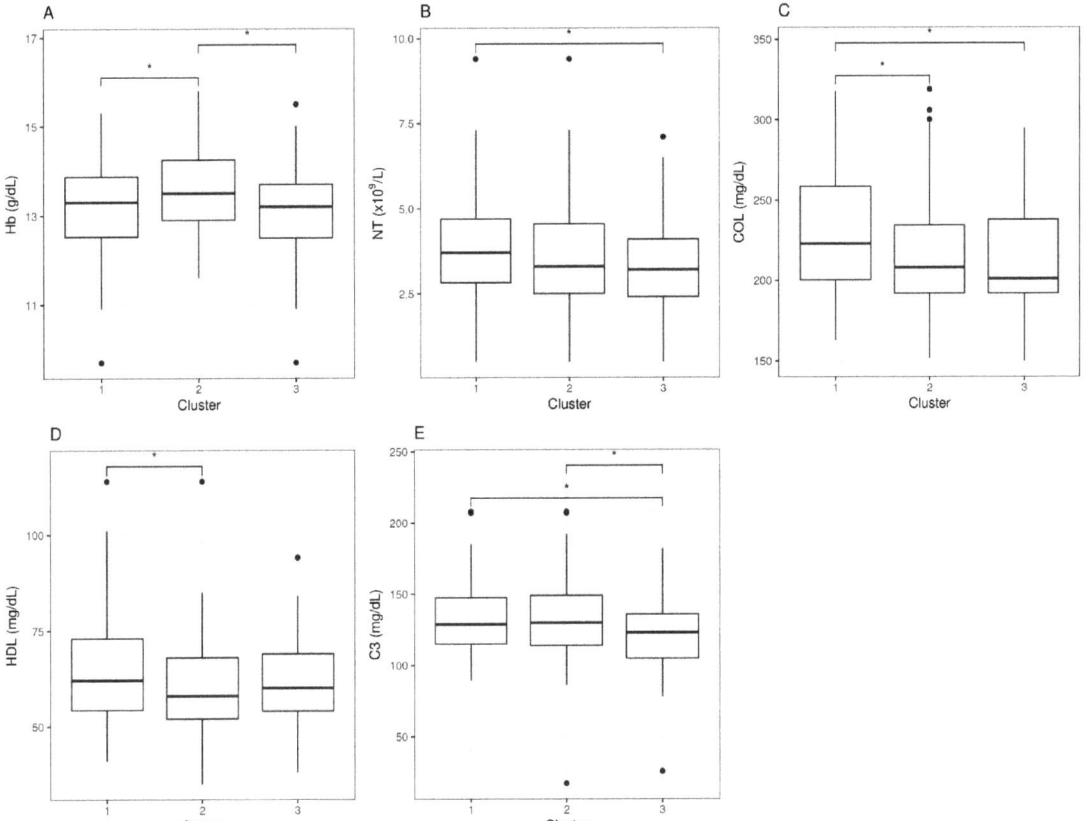

Figure 2. Blood analytic difference boxplots between ME/CFS symptom-based clusters. Abbreviations: Hb, hemoglobin; NT, neutrophil counts; COL, cholesterol; HDL, high-density lipoprotein; C3, complement 3. The significance level was set at * $p < 0.05$. Data beyond 1.5 inter-quartile range values, representing potential outliers, are plotted as individual dots.

In conclusion, symptom-based case clustering followed by differential blood analytics was inefficient for detecting robust single blood variables correlated with case health severity, as defined in these three clusters. It is, however, interesting that some of these blood parameters could, to some extent, differentiate between clusters, the significance of which is not understood at present.

3.4. Stratified Analysis

As an additional attempt to detect patient subgroups that could help refine current diagnosis methods, we evaluated sets of cases presenting abnormal blood parameter values for stratification purposes.

3.4.1. Outstanding Blood Parameters with Abnormal Values

Top analytic variable values deviating from established healthy population reference ranges were vit D (60.4%) mostly represented by deficiency, LDL (55.6%), complement factor C1q (42.8%), and cholesterol (26.4%), all showing increased values overall. Platelet mean volume values appeared both increased and decreased (Table 4 and Supplementary Figure S1).

Table 4. Top blood analytic variables showing abnormal values with respect to reference values in our cohort (n = 250). The number of cases with abnormal values with respect to reference values and percentages (%) are shown.

Variables	n (%)
25(OH).Vit.D3	151 (60.4)
LDL	140 (56)
C1q	107 (42.8)
25(OH).Vit.D3, LDL	81 (32.4)
25(OH).Vit.D3, C1q	72 (28.8)
COL	66 (26.4)
C1q, LDL	60 (24)
COL, LDL	58 (23.2)
PMV	56 (22.4)

Abbreviations: 25(OH) Vit.D3, vitamin D; LDL, low-density lipoprotein; C1q, complement factor C1q; COL, cholesterol; PMV, platelet mean volume.

Combinations of these five blood analytical variables which included at least 20% of the cases in our cohort showed that vitamin D and LDL were both abnormal in 32.4% of the participants. Other combinations, such as vitamin D deficiency and increment of C1q, or increased LDL with C1q or cholesterol involved over 20% of the participants (>50 cases). Since vitamin D reference values are widely influenced by genetic and environmental factors, and the assays to quantitate its levels typically show variability over ±10% [20,21], leading to a lack of consensus global reference values [22,23], we decided to exclude this variable from our stratified downstream analysis.

Similarly, since differences found in LDL and cholesterol are nonspecifically associated with disease, sometimes appearing together with vitamin D deficiency [22,23], they were not further pursued, meaning that they were not used to set stratification conditions of our cohort. The unexpected finding of a quite significant proportion of ME/CFS cases showing increased levels of C1q and decreased C1 inhibitor (42.8% and 8.8%, respectively) (Supplementary Table S1), together with the C1q deficiency being associated with autoimmune diseases such as systemic lupus erythematosus [24], motivated our interest to hypothesize C1q as a potential biomarker for ME/CFS subtyping.

3.4.2. Symptom Differences across C1q Case Clusters

Downstream analysis after a conservative 5% cutoff above C1q maximum normal value stratification (samples with C1q > 26.05 mg/dL, cluster 1, with n = 90; samples with C1q < 26.05 mg/dL, cluster 2, with n = 160), however, showed no significant differences in any symptom score, with the only exception of a tendency for bodily pain (p = 0.09), suggesting perhaps increased pain in the group with high C1q levels (mean values were 14.24 vs. 17.33, respectively) (Table 5).

Table 5. Symptom differences between case clusters with increased C1q values (cluster1) (>26.05 mg/dL) or within range (C1q < 26.05 mg/dL). Group mean values and standard deviations are shown.

	Cluster 1	Cluster 2	p-Value
Total FIS	132.6 (22.83)	133.56 (18.81)	0.7358
Total COMPASS	54.96 (16.84)	52.88 (15.94)	0.3401
Total PSQI	14.29 (4.06)	13.67 (4.21)	0.2544
Physical functioning	27.5 (18.36)	26.57 (16.56)	0.6907
Bodily pain	14.24 (13.63)	17.32 (13.95)	0.0906
Size	90	160	

3.4.3. Blood analytic Differences across C1q Case Clusters

To evaluate whether the group of cases presenting increased C1q levels (cluster 1, n = 90) could, at the same time, present with additional blood parameter differences, even when being within normal reference values for the group showing normal C1q values (cluster 2, n = 160), we applied a statistic test after cohort stratification, as detailed in Section 2. The results showed significant differences in seven blood parameters ($p < 0.05$), as shown in Table 6.

Table 6. Blood analytic differences between C1q case clusters. Group means and standard deviations are shown.

	Cluster 1	Cluster 2	p-Value
RBC ($\times 10^{12}$/L)	4.62 (0.32)	4.53 (0.38)	0.0431
PT (g/dL)	7.24 (0.39)	7.1 (0.42)	0.0093
IgG3/IgG	6.29 (3.64)	8.91 (13.47)	0.0219
IgG4/IgG	2.75 (1.7)	3.32 (2.56)	0.0343
C1$_{inh}$ (mg/dL)	25.56 (5.28)	27.56 (5.58)	0.0055
C3 (mg/dL)	137.44 (27.47)	125.43 (27.48)	0.0011
C4 (mg/dL)	30.73 (8.57)	27.7 (7.72)	0.006

Abbreviations: RBC, red blood cell; PT, total protein; IgG, immunoglobulin; C1$_{inh}$ complement 1 inhibitor; C, complement factor. Standard deviation values are shown between brackets.

Overall, the cluster with increased C1q levels presented with higher red blood cell counts, as well as total protein, C3, and C4 levels, and lower IgG3, IgG4, and C1$_{inh}$ concentrations, indicating pathways potentially connected with elevated C1q levels and, thus, potentially relevant for clinical treatment of an important subset of ME/CFS cases.

4. Discussion

As earlier mentioned, the use of standard blood tests to at least support a potential case of ME/CFS ("triage" diagnosis method) and/or differentiate case subgroups for therapeutic and research purposes would provide clear advantages. In fact, it may well constitute the key toward unveiling ME/CFS subgroup etiology and evolution.

Although clustering methods based on case symptoms have been useful in identifying autonomic phenotypes in CFS [25], they failed at detecting robust blood correlations between symptoms and individual blood parameters in our cohort (Figure 2). The approach did, however, show potential for differentiating cases with severe, moderate, or mild affection as defined by the five symptom scores used for clustering (Tables 2 and 3). The physiological significance of the findings, including the increased levels of C3 in severe and moderate with respect to mildly affected cases or the increased neutrophil count in severe ME/CFS by itself or in combination with LDL and cholesterol, as well as their involvement in symptom development or maintenance, remains to be elucidated.

Nevertheless, the presence of a large proportion of ME/CFS (42.8% or 107/250) cases with increased expression of C1q, for the first time, may importantly set the basis for future ME/CFS subtyping.

C1q acts as the first component in the classical complement pathway. The complement system is a central part of innate immunity with two important functions: serving as a defense system against invading pathogens and for the clearing of dead cells or debris [26,27]. C1q recognizes PAMPs (pathogen-associated molecular patterns), including LPS (lipopolysaccharide) and bacterial porins [28], in addition to recognizing molecules such as phosphatidylserine and dsDNA exposed on the surface of dying cells [29,30].

Thus, the detected increased levels of C1q and other complement components in a subgroup of ME/CFS cases may indicate a state of active efferocytosis toward fighting a subjacent infection or while clearing damaged tissue. Moreover, cases with chronic activation of the complement pathway may, for this reason, become particularly sensitive to PEM [4–7], a possibility that may be worth exploring.

It is well documented that, both inefficient and overstimulation of the complement system can be detrimental for the host, being associated with increased susceptibility to infections, autoimmunity, chronic inflammation, and thrombotic microangiopathy, among others [24,26,27,31]. Some of these processes have been associated with ME/CFS [32,33]. We, however, only found a few cases of positive self-antigen immunity across the 10-test run applied to the 250 participating cases (Supplementary Table S1).

The observation that, among the many blood parameters measured, those known to be related to C1q function, i.e., C1 inhibitors C3 and C4 showed significant differences between groups (Table 6) further supports a functional problem of the complement system in this subgroup of cases, perhaps with consequences in the process of coagulation. A prospective follow-up of coagulopathies in this subgroup of patients, thus, appears pertinent.

More recently, Benavente et al. showed that C1q acts as a ligand that can directly bind a series of receptors previously unidentified as partners of this molecule, including the following proteins: CD44, GPR62, BAI1, c-MET, and ADCY5, which trigger activation of downstream signaling pathways [34,35] and, thus, affect different aspects of neuroepithelial stem-cell biology. The finding by these authors that C1q is elevated upon nerve injury [34] and the emerging connections of C1q with neurodegenerative disease [36,37] open up the exciting possibility that increased levels of C1q may underlie ME/CFS cognitive problems [4–7]. C1q alters prion disease progression, regulates neuron pruning, and modulates the process of phagocytosis by microglia while responding to amyloid plaque formation [38–40]. Unfortunately, no specific instruments for detailed cognitive assessment of the participants or neuroimaging tools were used in this study.

Lastly, the fact that the two strata presenting normal vs. increased levels of C1q showed differences in pain may indicate a direct involvement of C1q in case symptoms. It may be relevant to include a more detailed assessment of this symptom by using pain-focused questionnaires, such as the FIQ (Fibromyalgia Impact Questionnaire) and/or others [41–43], in future studies of C1q's role in ME/CFS. Although the failure of questionnaires other than the SF-36 to detect symptom-related differences with C1q levels (Table 5) lead to us presuming no major involvement of C1q in this aspect of the disease, it seems curious that the plotting of the two clusters showed opposite trends in all five symptoms selected by the k-means screening method to set symptom-based clusters of the cohort (Figures 1 and 3).

Moreover, within the 94 cases in the "severe" group (cluster 1) of our symptom-based cluster analysis (Table 2), about 39% (37/94) presented increased C1q levels while 61% (57/94) showed normal levels; within the 107 cases of the "moderate" group (cluster 2), 35% (37/107) had increased C1q and 65% (70/107) normal C1q levels; within the 49 cases of the "mild" group (cluster 3), 33% (16/49) showed increased C1q levels and 67% (33/49) had C1q levels within normal reference values. This indicates a rough 1:2 overall ratio of cases with increased C1q levels in the "mild" group, with a slight increase in this ratio in the "moderate" and an even higher ratio (1:1.5) in the "severe" cluster, suggesting an increased prevalence of high C1q levels with case disease severity, despite the lack of significant correlations between individual symptom scores and C1q levels. A correlation of C1q levels with the chronicity status of cases could not be established either.

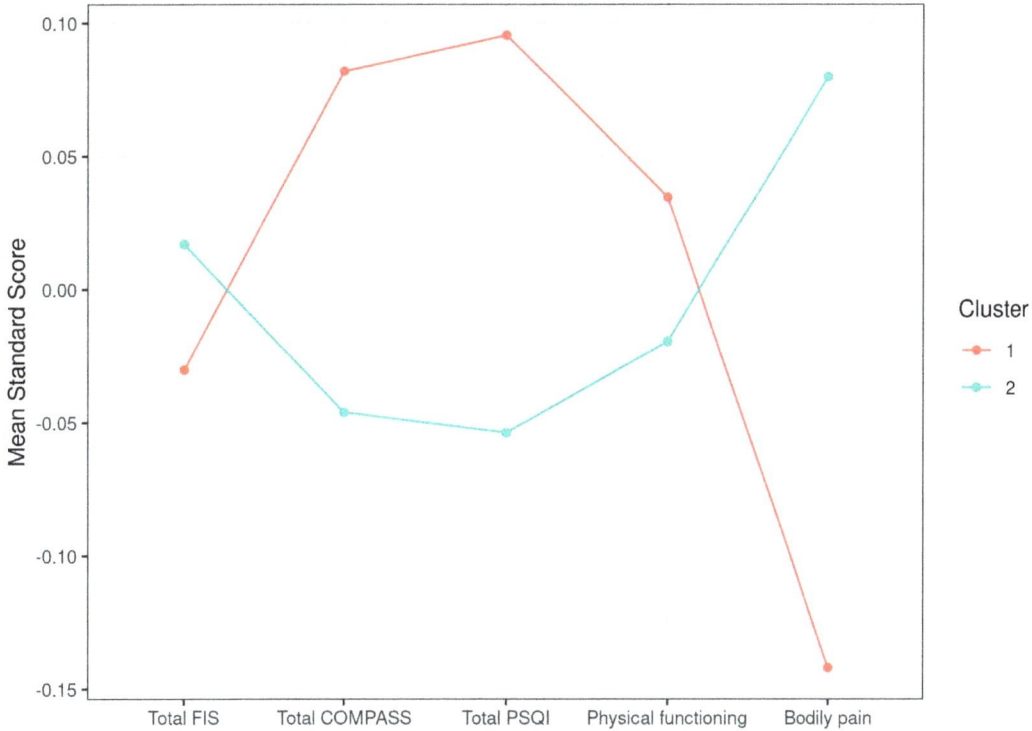

Figure 3. Graphic representation of ME/CFS symptom standard score differences in relation to C1q stratification.

Additional blood parameters that showed abnormal values in a large proportion of individuals in our cohort, such as vitamin D deficiency, LDL levels, cholesterol, C3 levels, or platelet mean value, may provide relevant information for treatment options, an aspect not well understood at present, which requires further monitoring in the future.

It should be mentioned that, although different reference values have been established for vitamin D deficiency, for example, the recommendations from the 2011 US Institute of Medicine (IOM) reported a minimal concentration of 52 nmol/L, while the US Endocrine Society guidelines stated a minimal concentration of 78 nmol/L [44,45], the applied range in this study was right below the lowest range (50 nmol/L, Supplementary Table S1), and yet a large proportion of cases (>60%) showed vitamin D deficiency (Table 4).

Additional Limitations

Although the cohort under study included a considerable number of subjects (n = 250), the external validity of the data remains limited to females. Random selection of participants can lead to more representative results population wise; however, subject heterogeneity translates into enhanced variability, compromising the establishment of robust differences, perhaps relevant to the diagnosis of ME/CFS. The lack of additional relevant differences across ME/CFS cases cannot be ruled out by the laborious, yet discrete analysis here performed.

5. Conclusions

In conclusion, this study identified a potential new player in the ME/CFS pathology, the C1q component of the complement system, affecting over 40% of cases. This finding paves the way for exploring a C1q-based standard lab assay to detect ME/CFS subtypes with relevant clinical and research implications. The understanding of the underlying pathomechanisms behind this finding is limited at present, granting further exploration of the observation.

Supplementary Materials: The following are available online at https://www.mdpi.com/article/10.3390/jcm10184171/s1, Figure S1: Box plots of top blood analytic variables showing off-normal reference values in our cohort (*n* = 250). Red lines indicate normal range values. Black line within the box is the median within quartile values. Normal values are shown in green while abnormal values are shown in red. Table S1: Cohort dataset.

Author Contributions: Conceptualization, J.C.-M. and E.O.; data gathering, J.C.-M. and J.A.-M.; data analysis and interpretation, J.C.-M., M.Z., E.A.-P. and E.O.; writing—original draft preparation, J.C.-M., M.Z. and E.O.; writing—review and editing, all authors; funding acquisition, J.C.-M., J.A.-M. and E.O. All authors have read and agreed to the published version of the manuscript..

Funding: This research was partially funded by the Association of Patients with ME/CFS and Fibromyalgia in Catalonia, Spain (ACAF; www.fibromyalgia.cat (accessed on 23 March 2019) to J.C.-M. and J.A.-M., and by a UCV 2020-270-001 grant to E.O.

Institutional Review Board Statement: The study protocol was conducted according to the guidelines of the Declaration of Helsinki and approved by the local Clinical Research Ethics Committee (Vall d'Hebron University Hospital, Barcelona, Spain; IRB reference number: CEIC/PR-AG-VITAE-2015, approved in June 2015).

Informed Consent Statement: Written informed consent was obtained from all subjects involved in the study.

Data Availability Statement: Datasets are provided as Supplementary Table S1.

Acknowledgments: The authors thank all the ME/CFS patients (Association of ME/CFS and Fibromyalgia in Catalonia, Spain) who took part for supporting this study. The authors are also particularly grateful to Ramon Sanmartin and Marta Musté for their administrative and technical support facilitating data acquisition from study participants. Vall d'Hebron Hospital Research Institute (VHIR) is a member of the CERCA program (Network of Excellence Research Centers of Catalonia, Spain).

Conflicts of Interest: The authors declare no conflict of interest. The funder had no role in the design of the study; in the collection, analyses, or interpretation of data, in the writing of the manuscript, or in the decision to publish the results.

References

1. WHO. *ICD-10: International Classification of Statistical Classification of Diseases and Related Health Problems*; World Health Organization: Geneva, Switzerland, 2004.
2. World Health Organization; Committee on the Diagnostic Criteria for Myalgic Encephalomyelitis/Chronic Fatigue Syndrome; Board on the Health of Select Populations; Institute of Medicine. *Beyond Myalgic Encephalomyelitis/Chronic Fatigue Syndrome: Redefining an Illness*; National Academies Press: Washington, DC, USA, 2015.
3. Estévez-López, F.; Castro-Marrero, J.; Wang, X.; Bakken, I.J.; Ivanovs, A.; Nacul, L.; Sepúlveda, N.; Strand, E.B.; Pheby, D.; Alegre, J.; et al. European Network on ME/CFS (EUROMENE). Prevalence and incidence of myalgic encephalomyelitis/chronic fatigue syndrome in Europe: The Euro-EpiME study from the European network on ME/CFS (EUROMENE): A protocol for a systematic review. *BMJ Open* **2018**, *8*, e020817. [CrossRef] [PubMed]
4. Clayton, E.W. Beyond myalgic encephalomyelitis/chronic fatigue syndrome: An IOM report on redefining an illness. *JAMA* **2015**, *313*, 1101–1102. [CrossRef] [PubMed]
5. Fukuda, K.; Straus, S.E.; Hickie, I.; Sharpe, M.C.; Dobbins, J.G.; Komaroff, A.; Schluederberg, A.; Jones, J.F.; Lloyd, A.R.; Wessely, S.; et al. The chronic fatigue syndrome: A comprehensive approach to its definition and study. *Ann. Intern. Med.* **1994**, *121*, 953–959. [CrossRef] [PubMed]
6. Carruthers, B.M.; Jain, A.K.; De Meirleir, K.L.; Peterson, D.L.; Klimas, N.G.; Lerner, A.; Bested, A.C.; Flor-Henry, P.; Joshi, P.; Powles, A.C.P.; et al. Myalgic encephalomyelitis/chronic fatigue syndrome: Clinical working case definition, diagnostic and treatment protocols. *J. Chron. Fatigue Syndr.* **2003**, *11*, 7–115. [CrossRef]
7. Carruthers, B.M.; van de Sande, M.I.; De Meirleir, K.L.; Klimas, N.G.; Broderick, G.; Mitchell, T.; Staines, D.; Powles, A.C.P.; Speight, N.; Vallings, R.; et al. Myalgic encephalomyelitis: International Consensus Criteria. *J. Intern. Med.* **2011**, *270*, 3273–3278. [CrossRef]
8. Lidbury, B.A.; Fisher, P.R. Biomedical Insights that Inform the Diagnosis of ME/CFS. *Diagnostics* **2020**, *10*, 92. [CrossRef]

9. Nacul, L.; de Barros, B.; Kingdon, C.C.; Cliff, J.M.; Clark, T.G.; Mudie, K.; Dockrell, H.M.; Lacerda, E.M. Evidence of Clinical Pathology Abnormalities in People with Myalgic Encephalomyelitis/Chronic Fatigue Syndrome (ME/CFS) from an Analytic Cross-Sectional Study. *Diagnostics* **2019**, *9*, 41. [CrossRef]
10. Almenar-Pérez, E.; Sarria, L.; Nathanson, L.; Oltra, E. Assessing diagnostic value of microRNAs from peripheral blood mononuclear cells and extracellular vesicles in Myalgic Encephalomyelitis/Chronic Fatigue Syndrome. *Sci. Rep.* **2020**, *10*, 2064. [CrossRef]
11. Kitami, T.; Fukuda, S.; Kato, T.; Yamaguti, K.; Nakatomi, Y.; Yamano, E.; Kataoka, Y.; Mizuno, K.; Tsuboi, Y.; Kogo, Y.; et al. Deep phenotyping of myalgic encephalomyelitis/chronic fatigue syndrome in Japanese population. *Sci. Rep.* **2020**, *10*, 19933. [CrossRef]
12. Fisk, J.D.; Ritvo, P.G.; Ross, L.; Haase, D.A.; Marrie, T.J.; Schlech, W.F. Measuring the functional impact of fatigue: Initial validation of the fatigue impact scale. *Clin. Infect. Dis.* **1994**, *18*, S79–S83. [CrossRef] [PubMed]
13. Sletten, D.M.; Suarez, G.A.; Low, P.A.; Mandrekar, J.; Singer, W. COMPASS 31: A refined and abbreviated Composite Autonomic Symptom Score. *Mayo. Clin. Proc.* **2012**, *87*, 1196–1201. [CrossRef]
14. Buysse, D.J.; Reynolds, C.F.; Monk, T.H.; Berman, S.R.; Kupfer, D.J. The Pittsburgh Sleep Quality Index: A new instrument for psychiatric practice and research. *Psychiatry Res.* **1989**, *28*, 193–213. [CrossRef]
15. Alonso, J.; Prieto, L.; Antó, J.M. The Spanish version of the SF-36 Health Survey: An instrument for measuring clinical results. *Med. Clin.* **1995**, *104*, 771–776.
16. Ward, J.H., Jr. Hierarchical Grouping to Optimize an Objective Function. *J. Am. Stat. Assoc.* **1963**, *58*, 236–244. [CrossRef]
17. R Core Team. *R: A Language and Environment for Statistical Computing*; R Foundation for Statistical Computing: Vienna, Austria, 2019. Available online: https://www.R-project.org (accessed on 4 September 2020).
18. Wickham, H. *ggplot2: Elegant Graphics for Data Analysis*; Springer: New York, NY, USA, 2016.
19. Obese Chooi, Y.C.; Ding, C.; Magkos, F. The epidemiology of obesity. *Metabolism* **2019**, *92*, 6–10. [CrossRef] [PubMed]
20. Ferrari, D.; Lombardi, G.; Banfi, G. Concerning the vitamin D reference range: Pre-analytical and analytical variability of vitamin D measurement. *Biochem. Med.* **2017**, *27*, 030501. [CrossRef]
21. Nikolac Gabaj, N.; Unic, A.; Miler, M.; Pavicic, T.; Culej, J.; Bolanca, I.; Herman Mahecic, D.; Milevoj Kopcinovic, L.; Vrtaric, A. In sickness and in health: Pivotal role of vitamin D. *Biochem Med.* **2020**, *30*, 020501. [CrossRef]
22. Surdu, A.M.; Pînzariu, O.; Ciobanu, D.M.; Negru, A.G.; Căinap, S.S.; Lazea, C.; Iacob, D.; Săraci, G.; Tirinescu, D.; Borda, I.M.; et al. Vitamin D and Its Role in the Lipid Metabolism and the Development of Atherosclerosis. *Biomedicines* **2021**, *9*, 172. [CrossRef] [PubMed]
23. Yarparvar, A.; Elmadfa, I.; Djazayery, A.; Abdollahi, Z.; Salehi, F. The Association of Vitamin D Status with Lipid Profile and Inflammation Biomarkers in Healthy Adolescents. *Nutrients* **2020**, *12*, 590. [CrossRef]
24. Trendelenburg, M. Autoantibodies against complement component C1q in systemic lupus erythematosus. *Clin. Transl. Immunol.* **2021**, *10*, e1279. [CrossRef]
25. Słomko, J.; Estévez-López, F.; Kujawski, S.; Zawadka-Kunikowska, M.; Tafil-Klawe, M.; Klawe, J.J.; Morten, K.J.; Szrajda, J.; Murovska, M.; Newton, J.L.; et al. Autonomic Phenotypes in Chronic Fatigue Syndrome Are Associated with Illness Severity: A Cluster Analysis. *J. Clin. Med.* **2020**, *9*, 2531. [CrossRef]
26. Merle, N.S.; Church, S.E.; Fremeaux-Bacchi, V.; Roumenina, L.T. Complement System Part I—Molecular Mechanisms of Activation and Regulation. *Front Immunol.* **2015**, *6*, 262. [CrossRef]
27. Merle, N.S.; Noe, R.; Halbwachs-Mecarelli, L.; Fremeaux-Bacchi, V.; Roumenina, L.T. Complement System Part II: Role in Immunity. *Front. Immunol.* **2015**, *6*, 257. [CrossRef]
28. Roumenina, L.T.; Popov, K.T.; Bureeva, S.V.; Kojouharova, M.; Gadjeva, M.; Rabheru, S.; Thakrar, R.; Kaplun, A.; Kishore, U. Interaction of the globular domain of human C1q with *Salmonella typhimurium* lipopolysaccharide. *Biochim. Biophys. Acta* **2008**, *1784*, 1271–1276. [CrossRef]
29. Gaboriaud, C.; Frachet, P.; Thielens, N.M.; Arlaud, G.J. The human c1q globular domain: Structure and recognition of non-immune self-ligands. *Front Immunol.* **2012**, *2*, 92. [CrossRef]
30. Païdassi, H.; Tacnet-Delorme, P.; Lunardi, T.; Arlaud, G.J.; Thielens, N.M.; Frachet, P. The lectin-like activity of human C1q and its implication in DNA and apoptotic cell recognition. *FEBS Lett.* **2008**, *582*, 3111–3116. [CrossRef] [PubMed]
31. Defendi, F.; Thielens, N.M.; Clavarino, G.; Cesbron, J.Y.; Dumestre-Pérard, C. The Immunopathology of Complement Proteins and Innate Immunity in Autoimmune Disease. *Clin. Rev. Allergy Immunol.* **2020**, *58*, 229–251. [CrossRef]
32. Morris, G.; Berk, M.; Galecki, P.; Maes, M. The emerging role of autoimmunity in myalgic encephalomyelitis/chronic fatigue syndrome (ME/CFS). *Mol Neurobiol.* **2014**, *49*, 741–756. [CrossRef] [PubMed]
33. Morris, G.; Berk, M.; Klein, H.; Walder, K.; Galecki, P.; Maes, M. Nitrosative Stress, Hypernitrosylation, and Autoimmune Responses to Nitrosylated Proteins: New Pathways in Neuroprogressive Disorders Including Depression and Chronic Fatigue Syndrome. *Mol. Neurobiol.* **2017**, *54*, 4271–4291. [CrossRef] [PubMed]
34. Benavente, F.; Piltti, K.M.; Hooshmand, M.J.; Nava, A.A.; Lakatos, A.; Feld, B.G.; Creasman, D.; Gershon, P.D.; Anderson, A. Novel C1q receptor-mediated signaling controls neural stem cell behavior and neurorepair. *Elife* **2020**, *9*, e55732. [CrossRef] [PubMed]
35. Noble, M.; Pröschel, C. The many roles of C1q. *Elife* **2020**, *9*, e61599. [CrossRef] [PubMed]
36. Kouser, L.; Madhukaran, S.P.; Shastri, A.; Saraon, A.; Ferluga, J.; Al-Mozaini, M.; Kishore, U. Emerging and Novel Functions of Complement Protein C1q. *Front. Immunol.* **2015**, *6*, 317. [CrossRef]

37. Cho, K. Emerging Roles of Complement Protein C1q in Neurodegeneration. *Aging Dis.* **2019**, *10*, 652–663. [CrossRef] [PubMed]
38. Bialas, A.R.; Stevens, B. TGF-β signaling regulates neuronal C1q expression and developmental synaptic refinement. *Nat. Neurosci.* **2013**, *16*, 1773–1782. [CrossRef] [PubMed]
39. Färber, K.; Cheung, G.; Mitchell, D.; Wallis, R.; Weihe, E.; Schwaeble, W.; Kettenmann, H. C1q, the recognition subcomponent of the classical pathway of complement, drives microglial activation. *J. Neurosci. Res.* **2009**, *87*, 644–652. [CrossRef] [PubMed]
40. Lynch, N.J.; Willis, C.L.; Nolan, C.C.; Roscher, S.; Fowler, M.J.; Weihe, E.; Ray, D.E.; Schwaeble, W.J. Microglial activation and increased synthesis of complement component C1q precedes blood-brain barrier dysfunction in rats. *Mol. Immunol.* **2004**, *40*, 709–716. [CrossRef]
41. Burckhardt, C.S.; Clark, S.R.; Bennett, R.M. The fibromyalgia impact questionnaire: Development and validation. *J. Rheumatol.* **1991**, *18*, 728–733. [PubMed]
42. Rivera, J.; González, T. The Fibromyalgia Impact Questionnaire: A validated Spanish version to assess the health status in women with fibromyalgia. *Clin. Exp. Rheumatol.* **2004**, *22*, 554–560.
43. Patel, K.V.; Amtmann, D.; Jensen, M.P.; Smith, S.M.; Veasley, C.; Turk, D.C. Clinical outcome assessment in clinical trials of chronic pain treatments. *Pain Rep.* **2021**, *6*, e784. [CrossRef]
44. Holick, M.F.; Binkley, N.C.; Bischoff-Ferrari, H.A.; Gordon, C.M.; Hanley, D.A.; Heaney, R.P.; Murad, M.H.; Weaver, C.M. Evaluation, treatment, and prevention of vitamin D deficiency: An Endocrine Society clinical practice guideline. *J. Clin. Endocrinol. Metab.* **2011**, *96*, 1911–1930. [CrossRef]
45. Ross, A.C.; Manson, J.E.; Abrams, S.A.; Aloia, J.F.; Brannon, P.M.; Clinton, S.K.; Durazo-Arvizu, R.A.; Gallagher, J.C.; Gallo, R.L.; Jones, G.; et al. The 2011 report on dietary reference intakes for calcium and vitamin D from the Institute of Medicine: What clinicians need to know. *J. Clin. Endocrinol. Metab.* **2011**, *96*, 53–58. [CrossRef] [PubMed]

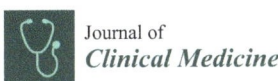

Article

Effects of Non-Pharmacological Treatment on Pain, Flexibility, Balance and Quality of Life in Women with Fibromyalgia: A Randomised Clinical Trial

Juan Rodríguez-Mansilla [1], Abel Mejías-Gil [1], Elisa María Garrido-Ardila [1,*], María Jiménez-Palomares [1], Jesús Montanero-Fernández [2] and María Victoria González-López-Arza [1]

1 ADOLOR Research Group, Department of Medical-Surgical Therapy, Faculty of Medicine and Health Sciences, Extremadura University, 06006 Badajoz, Spain; jrodman@unex.es (J.R.-M.); abel_mejias@hotmail.com (A.M.-G.); mariajp@unex.es (M.J.-P.); mvglez@unex.es (M.V.G.-L.-A.)
2 Mathematics Department, Faculty of Medicine and Health Sciences, Extremadura University, 06006 Badajoz, Spain; jmf@unex.es
* Correspondence: egarridoa@unex.es; Tel.: +34-653369655

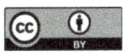

Citation: Rodríguez-Mansilla, J.; Mejías-Gil, A.; Garrido-Ardila, E.M.; Jiménez-Palomares, M.; Montanero-Fernández, J.; González-López-Arza, M.V. Effects of Non-Pharmacological Treatment on Pain, Flexibility, Balance and Quality of Life in Women with Fibromyalgia: A Randomised Clinical Trial. *J. Clin. Med.* **2021**, *10*, 3826. https://doi.org/10.3390/jcm10173826

Academic Editors: Giovanni Ricevuti and Lorenzo Lorusso

Received: 30 July 2021
Accepted: 25 August 2021
Published: 26 August 2021

Publisher's Note: MDPI stays neutral with regard to jurisdictional claims in published maps and institutional affiliations.

Copyright: © 2021 by the authors. Licensee MDPI, Basel, Switzerland. This article is an open access article distributed under the terms and conditions of the Creative Commons Attribution (CC BY) license (https://creativecommons.org/licenses/by/4.0/).

Abstract: Background: The functional deficits in people with fibromyalgia can be related to the level of physical activity performed. This study investigated the effectiveness of an active exercise programme versus exercise for well-being improving pain, flexibility, static balance, perceived exertion and quality of life of women with fibromyalgia; Methods: A randomised, single-blind, controlled trial was conducted. A total of 141 of women diagnosed with fibromyalgia were enrolled and randomised to an active exercise program group ($n = 47$), where they performed physical active exercises, an exercise for well-being group ($n = 47$), which performed the Qi Gong exercises named 'the twenty Wang Ziping figures for health and longevity', and a control group ($n = 47$), which did not receive any intervention, for a period of 4 weeks. Measures were taken at baseline and after the treatment. The primary outcome measures were static balance and centre of gravity (Wii-Fit Nintendo ©), flexibility (test de Wells and Dillon), pain (Visual Analogue Scale) and quality of life (Spanish-Fibromyalgia Impact Questionnaire). The secondary outcome measure was the perceived exertion during activity (BORG Scale). Results: In total, 93 participants completed the study. The mean value of the age was 52.24 ± 6.19. The post intervention results showed statistically significant improvements in the exercise for well-being and the active exercise programme groups vs. the control group in relation to pain ($p = 0.006$ active exercise programme group, $p = 0.001$ exercise for well-being group), static balance ($p < 0.001$ active exercise programme group) and quality of life ($p < 0.001$ active exercise programme group, $p = 0.002$ exercise for well-being group). In addition, the mean scores related to perceived fatigue during the sessions were 6.30 ± 1.88 for the active exercise programme group and 5.52 ± 1.55 for the exercise for well-being group. These differences were not significant. Conclusions: The active exercise program and exercise for well-being improved flexibility, static balance, pain and quality of life of women with fibromyalgia. The participants of the active exercise programme achieved better results that those of the exercise for well-being.

Keywords: fibromyalgia; exercise for well-being; active exercise program; flexibility; static balance; pain; quality of life

1. Introduction

The main clinical manifestation of Fibromyalgia is diffuse and widespread pain in combination with the presence of multiple tender points [1]. In addition to pain, these patients have sensory symptoms, such as paraesthesia, motor symptoms, such as muscle stiffness, contractures and tremors, and vegetative symptoms, such as tingling sensations [2].

Different authors have suggested that these symptoms can affect the functional capacity of these patients [3,4]. This is based on the association between symptoms, flexibility and balance impairments [3,4]. Moreover, balance impairment is a very frequent sign in persons with fibromyalgia and it is considered one of the 10 most disabling symptoms, with a prevalence between 45% and 68% [5]. In addition, it has been shown that these impairments often appear in persons with the same conditions, such as chronic fatigue syndrome, especially the loss of static and dynamic balance [6], which can lead to impaired mobility [7]. Vestibular function may be impaired in patients with chronic fatigue syndrome who also have fibromyalgia but not in those with chronic fatigue syndrome alone [8].

A study conducted by Jones et al. [5] showed how persons with fibromyalgia had significant inferior scores on different balance aspects and had six times more falls when compared with healthy subjects. Balance impairments and functional capacity are closely related [9] and have a significant impact in the quality of life of people with fibromyalgia [2].

These abilities are diminished or altered in patients with fibromyalgia compared to healthy subjects [10–14]. This can lead to limited or difficult mobility, which can increase the risk of falls [15,16], and consequently, it can have a negative impact on the quality of life of these patients [2].

According to the scientific evidence, these functional deficits in people with fibromyalgia are related to the level of physical activity performed [9]. Several systematic reviews analyse the efficacy of physical exercise programmes, either alone or in combination with other forms of physical or cognitive intervention [17–19]. All of them conclude that physical exercise improves the quality of life of these patients. In this regard, a literature review on the benefits of exercise in fibromyalgia published in 2019 [20] concluded that exercise also improves physical function and fatigue. However, further studies and research are needed to analyse this further [20].

Complementary and alternative therapies are currently being used as a non-pharmacological intervention for the management of fibromyalgia [21]. The World Health Organisation defines exercise for well-being (Qi Gong) as: "A component of traditional Chinese medicine that combines movement, meditation and breathing regulation to improve the flow of vital energy in the body (Qi), to improve circulation and immune function" [22].

The available literature supports that exercise for well-being improves pain management [23,24] and physical function [24] in patients with fibromyalgia. In addition, some clinical trials have shown that this treatment technique also improves balance and prevents falls [25]. Qi Gong is an aerobic exercise, which involves mental concentration, breathing that accompanies the movement, static postures and dynamic movements which combine stretching and activation of the muscle chains through isometric and isotonic contractions. It also includes self-massage movements and flexibility, strength, proprioception, coordination and balance work [26–28]. Qi Gong also corrects the posture of the spine and the pelvis and prevents stagnation of the energy in the joints [29]. On this basis, scientific research suggests that low-intensity aerobic exercise and meditative movement therapies, such as Qi Gong, are recommended for the treatment of fibromyalgia patients, as they improve their symptoms and quality of life [30–32].

However, the research conducted on this topic is scarce and the existing studies agree that further research on the effects of these alternative therapies in patients with fibromyalgia is needed. In the literature consulted, no studies that analyse these variables and compare both treatments, physical exercise or an active exercise programme and exercise for well-being, have been found.

Based on all this, the aim of this study was to evaluate the effectiveness of an active exercise programme and exercise for well-being exercise programme improving pain, flexibility, static balance and quality of life in patients with fibromyalgia, comparing both treatment approaches between them and with a control group.

2. Materials and Methods

This was a single-blind randomised clinical controlled trial. The CONSORT statements were used to conduct and report the trial. Ethical approval was granted by the Bioethical

Commission of the University of Extremadura in Spain (Reference number: 11/2012). The trial was retrospectively registered with the ClinicalTrials.gov registry (Study Identifier: NCT04328142). All the participants signed a written informed consent prior to their participation in the study.

The target population was women diagnosed with fibromyalgia from the Fibromyalgia Associations from Badajoz and Olivenza in Extremadura (Spain). The recruitment period took place from March to October 2012.

The inclusion criteria were: women between 30 and 65 years old, diagnosed with fibromyalgia [1] by a specialised physician at least one year before the study began. Potential participants were excluded if they had been prescribed with active exercise treatment previous to the study, they did regular physical exercise or aerobic training, they had previous knowledge of exercise for well-being or they had mobility impairments or absence of any limb.

An independent researcher who was unrelated to any aspect of the trial was responsible for the randomisation. A total of 141 participants were randomly allocated to an active exercise programme experimental group, an exercise for well-being experimental group or a control group (Figure 1). A total of 141 sealed envelopes containing the group names were put in an opaque bag. The independent researcher kept the bag closed during the randomisation process. The participant was in charge of opening the bag and the envelope during this process. After the first assessment, the researcher informed the participants to which group they were allocated to. The allocation of each participant was concealed at all times until assignment. No one directly involved in the study had access to the randomisation process or the list.

The study was conducted over six weeks: four weeks of treatment and two weeks of measurements. All participants were requested to attend two measurement sessions: the baseline assessment and the post intervention assessment. The University of Extremadura laboratories were the location where all measurement sessions took place. The assessor was blinded to the group allocation. He was independent to the study and was not aware of the treatments applied. Neither the participants nor their therapists were blind to the group assignment. Due to the nature of the treatment, they could clearly see to which group the participant was allocated.

The following variables were measured through a data collection protocol: sociodemographic data: age, education, working status and marital status.

Outcome measures: The primary outcome measures were static balance, flexibility, pain and quality of life. The secondary outcome measure was the perceived exertion during activity. The measurement tools used were as described below.

Balance test: A plantar pressure platform with optical sensors (Wii-Fit Nintendo ©) was used to assess balance. The patients, standing on the platform and with their feet on the specified marks, had to maintain a standing posture while their centre of gravity was being recorded. The displacements to the left and right were assessed as deviations in percentages. Subsequently, stabilometry was carried out by means of the one-leg stand test with a duration of 30 s. The value in percentage (0–100%) of their stability was obtaining with this test. The higher the value achieved, the better the balance.

Wells and Dillon *Test or Sit and Reach Test*: This test assesses the trunk flexion flexibility [33]. It has a relative intra-examiner reliability (0.89–0.99) and moderate validity that oscillates between $r = 0.37$–0.77 for men and $r = 0.37$–0.85 for women [34]. This test is performed with the aid of a measuring box which has on its front the numerical measurement values that correspond to a metre.

The patient is placed in a sitting position on the measuring box with feet together at a right angle. In this position, the patient is asked to make a maximum flexion of the trunk, with the knees extended and the upper limbs in full extension, using the palms of the hands and pushing a ruler until they have reached the maximum possible distance. The distance achieved by pushing with the fingers is measured in centimetres. As the patient moves away from zero, the centimetres achieved are noted with a positive sign. If, on the other hand, the person does not reach the tip of the toes, the remaining centimetres to zero are marked with a negative sign. The higher the positive value, the better the results. We quantified the improvement as the greater number of centimetres achieved.

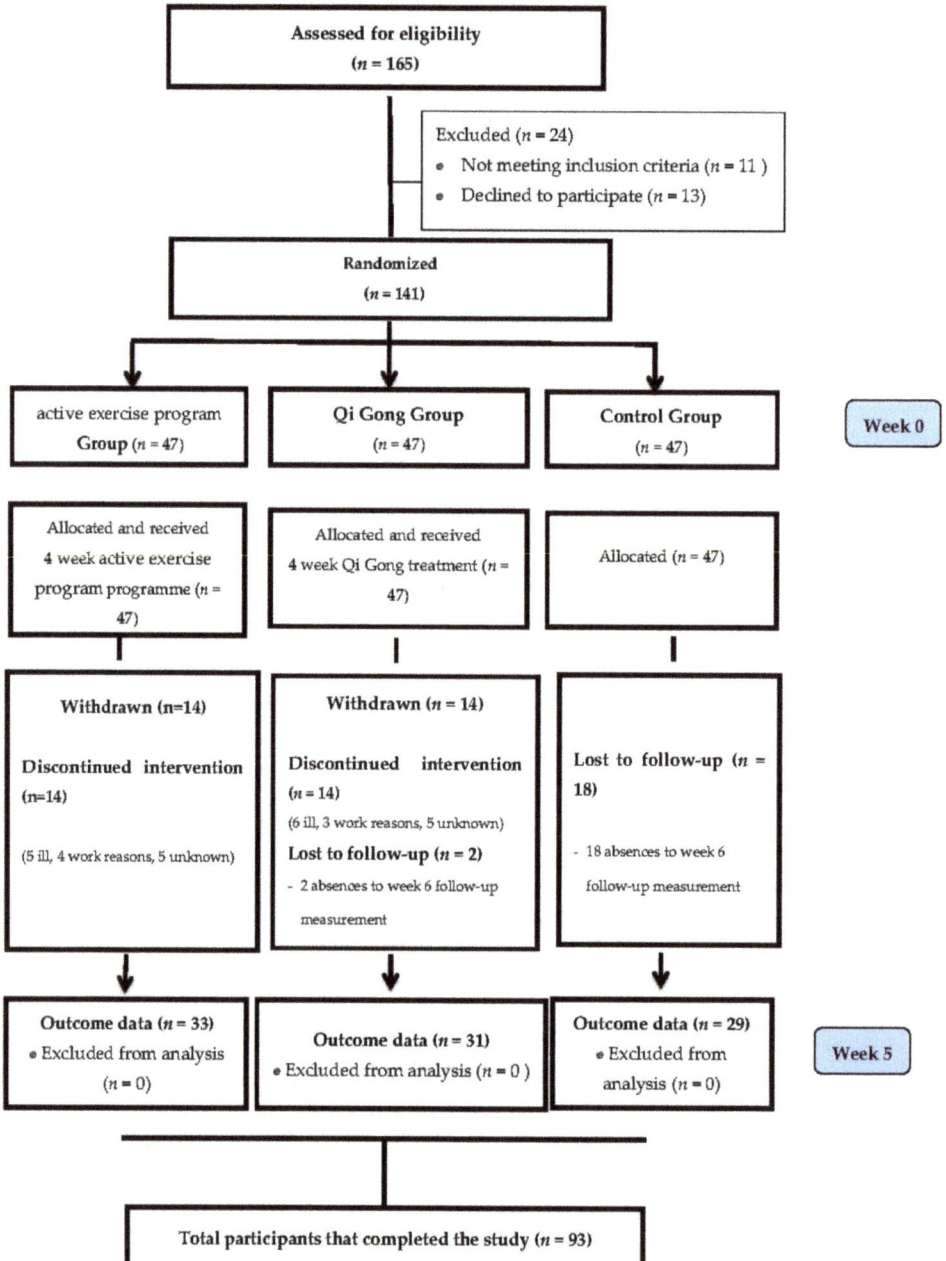

Figure 1. Flow diagram of study participation.

Visual Analogue Scale (VAS) of pain: This scale is a valid and reliable measure for the assessment of pain. It has proved its validity with high correlations with other pain measures (r = 0.62 to 0.91) and its reliability with a good test-retest (r = 0.94 to 0.71) [35]. Participants were asked to rate their worst pain intensity during the last week using a 100-mm VAS, with 0 denoting "no pain" and 100 denoting "extreme and unbearable pain" [36].

Quality of life: The impact of the condition on the patient's quality of life was assessed with the Spanish Fibromyalgia Impact Questionnaire (S-FIQ) [37]. This is the Spanish adaptation of the Fibromyalgia Impact Questionnaire [38]. The S-FIQ has a reliability coefficient of 0.81. The maximum score is 100 and the higher the result obtained, the higher the impact of the condition on the person.

Borg Scale of Perceived Exertion: This scale is a very useful tool to measure the perceived effort made in an activity. The Borg Scale of Perceived Exertion has an acceptable validity and reliability. Correlation coefficients between scale scores and heart rate, as well as test and post-test, are greater than 0.70 [39]. It consists of 10 numerical levels of dyspnoea ranging from 0 to 10 points: 0, rest; 1, very mild; 2, mild; 3, moderate; 4, somewhat hard; 5 and 6, hard; 7, 8 and 9, very hard; 10, maximum [40].

The sample was allocated to three groups: the experimental active exercise programme group, which completed an active physical exercise treatment programme, the experimental exercise for well-being group, which received exercise for well-being treatment, and the control group, which did not receive any treatment. Each group had 47 participants.

The study was conducted over 6 weeks: 4 weeks of treatment and 2 weeks of assessments. The measurements were done at baseline, the week before the beginning of the treatments and post intervention, the week after the treatments were completed.

The participants that were allocated to the active exercise programme group completed an active exercise programme, which was guided by a qualified physiotherapist, who is a member of the Spanish Chartered Society of Physiotherapists and is trained in exercise for fibromyalgia. The exercise programme aimed to work on all the musculoskeletal system. Therefore, it included a warm up of 3 to 5 min of walking, active mobilisation exercises of the shoulders, spine and hips, static balance exercises and stretches. The shoulder, hip and cervical spine exercises were performed in a standing posture. The thoracic spine and lumbar spine were done on an exercise mat. All exercises were performed in coordination with controlled gentle breathing. Each mobilisation exercise was done at maximum range of movement, was maintained for 10 s and repeated six times with eyes open and closed. All movements were done slowly and pain and fatigue were avoided.

The exercise for well-being was guided by an exercise for well-being teacher with 20 years of experience and qualified by the International Institute of Exercise for Well-Being (funded by Yes Requena). The exercises performed during the sessions were the 'twenty Wang Ziping figures for health and longevity'. These exercises are based on centennial therapeutic exercises from Daoyin, Wiqinxi, Yijinjing and Baduanjin, which are transmitted orally from master to disciple. The figures combine mental concentration and abdominal breathing during the performance of balance, flexibility and coordinated body movements. Each figure was repeated six times.

The active exercise program sessions as well as the exercise for well-being sessions lasted for 45 min and were done twice a week. The control group did not receive any intervention. All participants continued with their routine medical complying with the beneficence and non-maleficence principles of bioethics. More detailed information on the exercise programmes can be found in Figures S1–S3.

Statistical Analysis

The sample size did not respond to a previous calculation since as many subjects as possible were recruited. Finally, approximately 30 participants could be randomly assigned to each experimental group. As a reference, with this sample size and for a significance level of 5%, a minimum power of 80% could be achieved if we aimed to detect an effect size of 0.5 by a *t*-paired test.

The sociodemographic characteristics of the patients were analysed and described. The baseline values of the main outcome measures were also described by groups. A one-way ANOVA was applied to verify the homogeneity of the three experimental groups. For each main outcome, a comparison of the evolution by group was carried out by a repeated measures model, considering the group (control group, active exercise group and exercise for well-being group) as an inter-group factor and pre-post outcomes as an intra-group factor. We focused on interaction results so that, when it was not significant, the comparison between groups was analysed. When it was significant, the Tukey HSD post hoc comparison for the full model was applied and significant results were highlighted (taking into account that, since it involves 15 different contrasts, it is a conservative procedure that tends to provide no significant results with samples of moderate size). Additionally, the size effect for interaction (partial η^2) was reported.

The correlations between the age and each of the main outcome measures were analysed and the correlation test was applied. Student's independent samples test was applied to conduct other contrasts with just two means involved. The analysis was performed with SPSS version 22 and jamovi 1.8.4.

3. Results

A total of 93 participants completed the study. The active exercise programme group had 33 participants, the exercise for well-being group had 31 and the control group had 29. During the intervention and the follow-up period, there were a total of 48 withdrawals. The corresponding data were excluded from the statistical analysis. A CONSORT flow diagram is given in Figure 1.

The mean value of age was 52.24 ± 6.19. The youngest woman in the study was 34 and the eldest was 65. As expected, age showed a significant correlation with the baseline scores in flexibility, as this outcome measure worsened with age. Nevertheless, we hardly found significant correlations between age and changes along the treatment (except for flexibility, which got better with age). The rest of the sociodemographic variables are described in Table 1.

Table 1. Socio-demographic characteristics of the sample.

	Outcomes	N
Working status	Housewife	41
	Unemployed	10
	Employed	23
	Incapacitated	18
	Retired	1
Marital status	Married	81
	Lives with her partner	2
	Single	2
	Separated	2
	Divorced	3
	Widow	3
Education level	With no studies	11
	Primary Education	40
	Secondary Education	23
	Bachelor's Degree	19
Smoking habits	No	25
	Yes	68

Baseline and post-intervention outcome measurements divided by intervention groups are summarised in Table 2. According to the results of the one-way ANOVA, there were no significant differences between groups for flexibility, centre of gravity, S-FIQ, VAS and one-leg stance test ($p = 0.379$, $p = 0.669$, $p = 0.667$, $p = 0.237$, $p = 0.103$, respectively). A repeated measures model was applied, and the p-value corresponding to the interaction between the inter-group factor and the intra-group factor is shown in Table 2. The pre-post intervention evolution for each outcome is illustrated in Figures 2–6.

Table 2. Baseline and results of the post-intervention outcome measures.

Baseline Outcomes		Mean ±SD			p-Value *
		CG (N = 29)	AEG (N = 33)	EWG (N = 31)	
Flexibility	Pre	−6.24 ± 11.01	−9.24 ± 9.37	−6.10 ± 9.96	0.193
	Post	−3.14 ± 9.08	−2.94 ± 10.51	−2.03 ± 10.80	
Centre of gravity	Pre	54.07 ± 3.58	53.39 ± 2.99	53.94 ± 2.93	0.184
	Post	53.10 ± 2.64	54.30 ± 5.78	52.74 ± 2.66	
S-FIQ	Pre	68.86 ± 13.34	67.21 ± 16.51	65.35 ± 14.95	0.002
	Post	69.45 ± 4.02	57.79 ± 17.95	57.71 ± 15.79	
VAS	Pre	7.34 ± 1.61	7.88 ± 1.58	7.16 ± 2.02	0.020
	Post	7.31 ± 1.93	6.79 ± 1.43	6.16 ± 2.56	
One-leg stance test	Pre	55.55 ± 21.35	45.82 ± 27.02	57.26 ± 19.20	0.002
	Post	55.38 ± 23.14	68.27 ± 18.08	62.81 ± 18.56	

Note: CG: Control group; AEG: Active exercise Group; EWG: Exercise for well-being group; S-FIQ: Spanish Fibromyalgia Impact Questionnaire; VAS: Visual analogue scale, pre: before intervention, post: after intervention. * p-value corresponding to interaction contrast, according to a repeated measures model. A significant result means that change pre–post depends on the treatment.

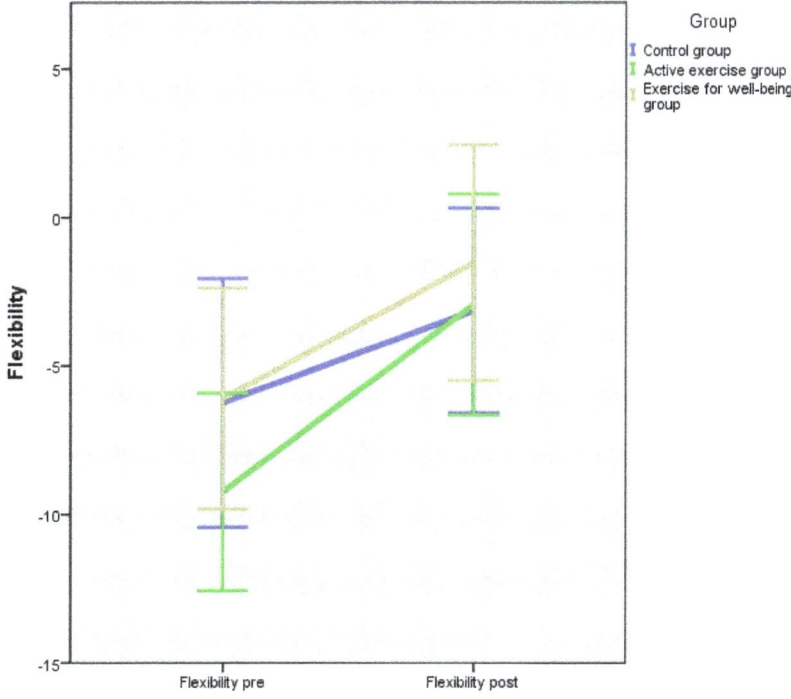

Figure 2. Changes in Flexibility.

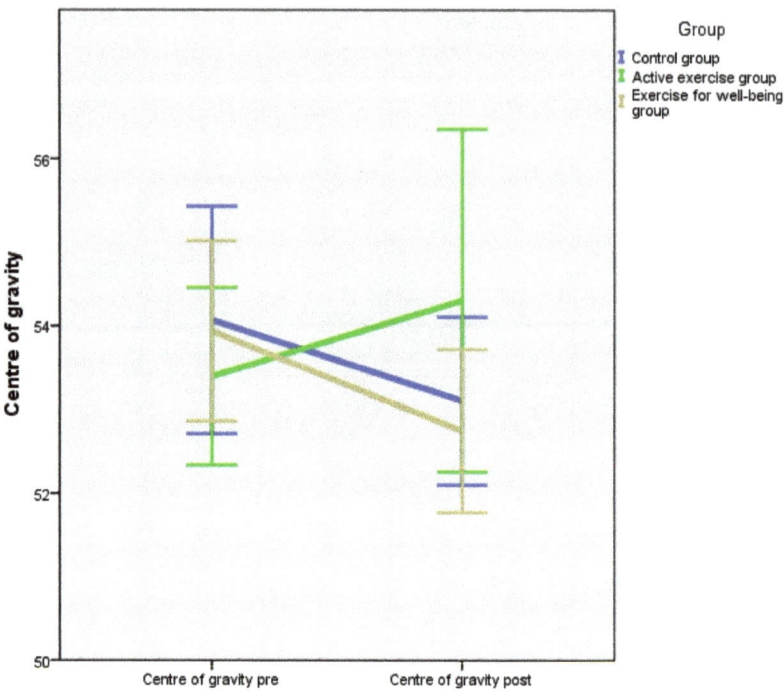

Figure 3. Changes in the centre of gravity.

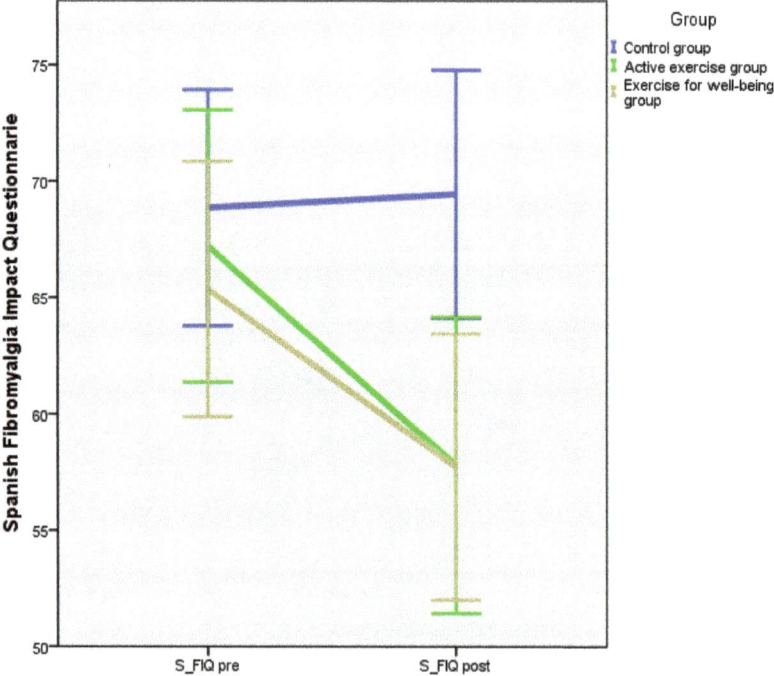

Figure 4. Changes in the Spanish Fibromyalgia Impact Questionnaire.

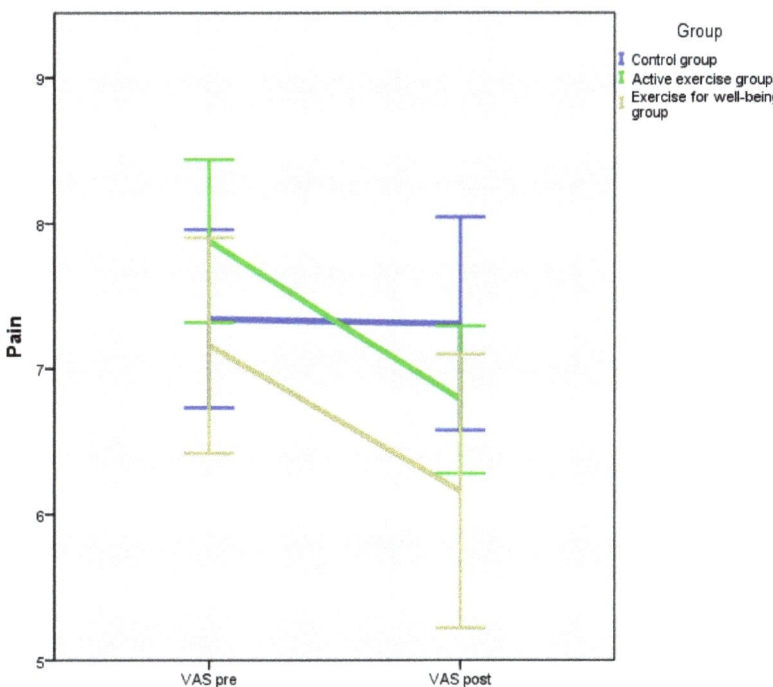

Figure 5. Changes in pain.

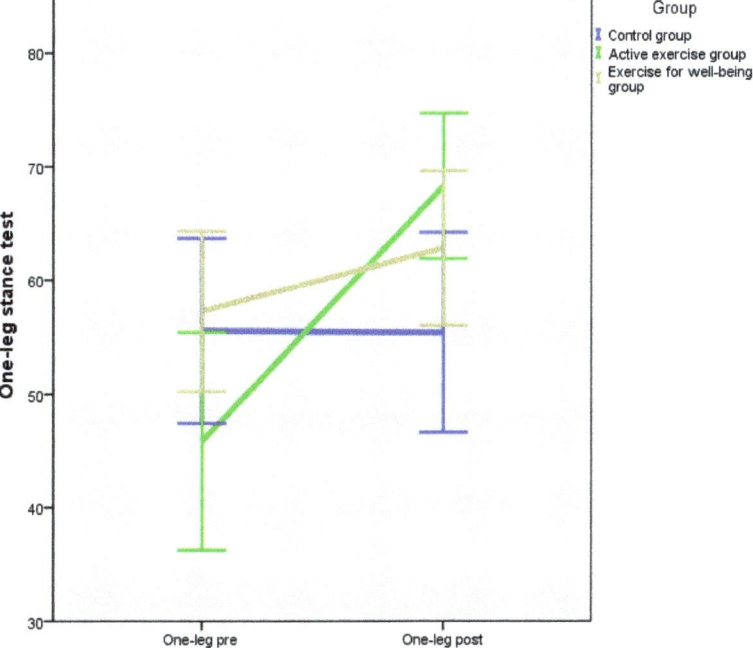

Figure 6. Changes in the one-leg stance test.

We observed a tendency to experience a slight or strong improvement in many outcomes, even for the control group. In other words, the patients seemed to perform spontaneously better at the second measurement. This could be explained by the training effect of the interventions. However, after applying a repeated measures model, no significant interactions between group and evolution for flexibility ($p = 0.193$) nor for centre of gravity ($p = 0.184$) were found. Moreover, the difference between groups was not significant ($p = 0.632$, $p = 0.745$, respectively).

However, we found a significant interaction for the S-FIQ ($p = 0.002$, $\eta^2 = 0.129$), the VAS ($p = 0.020$, $\eta^2 = 0.084$) and the one-leg stance test ($p = 0.002$, $\eta^2 = 0.132$). These results can be observed in Figures 4–6. In a deeper analysis performed with the Tukey HSD post hoc comparison, we could observe an evident improvement of the S-FIQ from baseline for the active exercise group ($p < 0.001$) and the exercise for well-being group ($p = 0.004$). Differences in post treatment measurements between these groups and the control group were close to significant ($p = 0.057$, $p = 0.061$, respectively). In the same way, the post hoc comparison showed significant improvement in the VAS for the active exercise group ($p = 0.002$) and the exercise for well-being group ($p = 0.006$). However, the differences in post intervention measurement in relation to the control group were not significant ($p = 0.911$, $p = 0.245$) according to the post-hoc comparison. Finally, according to the results of the Tukey method, there was a strong improvement in the one-leg stance test for the active exercise programme group ($p < 0.001$) and also a significant improvement for the exercise for well-being group ($p = 0.025$). The difference in the post-intervention measure in relation to the active exercise programme group were no significant ($p = 0.123$, $p = 0.702$).

When comparing the active exercise programme with the exercise for well-being, we observed (Table 2) a better performance of the first group, at least in descriptive terms. Nevertheless, we did not find any significant differences between both groups. It would be interesting to assess if the other observed differences would become significant with bigger samples.

Lastly, in the subjective assessment of fatigue experienced during the sessions, the mean for the active exercise programme group was 6.30 ± 1.88 and 5.52 ± 1.55 for the exercise for well-being group. These differences were not significant.

4. Discussion

The results of this study indicate that the active exercise programme and the exercise for well-being improve static balance, flexibility and pain in women with fibromyalgia compared to the control group. The most significant improvements were found in the active exercise programme group. In order to facilitate the discussion, this section is structured by the outcome measures analysed in the study.

4.1. Balance

The exercise for well-being group showed improvements in the final static balance scores (one leg stance test). However, these changes were not significant. In contrast, the active exercise programme group obtained significant improvements in static balance. We suspect that this improvement was due to the type of balance exercise performed. The women in the active exercise programme group did static balance exercises, maintaining equilibrium for 10 s. The active exercise programme group repeated the exercise slowly with eyes open and closed while the exercise for well-being exercises were performed with eyes open only.

With respect to the posturograph used (Wii-Fit, Nintendo ©), the results of the medical evidence have supported its use. In relation to its validity, several investigations can be highlighted. Holmes et al. [41] and Meldrum et al. [42] assessed balance in patients with neurological disease using the Wii-Fit (Nintendo ©). They concluded that the platform is a valid tool for the quantification of the postural stability, it is easy to use [41] and has no adverse effects when it is used to assess balance impairment [42]. Additionally, in agreement with Huurnink et al. [43], their results showed that it is a sufficiently accurate platform to quantify the centre of pressure trajectories in single-leg balance exercises.

Although there are few studies on active exercise programmes and balance in patients with fibromyalgia, the available literature has shown how physical therapy can improve balance in patients with this condition. The research conducted by Espí et al. [44] in 2016 analysed the effect of therapeutic aerobic exercise in women with fibromyalgia and concluded that exercise improves general discomfort. In addition, the authors observed that the effectiveness was greater when the exercise was combined with music therapy, which led to further improvements in quality of life and balance. Moreover, Kibar et al. [45] carried out an active exercise programme based on flexibility exercises to improve balance in these patients and observed a beneficial effect on static balance and functional levels. A study published in 2020 [46] analysed the effects of a 5-week core stability active exercise programme. The results showed that this exercise modality improved dynamic balance and postural control in women with fibromyalgia.

Based on the results of the present study and with those obtained by the mentioned authors, we consider that the active exercise interventions can improve balance in women with fibromyalgia.

As for exercise for well-being therapy, Roger et al. [25] specified that few studies applied this treatment approach and assessed its effects on balance of women with fibromyalgia. The authors observed that this treatment approach generally improved balance, but its potential to decrease falls had to be clarified.

However, there is evidence of the use of other exercise modalities for the improvement of balance, such as yoga or tai chi. Ulger et al. [47], in 2011, showed that yoga has a positive effect on women with balance and gait disorders due to musculoskeletal problems. In addition, Wong et al. [48] carried out a study in 2018, and showed how a 12-week tai chi intervention was effective in improving balance, fatigue, strength and flexibility in women with fibromyalgia.

As for the variable centre of gravity, we obtained non-significant results using the one leg stance test (Wii-Fit, Nintendo ©) after applying the experimental treatments. In the literature, we have not found any research assessing the changes of the centre of gravity in women with fibromyalgia nor studies that compared active exercise programmes or exercises for well-being. Only one study that analysed this variable and compared an active exercise programme with acupuncture and a control group was found [46]. The results coincide with ours, as the centre of gravity did not experience statistically significant improvements after both treatments. The authors concluded that neither the centre of gravity position nor the one-leg stance test were influenced by the intervention received in any of the groups.

4.2. Flexibility

The results of the Sit and Reach test showed a significant improvement in the flexibility of the participants of both experimental groups, the active exercise programme and the exercise for well-being groups. However, the improvements were more marked in the active exercise programme group. Our findings coincide with other research, such as that of Valencia et al. [49], who analysed the short- and medium-term effect of an active exercise programme on pain perception and muscle flexibility. Valencia et al. [49] showed how 20 women with fibromyalgia improved their level of flexibility and general well-being after an intervention based on kinesio-therapy and stretching exercises. The treatments were applied twice a week for 12 weeks and the outcome measurement were completed pre and post intervention and at 24 weeks of follow-up after the end of the treatments.

In the study conducted by Jones et al. [50], the objective was to assess the efficacy of a muscle strengthening programme compared to a stretching programme. A total of 68 women with fibromyalgia completed two weekly treatment sessions over 12 weeks. The authors found that flexibility improved with the stretching programme.

In addition, Ayan et al. [51] evaluated the long- and short-term effects of a multimodal programme (one hour every week for 3 months) combining muscular endurance and flexibility exercises with breathing and relaxation techniques plus a half-hour active exercise session. The sample consisted of 21 women with fibromyalgia that were assessed at baseline, post treatment and at 6 months of follow-up after the end of treatment. The authors demonstrated how flexibility exercises with breathing and relaxation techniques, in addition to active exercises, improved flexibility and reduced the impact of the disease. We consider it important to highlight that the duration of the treatment was longer in the studies conducted by Valencia et al. [49], Jones et al. [50] and Ayan et al. [51] than in our study, although the results related to flexibility coincide.

4.3. Perceived Exertion

No statistically significant changes were found in relation to the perceived exertion measured with the Borg scale or the subjective feeling of tiredness during the sessions. We were not able to conclude which experimental group (exercise for well-being or active exercise programme) had a significant lower level of perceived exertion. However, we found that the mean score for the exercise for well-being group was lower, 5.52 ± 1.55, (and therefore, better), than for the active exercise programme group.

The lower score obtained in the exercise for well-being group could be due to the fact that this therapy is carried out by the participants slowly, in a relaxed manner and with greater concentration. According to the bibliography consulted, there is no conclusive data in relation to the Borg scale in studies that carry out active exercise programmes and exercise for well-being treatments. There is scarce scientific evidence with a methodology similar to the one developed in our study. The study conducted by Nielens et al. [52] is one of them. The authors assessed the cardiorespiratory capacity and the perceived effort when performing a fitness programme, comparing 30 women with fibromyalgia syndrome and 67 healthy women. Nielens et al. [52] concluded that perceived exertion is greater in patients with fibromyalgia than in healthy patients. These results confirm that women with fibromyalgia have a higher perceived exertion than healthy patients.

4.4. Pain and Quality of Life

We believe that all the improvements in terms of flexibility and balance must have influenced the pain and improvement in the quality of life perceived by the patients, as the final pain scores obtained in both the active exercise programme group and the exercise for well-being group were lower. In this respect, we coincide with the studies carried out by Castro-Sánchez et al. [53], Kesiktas et al. [54] and Matsutani et al. [55]. All of them showed how stretching is effective for pain relief in patients with fibromyalgia. Moreover, Busch et al. [17] concluded that short-term aerobic exercise in fibromyalgia patients improves pain, global sense of well-being and physical function. Other studies confirmed that low-intensity, individualised physical exercise improves function and reduces symptoms of fibromyalgia [18]. In addition, Hooten et al. [56] demonstrated that, in two groups of 36 fibromyalgia patients, 3 weeks of aerobic exercise and strengthening exercise had similar effects on pain relief.

A study that was carried out by Yang et al. a [57] showed how a 4-week exercise for well-being programme (a treatment period that coincides with our study) helped to improve chronic pain and mood disorders.

Chen et al. [58] showed how exercise for well-being treatment can be very effective in treating pain and associated symptoms in fibromyalgia patients. Ten women who completed 5 to 7 exercise for well-being sessions of 40 min duration for more than 3 weeks were evaluated at baseline, post treatment and at 3 months of follow-up after the end of treatment. However, the methodological quality is questionable as the sample size was very small and had no control group.

In any future research, we would recommend that active exercise and exercise for well-being were combined to assess whether better improvements could be achieved. We would suggest increasing the duration of the treatment and including a follow-up period. It would also be interesting to carry out studies in which different types of exercise for well-being, such as tai chi or yoga, are practised. This would allow us to ascertain their effects on the variables studied in this population. On the other hand, it would be advisable in future studies to take into account variables such as body mass index and to monitor the presence of menopause. Research has shown that age [59] and body mass index [60] can influence musculoskeletal symptoms. In this regard, the prevalence of musculoskeletal disorders increases with age and appears to be associated with menopause [61]. On the other hand, a higher body mass index may be associated with greater pain and disease severity in patients with musculoskeletal disorders associated to fibromyalgia. It would also be interesting to provide a correlation with the pressure pain thresholds according to the American College of Rheumatology criteria.

4.5. Limitations of the Study

One limitation was the difficulty of learning each of the exercises to be performed. In the case of the exercise for well-being group, as this exercise is still quite unknown in our environment, it was necessary to explain the three essential aspects of its practice. These include the control of the position of the body and breathing as well as the regulation of the mind. Additionally, each exercise needed to be repeated during the learning process, and sometimes, it was necessary to rest during the practice of the exercises. Therefore, we consider that the four weeks of duration of the experimental treatment may be insufficient to obtain all the expected benefits, and perhaps a previous learning period would have been necessary.

However, if the treatment period was lengthened, the non-compliance with the programme could increase. Our research group has conducted a previous a study, with the same fibromyalgia associations, which studied the effects of the moderate consumption of red wine in these patients [62]. Out of 80 participants, there were 33 losses due to non-compliance (20 in the control group and 23 in the experimental group) in a 4-week intervention. Likewise, in the literature, we found studies carried out with this population [63,64] which had patient participation and follow-up dropout rates similar to the data provided in our research. The losses are generally due to the fluctuation of symptoms and the effects of different factors that can affect the condition [65]. Therefore, the longer the treatment period is, the higher the possibility that a participant stops the treatment or does not attend the measurement sessions. However, in this study, we have a final sample number of 93 women diagnosed with fibromyalgia, which is higher than the studies cited above.

5. Conclusions

The results of the present study indicate that active exercise and exercise for well-being improve pain, flexibility, static balance and quality of life in women with fibromyalgia. However, the active exercise programme achieved better results than the exercise for well-being. No statistically significant differences were found between groups in relation to the perceived feeling of tiredness during the sessions.

Supplementary Materials: The following are available online at https://www.mdpi.com/article/10.3390/jcm10173826/s1, Figure S1: Exercise 14: The carpenter handles a drill, Figure S2: Exercise 17: The white crane circles its knees, Figure S3: Active exercise programme.

Author Contributions: Conceptualisation, A.M.-G., J.R.-M. and E.M.G.-A.; methodology, A.M.-G., J.R.-M. and M.V.G.-L.-A.; formal analysis, J.M.-F., M.J.-P. and J.R.-M.; investigation, A.M.-G., J.R.-M. and M.V.G.-L.-A.; writing—original draft preparation, M.J.-P., E.M.G.-A. and J.R.-M.; writing—review and editing, E.M.G.-A., M.J.-P. and J.R.-M.; visualisation, M.J.-P., E.M.G.-A. and J.R.-M.; supervision, all authors. All authors have read and agreed to the published version of the manuscript.

Funding: This research received no external funding.

Institutional Review Board Statement: The study was conducted according to the guidelines of the Declaration of Helsinki and was approved by the Institutional Ethics Committee of the University of Extremadura (protocol code 11/2012 and date of approval: 8 February 2012).

Informed Consent Statement: Informed consent was obtained from all subjects involved in the study.

Data Availability Statement: The data underlying this article cannot be shared publicly to maintain the privacy of individuals that participated in the study. The data will be shared on reasonable request to the corresponding author.

Conflicts of Interest: The authors declare no conflict of interest.

References

1. Wolfe, F.; Clauw, D.J.; Fitzcharles, M.-A.; Goldenberg, D.L.; Häuser, W.; Katz, R.L.; Mease, P.J.; Russell, A.S.; Russell, I.J.; Walitt, B. 2016 Revisions to the 2010/2011 fibromyalgia diagnostic criteria. *Semin. Arthritis Rheum.* **2016**, *46*, 319–329. [CrossRef]
2. Rivera, J.; Alegre, C.; Ballina, F.J.; Carnonell, J.; Carmoa, L.; Castel, B.; Collado, A.; Esteve, J.J.; Martínez, F.G.; Tornero, J.; et al. Documento de consenso de la Sociedad Española de Reumatología sobre la fibromialgia. *Reumatol. Clín.* **2006**, *2*, s55–s65. [CrossRef]
3. Derek, J.; Panton, L.; Toole, T.; Sirithienthad, P.; Mathis, R.; McMillan, V. The effects of a 12-week strength-training program on strength and functionality in women with fibromialgia. *Arch. Phys. Med. Rehabil.* **2005**, *86*, 1713–1721. [CrossRef]
4. Assumpção, A.; Sauer, J.F.; Mango, P.C.; Pascual, A. Physical function interfering with pain and symptoms in fibromyalgia patients. *Clin. Exp. Rheumatol.* **2010**, *28*, S57–S63. [PubMed]
5. Jones, K.D.; Horak, F.B.; Winters-Stone, K.; Irvine, J.M.; Bennett, R.M. Fibromyalgia is associated with impaired balance and falls. *J. Clin. Rheumatol.* **2009**, *15*, 16–21. [CrossRef]
6. Rasouli, O.; Stensdotter, A.; Van, A. TauG-guidance of dynamic balance control during gait initiation in patients with chronic fatigue syndrome and fibromialgia. *Clin. Biomech.* **2016**, *37*, 147–152. [CrossRef]
7. Paul, L.M.; Wood, L.; Maclaren, W. The effect of exercise on gait and balance in patients with chronic fatigue síndrome. *Gait Posture* **2001**, *14*, 19–27. [CrossRef]
8. Serrador, J.; Quigley, K.; Zhao, C.; Findley, T.; Natelson, B. Balance deficits in Chronic Fatigue Syndrome with and without fibromialgia. *Neuro Rehabil.* **2018**, *42*, 235–246. [CrossRef]
9. Jones, C.J.; Rutledge, D.N.; Aquino, J. Predictors of physical performance and functional ability in people 50+ with and without fibromialgia. *J. Aging Phys. Act.* **2010**, *18*, 353–368. [CrossRef]
10. Valim, V.; Oliveira, L.M.; Suda, A.L.; Silva, L.E.; Faro, M.; Neto, T.L.B.; Feldman, D.; Natour, J. Peak oxygen uptake and ventilatory anaerobic threshold in fibromyalgia. *J. Rheumatol.* **2002**, *29*, 353–357. [PubMed]
11. Mannerkorpi, K.; Burckhardt, C.S.; Bjelle, A. Physical performance characteristics of women with fibromyalgia. *Arthritis Care Res.* **1994**, *7*, 123–129. [CrossRef]
12. Holland, G.J.; Tanaka, K.; Shigematsu, R.; Nakagaichi, M. Flexibility and physical functions of older adults: A review. *J. Aging Phys. Act.* **2002**, *10*, 169–206. [CrossRef]
13. Heredia, J.M.; Aparicio, V.A.; Porres, J.M.; Delgado, M.; Soto, V. Spatial-temporal parameters of gait in women with fibromyalgia. *Clin. Rheumatol.* **2009**, *28*, 595–598. [CrossRef]
14. Villafaina, S.; Gusi, N.; Rodriguez, S.; Martin, J.D.; Fuentes, J.P.; Collado, D. Influence of a Cell-Phone Conversation on Balance Performance in Women with Fibromyalgia: A Cross-Sectional Descriptive Study. *BioMed Res. Int.* **2019**, *2019*, 5132802. [CrossRef] [PubMed]
15. Rutledge, D.N.; Martinez, A.; Traska, T.K.; Rose, D.J. Fall experiences of persons with fibromyalgia over 6 months. *J. Adv. Nurs.* **2013**, *69*, 435–448. [CrossRef] [PubMed]
16. Collado, D.; Gallego, J.M.; Adsuar, J.C.; Dominguez, F.; Olivares, P.; Gusi, N. Fear of falling in women with fibromyalgia and its relation with number of falls and balance performance. *BioMed Res. Int.* **2015**, *2015*, 589014. [CrossRef]
17. Busch, A.J.; Barber, K.A.; Overend, T.J.; Peloso, P.M.; Schachter, C.L. Exercise for treating fibromyalgia syndrome. *Cochrane Database Syst. Rev.* **2007**, CD003786. [CrossRef]
18. Jones, K.D.; Adams, D.; Winters-Stone, K.; Burckhardt, C.S. A comprehensive review of 46 exercise treatment studies in fibromyalgia (1988–2005). *Health Qual. Life Outcomes* **2006**, *4*, 67. [CrossRef]
19. Häuser, W.; Klose, P.; Langhorst, J.; Moradi, B.; Steinbach, M.; Schiltenwolf, M.; Busch, A. Efficacy of different types of aerobic exercise in fibromyalgia syndrome: A systematic review and meta-analysis of randomised controlled trials. *Arthritis Res. Ther.* **2010**, *12*, R79. [CrossRef]
20. Bidonde, J.; Busch, A.J.; Schachter, C.L.; Webber, S.; Musselman, K.E.; Overend, T.J.; Góes, S.M.; Bello-Haas, V.D.; Boden, C. Mixed exercise training for adults with fibromyalgia. *Cochrane Database Syst. Rev.* **2019**, *5*, CD013340. [CrossRef]
21. Jiao, J.; Russell, I.J.; Wang, W.; Wang, J.; Zhao, Y.-Y.; Jiang, Q. Ba-Duan-Jin alleviates pain and fibromyalgia-symptoms in patients with fibromyalgia: Results of a randomised controlled trial. *Clin. Exp. Rheumatol.* **2019**, *37*, 953–962.

22. Estrategia de La OMS Sobre Medicina Tradicional 2002–2005. Organización Mundial de la Salud: Geneva, Switzerland, 2002. Available online: http://apps.who.int/iris/bitstream/handle/10665/67314/WHO_EDM_TRM_2002.1_spa.pdf;jsessionid=BD142DC22F7C85ADCB84488FAE99A7ED?sequence=1 (accessed on 20 May 2021).
23. Scott, D.; Firestone, K.; Dupree, K. Complementary and alternative exercise for fibromyalgia: A meta-analysis. *J. Pain Res.* **2013**, *6*, 247–260. [CrossRef]
24. Sawynok, J.; Lynch, M.E. Qigong and Fibromyalgia circa 2017. *Medicines* **2017**, *4*, 37. [CrossRef] [PubMed]
25. Jahnke, R.; Larkey, L.; Rogers, C.; Etnier, J.; Lin, F. A Comprehensive Review of Health Benefits of Qigong and Tai Chi. *Am. J. Health Promot.* **2010**, *24*, e1–e25. [CrossRef]
26. Park, K.S.; Jeong, H.Y.; Kim, Y.H. The effects of Qi-gong exercise on the health of the elderly-with respect to the physical health status, the fear of falling, balance efficacy, and Hwa-Byung. *J. Orient. Neuropsychiatr.* **2016**, *27*, 207–214. [CrossRef]
27. Shin, H.S.; Sok, S.R.; Yoo, J.H.; Im, Y.J.; Jang, M.H.; Jang, A.K.; Jang, A.K.; Jeong, Y.H.; Kang, Y.M.; Kim, Y.J.; et al. *Understanding and Practice in Oriental Nursing: Kyung Hee University, College of Nursing Science*; Su Moon Sa Press: Seoul, Korea, 2018.
28. Requena, Y. *Qigong: Gimnasia China Para la Salud y Longevidad*; La Liebre de Marzo: Barcelona, Spain, 2013.
29. Ahn, Y.J.; Jo, S.H.; Lee, S.H.; Lim, J.H. The review study on Yoga, Qigong, and Tai Chi interventions for anxiety: Based on Korean journal articles from 2009 to 2015. *J. Orient. Neuropsychiatr.* **2016**, *27*, 23–31. [CrossRef]
30. Hauser, W. Fibromyalgia syndrome: Basic knowledge, diagnosis and treatment. *Med. Mon. Pharm.* **2016**, *39*, 504–511.
31. Francielle, B.; Mendes, R.; Yukio, L.; Okino, L.; Goulart, I.; Okino, N. Benefits of Qigong as an integrative and complementary practice for health: A systematic review. *Rev. Lat.-Am. Enferm.* **2020**, *28*, e3317. [CrossRef]
32. Langhorst, J.; Heldmann, P.; Henningsen, P.; Kopke, K.; Krumbein, L.; Lucius, H.; Winkelmann, A.; Wolf, B.; Häuser, W. Complementary and alternative procedures for fibromyalgia syndrome: Updated guidelines 2017 and overview of systematic review articles. *Schmerz* **2017**, *31*, 289–295. [CrossRef] [PubMed]
33. Wells, K.F.; Dillon, E.K. The sit and reach. A test of back and leg flexibility. *Res. Q. Exerc. Sport* **2013**, *23*, 115–118. [CrossRef]
34. Avala, F.; Sainz, P.; Ste, M.; Santonja, F. Fiabilidad y validez de las pruebas sit-and-reach, revisión sistemática. *Rev. Andal. Med. Deporte* **2012**, *5*, 57–66. [CrossRef]
35. Scott, J.; Huskisson, E.C. Vertical or horizontal visual analogue scales. *Ann. Rheum. Dis.* **1979**, *38*, 560. [CrossRef]
36. Hawker GAMian, S.; Kendzerska, T.; French, M. Measures of adult pain: Visual Analog Scale for Pain (VAS Pain), Numeric Rating Scale for Pain (NRS Pain), McGill Pain Questionnaire (MPQ), Short-Form McGill Pain Questionnaire (SF-MPQ), Chronic Pain Grade Scale (CPGS), Short Form-36 Bodily Pain Scale (SF-36 BPS), and Measure of Intermittent and Constant Osteoarthritis Pain (ICOAP). *Arthritis Care Res.* **2011**, *63*, S240–S252. [CrossRef]
37. Monterde, S.; Salvat, I.; Montull, S.; Fernández-Ballart, J. Validación de la versión española del Fibromyalgia Impact Questionnaire. *Rev. Esp. Reumatol.* **2004**, *31*, 507–513.
38. Burckhardt, C.S.; Clark, S.R.; Bennet, R.M. The Fibromyalgia Impact Questionnaire: Development and validation. *J. Rheumatol.* **1991**, *18*, 728–733.
39. Castellanos, R.; Pulido, M.A. Validity and reliability of Borg's Perceived Exertion Scale. *Enseñanza E Investig. En Psicol.* **2009**, *14*, 169–177.
40. Borg, G. Psychophysical scaling with applications in physical work and the perception of exertion. *Scand. J. Work Environ. Health* **1990**, *16*, 55–58. [CrossRef]
41. Holmes, J.D.; Jenkins, M.E.; Johnson, A.M.; Hunt, M.; Clark, R. Validity of the Nintendo Wii(R) balance board for the assessment of standing balance in Parkinson's disease. *Clin. Rehabil.* **2012**, *27*, 361–366. [CrossRef] [PubMed]
42. Meldrum, D.; Glennon, A.; Herdman, S.; Murray, D.; McConn, R. Virtual reality rehabilitation of balance: Assessment of the usability of the Nintendo Wii (®) Fit Plus. *Disabil. Rehabil. Assist. Technol.* **2011**, *7*, 205–210. [CrossRef] [PubMed]
43. Huurnink, A.; Fransz, D.P.; Kingma, I.; van Dieen, J. Comparison of a laboratory grade force platform with a Nintendo Wii Balance Board on measurement of postural control in single-leg stance balance tasks. *J. Biomech.* **2013**, *46*, 1392–1395. [CrossRef]
44. Espí, G.V.; Inglés, M.; Ruescas, M.A.; Moreno, N. Effect of low-impact aerobic exercise combined with music therapy on patients with fibromyalgia. A pilot study. *Complement. Ther. Med.* **2016**, *28*, 1–7. [CrossRef]
45. Kibar, S.; Yıldız, H.E.; Ay, S.; Evcik, D.; Sureyya, E. New Approach in Fibromyalgia Exercise Program: A Preliminary Study Regarding the Effectiveness of Balance Training. *Arch. Phys. Med. Rehabil.* **2015**, *96*, 1576–1582. [CrossRef] [PubMed]
46. Garrido, E.M.; González, M.V.; Jiménez, M.; García, A.; Rodríguez, J. Effectiveness of acupuncture vs. core stability training in balance and functional capacity of women with fibromyalgia: A randomized controlled trial. *Clin. Rehabil.* **2020**, *34*, 630–645. [CrossRef]
47. Ulger, O.; Yağlı, N.V. Effects of Yoga on balance and gait properties in women with musculoskeletal problems: A pilot study. *Complement. Ther. Clin. Pract.* **2011**, *17*, 13–15. [CrossRef]
48. Wong, A.; Figueroa, A.; Sanchez, M.A.; Mok, W.; Chernykh, O.; Young, S. Effectiveness of Tai Chi on Cardiac Autonomic Function and Symptomatology in Women With Fibromyalgia: A Randomized Controlled Trial. *J. Aging Phys. Act.* **2018**, *26*, 214–221. [CrossRef] [PubMed]
49. Valencia, M.; Alonso, B.; Alvarez, M.J.; Barrientos, M.J.; Ayán, C.; Martín, V. Effects of 2 physiotherapy programs on pain perception, muscular flexibility, and illness impact in women with fibromyalgia: A pilot study. *J. Manip. Physiol. Ther.* **2009**, *32*, 84–92. [CrossRef] [PubMed]

50. Jones, K.D.; Burckhardt, C.S.; Clark, S.R.; Bennett, R.M.; Potempa, K.M. A randomized controlled trial of muscle strengthening versus flexibility training in fibromyalgia. *J. Rheumatol.* **2002**, *29*, 1041–1048. [PubMed]
51. Ayan, C.; Alvarez, M.J.; Alonso, B.; Barrientos, M.J.; Valencia, M.; Martín, V. Health education home-based program in females with fibromyalgia: A pilot study. *J. Back Musculoskelet. Rehabil.* **2009**, *22*, 99–105. [CrossRef] [PubMed]
52. Nielens, H.; Boisset, V.; Masquelier, E. Fitness and perceived exertion in patients with fibromyalgia syndrome. *Clin. J. Pain* **2000**, *16*, 209–213. [CrossRef]
53. Castro, A.M.; Matarán, G.A.; Arroyo, M.; Saavedra, M.; Fernández, C.; Moreno, C. Effects of myofascial release techniques on pain, physical function, and postural stability in patients with fibromyalgia: A randomized controlled trial. *Clin. Rehabil.* **2011**, *25*, 800–813. [CrossRef]
54. Kesiktas, N.; Karagülle, Z.; Erdogan, N.; Yazicioglu, K.; Yilmaz, H.; Paker, N. The efficacy of balneotherapy and physical modalities on the pulmonary system of patients with fibromialgia. *J. Back Musculoskelet. Rehabil.* **2011**, *24*, 57–65. [CrossRef]
55. Matsutani, L.A.; Marques, A.P.; Ferreira, E.A.; Assumpção, A.; Lage, L.V.; Casarotto, R.A.; Pereira, C.A.D.B. Effectiveness of muscle stretching exercises with and without laser therapy at tender points for patients with fibromyalgia. *Clin. Exp. Rheumatol.* **2007**, *25*, 410–415. [PubMed]
56. Hooten, W.M.; Qu, W.; Townsend, C.O.; Judd, J.W. Effects of strength vs aerobic exercise on pain severity in adults with fibromyalgia: A randomized equivalence trial. *Pain* **2012**, *153*, 915–923. [CrossRef]
57. Yang, K.H.; Kim, Y.H.; Lee, M.S. Efficacy of Qi-therapy (external Qigong) for elderly people with chronic pain. *Int. J. Neurosci.* **2005**, *115*, 949–963. [CrossRef] [PubMed]
58. Chen, K.W.; Hassett, A.L.; Hou, F.; Staller, J.; Lichtbroun, A.S. A pilot study of external qigong therapy for patients with fibromialgia. *J. Altern. Complement. Med.* **2006**, *12*, 851–856. [CrossRef] [PubMed]
59. Chaparro, M.; Diaz, V.; Gonzalez, J. Fibromialgia y osteoporosis. *Rev. Osteoporos. Metab. Miner.* **2011**, *3*, 113–118.
60. Aparicio, A.; Ortega, F.; Herediaa, J.; Carbonell, A.; Delgado, M. Analysis of the body composition of Spanish women with fibromialgia. *Reumatol. Clin.* **2011**, *7*, 7–12. [CrossRef]
61. Neyro, J.L.; Franco, R.; Rodriguez, E.; Carrero, A.; Palacios, S. Fibromialgia y climaterio: ¿Asociación o coincidencia? *Ginecol. Obstet. Mex.* **2011**, *79*, 572–578.
62. Vicente, T.P.J. Estudio Sobre Los Efectos Del Consumo Moderado de Vino Tinto en Mujeres Diagnosticadas de Fibromialgia (Study on the Effects of Moderate Consumption of Red Wine in Women Diagnosed with Fibromialgia). Ph.D. Thesis, University of Extremadura, Badajoz, Spain, 2009.
63. Bosch, E.; Sáenz, N.; Valls, M.; Viñolas, S. Estudio de la calidad de vida en pacientes con fibromialgia: Impacto de un programa de educación sanitaria. *Aten Primaria* **2002**, *30*, 16–21. [CrossRef]
64. Gelmana, S.M.; Lerab, S.; Caballero, F.; López, M.J. Tratamiento multidisciplinario de la fibromialgia. Estudio piloto prospectivo controlado. *Rev. Esp. Reumatol.* **2002**, *29*, 323–329.
65. Bennett, R.M. Clinical manifestations and diagnosis of fibromyalgia. *Rheum. Dis. Clin. N. Am.* **2009**, *35*, 215–232. [CrossRef] [PubMed]

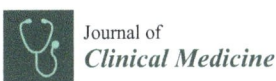

Article

Autoantibodies to Vasoregulative G-Protein-Coupled Receptors Correlate with Symptom Severity, Autonomic Dysfunction and Disability in Myalgic Encephalomyelitis/Chronic Fatigue Syndrome

Helma Freitag [1,*,†], Marvin Szklarski [1,†], Sebastian Lorenz [1], Franziska Sotzny [1], Sandra Bauer [1], Aurélie Philippe [2], Claudia Kedor [1], Patricia Grabowski [1], Tanja Lange [3], Gabriela Riemekasten [3], Harald Heidecke [4] and Carmen Scheibenbogen [1,5]

[1] Institute of Medical Immunology, Charité—Universitätsmedizin Berlin, 13353 Berlin, Germany; marvin.szklarski@charite.de (M.S.); sebastian.lorenz@charite.de (S.L.); franziska.sotzny@charite.de (F.S.); sandra.bauer@charite.de (S.B.); claudia.kedor@charite.de (C.K.); patricia.grabowski@charite.de (P.G.); carmen.scheibenbogen@charite.de (C.S.)
[2] Department of Nephrology and Critical Care Medicine, Charité—Universitätsmedizin Berlin, 13353 Berlin, Germany; aurelie.philippe@charite.de
[3] Department of Rheumatology and Clinical Immunology, University of Lübeck, 23538 Lübeck, Germany; tanja.lange@uksh.de (T.L.); Gabriela.Riemekasten@uksh.de (G.R.)
[4] CellTrend GmbH, 14943 Luckenwalde, Germany; heidecke@celltrend.de
[5] Berlin Institute of Health Center for Regenerative Therapies (BCRT), Charité—Universitätsmedizin Berlin, 10117 Berlin, Germany
* Correspondence: helma.freitag@charite.de
† These authors share first authorship.

Abstract: Background: Myalgic Encephalomyelitis/Chronic Fatigue Syndrome (ME/CFS) is an acquired complex disease with patients suffering from the cardinal symptoms of fatigue, post-exertional malaise (PEM), cognitive impairment, pain and autonomous dysfunction. ME/CFS is triggered by an infection in the majority of patients. Initial evidence for a potential role of natural regulatory autoantibodies (AAB) to beta-adrenergic (AdR) and muscarinic acetylcholine receptors (M-AChR) in ME/CFS patients comes from a few studies. Methods: Here, we analyzed the correlations of symptom severity with levels of AAB to vasoregulative AdR, AChR and Endothelin-1 type A and B (ETA/B) and Angiotensin II type 1 (AT1) receptor in a Berlin cohort of ME/CFS patients ($n = 116$) by ELISA. The severity of disease, symptoms and autonomic dysfunction were assessed by questionnaires. Results: We found levels of most AABs significantly correlated with key symptoms of fatigue and muscle pain in patients with infection-triggered onset. The severity of cognitive impairment correlated with AT1-R- and ETA-R-AAB and severity of gastrointestinal symptoms with alpha1/2-AdR-AAB. In contrast, the patients with non-infection-triggered ME/CFS showed fewer and other correlations. Conclusion: Correlations of specific AAB against G-protein-coupled receptors (GPCR) with symptoms provide evidence for a role of these AAB or respective receptor pathways in disease pathomechanism.

Keywords: adrenergic receptors; autoantibodies; myalgic encephalomyelitis; chronic fatigue syndrome; autoimmunity; vasoregulation; G-protein-coupled receptor

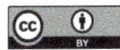

1. Introduction

Myalgic Encephalomyelitis/Chronic Fatigue Syndrome (ME/CFS) is an acquired complex disease with cardinal symptoms of fatigue, post-exertional malaise (PEM), cognitive dysfunction and pain [1]. The estimated prevalence is up to 0.86%, with peaks in teenage years and middle age [2,3]. ME/CFS is triggered by an infection in the majority of patients [4]. Although the pathogenesis is still unknown, there is ample evidence of immune and autonomic dysregulation [5].

There is increasing evidence that vascular dysfunction and hypoperfusion play an important role in ME/CFS. A diminished oxygen supply in muscles upon exercise was shown in several studies in ME/CFS patients [6,7]. In line with this, metabolic changes in ME/CFS indicate hypoxia and ischemia [8]. Several studies showed a decrease in cerebral blood flow upon orthostatic challenge [9,10]. Thus, hypoperfusion, which is aggravated upon exertion, may cause mental and skeletal muscle fatigue that are hallmarks of ME/CFS [11].

For the regulation of blood flow, G-protein-coupled receptors (GPCR) for vasoactive hormones, such as catecholamines, acetylcholine, angiotensin II and endothelin 1, play an important role [12]. Regulatory autoantibodies (AAB) targeting GPCR are involved in the pathogenesis of many diseases. Anti-GPCR AAB bind to their corresponding receptors, which can result in both agonistic and antagonistic effects [13]. Among the first AAB to GPCR described were those to beta1 adrenergic receptor (AdR) in dilated cardiomyopathy and to angiotensin II type 1 receptor (AT1-R), mediating vasoconstriction as risk factors for renal transplant rejection [14,15]. AAB against GPCR has been found in many rheumatic diseases as well [16]. These AAB belong to a regulatory network, which is dysregulated in many diseases [17].

There is evidence that AdR and muscarinic acetylcholine receptors (M-AChR)-AAB play a role in ME/CFS, too. Tanaka et al. were the first to describe elevated M-AChR-AAB in ME/CFS and their association with muscle weakness and neurocognitive impairment [18]. In a previous study, we found elevated AAB against beta2-AdR as well as M3/M4-AChR in a subgroup of ME/CFS patients [19]. Bynke et al. were able to verify these findings detecting elevated AAB against beta1/2-AdR and M3/M4-AChR in serum but not in cerebrospinal fluid of ME/CFS patients [20]. Beta1/2-AdR-AAB levels in blood correlated with structural alterations in the brain related to pain modulation [21]. Recently, we found agonistic beta2-AdR-AAB in healthy controls and in ME/CFS patients, stimulating the beta2-AdR on immune cells and reporter cell lines. Importantly, this agonistic function was attenuated in ME/CFS [22]. When performing immunoadsorption to remove AAB from circulation, we observed short-term clinical improvement in most patients [23,24]. For ME/CFS patients receiving rituximab, we documented a sustained decline of pretreatment elevated beta2-AdR-AAB levels in clinical responders to rituximab treatment [19].

The aim of this study was to investigate correlations between levels of AAB binding to vasoregulative GPCR and the severity of clinical symptoms in ME/CFS. As AAB responses are frequently activated by infections, we distinguished between patients with and without infection triggered ME/CFS onset. In a recent study, we found an increased prevalence of the autoimmune associated single-nucleotide variants in CTLA4 and PTPN22 in ME/CFS patients with infectious disease onset only [25]. Catecholamines binding to alpha1/2-AdR on vascular smooth muscle cells cause vasoconstriction, while they mediate vasodilation via beta2-AdR. Angiotensin II binding to AT1-R and endothelin-1 to endothelin-1 type A and B receptor (ETA/B-R) both activate important vasoconstrictive pathways. These ligands are increased by physical exertion [12]. Protease-activated receptors (PAR) play a role in vasoregulation during inflammation. Activation of PAR-1 by thrombin was shown to induce vascular constriction [26,27]. PAR-2 activated by trypsin can mediate inflammatory cell adhesion to the endothelium [28]. Acetylcholine can mediate vasodilatation via M3-AChR dependent release of nitric oxide [29]. M4-AChR expression was described in the brain microvascular system [30]. We expected that if vasoregulative AAB levels play a role in the pathomechanism of ME/CFS, they should correlate with the severity of key symptoms and disability.

2. Materials and Methods

2.1. Patients

A total of 116 patients were diagnosed at the outpatient clinic for immunodeficiencies at the Institute for Medical Immunology at the Charité Universitätsmedizin Berlin between October 2016 and May 2017. Diagnosis of ME/CFS in all patients was based on the 2003 Canadian Consensus Criteria and exclusion of other medical or neurological diseases that may cause fatigue by a comprehensive clinical and laboratory evaluation [1]. All patients received a cardiopulmonary workup prior to referral. In case of suspected rheumatic, gastrointestinal or neurological disease, patients were referred to specialists before the diagnosis ME/CFS was given. The study was approved by the Ethics Committee of Charité Universitätsmedizin Berlin (EA4/090/10) in accordance with the 1964 Declaration of Helsinki and its later amendments. All patients gave informed consent.

2.2. Determination of Autoantibody Levels and Laboratory Blood Data

CellTrend GmbH, Luckenwalde, Germany, analyzed serum levels of AAB against alpha1-, alpha2-, beta1-, beta2-, beta3-AdR, M3- and M4-AChR; AT1-R, ETA-R and ETB-R; PAR1/2. Whole blood samples from each subject were allowed to clot at room temperature and then centrifuged at $2000 \times g$ for 15 min in a refrigerated centrifuge. The serum was purified and stored at $-35\,^\circ$C. The AAB were measured in serum samples using a sandwich ELISA kit (CellTrend GmbH, Luckenwalde, Germany). The microtiter 96-well polystyrene plates were coated with full-length receptor proteins. To maintain the conformational epitopes of the receptor, 1 mM calcium chloride was added to every buffer. Duplicate samples of a 1:100 serum dilution were incubated at $4\,^\circ$C for 2 h. After washing steps, plates were incubated for 60 min with a 1:20,000 dilution of horseradish-peroxidase labelled goat anti-human IgG used for detection. In order to obtain a standard curve, the plates were incubated with test serum from a GPCR AAB-positive index patient. The ELISAs were validated according to the FDA's "Guidance for industry: Bioanalytical method validation". The concentration of serum IgG, IgA, IgM, IgE and IgG subclasses were determined at Charité diagnostics laboratory Labor Berlin GmbH.

2.3. Questionnaires for Symptom Scoring

The presence and severity of symptoms in patients with ME/CFS were assessed based on the 2003 Canadian Consensus Criteria [1,31]. Cardinal symptoms of fatigue, muscle pain, immune symptoms (mean of the 3 symptoms painful lymph nodes, sore throat and flu-like symptoms) and cognitive impairment (mean of the 3 symptoms memory disturbance, concentration ability and mental tiredness) were scored between 1 (no symptoms) and 10 (most severe symptoms) by the patients. Symptoms of autonomic dysfunction were assessed by the Composite Autonomic Symptom Score 31 (COMPASS 31) [32]. In addition, disability was examined using the Bell score focusing on the level of restriction in daily functioning [33] and fatigue using Chalder Fatigue Score [34]. Physical activities of daily life were assessed via the Short Form Health Survey 36 (SF-36) [35].

2.4. Statistical Analysis

Statistical data analyses were performed using IBM SPSS Statistics 22.0 (New York, NY, USA), GraphPad Prism 6.0 (San Diego, CA, USA) and R 4.0 (R Foundation for Statistical Computing, Vienna, Austria, http://www.R-project.org, accessed on 9 July 2021). All data were presented as median and interquartile range (IQR), mean and standard deviation (SD) or frequency (n) and percentage where appropriate. Comparisons of quantitative parameters between two groups were performed using the nonparametric Mann–Whitney test. Categorical parameters were compared between subgroups applying the Pearson's χ_2-test. Correlation analysis was performed using the nonparametric Spearman coefficient. Due to multiple testing, Benjamini–Hochberg (BH) correction was applied, aiming to control a false discovery rate of 5%. Adjusted p-values < 0.05 were considered to provide evidence for a statistically significant result.

3. Results

3.1. Cohort Characteristics

We analyzed a cohort of 116 ME/CFS patients for correlation of AAB levels with symptom severity. Patient characteristics are shown in Table 1. The median age was 43 years (IQR: 31–50), and the previous median duration of disease at the time of analysis was four years (IQR: 2–9). A total of 83 of the 116 patients (72%) were female, and 86 (74%) reported an infection-triggered onset of disease. Patients with infection-triggered onset were younger by a median difference of ten years ($p = 0.005$) and reported shorter disease duration ($p = 0.022$). There were no differences in symptom severity, Bell disability scale, SF-36 physical function and COMPASS 31-assessed autonomic dysfunction (Table 1) nor in AAB levels (Table 2) between these groups.

Table 1. Clinical characteristics. Asterisks mark significant differences between groups (Mann–Whitney test, * $p < 0.05$, ** $p < 0.01$).

	Whole Cohort (n = 116, Median with IQR)	w/Infection-Triggered Onset (n = 86, Median with IQR)	w/o Infection-Triggered Onset (n = 30, Median with IQR)	Inf. vs. Non-Inf.
Age	42.5a (31–50)	39a (31–47)	49a (40–54)	p: 0.005 **
Disease duration	4a (2–9)	3a (1–8)	6.50a (2.00–14.25)	p: 0.022 *
Sex (f/m)	83/33 (72%/28%)	64/22 (74%/26%)	19/11 (63%/37%)	p: 0.247
Fatigue	8 (7–9)	8 (7–9)	8.50 (8–10)	p: 0.113
Cognitive-score	7 (5.67–8.00)	7.21 (5.92–8.00)	6.84 (5.67–7.96)	p: 0.351
Muscle pain	7 (5–8)	7 (5–8)	8 (6.00–8.38)	p: 0.187
Immune-score	5.33 (4.00–6.67)	5.66 (4.17–7.00)	5.17 (3.67–5.96)	p: 0.226
Bell-Score	30 (30–40)	30 (30–40)	30 (30–40)	p: 0.560
Chalder-Fatigue Score	27 (25–30)	28 (25.88–30)	26 (24–30)	p: 0.130
SF-36 Score physical function	45 (20–55)	45 (18.75–61.25)	40 (30–50)	p: 0.834
COMPASS 31 total score	45.70 (35.18–55.42)	45.47 (34.36–55.34)	46.37 (39.28–56.13)	p: 0.687
COMPASS 31 orthostatic score	28 (20–32)	28 (20–32)	28 (20–32)	p: 0.954
COMPASS 31 vasomotoric score	0 (0–3)	0 (0–3)	0 (0–3)	p: 0.646
COMPASS 31 secretomotoric score	6.42 (3.75–8.56)	6.42 (2.14–8.56)	6.42 (4.28–8.56)	p: 0.294
COMPASS 31 gastrointestinal score	8.90 (6.90–12.46)	8.90 (6.23–12.46)	8.90 (7.12–12.02)	p: 0.932
COMPASS 31 bladder score	1.10 (0–2.20)	1.10 (0–2.20)	0 (0–2.20)	p: 0.369
COMPASS 31 pupillomotoric score	2.40 (1.43–3.00)	2.40 (1.50–3.00)	2.40 (1.20–3.00)	p: 0.772

Table 2. AAB levels and AAB/IgG-ratios. Differences between groups analyzed using Mann–Whitney test.

	Whole Cohort (n = 116, Median with IQR)	w/Infection-Triggered Onset (n = 86, Median with IQR)	w/o Infection-Triggered Onset (n = 30, Median with IQR)	Inf. vs. Non-Inf.
alpha1-AdR-AAB	8.71 U/l (7.24–11.65)	8.66 U/l (7.30–11.86)	8.83 U/l (6.85–10.02)	p: 0.400
alpha2-AdR-AAB	7.36 U/l (6.06–9.11)	7.37 U/l (6.05–9.65)	7.34 U/l (6.07–8.97)	p: 0.709
beta1-AdR-AAB	10.30 U/l (7.86–15.20)	9.88 U/l (7.61–16.20)	10.67 U/l (8.48–13.44)	p: 0.902
beta2-AdR-AAB	6.74 U/l (4.76–11.26)	6.74 U/l (4.75–11.55)	6.59 U/l (4.67–10.37)	p: 0.622
beta3-AdR-AAB	8.93 U/l (6.10–13.31)	9.45 U/l (6.29–13.68)	8.70 U/l (5.72–13.20)	p: 0.824
M3-AChR-AAB	4.74 U/l (3.41–6.10)	4.77 U/l (3.44–7.01)	4.45 U/l (3.37–5.62)	p: 0.293
M4-AChR-AAB	6.50 U/l (5.16–8.33)	6.50 U/l (5.20–9.11)	6.59 U/l (5.08–7.98)	p: 0.660
AT1-R-AAB	11.28 U/l (8.52–16.38)	11.62 U/l (8.50–17.05)	10.49 U/l (8.68–16.13)	p: 0.474
ETA-R-AAB	9.03 U/l (7.65–12.45)	8.98 U/l (7.60–12.79)	9.77 U/l (7.87–11.46)	p: 0.774
ETB-R-AAB	13.05 U/l (10.00–19.67)	13.05 U/l (10.03–19.87)	13.06 U/l (9.71–17.48)	p: 0.750
PAR1-AAB	4.52 U/l (3.14–5.96)	4.76 U/l (3.26–6.31)	3.49 U/l (3.07–4.91)	p: 0.102
PAR2-AAB	12.80 U/l (9.33–21.48)	12.12 U/l (8.46–22.08)	14.63 U/l (10.68–18.50)	p: 0.535
alpha1-AdR-AAB/IgG	0.90 U/g (0.78–1.20)	0.90 U/g (0.78–1.21)	0.90 U/g (0.77–1.13)	p: 0.626
alpha2-AdR-AAB/IgG	0.75 U/g (0.64–0.98)	0.74 U/g (0.63–0.99)	0.78 U/g (0.65–0.98)	p: 0.969
beta1-AR-AAB/IgG	1.06 U/g (0.82–1.54)	1.02 U/g (0.80–1.47)	1.14 U/g (0.86–1.57)	p: 0.595
beta2-AdR-AAB/IgG	0.71 U/g (0.49–1.12)	0.70 U/g (0.49–1.11)	0.78 U/g (0.44–1.15)	p: 0.897
beta3-AdR-AAB/IgG	0.88 U/g (0.66–1.31)	0.88 U/g (0.66–1.28)	0.89 U/g (0.67–1.49)	p: 0.989
M3-AChR-AAB/IgG	0.48 U/g (0.37–0.64)	0.48 U/g (0.37–0.66)	0.46 U/g (0.33–0.62)	p: 0.479
M4-AChR-AAB/IgG	0.69 U/g (0.51–0.87)	0.69 U/g (0.51–0.88)	0.68 U/g (0.52–0.88)	p: 0.984
AT1-R-AAB/IgG	1.16 U/g (0.92–1.73)	1.19 U/g (0.93–1.77)	1.14 U/g (0.85–1.47)	p: 0.414
ETA-R-AAB/IgG	0.95 U/g (0.77–1.29)	0.93 U/g (0.76–1.34)	1.03 U/g (0.81–1.18)	p: 0.812
ETB-R-AAB/IgG	1.29 U/g (1.02–1.93)	1.31 U/g (1.02–2.00)	1.29 U/g (1.00–1.82)	p: 0.707
PAR1-AAB/IgG	0.45 U/g (0.35–0.59)	0.45 U/g (0.36–0.66)	0.36 U/g (0.31–0.52)	p: 0.067
PAR2-AAB/IgG	1.37 U/g (0.96–1.99)	1.36 U/g (0.92–1.98)	1.55 U/g (1.15–2.16)	p: 0.398
total IgG	9.73 g/l (8.39–11.10)	9.79 g/l (8.41–11.09)	9.63 g/l (8.36–11.51)	p: 0.969

3.2. Correlation of AAB with Total IgG and Age

As we already observed in a previous study [19], most of the AAB levels showed a positive correlation with total IgG and IgG-subclasses, predominantly with IgG1 and IgG3 (Table S1). As the GPCR AAB belong to a regulatory network of AAB, their level may depend on total IgG levels. Further, we observed an inverse correlation with age for some AAB (Table S1), as well as between age and total IgG (whole cohort: r = −0.2526; p = 0.007, n = 114). Therefore, we calculated AAB/IgG ratios to correct for the effect of age (Table 2 and Table S2).

3.3. Correlation of AAB with Clinical Symptom Scores

Levels of various AAB correlated with symptom severity (Table S3). Further, we observed a positive correlation of alpha1/2-AdR, M4-AChR and ETA-R with disease duration (Table S2). Minimizing the effect of age by using AAB/IgG ratios for correlation analyses led, in general, to higher correlation estimates (r) and more correlations reached a level of significance (Table S4). We analyzed patient cohorts according to the type of disease onset. As 74% of patients reported an infectious onset, this group was much larger than the non-infectious onset group. Correlations of symptom severity with AAB/IgG ratios stratified according to disease onset are shown as Spearman's correlation coefficient values in Figure 1, and correlations of clinical symptoms with absolute AAB levels are shown in Figure S1. The most correlations were found in patients with infection-triggered onset only, while fewer and other correlations were found in those with non-infection-triggered onset (Tables S3 and S4).

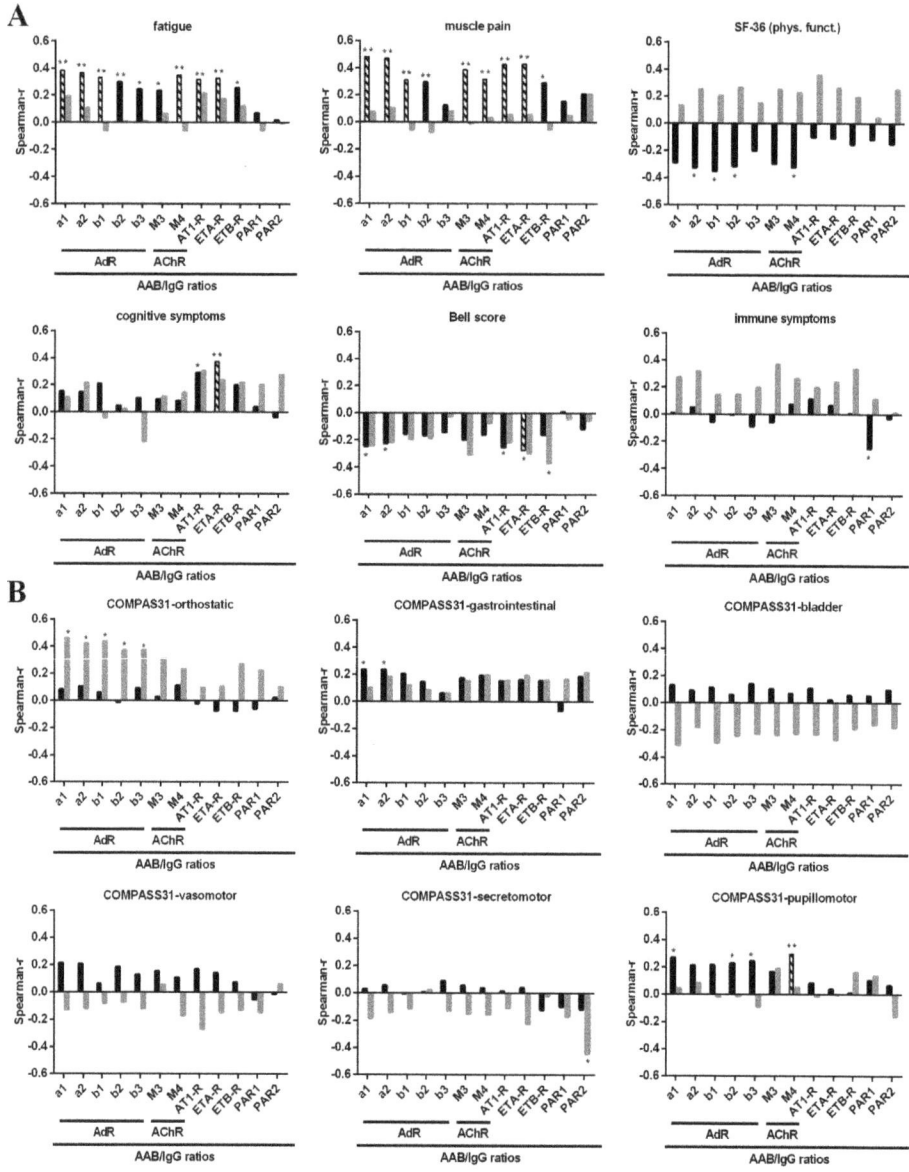

Figure 1. Correlations between symptom severity and AAB/IgG ratios. Correlation analysis of AAB/IgG ratios with the severity of (**A**) fatigue, muscle pain, cognitive and immune symptom scores, physical functioning (SF-36) and Bell disability score and (**B**) with COMPASS 31 subdomains. Spearman correlation coefficients (r) are shown for patients with infection-triggered onset (black bars) and patients without infection-triggered onset (grey bars). Significant correlations prior to BH-correction are marked with asterisks (* $p < 0.05$, ** $p < 0.01$), correlations that remained significant after BH-correction are indicated by black-and-white striped bars.

In patients with infection-triggered onset ($n = 86$), severity of fatigue correlated positively with most AAB/IgG ratios, including those against alpha1/2-AdR, beta1/2/3-AdR, M3/4-AChR, AT1-R, ETA-R and ETB-R, but not PAR-1/2 (Figure 1A, black bars). Muscle pain severity showed similar correlations to fatigue, except for beta3-AdR-AAB/IgG.

The SF-36 physical function showed a correlation pattern similar to fatigue and muscle pain with significant negative correlations (due to lower scores indicating more severe impairment) with alpha2-AdR-, beta1/2-AdR- and M4-ACh-AAB/IgG. In contrast, the severity of cognitive symptoms correlated positively with AT1-R- and ETA-R-AAB/IgG only. The severity of the Bell disability score showed a similar negative correlation with AT1-R- and ETA-R-, and with alpha1/2-AdR-AAB/IgG. For the immune score, only an inverse correlation with PAR1 was found. The Chalder Fatigue Score did not correlate with AAB/IgG (not shown). Scatter plots for significant correlations are shown in Figures S2–S5.

None of these significant correlations of fatigue and muscle pain were found in patients without infection-triggered onset (Figure 1A, grey bars). Correlations between most AAB/IgG and SF-36 physical function scores were even opposite to those of patients with infection-triggered onset. However, the correlation estimates (r) between AT1-R-AAB/IgG and cognitive symptoms and between AT1-R- and ETA-R-AAB/IgG and the Bell score were similar to those of patients with infection-triggered onset. As this subgroup was much smaller (n = 30), this may explain a lack of significance. Further, we found a significant negative correlation of ETB-R-AAB/IgG and the Bell score in this group only.

Interesting correlation patterns were also found for AAB/IgG and the three domains of orthostatic, gastrointestinal and pupillomotor function assessed by the COMPASS 31 questionnaire (Figure 1B). In patients with infection-triggered onset, the gastrointestinal symptoms correlated positively with alpha1/2-AdR- and the pupillomotor symptoms with alpha1-, beta2/3-AdR- and M4-AChR-AAB/IgG ratios. In contrast, the non-infection-triggered onset group showed strong correlations of alpha1/2-AdR- and beta1/2/3-AdR-AAB/IgG with orthostatic symptoms and an inverse correlation of PAR2-AAB/IgG with secretomotor symptoms, which are absent in the other subgroup. We did not observe any of these correlations with total IgG (not shown). Patients without infection-triggered onset had a significantly longer disease duration prior to these analyses (Table 1). As we observed higher alpha1/2-AdR, M4-AChR and ETA-R-AAB/IgG ratios to be associated with longer disease duration (Table S2), this may have an impact on the correlations of alpha1/2-AdR/IgG with orthostatic symptoms.

In patients with infection-triggered onset, most of the AAB/IgG ratio correlations with fatigue, muscle pain and cognitive symptoms, as well as Bell score with ETA-R-AAB/IgG, remained significant after BH-correction (Table 3 and Figure 1). In addition, the association of pupillomotor symptoms with M4-AChR-AAB/IgG remained significant. After BH correction, none of the correlations observed in patients without infection-triggered onset remained significant.

Table 3. Significant clinical correlations with AAB/IgG ratios after BH-correction in patients with infection-triggered onset (Spearman correlation coefficient and Benjamini–Hochberg corrected p-value; significant correlations marked with asterisks: * $p < 0.05$, ** $p < 0.01$).

	alpha1-AdR-AAB/IgG	alpha2-AdR-AAB/IgG	beta1-AdR-AAB/IgG	M3-AChR-AAB/IgG	M4-AChR-AAB/IgG	AT1-R-AAB/IgG	ETA-R-AAB/IgG
Fatigue	r: 0.383 p: 0.004 **	r: 0.363 p: 0.009 **	r: 0.331 p: 0.045 *	r: 0.234 p: 0.280	r: 0.349 p: 0.028 *	r: 0.317 p: 0.035 *	r: 0.328 p: 0.017 *
Muscle pain	r: 0.482 p: <0.001 **	r: 0.471 p: <0.001 **	r: 0.310 p: 0.045 *	r: 0.386 p: 0.008 **	r: 0.319 p: 0.035 *	r: 0.427 p: 0.002 **	r: 0.429 p: 0.001 **
Cognitive score	r: 0.152 p: 0.303	r: 0.144 p: 0.306	r: 0.209 p: 0.132	r: 0.095 p: 0.583	p: 0.084 p: 0.589	r: 0.290 p: 0.051	r: 0.371 p: 0.007 **
Bell Score	r: −0.244 p: 0.099	r: −0.223 p: 0.105	r: −0.154 p: 0.270	r: −0.196 p: 0.280	r: −0160 p: 0.308	r: −0.250 p: 0.083	r: −0.273 p: 0.045 *
COMPASS 31 pupillomotoric score	r: 0.268 p: 0.082	r: 0.212 p: 0.123	r: 0.215 p: 0.132	r: 0.166 p: 0.298	r: 0.294 p: 0.042 *	r: 0.084 p: 0.590	r: 0.039 p: 0.791

4. Discussion

There is increasing evidence for a role of vascular dysfunction in ME/CFS that shows associations with key symptoms [11]. In this study, we found several remarkable correlations of vasoregulative AAB with clinical symptoms in ME/CFS. The dependence between the measured biologic gradient of AAB and the severity of symptoms suggests a causal pathomechanistic connection.

Due to a correlation of natural regulative AAB with total IgG [19] and dependence of IgG levels on age [36], AAB/IgG ratios were used in our analyses in order to correct for the influence of age. Using the AAB/IgG ratios instead of absolute AAB levels revealed stronger and more correlations, and more p-values reached a level of significance.

In line with our hypothesis of a role of vasoactive AAB in ME/CFS, we found that levels of alpha1/2- and beta1/2/3-AdR-, M3/4-AChR-, and AT1-R-, ETA/B-R-AAB/IgG ratios all significantly correlate with the severity of fatigue and, with the exception of beta3-AdR-AAB/IgG, with muscle pain. The same AAB alpha2-AdR-, beta1/2-AdR- and M4-AChR- (but not AT1-R-, ETA/B-R-) correlated with SF-36 physical function. Tanaka et al. already described the levels of M-AChR-AAB (without data on the M subtype) in ME/CFS to be associated with muscle weakness [18]. Bynke et al. could not show an association of AAB against beta1/2-AdR and M3/M4-AChR with various health-related questionnaires, but their cohort was rather small, and key symptoms including fatigue, muscle pain, cognitive and autonomous symptoms were not separately assessed [20]. We found elevated AAB against beta2-AdR, as well as M3 and M4-AChR, in ME/CFS patients in our previous study [19]. In this study, the severity of symptoms was not determined. In patients with postural tachycardia syndrome (POTS), one study reported elevated levels of AAB against alpha1-AdR and M4-AChR to correlate with symptom severity [37], while another demonstrated elevated levels of AAB against beta1-AdR- and beta2-AdR to correlate with symptom severity [38].

We observed a distinct pattern for cognitive impairment, which was associated with ETA-R and AT1-R-AAB. Of interest, ETA/B-R-, AT1-R- and further alpha1/2-AdR AAB/IgG correlated with the severity of Bell disability score, too, capturing exertion induced symptoms and ability to work. ETA-R-, AT1-R- and alpha1/2-AdR all activate strong vasoconstrictor pathways stimulated by physical exertion [12]. Enhanced levels of AT1-R-AAB are a well-established risk factor for renal transplant rejection [14]. In hypertension, elevated AT1-R-AAB and alpha1-AdR-AAB have been described suggesting an agonistic effect on their receptors [39]. Furthermore, AT1-R-AAB were associated with vascular aging and arterial stiffness [40,41]. The role of ETA-R-AAB was described in autoimmune-related pulmonary arterial hypertension in both systemic lupus erythematosus and systemic sclerosis [42,43]. Our concept of higher ETA-R and AT1-R AAB/IgG to correlate with cognitive impairment due to vasoconstriction is in line with the recent studies by van Campen et al., showing both cerebral hypoperfusion and a decline in cognitive function in ME/CFS upon orthostatic stress [9,10].

Interesting correlation patterns were found for AAB/IgG ratios and gastrointestinal and pupillomotor function in the infection-triggered onset group as well. The gastrointestinal symptoms correlated with alpha1/2-AdR-ABB/IgG. This finding is in line with a study showing that colorectal motility is mediated by alpha1-AdR [44]. Pupillomotor symptoms correlated with alpha1-AdR-, beta2/3-AdR- and M4-AChR-ABB/IgG. Upon BH correction, the association of pupillomotor symptoms with M4-AChR-ABB/IgG remained significant. M4-AChR expression was described in the brain microvascular system and corneal endothelium [30,45].

Remarkably, we found no significant correlations of AAB/IgG against AdR, AChR and AT1-R/ET-R with fatigue, muscle pain and of AdR- and AChR-ABB/IgG with SF-36 physical function in patients without an infection-triggered onset of disease. However, similar estimates for correlations of AAB/IgG ratios to AT1-R/ETA-R and alpha1/2-AdR with cognition and Bell Score were found, which were not significant, likely related to the three-fold lower number of patients in this group. Only in patients with non-infectious disease onset significant correlations of symptoms of orthostatic intolerance with all AdR-AAB/IgG were seen. Further, an inverse correlation of PAR2-AAB/IgG with secretomotor symptoms was found. PAR2 activated by trypsin was shown to mediate salivary secretion [46].

GPCR AAB are different from classical autoantibodies that frequently activate, complement and can mediate inflammation and destruction [47]. No cytotoxic effect or complement activation of GPCR AAB has been reported so far. GPCR AAB specifically bind to their corresponding receptors, which can have functional consequences. Both stimulating agonistic and inhibiting antagonistic effects were described [13,15,48]. Considering an agonistic function, several associations of AAB with symptoms that we found are plausible. Elevated levels of agonistic AT1-R/ETA-R AAB could well explain the association with more cognitive dysfunction due to their effect on vasoconstriction described in several other diseases [49]. In a similar manner, enhanced PAR2 activity could explain fewer secretomotor symptoms and enhanced alpha1-AdR activity more gastrointestinal symptoms [44]. The inverse correlation of immune score with PAR1-AAB/IgG could be explained by lower levels of PAR1-AAB, resulting in less vascular constriction [26,27]. The associations of elevated levels of both alpha- and beta-AdR-AAB with more severe fatigue and muscle pain in post-infectious ME/CFS could point to overactivity of vasoconstrictive alpha-AdR-AAB or an impaired function of vasodilatative beta2-AdR-AAB. Previously, we found an impaired agonistic beta2-AdR-AAB function in immune and reporter cell line assays in ME/CFS patients with higher AAB levels [22]. AAB against beta1-AdR were shown to impair both beta1-AdR- and beta3-AdR-mediated vasorelaxation in rats [50]. The AdR dysfunction may specifically play a role upon exertion with enhanced release of epinephrine and norepinephrine, resulting in enhanced vasoconstriction and hypoperfusion with consecutive fatigue and muscle pain. Autoimmune mechanisms are likely in post-infectious ME/CFS [25]. As all these AAB are natural regulatory, AAB dysfunction may evolve during infection by bystander activation and somatic hypermutation resulting in AAB with a stronger or altered antigen binding to GPCR or in epitope spreading. With respect to AdR such a scenario would be in line with patients frequently reporting that an infection in a stressful situation, presumably going along with a stress-induced activation of AdR, triggered the disease onset.

The most discrepant patterns we observed between the patient subgroups are the correlations of all AdR-AAB with orthostatic dysfunction in non-infection-triggered disease but with fatigue, muscle pain and SF-36 in post-infectious ME/CFS. Since absolute AAB levels, as well as AAB/IgG ratios, did not differ between the two patient subgroups, this implicates that not merely the AAB level but rather the function of the AAB or of the receptors are different in these patient subgroups. To further follow this hypothesis, in patients with non-infection-triggered onset, the function of AdR-AAB responses may not be altered, but correlations here could reflect an adaptive response. For example, patients with connective tissue diseases, such as Ehlers Danlos syndrome (EDS), are at higher risk to develop ME/CFS. Here the vasculature is more elastic, leading to lower systolic and diastolic blood pressure, tachycardia and often POTS. Patients have an autonomic dysfunction with gastrointestinal problems and disturbed bladder function as well. There is evidence that patients with EDS have heightened vasoconstriction due to adrenergic hyper-responsiveness [51]. It is tempting to speculate that in these patients, elevated AdR-AAB are reflecting this compensatory overactivity of the adrenergic system. In line with this concept, in patients with POTS, elevated levels of AAB against alpha1-AdR and M4-AChR correlated with symptom severity [37].

A limitation of this study is that several correlations were no longer evident after correction for multiple testing due to the many parameters analyzed in our study. We provided both the corrected and the uncorrected correlations in order to address a possible unnecessary rejection of true findings upon adjustment for multiple testing [52]. The interpretation of the findings in the cohort without infection-triggered onset is based on a smaller number of patients and some non-significant findings. We did not increase the number of patients with non-infection triggered ME/CFS because we did not want to add a patient group diagnosed and analyzed at a later time point. In addition, disease onset is self-reported, and some patients may be wrongly classified. The symptom severity is self-reported and a subjective measure, leading to a wide distribution. As sleep disturbances are a key symptom in ME/CFS too, and sleep is associated with the parasympathetic system, a sleep score should be assessed in further studies. Further, we did not analyze a healthy control cohort in this study. In previous and ongoing unpublished studies, we constantly found that a subgroup of approximately one-third of ME/CFS patients has higher AAB against beta2-AdR as well as M3/M4-AChR compared to healthy controls [19,20]. Findings from our recent functional study suggest that the agonistic function of beta2-AdR AAB may be attenuated in ME/CFS patients, too, despite normal AAB levels [22].

In conclusion, our study provides evidence that AAB and/or the receptor pathways of AdR, AChR as well as AT1-R and ET-R play a role in ME/CFS due to the association with symptom severity. Thus, it is conceivable that various symptoms of ME/CFS, including fatigue, muscle pain, cognitive impairment and autonomic dysregulation, could be mediated or aggravated by these AAB. Further studies are required to decipher the mechanism and binding specificity of these GPCR-AAB, and their effect of on vascular function in ME/CFS, and how this may be translated into therapeutic concepts. In the case of dysfunctional AAB, therapies targeting AAB, such as immunoadsorption or rituximab, would be warranted and were shown to be effective in a subset of ME/CFS patients (reviewed in [5]). Further specific targeting of dysfunctional or regulative AAB may be developed as treatment strategies in ME/CFS.

5. Patents

CellTrend GmbH holds a patent for the use of beta-adrenergic receptor antibodies in the diagnosis of CFS.

Supplementary Materials: The following are available online at https://www.mdpi.com/article/10.3390/jcm10163675/s1, Table S1: AAB para-clinical correlations, Table S2: AAB/IgG ratio para-clinical correlations, Table S3: AAB clinical correlations of AdR-, AChR- and other AAB; onset-stratified, Table S4: Clinical correlations of AdR-, AChR- and other AAB/IgG ratio; onset-stratified, Figure S1: Correlations between symptom severity and AAB, Figure S2: Correlations with fatigue in patients with infection-triggered onset, Figure S3: Correlations with muscle pain, cognitive and immune symptoms in patients with infection-triggered onset, Figure S4: Correlations with Bell score, physical functioning and symptoms of autonomic dysfunction in patients with infection-triggered onset, Figure S5: Correlations in patients without infection-triggered onset.

Author Contributions: Conceptualization, C.S. methodology, M.S., S.L., H.F. and H.H.; validation, M.S., H.F., S.B. and F.S.; formal analysis, M.S.; investigation, S.B., C.K., P.G. and H.H.; resources, C.K. and P.G.; data curation, M.S., S.L. and T.L.; writing—original draft preparation, M.S., H.F. and C.S.; writing—review and editing, S.L., F.S., S.B., A.P., C.K., P.G., T.L., G.R. and H.H.; visualization, H.F. and M.S.; supervision, C.S.; project administration, C.S.; funding acquisition, C.S. All authors have read and agreed to the published version of the manuscript.

Funding: This research was funded by the Weidenhammer-Zöbele Foundation, M.S. received a scholarship from the Lost Voices Foundation.

Institutional Review Board Statement: The study was conducted according to the guidelines of the Declaration of Helsinki and approved by the Ethics Committee of Charité Universitätsmedizin Berlin (protocol code EA4/090/10, date of approval 11 December 2012).

Informed Consent Statement: Informed consent was obtained from all subjects involved in the study.

Data Availability Statement: The data presented in this study are available on reasonable request from the corresponding author.

Acknowledgments: The support in patient care and data management by Silvia Thiel is acknowledged. Further, we thank all patients who trustfully donated the blood samples and agreed to participate in this research project.

Conflicts of Interest: H.H., managing director of CellTrend GmbH, holds a patent for the use of beta-adrenergic receptor antibodies in diagnosis of CFS. All other authors declare no conflict of interest. The funders had no role in the design of the study; in the collection, analyses, or interpretation of data; in the writing of the manuscript, or in the decision to publish the results.

References

1. Carruthers, B.M.; Jain, A.K.; De Meirleir, K.L.; Peterson, D.L.; Klimas, N.G.; Lerner, A.M.; Bested, A.C.; Flor-Henry, P.; Joshi, P.; Powles, A.C.P.; et al. Myalgic Encephalomyelitis/Chronic Fatigue Syndrome. *J. Chronic Fatigue Syndr.* **2003**, *11*, 7–115. [CrossRef]
2. Bakken, I.J.; Tveito, K.; Gunnes, N.; Ghaderi, S.; Stoltenberg, C.; Trogstad, L.; Haberg, S.E.; Magnus, P. Two age peaks in the incidence of chronic fatigue syndrome/myalgic encephalomyelitis: A population-based registry study from Norway 2008–2012. *BMC Med.* **2014**, *12*, 167. [CrossRef]
3. Valdez, A.R.; Hancock, E.E.; Adebayo, S.; Kiernicki, D.J.; Proskauer, D.; Attewell, J.R.; Bateman, L.; DeMaria, A., Jr.; Lapp, C.W.; Rowe, P.C.; et al. Estimating Prevalence, Demographics, and Costs of ME/CFS Using Large Scale Medical Claims Data and Machine Learning. *Front. Pediatrics* **2018**, *6*, 412. [CrossRef] [PubMed]
4. Chu, L.; Valencia, I.J.; Garvert, D.W.; Montoya, J.G. Onset Patterns and Course of Myalgic Encephalomyelitis/Chronic Fatigue Syndrome. *Front. Pediatrics* **2019**, *7*, 12. [CrossRef] [PubMed]
5. Sotzny, F.; Blanco, J.; Capelli, E.; Castro-Marrero, J.; Steiner, S.; Murovska, M.; Scheibenbogen, C.; European Network on, M.C. Myalgic Encephalomyelitis/Chronic Fatigue Syndrome—Evidence for an autoimmune disease. *Autoimmun. Rev.* **2018**, *17*, 601–609. [CrossRef]
6. Vermeulen, R.C.; Kurk, R.M.; Visser, F.C.; Sluiter, W.; Scholte, H.R. Patients with chronic fatigue syndrome performed worse than controls in a controlled repeated exercise study despite a normal oxidative phosphorylation capacity. *J. Transl. Med.* **2010**, *8*, 93. [CrossRef] [PubMed]
7. Keller, B.A.; Pryor, J.L.; Giloteaux, L. Inability of myalgic encephalomyelitis/chronic fatigue syndrome patients to reproduce VO(2)peak indicates functional impairment. *J. Transl. Med.* **2014**, *12*, 104. [CrossRef] [PubMed]
8. Germain, A.; Barupal, D.K.; Levine, S.M.; Hanson, M.R. Comprehensive Circulatory Metabolomics in ME/CFS Reveals Disrupted Metabolism of Acyl Lipids and Steroids. *Metabolites* **2020**, *10*, 34. [CrossRef]
9. van Campen, C.; Rowe, P.C.; Verheugt, F.W.A.; Visser, F.C. Cognitive Function Declines Following Orthostatic Stress in Adults With Myalgic Encephalomyelitis/Chronic Fatigue Syndrome (ME/CFS). *Front. Neurosci.* **2020**, *14*, 688. [CrossRef]
10. van Campen, C.; Verheugt, F.W.A.; Rowe, P.C.; Visser, F.C. Cerebral blood flow is reduced in ME/CFS during head-up tilt testing even in the absence of hypotension or tachycardia: A quantitative, controlled study using Doppler echography. *Clin. Neurophysiol. Pr.* **2020**, *5*, 50–58. [CrossRef]
11. Wirth, K.; Scheibenbogen, C. A Unifying Hypothesis of the Pathophysiology of Myalgic Encephalomyelitis/Chronic Fatigue Syndrome (ME/CFS): Recognitions from the finding of autoantibodies against ss2-adrenergic receptors. *Autoimmun. Rev.* **2020**, *19*, 102527. [CrossRef]
12. Holwerda, S.W.; Restaino, R.M.; Fadel, P.J. Adrenergic and non-adrenergic control of active skeletal muscle blood flow: Implications for blood pressure regulation during exercise. *Auton. Neurosci.* **2015**, *188*, 24–31. [CrossRef]
13. Dragun, D.; Philippe, A.; Catar, R.; Hegner, B. Autoimmune mediated G-protein receptor activation in cardiovascular and renal pathologies. *Thromb. Haemost.* **2009**, *101*, 643–648.
14. Dragun, D.; Muller, D.N.; Brasen, J.H.; Fritsche, L.; Nieminen-Kelha, M.; Dechend, R.; Kintscher, U.; Rudolph, B.; Hoebeke, J.; Eckert, D.; et al. Angiotensin II type 1-receptor activating antibodies in renal-allograft rejection. *N. Engl. J. Med.* **2005**, *352*, 558–569. [CrossRef]
15. Wallukat, G.; Muller, J.; Podlowski, S.; Nissen, E.; Morwinski, R.; Hetzer, R. Agonist-like beta-adrenoceptor antibodies in heart failure. *Am. J. Cardiol.* **1999**, *83*, 75H–79H. [CrossRef]
16. Cabral-Marques, O.; Riemekasten, G. Functional autoantibodies targeting G protein-coupled receptors in rheumatic diseases. *Nat. Rev. Rheumatol.* **2017**, *13*, 648–656. [CrossRef] [PubMed]
17. Cabral-Marques, O.; Marques, A.; Giil, L.M.; De Vito, R.; Rademacher, J.; Gunther, J.; Lange, T.; Humrich, J.Y.; Klapa, S.; Schinke, S.; et al. GPCR-specific autoantibody signatures are associated with physiological and pathological immune homeostasis. *Nat. Commun.* **2018**, *9*, 5224. [CrossRef]
18. Tanaka, S.; Kuratsune, H.; Hidaka, Y.; Hakariya, Y.; Tatsumi, K.I.; Takano, T.; Kanakura, Y.; Amino, N. Autoantibodies against muscarinic cholinergic receptor in chronic fatigue syndrome. *Int. J. Mol. Med.* **2003**, *12*, 225–230. [CrossRef]
19. Loebel, M.; Grabowski, P.; Heidecke, H.; Bauer, S.; Hanitsch, L.G.; Wittke, K.; Meisel, C.; Reinke, P.; Volk, H.D.; Fluge, O.; et al. Antibodies to beta adrenergic and muscarinic cholinergic receptors in patients with Chronic Fatigue Syndrome. *Brain Behav. Immun.* **2016**, *52*, 32–39. [CrossRef] [PubMed]
20. Bynke, A.J.P.; Gottfries, C.F.; Heidecke, H.; Scheibenbogen, C.; Bergquist, J. Autoantibodies to beta-adrenergic and muscarinic cholinergic receptors in Myalgic Encephalomyelitis (ME) patients—A validation study in plasma and cerebrospinal fluid from two Swedish cohorts. *Brain Behav. Immun.-Health* **2020**, *7*, 100107. [CrossRef]
21. Fujii, H.; Sato, W.; Kimura, Y.; Matsuda, H.; Ota, M.; Maikusa, N.; Suzuki, F.; Amano, K.; Shin, I.; Yamamura, T.; et al. Altered Structural Brain Networks Related to Adrenergic/Muscarinic Receptor Autoantibodies in Chronic Fatigue Syndrome. *J. Neuroimaging Off. J. Am. Soc. Neuroimaging* **2020**, *30*, 822–827. [CrossRef]

22. Hartwig, J.; Sotzny, F.; Bauer, S.; Heidecke, H.; Riemekasten, G.; Dragun, D.; Meisel, C.; Dames, C.; Grabowski, P.; Scheibenbogen, C. Research article IgG stimulated β2 adrenergic receptor activation is attenuated in patients with ME/CFS. *Brain Behav. Immun.-Health* **2020**, *3*, 100047. [CrossRef]
23. Scheibenbogen, C.; Loebel, M.; Freitag, H.; Krueger, A.; Bauer, S.; Antelmann, M.; Doehner, W.; Scherbakov, N.; Heidecke, H.; Reinke, P.; et al. Immunoadsorption to remove ss2 adrenergic receptor antibodies in Chronic Fatigue Syndrome CFS/ME. *PLoS ONE* **2018**, *13*, e0193672. [CrossRef]
24. Tolle, M.; Freitag, H.; Antelmann, M.; Hartwig, J.; Schuchardt, M.; van der Giet, M.; Eckardt, K.U.; Grabowski, P.; Scheibenbogen, C. Myalgic Encephalomyelitis/Chronic Fatigue Syndrome: Efficacy of Repeat Immunoadsorption. *J. Clin. Med.* **2020**, *9*, 2443. [CrossRef] [PubMed]
25. Steiner, S.; Becker, S.C.; Hartwig, J.; Sotzny, F.; Lorenz, S.; Bauer, S.; Lobel, M.; Stittrich, A.B.; Grabowski, P.; Scheibenbogen, C. Autoimmunity-Related Risk Variants in PTPN22 and CTLA4 Are Associated With ME/CFS With Infectious Onset. *Front. Immunol.* **2020**, *11*, 578. [CrossRef] [PubMed]
26. Tognetto, M.; D'Andrea, M.R.; Trevisani, M.; Guerrini, R.; Salvadori, S.; Spisani, L.; Daniele, C.; Andrade-Gordon, P.; Geppetti, P.; Harrison, S. Proteinase-activated receptor-1 (PAR-1) activation contracts the isolated human renal artery in vitro. *Br. J. Pharm.* **2003**, *139*, 21–27. [CrossRef] [PubMed]
27. Kuwabara, Y.; Tanaka-Ishikawa, M.; Abe, K.; Hirano, M.; Hirooka, Y.; Tsutsui, H.; Sunagawa, K.; Hirano, K. Proteinase-activated receptor 1 antagonism ameliorates experimental pulmonary hypertension. *Cardiovasc. Res.* **2019**, *115*, 1357–1368. [CrossRef] [PubMed]
28. Tennant, G.M.; Wadsworth, R.M.; Kennedy, S. PAR-2 mediates increased inflammatory cell adhesion and neointima formation following vascular injury in the mouse. *Atherosclerosis* **2008**, *198*, 57–64. [CrossRef]
29. Rhoden, A.; Speiser, J.; Geertz, B.; Uebeler, J.; Schmidt, K.; de Wit, C.; Eschenhagen, T. Preserved cardiovascular homeostasis despite blunted acetylcholine-induced dilation in mice with endothelial muscarinic M3 receptor deletion. *Acta Physiol.* **2019**, *226*, e13262. [CrossRef]
30. Radu, B.M.; Osculati, A.M.M.; Suku, E.; Banciu, A.; Tsenov, G.; Merigo, F.; Di Chio, M.; Banciu, D.D.; Tognoli, C.; Kacer, P.; et al. All muscarinic acetylcholine receptors (M1-M5) are expressed in murine brain microvascular endothelium. *Sci. Rep.* **2017**, *7*, 5083. [CrossRef]
31. Fluge, O.; Risa, K.; Lunde, S.; Alme, K.; Rekeland, I.G.; Sapkota, D.; Kristoffersen, E.K.; Sorland, K.; Bruland, O.; Dahl, O.; et al. B-Lymphocyte Depletion in Myalgic Encephalopathy/Chronic Fatigue Syndrome. An Open-Label Phase II Study with Rituximab Maintenance Treatment. *PLoS ONE* **2015**, *10*, e0129898. [CrossRef]
32. Sletten, D.M.; Suarez, G.A.; Low, P.A.; Mandrekar, J.; Singer, W. COMPASS 31: A refined and abbreviated Composite Autonomic Symptom Score. *Mayo Clin. Proc.* **2012**, *87*, 1196–1201. [CrossRef]
33. Bell, D.S. *The Doctor's Guide to Chronic Fatigue Syndrome: Understanding, Treating and Living with CFIDS*; Da Capo Lifelong Books: Boston, MA, USA, 1995.
34. Cella, M.; Chalder, T. Measuring fatigue in clinical and community settings. *J. Psychosom. Res.* **2010**, *69*, 17–22. [CrossRef]
35. Ware, J.E., Jr.; Sherbourne, C.D. The MOS 36-item short-form health survey (SF-36). I. Conceptual framework and item selection. *Med. Care* **1992**, *30*, 473–483. [CrossRef]
36. Lock, R.J.; Unsworth, D.J. Immunoglobulins and immunoglobulin subclasses in the elderly. *Ann. Clin. Biochem.* **2003**, *40*, 143–148. [CrossRef] [PubMed]
37. Gunning, W.T., 3rd; Kvale, H.; Kramer, P.M.; Karabin, B.L.; Grubb, B.P. Postural Orthostatic Tachycardia Syndrome Is Associated With Elevated G-Protein Coupled Receptor Autoantibodies. *J. Am. Heart Assoc.* **2019**, *8*, e013602. [CrossRef]
38. Li, H.; Yu, X.; Liles, C.; Khan, M.; Vanderlinde-Wood, M.; Galloway, A.; Zillner, C.; Benbrook, A.; Reim, S.; Collier, D.; et al. Autoimmune basis for postural tachycardia syndrome. *J. Am. Heart Assoc.* **2014**, *3*, e000755. [CrossRef] [PubMed]
39. Liao, Y.H.; Wei, Y.M.; Wang, M.; Wang, Z.H.; Yuan, H.T.; Cheng, L.X. Autoantibodies against AT1-receptor and alpha1-adrenergic receptor in patients with hypertension. *Hypertens. Res.* **2002**, *25*, 641–646. [CrossRef] [PubMed]
40. Wang, M.; Yin, X.; Zhang, S.; Mao, C.; Cao, N.; Yang, X.; Bian, J.; Hao, W.; Fan, Q.; Liu, H. Autoantibodies against AT1 Receptor Contribute to Vascular Aging and Endothelial Cell Senescence. *Aging Dis.* **2019**, *10*, 1012–1025. [CrossRef] [PubMed]
41. Li, G.; Cao, Z.; Wu, X.W.; Wu, H.K.; Ma, Y.; Wu, B.; Wang, W.Q.; Cheng, J.; Zhou, Z.H.; Tu, Y.C. Autoantibodies against AT1 and alpha1-adrenergic receptors predict arterial stiffness progression in normotensive subjects over a 5-year period. *Clin. Sci.* **2017**, *131*, 2947–2957. [CrossRef] [PubMed]
42. Guo, L.; Li, M.; Chen, Y.; Wang, Q.; Tian, Z.; Pan, S.; Zeng, X.; Ye, S. Anti-Endothelin Receptor Type A Autoantibodies in Systemic Lupus Erythematosus-Associated Pulmonary Arterial Hypertension. *Arthritis Rheumatol.* **2015**, *67*, 2394–2402. [CrossRef]
43. Becker, M.O.; Kill, A.; Kutsche, M.; Guenther, J.; Rose, A.; Tabeling, C.; Witzenrath, M.; Kuhl, A.A.; Heidecke, H.; Ghofrani, H.A.; et al. Vascular receptor autoantibodies in pulmonary arterial hypertension associated with systemic sclerosis. *Am. J. Respir. Crit. Care Med.* **2014**, *190*, 808–817. [CrossRef]
44. Naitou, K.; Shiina, T.; Kato, K.; Nakamori, H.; Sano, Y.; Shimizu, Y. Colokinetic effect of noradrenaline in the spinal defecation center: Implication for motility disorders. *Sci. Rep.* **2015**, *5*, 12623. [CrossRef] [PubMed]
45. Grub, M.; Mielke, J.; Rohrbach, J.M. [m4 muscarinic receptors of the cornea: Muscarinic cholinoceptor-stimulated inhibition of the cAMP-PKA pathway in corneal epithelial and endothelial cells]. *Ophthalmologe* **2011**, *108*, 651–657. [CrossRef] [PubMed]

46. Nishiyama, T.; Nakamura, T.; Obara, K.; Inoue, H.; Mishima, K.; Matsumoto, N.; Matsui, M.; Manabe, T.; Mikoshiba, K.; Saito, I. Up-regulated PAR-2-mediated salivary secretion in mice deficient in muscarinic acetylcholine receptor subtypes. *J. Pharm. Exp.* **2007**, *320*, 516–524. [CrossRef]
47. Ludwig, R.J.; Vanhoorelbeke, K.; Leypoldt, F.; Kaya, Z.; Bieber, K.; McLachlan, S.M.; Komorowski, L.; Luo, J.; Cabral-Marques, O.; Hammers, C.M.; et al. Mechanisms of Autoantibody-Induced Pathology. *Front. Immunol.* **2017**, *8*, 603. [CrossRef] [PubMed]
48. Riemekasten, G.; Petersen, F.; Heidecke, H. What Makes Antibodies Against G Protein-Coupled Receptors so Special? A Novel Concept to Understand Chronic Diseases. *Front. Immunol.* **2020**, *11*, 564526. [CrossRef]
49. Lukitsch, I.; Kehr, J.; Chaykovska, L.; Wallukat, G.; Nieminen-Kelha, M.; Batuman, V.; Dragun, D.; Gollasch, M. Renal ischemia and transplantation predispose to vascular constriction mediated by angiotensin II type 1 receptor-activating antibodies. *Transplantation* **2012**, *94*, 8–13. [CrossRef]
50. Abdelkrim, M.A.; Leonetti, D.; Montaudon, E.; Chatagnon, G.; Gogny, M.; Desfontis, J.C.; Noireaud, J.; Mallem, M.Y. Antibodies against the second extracellular loop of beta(1)-adrenergic receptors induce endothelial dysfunction in conductance and resistance arteries of the Wistar rat. *Int. Immunopharmacol.* **2014**, *19*, 308–316. [CrossRef]
51. Gazit, Y.; Nahir, A.M.; Grahame, R.; Jacob, G. Dysautonomia in the joint hypermobility syndrome. *Am. J. Med.* **2003**, *115*, 33–40. [CrossRef]
52. Althouse, A.D. Adjust for Multiple Comparisons? It's Not That Simple. *Ann. Thorac. Surg.* **2016**, *101*, 1644–1645. [CrossRef] [PubMed]

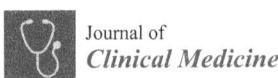

Article

Health, Wellbeing, and Prognosis of Australian Adolescents with Myalgic Encephalomyelitis/Chronic Fatigue Syndrome (ME/CFS): A Case-Controlled Follow-Up Study

Elisha K. Josev [1,2,*], Rebecca C. Cole [1], Adam Scheinberg [1,2,3,4], Katherine Rowe [5], Lionel Lubitz [5] and Sarah J. Knight [1,2,4]

1. Neurodisability and Rehabilitation, Murdoch Children's Research Institute, Royal Children's Hospital, Melbourne 3052, Australia; beccole26@gmail.com (R.C.C.); adam.scheinberg@rch.org.au (A.S.); sarah.knight@mcri.edu.au (S.J.K.)
2. Department of Paediatrics, University of Melbourne, Melbourne 3052, Australia
3. Department of Paediatrics, Monash University, Melbourne 3800, Australia
4. Victorian Paediatric Rehabilitation Service, Royal Children's Hospital, Melbourne 3052, Australia
5. Department of General Medicine, Royal Children's Hospital, Melbourne 3052, Australia; kathy@roweresearch.com (K.R.); lubitz@bigpond.net.au (L.L.)
* Correspondence: elisha.josev@mcri.edu.au

Citation: Josev, E.K.; Cole, R.C.; Scheinberg, A.; Rowe, K.; Lubitz, L.; Knight, S.J. Health, Wellbeing, and Prognosis of Australian Adolescents with Myalgic Encephalomyelitis/ Chronic Fatigue Syndrome (ME/CFS): A Case-Controlled Follow-Up Study. *J. Clin. Med.* **2021**, *10*, 3603. https://doi.org/10.3390/jcm10163603

Academic Editor: Giovanni Ricevuti

Received: 30 June 2021
Accepted: 9 August 2021
Published: 16 August 2021

Publisher's Note: MDPI stays neutral with regard to jurisdictional claims in published maps and institutional affiliations.

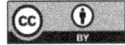

Copyright: © 2021 by the authors. Licensee MDPI, Basel, Switzerland. This article is an open access article distributed under the terms and conditions of the Creative Commons Attribution (CC BY) license (https://creativecommons.org/licenses/by/4.0/).

Abstract: Background: The purpose of this study was to follow-up an Australian cohort of adolescents newly-diagnosed with ME/CFS at a tertiary paediatric ME/CFS clinic and healthy controls over a mean period of two years (range 1–5 years) from diagnosis. Objectives were to (a) examine changes over time in health and psychological wellbeing, (b) track ME/CFS symptomatology and fulfillment of paediatric ME/CFS diagnostic criteria over time, and (c) determine baseline predictors of ME/CFS criteria fulfilment at follow-up. Methods: 34 participants aged 13–18 years (25 ME/CFS, 23 controls) completed standardised questionnaires at diagnosis (baseline) and follow-up assessing fatigue, sleep quality and hygiene, pain, anxiety, depression, and health-related quality of life. ME/CFS symptomatology and diagnostic criteria fulfilment was also recorded. Results: ME/CFS patients showed significant improvement in most health and psychological wellbeing domains over time, compared with controls who remained relatively stable. However, fatigue, pain, and health-related quality of life remained significantly poorer amongst ME/CFS patients compared with controls at follow-up. Sixty-five percent of ME/CFS patients at baseline continued to fulfil ME/CFS diagnostic criteria at follow-up, with pain the most frequently experienced symptom. Eighty-two percent of patients at follow-up self-reported that they still had ME/CFS, with 79% of these patients fulfilling criteria. No significant baseline predictors of ME/CFS criteria fulfilment at follow-up were observed, although pain experienced at baseline was significantly associated with criteria fulfilment at follow-up ($R = 0.6$, $p = 0.02$). Conclusions: The majority of Australian adolescents with ME/CFS continue to fulfil diagnostic criteria at follow-up, with fatigue, pain, and health-related quality of life representing domains particularly relevant to perpetuation of ME/CFS symptoms in the early years following diagnosis. This has direct clinical impact for treating clinicians in providing a more realistic prognosis and highlighting the need for intervention with young people with ME/CFS at the initial diagnosis and start of treatment.

Keywords: chronic fatigue syndrome; myalgic encephalomyelitis; follow-up; adolescence; health; wellbeing; diagnostic criteria

1. Introduction

Paediatric myalgic encephalomyelitis/chronic fatigue syndrome (ME/CFS) is a disabling condition of unknown etiology. It causes significant and well-documented adverse effects in physical and psychological functioning, school attendance and participation, and quality of life [1–4]. Less documented are the longer-term impacts on health and wellbeing for young people with ME/CFS in the years following diagnosis, in comparison with their healthy peers. Such information is invaluable for understanding illness course, prognosis, and potential targets for management and treatment of paediatric ME/CFS. It may also help identify potentially diverging developmental trajectories for patients with ME/CFS during adolescence and young adulthood; a period already characterised by considerable transition and change.

Significant change in emotional, social, hormonal, and physical functioning is typical in the transition from childhood to early adulthood [5]. Onset of paediatric ME/CFS during this period can therefore pose a diagnostic challenge. Indeed, paediatric ME/CFS is known to be associated with compromised physical health and psychological health and wellbeing, including greater fatigue, pain, anxiety and depressive symptoms, and poorer sleep quality and quality of life [6–13]. However, fatigue and insufficient, poor quality sleep is also prevalent amongst healthy high-school-aged Australians [14,15], rates of anxiety and depression tend to increase across mid to late adolescence [16–18], and health-related quality of life declines from 12 years of age onwards at a population level [19–21]. In order to quantify the impacts of paediatric ME/CFS on fatigue, sleep, emotional problems and health related quality of life, there is a need to compare the trajectories of these outcomes in both adolescents with ME/CFS and healthy adolescents using a longitudinal standardised design. Tracking specific ME/CFS symptomatology in the same patients over time using the same standardised measures has the benefit of identifying which illness aspects are endorsed most frequently (and perhaps, the ones that carry the most burden), as well as understanding the factors that might predict patients' future wellbeing and health status.

While there are relatively few longitudinal studies assessing follow-up of adolescent patients with ME/CFS, the limited evidence available suggests that improvement and recovery are more likely in paediatric ME/CFS compared with adult ME/CFS [1]. To date, paediatric ME/CFS follow-up studies (ranging from 1 to 21 years follow-up) have reported recovery rates of between 5% and 83% [11,12,22–30], although there is variability in how recovery is defined across studies. Research has tended to use individuals' self-defined recovery in the common domains of fatigue, physical functioning, and school attendance [30]. The latter measure may be problematic, however, for older adolescents who had already finished schooling at the follow-up time point, or for younger adolescents who are attending school but not functioning well due to ongoing cognitive disturbances.

Surprisingly few studies have focused on the health factors that may predict longer-term outcomes such as persistence of diagnostic symptoms, with studies tending to focus on risk factors for new-onset ME/CFS [15,31]. The few studies that have assessed these factors have been inconclusive. For example, studies of adolescents with ME/CFS-like symptoms have shown that baseline anxiety and depression predicts future fatigue persistence [32,33]. In contrast, subsequent studies have found no association between baseline depression and anxiety and recovery from paediatric ME/CFS at follow-up [11,26]. Other methodological factors have limited the ability to predict patients' ME/CFS clinical status and symptom persistence at follow-up, such as the inclusion of patients whose baseline ME/CFS status was unable to be verified by a physician's clinical diagnosis or did not fulfil diagnostic ME/CFS criteria, and/or the use of different tools or methods to measure patients' symptoms at baseline and follow-up [12,28,34]. Understanding the relative importance of physical and psychological health factors to patients' long-term outcome is, therefore, important for guiding future preventative, management and treatment approaches.

There were three mains aims for this study. First, we aimed to examine the change over time in factors associated with health and psychological wellbeing (i.e., fatigue, sleep quality and hygiene, pain, anxiety, depression, and HRQOL) in newly-diagnosed adolescents with ME/CFS relative to healthy adolescents, across a mean follow-up period of two years from diagnosis (and study enrolment). Second, we aimed to track patients' ME/CFS symptomatology over time to determine the type and frequency of symptoms experienced, and fulfilment of paediatric ME/CFS diagnostic criteria at follow-up (i.e., prognosis). Finally, the third aim was to determine which aspects of health and psychological wellbeing at diagnosis best predicted ME/CFS criteria fulfilment at follow-up.

2. Materials and Methods

2.1. Participants

This study represents a follow-up of a wider study that investigated brain structure and function, cognition, and psychological wellbeing in adolescents first diagnosed with ME/CFS and healthy adolescent controls [35]. A total of 48 participants (25 with ME/CFS and 23 healthy controls) participated in the original study. Inclusion and exclusion criteria for this study have been described in detail previously [35]. Participants included adolescents aged 13–18 years diagnosed with ME/CFS by a paediatrician specialising in ME/CFS at an Australian tertiary children's hospital using the Canadian Criteria adapted for paediatrics [36,37] and healthy adolescent controls aged 13–18 with no history of ME/CFS or other chronic illnesses. Exclusion criteria at study enrolment were insufficient English to complete the questionnaires, major depression or anxiety disorder, history of psychosis or bipolar disorder, pre-existing developmental disability or brain injury, and current use of any medication that may affect brain function.

All 48 participants were invited to participate in the follow-up study approximately two years after their participation in the original study when they were first diagnosed with ME/CFS. Ten participants (7 ME/CFS and 3 controls) could not be contacted despite multiple attempts, and 4 participants withdrew at follow-up (1 ME/CFS and 3 controls). Therefore, 34 participants (17 adolescents originally diagnosed with ME/CFS and 17 healthy controls) took part in both the original and follow-up studies and were included as part of the current investigation. Informed consent was obtained from all participants and their parents, and no compensation or incentives were offered to participate in the research. The study was approved by The Royal Children's Hospital Human Research Ethics Committee (HREC 32233, 37200).

2.2. Procedure

Original study at diagnosis (Baseline). Participants completed standardised questionnaires via REDCap Software (version 5.10.2, Vanderbilt University, Nashville, TN, USA, 2014; [38]). The questionnaires aimed to assess factors associated with health and psychological wellbeing, namely fatigue, sleep quality and hygiene, pain, anxiety, depression, and health-related quality of life. Questions regarding demographic characteristics were also completed, and for the ME/CFS cohort, additional clinical information was collected by their paediatrician in consultation with the family. This included illness characteristics such as time from symptom onset to diagnosis (study enrolment) (i.e., how long had symptoms been present when diagnosis was made) and perceived illness trigger, as well as diagnostic symptom criteria.

Follow-up study. Participants completed the same questionnaires administered at baseline. In addition, the adolescents originally diagnosed with ME/CFS were also asked to complete a health questionnaire about symptoms experienced over the past 3 months.

2.3. Measures

Health and psychological wellbeing measures across five domains were collected at both baseline and follow-up, and shown in Table 1. These were validated for use in children, adolescents and young people up to 25 years of age, and demonstrated good to excellent reliability, validity and internal consistency in adolescents with ME/CFS, other chronic health conditions, and healthy adolescents [8,29,39–46].

Table 1. Measures to evaluate health and psychological wellbeing in adolescents with ME/CFS and healthy controls.

Measure Domain	Name of Measure	Description of Measure
Fatigue	PedsQL™ Multidimensional Fatigue Scale [47,48]	18-item Likert-rated scale (from 'Never' or 0 to 'Almost always' or 4) that assesses level of subjective fatigue over the past month. Items reversed scored, linearly transformed to a 0–100 scale, and summed over the number of items answered to form a Total Fatigue score. Higher total fatigue scores reflected fewer problems related to fatigue.
Sleep quality and sleep hygiene	Adolescent Sleep Wake Scale (ASWS) and Adolescent Sleep Hygiene Scale (ASHS) [49]	Two 28-item instruments that assess aspects of sleep over past month: ASWS assesses subjective sleep quality including evaluation of sleep initiation and maintenance; ASHS assesses sleep hygiene and sleep practices. Items measured on a 6-point Likert scale (1 = always; 6 = never). Higher total scores indicate better sleep quality and hygiene.
Pain	PedsQL™ Pediatric Pain Questionnaire Visual Analogue Scale [50]	Self-rated 100 mm scale to measure intensity of present pain, from 'not hurting' or 'no pain' (0) to 'hurting a whole lot' or 'severe pain' (100).
Depression and Anxiety	Hospital Anxiety and Depression Scale [51]	Consists of 14 items (7 in each subscale) and each item is scored from 0 to 3. Higher total scores indicate greater levels of depression and anxiety.
Health-related quality of life (HRQOL)	PedsQL™ Core Generic Module [46,47]	Widely-used measure of health-related quality of life (HRQOL) assessing subjective impact of health status on wellbeing and life satisfaction. Respondents rate 23 items on 5-point Likert scale (0 = never a problem; 4 = almost always a problem) according to how much of a problem each item has been over the previous month. Items reversed scored and linearly transformed to create a total score ranging between 0 and 100. Higher total scores indicate better perceived HRQOL.

A short researcher-designed health questionnaire for the ME/CFS cohort was administered at baseline and follow-up, based on the diagnostic criteria for the paediatric case definition of ME/CFS and developed by the Pediatric ME/CFS Case Definition Working Group [36,37,52]. At baseline, the health questionnaire was completed by the ME/CFS patient's paediatrician who specialised in ME/CFS, and at follow-up the questionnaire completed by the adolescent with ME/CFS (some words were rephrased to be understood by a younger audience, see Supplementary Table S1 for comparison).

Two main measures were obtained from the health questionnaire: (a) fulfilment of ME/CFS diagnostic criteria (including 'severe', 'moderate', or 'atypical' ME/CFS, [36,37,53]), and (b) whether patients subjectively perceived they had ME/CFS at follow-up ('Do you still have ME/CFS? Yes or No.'). As defined in the paediatric case definition [37], 'severe ME/CFS' participants had to meet all six classic symptom criteria, including at least one symptom from two of the three categories of autonomic, neuroendocrine, and immune manifestations. 'Moderate ME/CFS' participants were defined as meeting five out of the six classic symptom criteria, including at least one symptom in any of the three autonomic, neuroendocrine, and immune categories. 'Atypical ME/CFS' participants were defined as meeting two to four of the classic six symptom categories. At follow-up, the questionnaire relied on self-report rather than medical consultation and examination with their clinician and, as such, the case definition criteria for exclusionary conditions and concomitant disorders and ratings of severity were not included. At follow-up, the questionnaire also asked about the types of health professional/s seen for management of the participant's condition, the number of visits to that/those health professionals since baseline, and the impact of their ME/CFS on their participation in school, university or employment ('a lot', 'a little', or 'not at all').

Finally, participants completed the *Wechsler Abbreviated Scale of Intelligence—Second Edition (WASI-II): Two-subtest Full Scale Intellectual Quotient* (Vocabulary and Matrix Reasoning subtests) at baseline and follow-up to obtain an estimation of their general intellectual ability, or FSIQ [54]. Standardised scores were reported ($M = 100$, $SD = 15$).

2.4. Statistical Analysis

All data were analysed using the statistical analysis program Stata 16.0 (StataCorp Release 16, College Station, TX, USA: StataCorp LLC, 2019), and screened for violations of statistical assumptions. The sample characteristics were summarised using descriptive statistics. Independent samples *t*-tests and chi-square tests were used to assess group differences at baseline and follow-up.

For the first aim, analysis of group differences in aspects of health and psychological wellbeing over time involved a single linear mixed-effects regression model for each outcome (dependent variable). Models included time (baseline vs. follow-up) and group (ME/CFS vs. control) as predictors, an interaction term between group and time, a random intercept for each participant to allow for clustering of observations within a participant, and follow-up time interval in years as a covariate (i.e., time since participation in original study). The linear mixed-effects regression results were presented as estimated mean differences (fixed main effects and pairwise contrasts of the dependent variable); that is, unstandardised regression coefficients (b) with their 95% confidence intervals (CIs), and associated standard errors (SE). A significance level of 0.05 was used for all models, and rather than relying solely on p values, Cohen's d was calculated to determine the magnitude of the effect and interpreted according to Cohen's [55] and Sawilowsky's [56] guidelines (0.20 and below = small, 0.50 = moderate, 0.80 = large, 1.20 and above = very large). Moderate to large values were considered clinically meaningful.

For the second aim, frequency statistics and percentages were used to summarise participants' responses to the health questionnaire; namely, (a) the proportion that fulfilled paediatric ME/CFS diagnostic criteria [36,37], (b) frequency of reported ME/CFS symptoms, and (c) the proportion who perceived they still had ME/CFS at follow-up. Responses were dummy coded (1 = met criteria; 0 = did not meet criteria) and then summed, with a possible total score range of 0–6, to reflect the classic six paediatric ME/CFS case definition criteria.

For the third aim, multiple logistic mixed-effects regression models were performed to determine which baseline variables of health and psychological wellbeing best predicted fulfilment of ME/CFS diagnostic criteria at follow up (controlling for time interval between studies), via unstandardised regression coefficients, 95% CIs, and p values. ORs were used as the magnitude of the effect and were interpreted according to Rosenthal's [57] guidelines (1.5:1 = small, 2.5:1 = moderate, 4:1 = large, 10:1 = very large). Pearson correlations were also used to assess the strength and direction of the linear associations between the baseline and follow-up variables of health and psychological wellbeing and fulfilment of ME/CFS criteria at follow-up.

3. Results

3.1. Participant Characteristics

As shown in Table 2, there were no significant group differences in mean age, sex (proportion of females), socio-economic status, or FSIQ. Results remained unchanged when the analysis was repeated for participants at baseline who were lost to follow-up (ME/CFS group: n = 17 participated at follow-up, n = 8 lost to follow-up; Control group: n = 17 participated at follow-up, n = 6 lost to follow-up). Average time interval between baseline and follow-up was significantly longer for adolescents with ME/CFS compared with controls, so follow-up time interval was included as a covariate in subsequent mixed-effects regression analyses.

3.2. Group Differences in Trajectories of Health and Psychological Wellbeing from Baseline to Follow-Up

Estimated mean group differences (ME/CFS vs. control) over the approximate two-year period (baseline vs. follow-up) are shown in Table 3 and Figure 1. Raw means for each measure can be found in Table S2.

Table 2. Participant characteristics at baseline and follow-up.

Participant Characteristics	ME/CFS (n = 17)	Controls (n = 17)	Independent t-test	p-Value
Age in years ((M (SD; range))				
Baseline	15.99 (1.59; 13.42–18.92)	15.90 (1.60; 13.33–18.08)	0.17	0.86
Follow-up	18.78 (1.63; 15.5–21.58)	18.20 (1.56; 15.58–20.58)	1.07	0.29
Female sex (%, n)	82%, 14	65%, 11	$X^2 = 1.36$	0.24
Socio-economic Indexes for Areas (SEIFA) (M (range)) *	7.12 (1–10)	7.81 (1–10)	−0.73	0.47
Follow-up time interval in years (M (SD; range))	2.75 (0.81; 1.83–4.58)	2.27 (0.43; 1.67–3)	2.14	0.04
Estimated FSIQ (M (SD; range)) **				
Baseline	103.75 (13.67; 86–145)	107.71 (12.50; 89–130)	−0.87	0.39
Follow-up	105.56 (11.41; 90–136)	109.94 (12.98; 81–129)	−1.03	0.31
Time from symptom onset to diagnosis (study enrolment) (%, n)		-	-	-
3–6 months	24%, 4	-	-	-
7–12 months	29%, 5	-	-	-
13–24 months	24%, 4	-	-	-
>24 months	24%, 4	-	-	-
Perceived illness trigger at study enrolment (%, n) ** ˣ				
Infectious Illness	41%, 7	-	-	-
Accident	12%, 2	-	-	-
Severe stress	12%, 2	-	-	-
Immunisation	6%, 1	-	-	-
Trip or vacation	0%, 0	-	-	-
No identifiable trigger	24%, 4	-	-	-
Visited health professional or specialist between baseline and follow-up ˣ				
No	24%, 4			
Yes	76%, 13			
General Practitioner	47%, 8			
Paediatrician	41%, 7			
Physiotherapist	29%, 5			
Psychologist	29%, 5			
Cardiologist	12%, 2			
Gynaecologist	12%, 2			
Psychiatrist	6%, 1			
Neurologist	6%, 1			
Gastroenterologist	6%, 1			
Naturopath	6%, 1			
Number of visits to that health professional or specialist between baseline and follow-up				
0 visits	24%, 4			
1 visit	0%, 0			
2 visits	12%, 2			
3 visits	0%, 0			
>3 visits	65%, 11			

* Control n = 16; ** ME/CFS n = 16; ˣ Participants reported more than one trigger. For participant characteristics for the full cohort of 48 adolescents (25 ME/CFS, 23 controls) that participated in the original study, see [35].

Table 3. Estimated mean differences in health and psychological wellbeing over time (baseline vs. follow-up) and between groups (ME/CFS vs. Control).

Measures of Health and Psychological Wellbeing	Estimated Mean Difference (b) with 95% CIs	SE	p-Value	Effect Size (Cohen's d)
Fatigue				
Time	17.89 (8.83, 26.96)	4.62	<0.001	0.66
Group	41.62 (32.10, 51.14)	4.86	<0.001	1.47
Time × Group	−21.73 (−34.55, −8.91)	6.54	0.001	0.57
Sleep quality				
Time	0.24 (0.02, 0.45)	0.11	0.03	0.37
Group	0.66 (0.33, 0.99)	0.17	<0.001	0.67
Time × Group	−0.34 (−0.64, −0.03)	0.16	0.03	0.37
Sleep hygiene				
Time	0.05 (−0.13, 0.23)	0.09	0.60	0.09
Group	0.20 (−0.11, 0.50)	0.16	0.20	0.22
Time × Group	−0.29 (−0.55, −0.03)	0.13	0.03	0.38
Pain				
Time	−14.24 (−24.23, −4.24)	5.10	<0.01	0.48
Group	−33.97 (−48.14, −19.80)	7.23	<0.001	0.81
Time × Group	14.57 (0.33, 28.61)	7.21	0.045	0.34
Anxiety				
Time	−3.41 (−4.81, −2.02)	0.71	<0.001	0.82
Group	−4.35 (−6.42, −2.29)	1.05	<0.001	0.71
Time × Group	3.59 (1.62, 5.56)	1.01	<0.001	0.61
Depression				
Time	−0.35 (−2.18, 1.48)	0.93	0.71	0.06
Group	−2.00 (−4.84, 0.84)	1.45	0.17	0.24
Time × Group	1.59 (−1.00, 4.18)	1.32	0.23	0.21
HRQOL				
Time	13.19 (6.48, 19.91)	3.43	<0.001	0.66
Group	34.75 (24.95, 44.55)	5.00	<0.001	1.19
Time × Group	−18.43 (−27.93, −8.94)	4.84	<0.001	0.65

Fatigue. A significant main effect of group, time, and group by time interaction effect was observed. At baseline, the ME/CFS group had a significantly greater level of problems related to fatigue than controls (mean difference = 41.62, $p < 0.001$, $d = 1.47$). This group difference diminished over time, with the ME/CFS group reporting significant improvement in fatigue levels from baseline to follow-up (mean difference = 17.89, $p < 0.001$, $d = 0.66$), and the control group remaining relatively stable (mean difference = −3.84, $p > 0.05$, $d = 0.14$). At follow-up, the ME/CFS group still reported significantly greater fatigue than controls, although the magnitude of this effect was reduced compared to baseline (mean difference = 19.89, $p < 0.001$; $d = 0.70$).

Sleep quality. A significant main effect of group, time, and group by time interaction effect was observed. At baseline, the ME/CFS group reported significantly poorer sleep quality than controls (mean difference = 0.66, $p < 0.001$, $d = 0.67$). This magnitude of change over time in sleep quality differed between the groups, with the ME/CFS group reporting significant improvement from baseline to follow-up (mean difference = 0.24, $p = 0.03$, $d = 0.37$), and the control group remaining stable (mean difference = −0.10, $p > 0.05$, $d = 0.15$). At follow-up, there was no significant difference in sleep quality between the two groups (mean difference = 0.32, $p > 0.05$, $d = 0.33$).

Sleep hygiene. A significant time by group interaction effect was observed, however the individual effects of time and group were very small and did not reach significance. The groups showed similar levels of sleep hygiene at both baseline and follow-up, and the interaction effect appeared to be driven by a small decline in sleep hygiene in the control group over time (mean difference = −0.24, $p = 0.01$, $d = 0.44$).

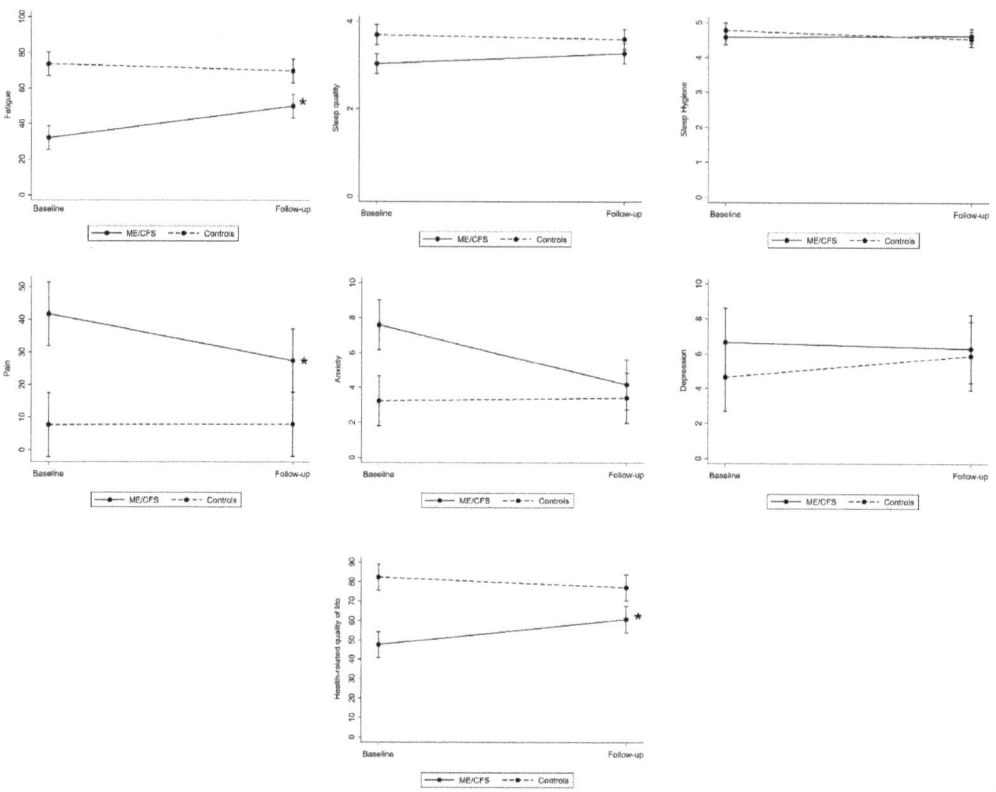

Figure 1. Estimated mean differences in measures of health and psychological wellbeing over time (baseline vs. follow-up) and between groups (ME/CFS vs controls). * Significant within-group change over time at 0.05 level and moderate to large Cohen's d effect sizes ≥ 0.5.

Pain. A significant effect of group, time, and group by time interaction effect was observed. At baseline, the ME/CFS group reported significantly greater severity of present pain than controls (mean difference = -33.97, $p < 0.001$, $d = 0.81$). Over time, the ME/CFS group reported a significant decline in pain from baseline to follow-up (mean difference = -14.24, $p < 0.01$, $d = 0.48$), and the control group remained stable (mean difference = 0.24, $p > 0.05$, $d = 0.01$). At follow-up, the ME/CFS group continued to report significantly greater pain than controls, although the magnitude of this effect was reduced compared to baseline (mean difference = -19.50, $p < 0.01$; $d = 0.46$).

Anxiety. A significant main effect of group, time, and group by time interaction effect was observed. At baseline, the ME/CFS group reported significantly greater levels of anxiety than the control group (mean difference = -4.35, $p < 0.001$, $d = 0.71$). Over time, anxiety levels significantly decreased for the ME/CFS group (mean difference = -3.41, $p < 0.001$, $d = 0.82$), but did not significantly change for controls (mean difference = -0.18, $p > 0.05$, $d = 0.04$), such that at follow-up there was no significant difference in anxiety levels between the two groups (mean difference = -0.76, $p > 0.05$, $d = 0.12$).

Depression. No significant main effects of time or group, nor a significant time by group interaction effect was observed (all $p > 0.05$). Mean group differences in depression from baseline to follow-up were associated with negligible effect sizes for both groups (both $p > 0.05$ and small d).

HRQOL. A significant main effect of group, time, and group by time interaction effect was observed. At baseline, the ME/CFS group reported significantly poorer HRQOL than controls (mean difference = 34.75, $p < 0.001$, $d = 1.19$). Over time, this magnitude of this group difference diminished, whereby HRQOL significantly improved for the ME/CFS group (mean difference = 13.19, $p < 0.001$, $d = 0.66$) but did not significantly change for the control group (mean difference = -5.24, $p > 0.05$, $d = 0.26$). At follow-up, the ME/CFS group still reported significantly worse HRQOL than controls, although the magnitude of the effect was reduced compared to baseline (mean difference = 16.32, $p = 0.001$, $d = 0.56$).

3.3. ME/CFS Symptomatology and Fulfilment of ME/CFS Diagnostic Criteria

At baseline, all 17 adolescents diagnosed with ME/CFS by their consultant ME/CFS specialist paediatrician fulfilled criteria for ME/CFS ('severe ME/CFS': 59%, $n = 10$; 'moderate ME/CFS': 41%, $n = 7$). At follow-up, 65% ($n = 11$) of participants fulfilled criteria for ME/CFS ('severe ME/CFS': 24%, n = 4; 'moderate ME/CFS': 18%, $n = 3$; 'atypical ME/CFS': 24%, $n = 4$). Of the 4 participants who met criteria for 'atypical ME/CFS' (i.e., only requiring 2 to 4 symptoms be endorsed) at follow-up, all 4 met criteria for the classic criteria of fatigue, sleep problems, and pain. Six of the 17 (35%) did not fulfil ME/CFS criteria at follow-up, and none of these endorsed persistent and unrelenting fatigue as a symptom.

Of the majority that self-reported as having ME/CFS at follow-up in response to the question 'do you still have ME/CFS?' (82%, $n = 14$), a greater proportion fulfilled criteria for ME/CFS than not (79% vs. 21%, respectively). Nine of the 14 participants reported that their ME/CFS had impacted 'a lot' on their participation in school, studies or employment, while 5 reported that it impacted 'a little'. All three participants who self-reported as not having ME/CFS at follow-up did not fulfill criteria for ME/CFS. Breakdown of participants who fulfilled paediatric ME/CFS diagnostic criteria at both time points is summarised in Table S3.

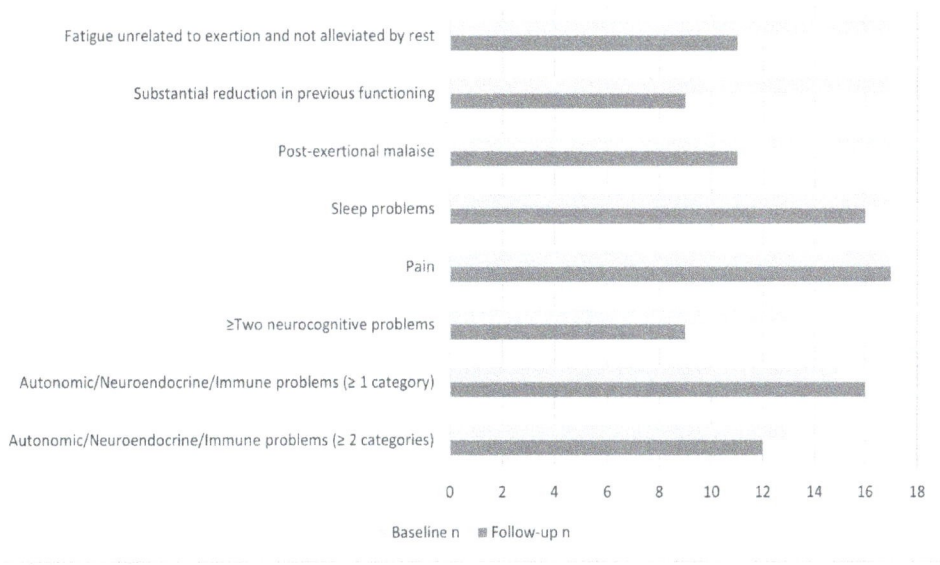

Figure 2. The number of participants who fulfilled each of the classic criteria for paediatric ME/CFS [36,37] for 3 or more months at baseline and follow-up ($n = 17$):(1) unexplained, persistent fatigue that is unrelated to exertion and not alleviated by rest, and represents a substantial reduction in previous functioning (criterion 1A, B, C), (2) post-exertional malaise (criterion 2), (3) sleep problems (criterion 3), (4) pain (criterion 4), (5) two or more neurocognitive problems (criterion 5), and (6) autonomic, immune, and/or neuroendocrine problems (criterion 6).

Figure 2 shows the number of participants who fulfilled each of the classic symptom criteria for paediatric ME/CFS at baseline and follow-up (*n* = 17). Pain was the most endorsed symptom at follow-up (100%), closely followed by sleep problems (94.1%) and one or more autonomic/neuroendocrine/immune problems (94.1%).

3.4. Predictors of ME/CFS Criteria Fulfilment at Follow-Up

None of the baseline variables of health and psychological wellbeing were significant predictors of fulfilment of ME/CFS diagnostic criteria at follow-up (all $p > 0.05$, d range = 0.02–0.33, OR range = 0.83–2.54). Pain experienced at baseline was close to reaching significance ($b = 0.05$, $p = 0.053$) and was associated with a moderate effect size ($d = 0.33$), but a small OR (OR = 1.05; SE(OR) = 0.02). For the Pearson correlation analysis, only pain experienced at baseline was significantly associated with ME/CFS criteria fulfilment at follow-up, with moderate effect ($R = 0.6$, $p = 0.02$). The Pearson correlation matrix for this analysis can be found in Table S4.

4. Discussion

This study aimed to examine trajectories of health and psychological wellbeing across an (approximately) two-year period in adolescents diagnosed with ME/CFS compared with their healthy peers. It also aimed to track patients' ME/CFS symptomatology and fulfillment of paediatric ME/CFS diagnostic criteria at follow-up, and determine whether ME/CFS criteria fulfilment at follow-up could be predicted by aspects of health and psychological wellbeing at diagnosis.

4.1. Trajectories of Health and Psychological Wellbeing from Baseline to Follow-Up

Greater levels of fatigue, pain, and anxiety, and lower levels of sleep quality and HRQOL were observed amongst adolescents with ME/CFS at baseline compared with their healthy peers. This is consistent with previous cross-sectional findings in adolescents with ME/CFS from our own team [3,9,43,58] and others [7,13,59–64]. This is perhaps unsurprising given that the cohort met paediatric case definition criteria for either severe (59%) or moderate (41%) severity ME/CFS at baseline, and the assessed domains of fatigue, pain, and sleep problems map onto the known clinical symptoms experienced in this condition. Importantly, the group disparity in these features of health and psychological wellbeing became less pronounced from diagnosis to follow-up, due to the significant improvement observed over time in the ME/CFS group, and the relative stability of the control group over time. Indeed, improvement in ME/CFS patient-reported outcomes have previously been shown in the domain of fatigue [12,65], with a recent systematic review showing recovery rates for paediatric ME/CFS of between 15% and 85% based on outcome measures of fatigue severity [30]. Fatigue and HRQOL have also been shown to co-vary in paediatric ME/CFS [43], which may account for the relative improvement being observed in both these domains over the follow-up period. Trends for a decline in the presence of pain or sleep disturbance over the follow-up period has also been noted in paediatric ME/CFS, regardless of intervention received [12]. The added value of the current study is that we were able to assess levels of severity within ME/CFS symptom domains using the same measures at baseline and follow-up. This allowed for a more comprehensive evaluation of change over time in comparison with healthy controls.

A positive finding from this study was that with significant improvement over time, adolescents with ME/CFS became comparable to their healthy peers at follow-up in their level of anxiety and sleep quality. The lack of follow-up studies assessing anxiety in paediatric ME/CFS make the reasons for this improvement in anxiety level unclear. It is possible that anxiety experienced at baseline related to the diagnosis itself and/or diagnostic and prognostic uncertainty, all of which may have reduced in impact over time. Gradual acceptance and better management of their chronic condition may also have played a role in improving anxiety and sleep quality, including multi-disciplinary input in the post-diagnosis period. Certainly, many participants with ME/CFS continued to be managed by a general practitioner (47% of the ME/CFS cohort), paediatrician (41%), psychologist (29%) and/or physiotherapist (29%) for more than 3 visits (71%) over the course of the study period. Inter-relatedness of the domains studied would also suggest that management, rehabilitation and improvement in one area would likely lead to symptom reduction in related domains (i.e., fatigue severity and anxiety have been shown to co-vary in adolescents with ME/CFS [7,32]).

More concerning was the finding that despite significant and clinically-meaningful improvement over time (with moderate to large effect sizes), adolescents with ME/CFS continued to show significantly greater fatigue, pain and poorer health-related quality of life than their healthy peers at follow-up. This observation is important for the treating clinician to understand so that a more realistic prognosis and need for intervention can be discussed with the young person and their family at the initial diagnosis and start of treatment. Van Geelen et al. [26] found considerable levels of fatigue in adolescents with ME/CFS at a similar follow-up timeframe to the current study (approximately 2 years), despite substantial health care use in the cohort, and this correlated with greater pain and poorer health and psychological wellbeing. We recognise that the patient cohorts from our (and Van Geelen's) study were comparatively early in their trajectory of recovery, with further improvement expected over time. Rowe [11] reported a mean paediatric ME/CFS illness duration of 5 years for those reporting recovery, but with a range of 1 to 15 years. In the current cohort, the mean two-year follow-up time interval from diagnosis had a range of 1 to 4 years, with the onset of symptoms prior to diagnosis ranging from 3 months to over 24 months. Our cohort may also have represented ME/CFS cases of greater severity and reduced functioning given they had been referred for specialist tertiary care.

Unlike previous studies [6,31,62,66], we did not find higher rates of depression in adolescents with ME/CFS compared with healthy controls, nor an increase in depression over time. However, our findings do support two recent paediatric ME/CFS follow-up studies showing stable depression levels over time [67,68]. Although Loades et al. [68] observed consistently higher levels of depression in the paediatric ME/CFS group than healthy controls, baseline ME/CFS depression was found to explain most of the variance in follow-up ME/CFS depression, which appears to suggest stable depression levels across time in paediatric ME/CFS. Of note, Loades et al.'s sample included a higher proportion of adolescents with depression compared with previous studies [6,66]. It may be that there is a subtype of ME/CFS that is particularly associated with comorbid depression [69], which was represented in Loades et al.'s [68] sample but not in our study. Major psychiatric illness that could adequately explain fatigue symptoms was an exclusionary criteria in our study, which would have played an additional role.

4.2. Fulfilment of Paediatric ME/CFS Diagnostic Criteria at Follow-Up

The main finding from the second aim of our study was that approximately two thirds (65%) of participants continued to fulfill paediatric ME/CFS diagnostic criteria at follow-up, which included cases of severe, moderate, and atypical severity. The remaining third (35%) were not classified as meeting criteria and more likely reflected a sub-clinical sample of individuals that had improved considerably since diagnosis, given that none reported unexplained, persistent fatigue that represented a substantial reduction in previous functioning. This 35% of participants could be interpreted as having improved clinical status since diagnosis, which would fall within the observed 'recovery' range in Moore et al.'s [30] systematic review of paediatric ME/CFS longitudinal studies (ranging from 5% to 83% recovery). However, there are obvious limitations in inferring recovery and when comparing results across these follow-up studies, given the variability in case definition, inclusion criteria, and definitions of recovery used. In the current study, follow-up diagnostic status was determined through self-report only. The known fluctuating nature and severity of ME/CFS experienced by patients, as well as our lack of diagnostic biomarker/s, also makes it more difficult to establish accurate diagnostic status at follow-up. This is supported by Rowe [11] who found 58% of paediatric ME/CFS patients had a fluctuating severity pattern of illness over the follow-up period, with 14% reporting a consistent level of severity, and 12% showing a relapsing and remitting pattern.

Consistent with the majority of patients fulfilling paediatric ME/CFS criteria at follow-up, the majority of patients (82%) self-identified as continuing to have the condition at follow-up. Of these patients, 79% did indeed fulfil criteria for ME/CFS, while 21% did not. On one hand, the disparity could be an issue of construct validity. Whilst the Canadian consensus criteria for paediatric ME/CFS is considered an improvement upon previous case definitions [70], greater sensitivity and specificity may be needed given the heterogeneity of the illness [71,72]. On the other hand, a disparity between adolescent-defined and criteria-defined clinical status could be a function of the dimensional nature of many ME/CFS symptoms, including pain, sleep problems and fatigue [73,74]. It is possible that adolescents interpret the persistence of their somatic symptoms as a sign of overall ME/CFS persistence, even if the more cardinal ME/CFS symptoms (e.g., post-exertional malaise) are no longer an issue and/or the severity of their somatic symptoms has lessened. This may be supported by the finding that pain was the most endorsed symptom at follow-up in the ME/CFS group (100% of the cohort). Whatever the cause, if there is a disparity between the subjective experience of paediatric ME/CFS and what is being captured by current criteria, this has ramifications for research and practice. It is recommended that future research increase the specificity of ME/CFS somatic symptom criteria by drawing upon up-to-date research in sleep, fatigue and pain, in addition to continuing to dedicate resources towards identifying diagnostic biomarkers for paediatric ME/CFS.

4.3. Predictors of ME/CFS Criteria Fulfilment

The main finding from the third aim of our study was that no aspects of baseline health and psychological wellbeing were found to significantly predict ME/CFS criteria fulfilment at follow-up, with any great effect. However, despite not reaching significance as a predictor (with moderate effect), pain at baseline was significantly and positively associated with meeting criteria at follow-up, and was also the most commonly endorsed symptom by patients at follow-up. This would suggest that the experience of pain early in illness course may be relevant to later diagnostic status in the wider paediatric ME/CFS population, which is supported by previous research [3,75].

Although many reports imply that the presence of poor health at ME/CFS onset influences future recovery [1,63,76], empirical support is lacking. In fact, investigations focused on anxiety and depression suggest otherwise. For example, Rowe [11] reported no association between baseline depression/anxiety and recovery, and whilst Rimes et al. [15] found an association between baseline anxiety/depression and *new onset* chronic fatigue, they found no association between baseline anxiety/depression and *persistent* chronic fatigue. Rowe [11] and Rimes et al. [15] findings are consistent with the present study's results. It is worth noting that previous follow-up studies have tended to identify demographic predictors (rather than health/psychological predictors) of future clinical status, namely: older age, female gender, higher IQ, higher BMI, and school absenteeism [12,15,24,76]. Those studies that *have* found associations between baseline health/psychological wellbeing—e.g., sleep quality [77], depression [28,78], anxiety and fatigue [32]—and follow-up recovery status have relied on a proxy for ME/CFS (e.g., "CFS-like symptoms", "Chronic Disabling Fatigue", etc.). Therefore, it remains to be seen whether baseline aspects of health and psychological wellbeing are useful prognostic indicators of future diagnostic status or recovery in adolescents who have been diagnosed by a paediatric ME/CFS specialist.

4.4. Study Limitations and Strengths

It is important to acknowledge the possibility that those adolescents with ME/CFS who were lost to follow-up (*n* = 8) may potentially have been more functionally impaired than those who participated at follow-up, thereby influencing the representativeness of our sample. Importantly, analysis comparing baseline data for those involved in and those lost to follow-up revealed no significant differences in demographic characteristics (age,

SEIFA, sex) or intellectual ability (FSIQ), which suggests these influences were minimal. Our study would also have benefited from the inclusion of a comparison group such as adolescents with fibromyalgia, and with a larger sample size, would have been powered to separate the cohort into subgroups of mild, moderate, and severe ME/CFS for analysis. This would have helped to offset any influence of regression toward the mean when evaluating change over time [79], and helped to improve our ability to detect significant associations between baseline health status and ME/CFS criteria fulfilment at follow-up. Given these considerations, caution should be taken when generalising the present study's findings to adolescents with severe ME/CFS or sufficiently poor health at diagnosis, with the view that they may overestimate improvement in long-term outcomes for this group. In addition, further information regarding types of medication and treatments over the course of the follow-up period would be beneficial for future evaluation of the factors that may influence longer-term outcomes in this population.

A key strength of this study was the use of a case-controlled, longitudinal design and a cohort of well-characterised adolescents with ME/CFS whose diagnosis was confirmed by a specialist paediatrician using consensus clinical criteria, and whose follow-up diagnostic status was recorded using the same criteria. While it is acknowledged that some diagnostic items assessed at follow-up had to be re-phrased for the younger patient audience, the content at both timepoints was the same (as seen in Supplementary Table S1) allowing for reasonable comparison across time. This is an improvement upon previous follow-up studies which have relied on a proxy for ME/CFS diagnosis [32,78,80] or have not included a control group for comparison [12,24,25]. Using the same measures at baseline and follow-up also allowed for direct comparisons over time, including measures of health and psychological wellbeing which are less often studied in longitudinal paediatric ME/CFS studies. To the authors' knowledge, this study represents one of the first case-controlled follow-up studies of adolescents with ME/CFS in terms of their health, well-being and longer-term prognosis of their condition.

4.5. Clinical Implications and Future Directions

Given the observed persistence of ME/CFS symptoms, poorer health and reduced psychological well-being at follow-up compared with healthy controls (i.e., fatigue, pain, and health-related quality of life problems), the current study highlights the need for early identification and targeted and intensive treatment in these domains that continues at least two years post-diagnosis, but ideally longer. The symptom domain of pain may be a particularly pertinent area of focus in the management of paediatric ME/CFS, given pain was most frequently endorsed at follow-up, and pain at baseline was significantly associated with fulfilment of ME/CFS criteria at follow-up. Clinical multidisciplinary strategies targeting pain relief and management including medication, physiotherapy, cognitive and behavioural techniques (i.e., meditation, mindfulness and acceptance and commitment therapy), and regular follow-up with the treating physician will be essential in this regard. The use of standardised and consistent measurement of symptomatology across illness course, including evidence-based consensus criteria, and person-centred measurements of recovery will also be important in tracking patients' clinical outcomes and wellbeing over time in a meaningful way. Based on our findings, future research must employ multiple follow-up time points over a longer time period (i.e., longer than 4 years) to accommodate and record the fluctuating nature of symptoms and illness severity over the ME/CFS illness course. Such information would be invaluable for understanding the different types of illness trajectories experienced by patients, and best predictors of recovery. It would also help clinicians, adolescent patients, and their families in preparing young people with ME/CFS for the potential transition from family-oriented paediatric health services to more independently-oriented adult health services if required.

Supplementary Materials: The following are available online at https://www.mdpi.com/article/10.3390/jcm10163603/s1, Supplementary Table S1: Classic ME/CFS diagnostic criteria of the Canadian Consensus Criteria adapted for pediatrics (left column), and how these were assessed at baseline (middle column) and follow-up (right column), Table S2: Raw means of measures of health and psychological wellbeing at baseline and follow-up for adolescents with ME/CFS and healthy controls, Table S3: Participants who fulfilled paediatric ME/CFS diagnostic criteria at baseline and follow-up, Table S4: Pearson correlation matrix between health and psychological wellbeing measures and fulfilment of paediatric ME/CFS diagnostic criteria

Author Contributions: Conceptualisation, E.K.J., A.S., K.R., L.L., S.J.K.; methodology, E.K.J., A.S., K.R., L.L., S.J.K.; validation, E.K.J., R.C.C., A.S., K.R., L.L., S.J.K.; formal analysis, E.K.J., R.C.C.; investigation, E.K.J., R.C.C., A.S., K.R., L.L., S.J.K.; resources, E.K.J., A.S., S.J.K.; data curation, E.K.J., R.C.C., S.J.K.; writing—original draft preparation, E.K.J., R.C.C.; writing—review and editing, E.K.J., R.C.C., A.S., K.R., L.L., S.J.K.; visualisation, E.K.J., R.C.C.; supervision, E.K.J., S.J.K.; project administration, E.K.J., R.C.C., S.J.K.; funding acquisition, E.K.J., A.S., S.J.K. All authors have read and agreed to the published version of the manuscript.

Funding: This research was supported by ME Research UK (SCIO charity number SCO36942, http://www.meresearch.org.uk/, accessed on 9 August 2021). The Judith Jane Mason and Harold Stannett Williams Memorial Foundation (Mason Foundation, ABN96140017725), the Murdoch Children's Research Institute, the Royal Children's Hospital, and the Victorian Government's Operational Infrastructure Support Program. The APC was funded by the Mason Foundation.

Institutional Review Board Statement: The study was conducted according to the guidelines of the Declaration of Helsinki, and approved by the Royal Children's Hospital Human Research Ethics Committee (HREC 32233, 37200).

Informed Consent Statement: Informed consent was obtained from all participants and their parents involved in this study.

Data Availability Statement: The data presented in this study are available in text and the supplementary material, in Josev et al. (2020), and on request from the corresponding author, and are not publicly available due to patient privacy and ethical restrictions.

Acknowledgments: We sincerely thank Cathriona Clarke, Ngoc Nguyen, and clinicians in the Royal Children's Hospital CFS Rehabilitation Clinic, and Department of General Medicine and Adolescent Health for their assistance with data collection, as well as the research participants and their families for generously donating their time to this research project.

Conflicts of Interest: The authors declare no conflict of interest. The funders had no role in the design of the study; in the collection, analyses, or interpretation of data; in the writing of the manuscript, or in the decision to publish the results.

References

1. Crawley, E. Pediatric chronic fatigue syndrome: Current perspectives. *Pediatric Health Med. Ther.* **2017**, *9*, 27. [CrossRef]
2. Kennedy, G.; Underwood, C.; Belch, J.J. Physical and functional impact of chronic fatigue syndrome/myalgic encephalomyelitis in childhood. *Pediatrics* **2010**, *125*, e1324–e1330. [CrossRef]
3. Knight, S.; Harvey, A.; Lubitz, L.; Rowe, K.; Reveley, C.; Veit, F.; Hennel, S.; Scheinberg, A. Paediatric chronic fatigue syndrome: Complex presentations and protracted time to diagnosis. *J. Paediatr. Child Health* **2013**, *49*, 919–924. [CrossRef]
4. Knight, S.; Politis, J.; Garnham, C.; Scheinberg, A.; Tollit, M. School functioning in adolescents with Chronic Fatigue Syndrome. *Front. Pediatrics* **2018**, *6*, 302. [CrossRef]
5. Ausubel, D.P. *Theory and Problems of Adolescent Development*; iUniverse: Bloomington, Indiana, 2002.
6. Bould, H.; Collin, S.; Lewis, G.; Rimes, K.; Crawley, E. Depression in paediatric chronic fatigue syndrome. *Arch. Dis. Child.* **2013**, *98*, 425–428. [CrossRef] [PubMed]
7. Crawley, E.; Hunt, L.; Stallard, P. Anxiety in children with CFS/ME. *Eur. Child Adolesc. Psychiatry* **2009**, *18*, 683. [CrossRef] [PubMed]
8. Davis, E.; Waters, E.; Mackinnon, A.; Reddihough, D.; Graham, H.K.; Mehmet-Radji, O.; Boyd, R. Paediatric quality of life instruments: A review of the impact of the conceptual framework on outcomes. *Dev. Med. Child Neurol.* **2006**, *48*, 311–318. [CrossRef]
9. Josev, E.; Jackson, M.; Bei, B.; Trinder, J.; Harvey, A.; Clarke, C.; Snodgrass, K.; Scheinberg, A.; Knight, S. Sleep quality in adolescents with chronic fatigue syndrome/myalgic encephalomyelitis (CFS/ME). *J. Clin. Sleep Med.* **2017**, *13*, 1057–1066. [CrossRef] [PubMed]

10. Parslow, R.M.; Anderson, N.; Byrne, D.; Shaw, A.; Haywood, K.L.; Crawley, E. Adolescent's descriptions of fatigue, fluctuation and payback in chronic fatigue syndrome/myalgic encephalopathy (CFS/ME): Interviews with adolescents and parents. *BMJ Paediatr. Open* **2018**, *2*, e000281. [CrossRef]
11. Rowe, K. Long Term Follow up of Young People with Chronic Fatigue Syndrome Attending a Pediatric Outpatient Service. *Front. Pediatrics* **2019**, *7*, 21. [CrossRef] [PubMed]
12. Sankey, A.; Hill, C.M.; Brown, J.; Quinn, L.; Fletcher, A. A follow-up study of chronic fatigue syndrome in children and adolescents: Symptom persistence and school absenteeism. *Clin. Child Psychol. Psychiatry* **2006**, *11*, 126–138. [CrossRef]
13. Winger, A.; Kvarstein, G.; Wyller, V.B.; Ekstedt, M.; Sulheim, D.; Fagermoen, E.; Småstuen, M.C.; Helseth, S. Health related quality of life in adolescents with chronic fatigue syndrome: A cross-sectional study. *Health Qual. Life Outcomes* **2015**, *13*, 96. [CrossRef] [PubMed]
14. Short, M.A.; Gradisar, M.; Lack, L.C.; Wright, H.R.; Dohnt, H. The sleep patterns and well-being of Australian adolescents. *J. Adolesc.* **2013**, *36*, 103–110. [CrossRef] [PubMed]
15. Rimes, K.A.; Goodman, R.; Hotopf, M.; Wessely, S.; Meltzer, H.; Chalder, T. Incidence, prognosis, and risk factors for fatigue and chronic fatigue syndrome in adolescents: A prospective community study. *Pediatrics* **2007**, *119*, e603–e609. [CrossRef] [PubMed]
16. Van Oort, F.; Greaves-Lord, K.; Verhulst, F.; Ormel, J.; Huizink, A. The developmental course of anxiety symptoms during adolescence: The TRAILS study. *J. Child Psychol. Psychiatry* **2009**, *50*, 1209–1217. [CrossRef]
17. Merikangas, K.R.; He, J.-p.; Burstein, M.; Swanson, S.A.; Avenevoli, S.; Cui, L.; Benjet, C.; Georgiades, K.; Swendsen, J. Lifetime prevalence of mental disorders in US adolescents: Results from the National Comorbidity Survey Replication–Adolescent Supplement (NCS-A). *J. Am. Acad. Child Adolesc. Psychiatry* **2010**, *49*, 980–989. [CrossRef]
18. Lawrence, D.; Johnson, S.; Hafekost, J.; de Haan, K.B.; Sawyer, M.; Ainley, J.; Zubrick, S.R. *The Mental Health of Children and Adolescents: Report on the Second Australian Child and Adolescent Survey of Mental Health and Wellbeing*; Department of Health: Canberra, Australia, 2015.
19. Bisegger, C.; Cloetta, B.; Von Bisegger, U.; Abel, T.; Ravens-Sieberer, U. Health-related quality of life: Gender differences in childhood and adolescence. *Soz.-Und Präventivmedizin* **2005**, *50*, 281–291. [CrossRef]
20. Goldbeck, L.; Schmitz, T.G.; Besier, T.; Herschbach, P.; Henrich, G. Life satisfaction decreases during adolescence. *Qual. Life Res.* **2007**, *16*, 969–979. [CrossRef] [PubMed]
21. Meuleners, L.B.; Lee, A.H. Adolescent quality of life: A school-based cohort study in Western Australia. *Pediatrics Int.* **2003**, *45*, 706–711. [CrossRef]
22. Smith, M.S.; Glover, D.; Mitchell, J.; McCauley, E.A.; Corey, L.; Gold, D.; Tenover, F.C. Chronic fatigue in adolescents. *Pediatrics* **1991**, *88*, 195–202.
23. Krilov, L.R.; Fisher, M.; Friedman, S.B.; Reitman, D.; Mandel, F.S. Course and outcome of chronic fatigue in children and adolescents. *Pediatrics* **1998**, *102*, 360–366. [CrossRef]
24. Bell, D.; Jordan, K.; Robinson, M. Thirteen-year follow-up of children and adolescents with chronic fatigue syndrome. *Pediatrics* **2001**, *107*, 994–998. [PubMed]
25. Andersen, M.; Permin, H.; Albrecht, F. Illness and disability in Danish chronic fatigue syndrome patients at diagnosis and 5-year follow-up. *J. Psychosom. Res.* **2004**, *56*, 217–229. [CrossRef]
26. van Geelen, S.M.; Bakker, R.J.; Kuis, W.; van de Putte, E.M. Adolescent chronic fatigue syndrome: A follow-up study. *Arch. Pediatrics Adolesc. Med.* **2010**, *164*, 810–814. [CrossRef]
27. Rangel, L.; Garralda, M.; Levin, M.; Roberts, H. The course of severe chronic fatigue syndrome in childhood. *J. R. Soc. Med.* **2000**, *93*, 129–134. [CrossRef] [PubMed]
28. Norris, T.; Collin, S.M.; Tilling, K.; Nuevo, R.; Stansfeld, S.A.; Sterne, J.A.; Heron, J.; Crawley, E. Natural course of chronic fatigue syndrome/myalgic encephalomyelitis in adolescents. *Arch. Dis. Child.* **2017**, *102*, 522–528. [CrossRef]
29. Lim, A.; Lubitz, L. Chronic fatigue syndrome: Successful outcome of an intensive inpatient programme. *J. Paediatr. Child Health* **2002**, *38*, 295–299. [CrossRef] [PubMed]
30. Moore, Y.; Serafimova, T.; Anderson, N.; King, H.; Richards, A.; Brigden, A.; Sinai, P.; Higgins, J.; Ascough, C.; Clery, P.; et al. Recovery from chronic fatigue syndrome: A systematic review—Heterogeneity of definition limits study comparison. *Arch. Dis. Child.* **2021**. Epub ahead of print: 12 April 2021. [CrossRef]
31. Crawley, E. The epidemiology of chronic fatigue syndrome/myalgic encephalitis in children. *Arch. Dis. Child.* **2014**, *99*, 171–174. [CrossRef]
32. ter Wolbeek, M.; Van Doornen, L.J.; Kavelaars, A.; Heijnen, C.J. Predictors of persistent and new-onset fatigue in adolescent girls. *Pediatrics* **2008**, *121*, e449–e457. [CrossRef]
33. Viner, R.M.; Clark, C.; Taylor, S.J.; Bhui, K.; Klineberg, E.; Head, J.; Booy, R.; Stansfeld, S.A. Longitudinal risk factors for persistent fatigue in adolescents. *Arch. Pediatrics Adolesc. Med.* **2008**, *162*, 469–475. [CrossRef]
34. Carter, B.D.; Marshall, G.S. New developments: Diagnosis and management of chronic fatigue in children and adolescents. *Curr. Probl. Pediatrics* **1995**, *25*, 281–293. [CrossRef]
35. Josev, E.K.; Malpas, C.B.; Seal, M.L.; Scheinberg, A.; Lubitz, L.; Rowe, K.; Knight, S.J. Resting-state functional connectivity, cognition, and fatigue in response to cognitive exertion: A novel study in adolescents with chronic fatigue syndrome. *Brain Imaging Behav.* **2020**, *14*, 1815–1830. [CrossRef]

36. Jason, L.; Jordan, K.; Miike, T.; Bell, D.; Lapp, C.; Torres-Harding, S.; Rowe, K.; Gurwitt, A.; De Meirleir, K.; Van Hoof, E. A pediatric case definition for myalgic encephalomyelitis and chronic fatigue syndrome. *J. Chronic Fatigue Syndr.* **2006**, *13*, 1–44. [CrossRef]
37. Jason, L.; Porter, N.; Shelleby, E.; Till, L.; Bell, D.; Lapp, C.; Rowe, K.; Meirleir, K.D. Examining criteria to diagnose ME/CFS in pediatric samples. *J. Behav. Health Med.* **2010**, *1*, 186. [CrossRef]
38. Harris, P.A.; Taylor, R.; Thielke, R.; Payne, J.; Gonzalez, N.; Conde, J.G. Research electronic data capture (REDCap)—A metadata-driven methodology and workflow process for providing translational research informatics support. *J. Biomed. Inform.* **2009**, *42*, 377–381. [CrossRef]
39. Cohen, L.L.; Lemanek, K.; Blount, R.L.; Dahlquist, L.M.; Lim, C.S.; Palermo, T.M.; McKenna, K.D.; Weiss, K.E. Evidence-based assessment of pediatric pain. *J. Pediatric Psychol.* **2008**, *33*, 939–957. [CrossRef]
40. Crichton, A.; Knight, S.; Oakley, E.; Babl, F.; Anderson, V. Fatigue in child chronic health conditions: A systematic review of assessment instruments. *Pediatrics* **2015**, *135*, e1015–e1031. [CrossRef]
41. Deale, A.; Wessely, S. Patients' perceptions of medical care in chronic fatigue syndrome. *Soc. Sci. Med.* **2001**, *52*, 1859–1864. [CrossRef]
42. Huber, N.L.; Nicoletta, A.; Ellis, J.M.; Everhart, D.E. Validating the Adolescent Sleep Wake Scale for use with young adults. *Sleep Med.* **2020**, *69*, 217–219. [CrossRef] [PubMed]
43. Knight, S.; Harvey, A.; Hennel, S.; Lubitz, L.; Rowe, K.; Reveley, C.; Dean, N.; Clarke, C.; Scheinberg, A. Measuring quality of life and fatigue in adolescents with chronic fatigue syndrome: Estimates of feasibility, internal consistency and parent–adolescent agreement of the PedsQL™. *Fatigue Biomed. Health Behav.* **2015**, *3*, 220–234. [CrossRef]
44. Storfer-Isser, A.; Lebourgeois, M.K.; Harsh, J.; Tompsett, C.J.; Redline, S. Psychometric properties of the Adolescent Sleep Hygiene Scale. *J. Sleep Res.* **2013**, *22*, 707–716. [CrossRef]
45. White, D.; Leach, C.; Sims, R.; Atkinson, M.; Cottrell, D. Validation of the Hospital Anxiety and Depression Scale for use with adolescents. *Br. J. Psychiatry* **1999**, *175*, 452–454. [CrossRef]
46. Varni, J.W.; Seid, M.; Kurtin, P.S. PedsQL™ 4.0: Reliability and validity of the Pediatric Quality of Life Inventory™ Version 4.0 Generic Core Scales in healthy and patient populations. *Med. Care* **2001**, *39*, 800–812. [CrossRef]
47. Varni, J.W.; Limbers, C.A. The PedsQL Multidimensional Fatigue Scale in young adults: Feasibility, reliability and validity in a University student population. *Qual. Life Res.* **2008**, *17*, 105–114. [CrossRef]
48. Varni, J.W.; Burwinkle, T.M.; Katz, E.R.; Meeske, K.; Dickinson, P. The PedsQL™ in pediatric cancer: Reliability and validity of the pediatric quality of life inventory™ generic core scales, multidimensional fatigue scale, and cancer module. *Cancer* **2002**, *94*, 2090–2106. [CrossRef] [PubMed]
49. LeBourgeois, M.K.; Giannotti, F.; Cortesi, F.; Wolfson, A.R.; Harsh, J. The relationship between reported sleep quality and sleep hygiene in Italian and American adolescents. *Pediatrics* **2005**, *115*, 257–265. [CrossRef] [PubMed]
50. Varni, J.W.; Thompson, K.L.; Hanson, V. The Varni/Thompson Pediatric Pain Questionnaire. I. Chronic musculoskeletal pain in juvenile rheumatoid arthritis. *Pain* **1987**, *28*, 27–38. [CrossRef]
51. Zigmond, A.S.; Snaith, R.P. The hospital anxiety and depression scale. *Acta Psychiatr. Scand.* **1983**, *67*, 361–370. [CrossRef]
52. Jason, L.; Evans, M.; Porter, N.; Brown, M.; Brown, A.; Hunnell, J.; Anderson, V.; Lerch, A.; Meirleir, K.D.; Friedberg, F. The Development of a Revised Canadian Myalgic Encephalomyelitis Chronic Fatigue Syndrome Case Definition. *Am. J. Biochem. Biotechnol.* **2010**, *6*, 120–135. [CrossRef]
53. Jason, L.; Porter, N.; Shelleby, E.; Till, L.; Bell, D.S.; Lapp, C.W.; Rowe, K.; De Meirleir, K. Severe Versus Moderate Criteria for the New Pediatric Case Definition for ME/CFS. *Child Psychiatry Hum. Dev.* **2009**, *40*, 609–620. [CrossRef]
54. Wechsler, D. *Wechsler Abbreviated Scale of Intelligence (WASI-II)*, 2nd ed.; The Psychological Corporation: San Antonio, TX, USA, 2011.
55. Cohen, J. *Statistical Power Analysis for the Behavioral Sciences*; Department of Psychology. New York University: New York, NY, USA, 1988; pp. 1–567.
56. Sawilowsky, S.S. New effect size rules of thumb. *J. Mod. Appl. Stat. Methods* **2009**, *8*, 26. [CrossRef]
57. Rosenthal, J.A. Qualitative Descriptors of Strength of Association and Effect Size. *J. Soc. Serv. Res.* **1996**, *21*, 37–59. [CrossRef]
58. Snodgrass, K.; Harvey, A.; Scheinberg, A.; Knight, S. Sleep disturbances in pediatric chronic fatigue syndrome: A review of current research. *J. Clin. Sleep Med.* **2015**, *11*, 757–764. [CrossRef] [PubMed]
59. Roma, M.; Marden, C.; Flaherty, M.; Jasion, S.; Cranston, E.; Rowe, P. Impaired health-related quality of life in adolescent myalgic encephalomyelitis/chronic fatigue syndrome: The impact of core symptoms. *Front. Pediatrics* **2019**, *7*, 26. [CrossRef]
60. Bell, D.; Bell, K.; Cheney, P. Primary juvenile fibromyalgia syndrome and chronic fatigue syndrome in adolescents. *Clin. Infect. Dis.* **1994**, *18*, S21–S23. [CrossRef]
61. Jackson, M.L.; Bruck, D. Sleep abnormalities in chronic fatigue syndrome/myalgic encephalomyelitis: A review. *J. Clin. Sleep Med.* **2012**, *8*, 719–728. [CrossRef]
62. Garralda, E.; Rangel, L.; Levin, M.; Roberts, H.; Ukoumunne, O. Psychiatric adjustment in adolescents with a history of chronic fatigue syndrome. *J. Am. Acad. Child Adolesc. Psychiatry* **1999**, *38*, 1515–1521. [CrossRef]
63. Smith, M.S.; Martin-Herz, S.P.; Womack, W.M.; Marsigan, J.L. Comparative study of anxiety, depression, somatization, functional disability, and illness attribution in adolescents with chronic fatigue or migraine. *Pediatrics* **2003**, *111*, e376–e381. [CrossRef]

64. van Middendorp, H.; Geenen, R.; Kuis, W.; Heijnen, C.J.; Sinnema, G. Psychological adjustment of adolescent girls with chronic fatigue syndrome. *Pediatrics* **2001**, *107*, E35. [CrossRef] [PubMed]
65. Sulheim, D.; Hurum, H.; Helland, I.B.; Thaulow, E.; Wyller, V.B. Adolescent chronic fatigue syndrome; a follow-up study displays concurrent improvement of circulatory abnormalities and clinical symptoms. *Biopsychosoc. Med.* **2012**, *6*, 10. [CrossRef] [PubMed]
66. Walford, G.; Nelson, W.; McCluskey, D. Fatigue, depression, and social adjustment in chronic fatigue syndrome. *Arch. Dis. Child.* **1993**, *68*, 384–388. [CrossRef] [PubMed]
67. Ali, S.; Adamczyk, L.; Burgess, M.; Chalder, T. Psychological and demographic factors associated with fatigue and social adjustment in young people with severe chronic fatigue syndrome/myalgic encephalomyelitis: A preliminary mixed-methods study. *J. Behav. Med.* **2019**, *42*, 898–910. [CrossRef]
68. Loades, M.E.; Rimes, K.A.; Ali, S.; Chalder, T. Depressive symptoms in adolescents with chronic fatigue syndrome (CFS): Are rates higher than in controls and do depressive symptoms affect outcome? *Clin. Child Psychol. Psychiatry* **2019**, *24*, 580–592. [CrossRef]
69. Williams, T.E.; Chalder, T.; Sharpe, M.; White, P.D. Heterogeneity in chronic fatigue syndrome–empirically defined subgroups from the PACE trial. *Psychol. Med.* **2017**, *47*, 1454–1465. [CrossRef]
70. Morris, G.; Maes, M. Case definitions and diagnostic criteria for Myalgic Encephalomyelitis and Chronic fatigue Syndrome: From clinical-consensus to evidence-based case definitions. *Neuroendocrinol. Lett.* **2013**, *34*, 185–199.
71. Collin, S.M.; Nuevo, R.; Van De Putte, E.M.; Nijhof, S.L.; Crawley, E. Chronic fatigue syndrome (CFS) or myalgic encephalomyelitis (ME) is different in children compared to in adults: A study of UK and Dutch clinical cohorts. *BMJ Open* **2015**, *5*, e008830. [CrossRef]
72. May, M.; Emond, A.; Crawley, E. Phenotypes of chronic fatigue syndrome in children and young people. *Arch. Dis. Child.* **2010**, *95*, 245–249. [CrossRef]
73. van de Putte, E.M.; Engelbert, R.; Kuis, W.; Kimpen, J.; Uiterwaal, C.S. How fatigue is related to other somatic symptoms. *Arch. Dis. Child.* **2006**, *91*, 824–827. [CrossRef]
74. Winger, A.; Kvarstein, G.; Wyller, V.B.; Sulheim, D.; Fagermoen, E.; Småstuen, M.C.; Helseth, S. Pain and pressure pain thresholds in adolescents with chronic fatigue syndrome and healthy controls: A cross-sectional study. *BMJ Open* **2014**, *4*, e005920. [CrossRef]
75. Nijhof, S.L.; Priesterbach, L.P.; Bleijenberg, G.; Engelbert, R.H.; van de Putte, E.M. Functional improvement is accompanied by reduced pain in adolescent chronic fatigue syndrome. *Pain Med.* **2013**, *14*, 1435–1438. [CrossRef] [PubMed]
76. Lievesley, K.; Rimes, K.A.; Chalder, T. A review of the predisposing, precipitating and perpetuating factors in Chronic Fatigue Syndrome in children and adolescents. *Clin. Psychol. Rev.* **2014**, *34*, 233–248. [CrossRef]
77. Collin, S.M.; Norris, T.; Gringras, P.; Blair, P.S.; Tilling, K.; Crawley, E. Childhood sleep and adolescent chronic fatigue syndrome (CFS/ME): Evidence of associations in a UK birth cohort. *Sleep Med.* **2018**, *46*, 26–36. [CrossRef] [PubMed]
78. Collin, S.M.; Norris, T.; Joinson, C.; Loades, M.E.; Lewis, G.; Stansfeld, S.A.; Crawley, E. Depressive symptoms at age 9–13 and chronic disabling fatigue at age 16: A longitudinal study. *J. Adolesc.* **2019**, *75*, 123–129. [CrossRef] [PubMed]
79. Barnett, A.G.; Van Der Pols, J.C.; Dobson, A.J. Regression to the mean: What it is and how to deal with it. *Int. J. Epidemiol.* **2005**, *34*, 215–220. [CrossRef]
80. Ter Wolbeek, M.; Van Doornen, L.J.; Kavelaars, A.; Tersteeg-Kamperman, M.D.; Heijnen, C.J. Fatigue, depressive symptoms, and anxiety from adolescence up to young adulthood: A longitudinal study. *Brain Behav. Immun.* **2011**, *25*, 1249–1255. [CrossRef]

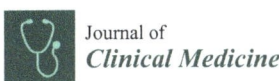

Article

Fibromyalgia Detection Based on EEG Connectivity Patterns

Ramón Martín-Brufau [1], Manuel Nombela Gómez [2], Leyre Sanchez-Sanchez-Rojas [3] and Cristina Nombela [4],*

[1] Unidad de Corta Estancia, Hospital Psiquiátrico Román Alberca, National Service of Health, 30120 Murcia, Spain; r.martinbrufau@um.es
[2] Research Support Service, University of Murcia, 30100 Murcia, Spain; manolonombela@gmail.com
[3] Regenerative Medicine and Advanced Therapies Lab., Instituto de Investigación Sanitaria San Carlos (IdISSC), Hospital Clínico San Carlos, 28040 Madrid, Spain; leyre.sanchez@salud.madrid.org
[4] Biological and Health Psychology, Autonomous University of Madrid (UAM), 28049 Madrid, Spain
* Correspondence: Cristina.nombela@uam.es; Tel.: +34-4975921

Abstract: Objective: The identification of a complementary test to confirm the diagnosis of FM. The diagnosis of fibromyalgia (FM) is based on clinical features, but there is still no consensus, so patients and clinicians might benefit from such a test. Recent findings showed that pain lies in neuronal bases (pain matrices) and, in the long term, chronic pain modifies the activity and dynamics of brain structures. Our hypothesis is that patients with FM present lower levels of brain activity and therefore less connectivity than controls. Methods: We registered the resting state EEG of 23 patients with FM and compared them with 23 control subjects' resting state recordings from the PhysioBank database. We measured frequency, amplitude, and functional connectivity, and conducted source localization (sLORETA). ROC analysis was performed on the resulting data. Results: We found significant differences in brain bioelectrical activity at rest in all analyzed bands between patients and controls, except for Delta. Subsequent source analysis provided connectivity values that depicted a distinct profile, with high discriminative capacity (between 91.3–100%) between the two groups. Conclusions: Patients with FM show a distinct neurophysiological pattern that fits with the clinical features of the disease.

Keywords: fibromyalgia; EEG; fast Fourier transform; diagnosis; ROC curve

1. Introduction

Fibromyalgia (FM) is a highly prevalent, painful disease, suffered by 2–4% of the population in the industrialized world, predominantly in women (ratio 9:1); it is very debilitating both physically and psychologically [1]. Current diagnosis criteria evaluate neither peripheral nor central functional deficiencies linked with the clinical symptoms, which complicates both the identification of the physiopathology of the disease and the search for adequate treatment [2].

In general terms, FM represents an enormous expenditure of resources, both direct (health care and medication) and indirect (e.g., loss of jobs and use of government aid) for the health, social and economic systems. The mean annual cost per patient in western countries ranged from US $2274 to $9573 in the central studies and even more in others, depending on the severity of symptoms and methods of cost calculation [3]. There exists, therefore, a need to identify a discriminative complementary method which, together with the description of the clinical symptoms, would help in the detection of FM [2]. Early diagnosis and treatment would reduce the burdens on patients, relatives, and society.

The feeling of pain is generated by a widely distributed brain network rather than by a direct sensory input evoked by a lesion or other pathology [4]. There are clear, substantial differences between (i) acute pain, which is evoked by specific noxious inputs, and whose sensory transmission mechanisms are well described, and (ii) chronic pain syndromes, which are often characterized by severe pain associated with little or no discernible injury or pathology, and are still not well understood [4]. In the last five years, some studies have shed some light on the cerebral mechanisms of chronic pain modulation [5], showing that subjective pain experience corresponds to a defined pattern of brain activity, in what is called the 'pain matrix' [6,7].

Such experience of pain has consequences that go further than temporary unpleasant feelings. Pain leaves a footprint: experiencing chronic pain can cause anatomical and functional reorganization of the brain [8], as shown in several disorders such as phantom pain, chronic back pain, irritable bowel syndrome, and FM (May, 2008). The morphological changes include the loss of gray matter volume [9], whereas the functional alterations include aberrant functional activity [10]. Recent reviews of the long-term effects of chronic pain have demonstrated the appearance of a "brain signature" [7,11]. The neural dynamics of the experience of pain follow specific processes related to coherence, activation, and deactivation of "core structures" in the default mode network, which are not linearly associated with stimulus intensity [12]. Such oscillations and the synchrony characteristics of pain can be measured by EEG and studied [13,14], including in clinical settings [15]. For example, Jensen et al. (2013) reported that the presence of specific EEG patterns might predict with 83% accuracy spinal cord injury patients' vulnerability to feelings of chronic pain [16], and Vuckovic et al. (2018) reported up to 85% accuracy in other studies [17]. A similar phenomenon takes place in healthy controls [15].

In the case of FM generalized pain, allodynia, and other neurological symptoms of central origin [18], result from deep tissue, like joints or muscles, in combination with central sensitization mechanisms. The nociceptive input may begin in peripheral tissue (e.g., by infection), generating allodynia or central sensitization. Those impairments in pain mechanisms might derive from long-term neuroplastic imbalances that the patients' antinociceptive capabilities cannot manage and result in ever-increasing pain sensitivity and dysfunction [19].

The physiopathology of the FM syndrome described in the literature is compatible with a central state of hyperexcitability of the nociceptive system [20,21], specifically, a persistent over-activation of Theta and Beta bands [22,23].

Complementary research indicates that both power band and power density differences exist between patients and matched controls. For example, Delta power density at temporal areas appears to be decreased in patients concerning controls, but Beta power reaches higher values in frontal and cingulate regions of patients with FM (Gonzalez-Roldan). Other types of analysis based on EEG data as source analysis have also indicated differences in the cingulate cortex. In particular, Vanneste et al. focused on both the degree of activation and the degree of integration and concluded that patients with FM showed decreased connectivity in the anterior cingulate cortex, which may affect the pain inhibitory pathway, mediating the pain feeling [24]. Pain experience correlates with a decreased level of Alpha-2 (11–12 Hz) in the posterior cortex [25] and decreased connectivity of the insula within the default mode network [26].

Other neuroimaging techniques, such as magnetoencephalography (MEG), have also shown disrupted connectivity at the Theta frequency for patients with FM compared with controls in the default mode network [27] and with resting state sequences [28]. However, there is little information comparing patients with FM with controls on electrical coherence between brain regions [24], and specific connections between regions have not yet been addressed. The analysis of such differences could, perhaps, be based on the EEG technique [29]. Working on EEG data, this study aims to describe the connectivity patterns in the default mode network in a group of patients to establish differential parameters and compare them with a sample of healthy controls. The hypothesis is that patients with fibromyalgia present significant differences from the controls in EEG activity and that this differential activity would be linked to a decrease in brain connectivity, as happens in other diseases related to chronic pain [30–33].

2. Materials and Methods

2.1. Sample

The sample consisted of 23 patients with FM and 23 healthy control subjects. The patients with FM were recruited via FIBROFAMUR (the association of patients with FM). They had all been diagnosed with FM by the Rheumatology Department of the Virgen de la Arrixaca University Hospital, Murcia) according to the American College of Rheumatology Diagnostic Criteria for fibromyalgia, with no record of epilepsy seizures or other neurological disorder in the sample. Recruiting, testing, and analysis of the data took place in 2017 and 2019.

The two groups were matched for age and gender. The mean age of the experimental group was 56 years (range 35–65). Seventy-seven percent had had the disease for more than 12 years. T-test analysis indicated no significant differences in age ($t(44) = 0.061$, $p = 0.54$) with the control group. The gender distribution was five males (21.8%) and eighteen females (78.2%) in each group. The control sample was randomly collected from the PhysioBank database, a public standard database available on the internet from the National Center for Research Resources of the National Institutes of Health [34]. It came from an experiment on motor movement/imagery, with a baseline of eyes closed EEG in resting state conditions, similar to the FM patients. A history of neurological or neuropsychiatric records or the use of drugs were exclusion criteria for participation in the control group. Accordingly, no pathological signals were found on the EEG registry of the control sample. Control sample registries undergo visual inspection to check the absence of pathological signs [35].

The Ethical Committee of the University of Murcia (Spain) approved the study. All procedures used followed the ethical standards of the responsible committee on human experimentation (institutional and national) and with the Helsinki Declaration of 1964 and its later amendments. All patients signed a written informed consent before their inclusion in the study.

2.2. Procedure

Twenty-one high-resolution EEG channels (NEURON-SPECTRUM-AM®) were used to record the data following 15 min eyes-closed resting state protocol. The sampling rate was 512 Hz. Guidelines to standard sample registration were followed (demographics, medical history, screening EEG, medication status) [36]. Data acquisition was conducted in complete silence, sitting in a comfortable and isolated room free from unpleasant stimuli. The disposition of electrodes followed the international 10–20 system with earlobes used as references and ground reference located in the Fpz location.

2.2.1. Data Preprocessing

Average reference, filtering, and analysis of the EEG signal were equal in both samples. A medical doctor with 50 years' experience in EEG ran a qualitative analysis by visual inspection of specific assemblies of bipolar montages. Segments of no less than 1 min of EEG free from artifacts were selected for analysis. The grapho-elements of pathological significance were registered (i.e., frequent posterior sharp waves) [37] since the morphological mapping tests of these patients usually show the presence of areas with atrophy [38,39], with signs of aging [40] or irrigation alterations [41] (Figure 1).

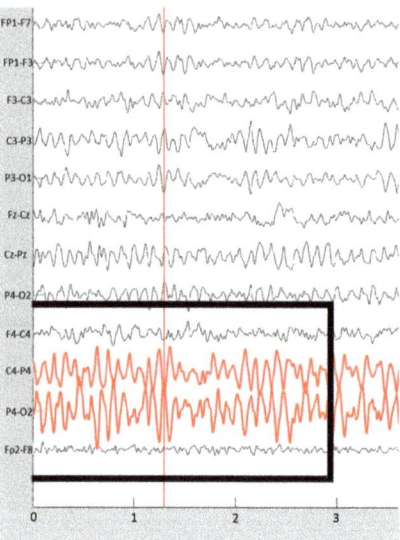

Figure 1. Example of EEG registry that presents abnormal activity (squared in black). Recording details: amplitude 70 microvolts, 10 s.

2.2.2. Data Analysis

Global EEG power was calculated with a weighted average across all channels with an average reference. Quantitative analyses (both fast Fourier transformation (FFT) and coherence analysis) were performed using the Brainstorm software [42] on MAT-LAB compiler runtime R2015b (MCR v9.0). The amplitude for each frequency band was calculated through the FFT and the functional connectivity through the coherence method (https://neuroimage.usc.edu/brainstorm/ Retrieved on 13 April 2021) previously used [43]. Relative amplitude was calculated as a percentage for each frequency band from the total absolute amplitude spectrum (from 1 to 32 Hz). The localization of the abnormal activity source required the standardized low-resolution brain electromagnetic tomography (sLORETA) method [44].

2.3. Statistical Analysis

The calculation of the mean amplitude and coherence differences for each group were obtained using the Student's T method. The 95% confidence intervals were estimated with a significance level of $p < 0.05$. The Bonferroni method was used to minimize errors arising from multiple comparisons.

Although we calculated several indices of functional association between pairs of electrodes that obtained good discriminative capacity, only significant ones are reported here. Their calculation was based on the sum of the coherences between the temporary locations (T3 and T4) with the Fz [index of functional discrimination between healthy and FM = (T3 − Fz coherence) + (T4− Fz coherence)].

To elucidate whether the connectivity pattern may serve to identify patients with fibromyalgia, we calculated ROC curves through the SPSS ROC curve calculation, obtaining sensitivity and specificity values and a total discrimination index. This index was used alongside the clinical diagnosis to calculate the sensitivity/susceptibility, $S = TP/(TP + FN)$, and the specificity, $E = TN/(FP + TN)$, of the EEG as a diagnostic tool, where TP means "true positive", TN "true negative", FN "false negative", and FP "False positive". ROC curves were used as an accuracy index to explore the discriminative validity of EEG parameters. Note that no machine learning methods were used. The discriminative capacity, following the ROC curve analysis, using 95% confidence intervals (CI), was calculated using the following formula: sensitivity − (1 − specificity) [45]. The software SPSS v.23 was used for statistical analysis.

3. Results

3.1. Frequency Analysis

The FM group had significantly lower amplitude values than the control group ($p < 0.001$). These differences appeared in all frequency bands and locations studied, except for the relative frequency of the Delta band (absolute and relative frequency values appear in Figure 2 and the statistical figures Table 1).

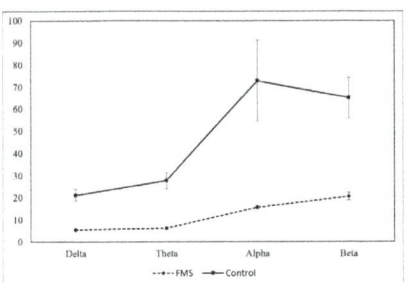

Figure 2. Absolute amplitude average of frequency bands (μV) in FMS and control groups ($p < 0.0001$ for all frequency bands comparisons).

Table 1. Differences in frequency bands between groups of absolute and relative mean frequencies for FM and control group * $p < 0.001$.

	FM (n = 23)		Control (n = 23)		
	Mean	SD	Mean	SD	p
ABSOLUTE					
Delta	5.59	0.42	21.22	2.69	0.000 *
Theta	6.32	0.50	27.88	3.75	0.000 *
Alpha	15.74	0.75	72.86	18.53	0.000 *
Beta	20.67	1.72	65.11	9.22	0.000*
RELATIVE					
Delta	11.57	0.49	11.57	2.07	0.991
Theta	13.08	0.65	15.02	1.55	0.000 *
Alpha	32.62	1.06	38.45	4.09	0.000 *
Beta	42.72	1.17	34.97	2.08	0.000 *

Analyzing each group, frequency maps of the FM sample showed greater activity in the right parietal region (location P4) for the other bands. This seems to agree with the presence of spike-type grapho-elements in the right parietal and occipital areas, mentioned earlier.

3.2. Sources by LORETAs

All EEG registries were visually checked. A higher frequency of spike-type grapho-elements was found in patients (17.8%) than in controls (0%), with potential symptomatic seizures from irritation of neighboring cerebral cortical tissue located on the right occipital and parietal regions [35]. This is a common finding, as nonepileptic seizures (PNES) are frequently found in FM patients [46–48].

By analyzing the location of sources using the sLORETA method we located anomalous activity (signs of irritation) on the bilateral precuneus, with right predominance, on the right inferior parietal cortex, bilateral prefrontal medial cortex, and right anterior Cingular cortex for patients with FM. Figure 3 shows the localization of the band activity.

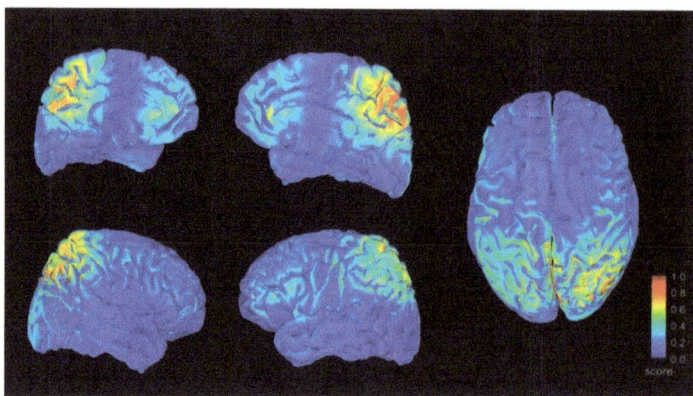

Figure 3. Source localization of abnormal activity in FMS patients.

3.3. Analysis of Coherence

In the FM group, we found that cortical interconnections in FM were very scarce during eyes-closed resting, especially for Delta and Beta frequencies. Those existing in the Alpha and Theta bands were only visible in frontotemporal regions ($p < 0.001$). These findings contrast strongly with the degree of interconnection shown by control subjects. In particular, the coherence analysis revealed greater functional connectivity between the insular regions and the frontal regions in the patients with FM, but not in the control sample ($p < 0.001$). The coherence measures for FM and control samples appear in Figure 4, where only coherences equal to or greater than 0.5 were included.

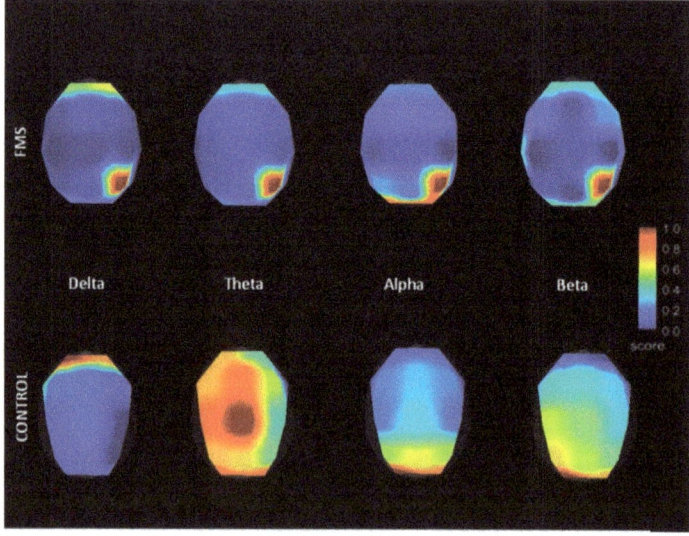

Figure 4. Grand average representation of FFT frequency bands for FMS and control subjects. Amplitude was reduced in FMS patients for all electrode positions.

3.4. Discriminatory Index

Finally, to distinguish patients with FM from controls, we analyzed a discrimination index using average amplitudes, the region of interest amplitude of P4, and functional connectivity between fronto-bitemporal locations. Statistical data appear in Table 2, showing good discrimination results with high accuracy (between 91.3–100%), and in Table 3, showing the area under the curve for ROC curves from frontal and temporal coherence values. The Theta band showed the best AUC with a sensitivity of cases of 100% and inclusion of 0% false cases. Frontotemporal functional connectivity showed a sensitivity of 91.3% and inclusion of 21.4% of false cases.

Table 2. Comparison between discriminative indexes for different EEG parameters. AUC = area under the curve.

FFT Amplitude	ROC (AUC)	Sensitivity/ 1 − Specificity	p [95% CI]
Delta (1–4 Hz)	0.618	0.643/0.609	0.234 (0.417, 0.819)
Theta (4–7 Hz)	1	1/0	0.000 (1, 1)
Alpha (7–14 Hz)	0.975	1/0.217	0.000 (1, 1)
Beta (15–32 Hz)	0.988	1/0.174	0.000 (0.960, 1)
Right Parieto-Occipital activity (P4)	0.984	1/0.217	0.000 (0.951, 1)
Frontotemporal functional connectivity	0.913	0.913/0.214	0.000 (0.816, 1)

Table 3. Accuracy index—area under the curve (AUC) for ROC curves calculated from coherence values. * $p < 0.05$; ** $p < 0.001$.

Derivations	Delta	Theta	Alpha	Beta
Fp1-Fp2	0.390	0.467	0.294	0.238
Fp2-T4	0.843 **	0.907 **	0.875 **	0.846 **
Fp1-T3	0.843 **	0.849 **	0.884 **	0.746 *
T3-T4	0.580	0.596	0.706	0.593
Fz-T3	0.712 *	0.684	0.780 *	0.765 *
Fz-T4	0.799 *	0.835 *	0.774 *	0.846 **
Fz-T3 + Fz-T4	0.877 **	0.794 *	0.788 *	0.822 *
Fp1-T3 + Fp2-T4	0.765 *	0.887 **	0.913 **	0.80 *

4. Discussion

In this study, we report the EEG data of a sample of 23 patients with FM and 23 matched controls to identify electrical differences between the two groups. The differential pattern of coherence, in the last instance, might work as a complementary method for FM diagnosis.

According to our results, patients with FM presented lower values than controls in all frequencies except for the Delta band. The frequency maps of the FM group indicated greater activity in parietal areas than in the rest of the scalp. Subsequent sources analysis indicated anomalous activity at the bilateral precuneus, with right predominance, on the right inferior parietal cortex, bilateral prefrontal medial cortex, and right anterior cingular cortex in the FM group. The coherence analysis of the brain signal showed clear differences between the groups, particularly in the bilateral frontotemporal region. Discriminatory analysis indicated a significant difference in interconnectivity patterns between patients and controls.

In general, we can state that frequency power was dramatically lower in the FM group than in the controls. These findings are compatible with the morphological findings reported by multiple authors using neuroimaging techniques [49]. The weight of the encephalon can be up to 3.3 times lower in chronic pain patients than in healthy subjects. In particular, this neuronal loss affects white matter, as evaluated by fractional anisotropy techniques [50]. With regard to location, studies by Kuchinad et al. (2007) showed that the most affected structures were the thalamus, medial posterior cingulate cortex, insula, prefrontal cortex, parahippocampus, hippocampus, anterior cingulate cortex, and striated nuclei [51]. A neuronal loss might explain the decrease in neuronal working synchrony, as a consequence of the communication defects caused by both the diffuse neuronal loss and the fibers of the white matter [52].

Deeper analysis of the affected bands shows that the most severe decrease took place in Alpha, Theta, and Beta frequency bands and was not significant in the Delta band. On the one hand, given that the first three bands depend on the cortical neuronal interaction and its networks, it is reasonable to link these alterations with the morphological impairments described above. On the other hand, Delta activity is more dependent on the somas of the deep pyramidal neurons affected in degeneration, usually by irrigation defects [53]. Other studies have reported similar differences between patients with FM and healthy controls while solving problems of various types. In global field power analysis, patients with FM presented lower modulation of Alpha and Theta, less synchronization, and lower spectral density, which indicates the presence of excessive neuronal noise [54]. According to fMRI research, patients with FM have to mobilize more cortical extension than healthy subjects, even in young patients aged between 25 and 40. This process may explain the presence of cognitive impairments. This reaction closely resembles the one in healthy elderly people, which is why some authors compare the consequences of fibromyalgia with an accelerated brain aging process.

Frequency mapping with a separate representation of the different frequency bands demonstrates that all bands showed their maximum amplitude in the right parieto-occipital region (Figure 5). This predominance may represent better conservation of the neuronal structure of the right parietal lobe than in other cortical areas (susceptible to potential irritative characters) [55]. This may also be related to the increase of glutamic acid and the decrease of gamma-aminobutyric acid described by Puiu et al. at the anterior cingular cortex, insula, and amygdaloid nucleus [56].

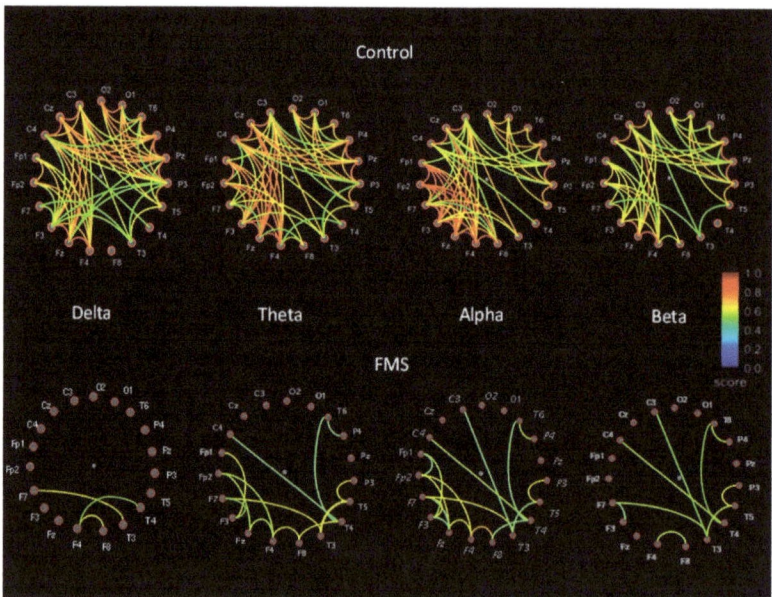

Figure 5. Functional connectivity comparison between control and FMS samples (connectivity between temporal and frontal locations).

Analysis of the source with the sLORETA system pointed to the bilateral precuneus, right inferior parietal cortex, bilateral medial prefrontal cortex, and right anterior cingular cortex. These cortical structures are part of the default mode network, except for the insula, which was not observed in our maps. The most activated structure was the anterior cingular cortex, the first structure affected in FM, and the one in which has been observed the most manifest excess of glutamic acid, reduction in gamma-aminobutyric acid, and neuronal loss [24]. This fact may help explain why some authors argue that the exacerbation of pain in FM results from the existence of hypersensitive neural networks which, with their explosive response to any stimulus, cause synchronizations of the most sensitive networks [57]. These authors found a positive relationship between the intensity of pain caused by any normal stimulus and the degree of explosive synchronization of the EEG in these patients. According to the results of the current study, the presence of EEG spikes could be an example of these explosive phenomena, although it can also only facilitate them.

Concerning connectivity patterns, the intercommunication at the Alpha and Theta frequencies were more abundant in patients with FM, but short association fiber between neighboring areas predominate in the bilateral frontotemporal region, suggesting better conservation of U-fibers than long fibers in the whole of the white substance (Table 3). This contrasts with recent findings in which long fibers appeared more connected than short ones in the Alpha band [54]. Other studies support our results about the significantly lower level of connectivity signal in the FM group than in controls during resting state, particularly in the Theta band [27,58,59]. These functional connectivity differences are related to differences in pain intensity between FM patients and controls [60].

It also seems that some treatments that reduce pain in FM produce a change in brain connectivity, including the insula and the cingulate cortex, as in our study [61]. Physical exercise interventions also seem to normalize aberrant resting state functional connectivity in FM patients and to be associated with pain improvement [62]. These patterns of altered connectivity have been found to be associated with altered integration of sensory information [63]. Other studies of functional connectivity have shown a reduced pattern of connectivity in FM, and it has been suggested that functional connectivity could have clinical implications if used as an objective measure of pain dysregulation [64].

Test Accuracy

The resulting patterns demonstrated high discriminability between patients and controls, predominantly in the Theta band and right frontotemporal regions (Table 3), agreeing with Ichesco [65]. A variety of methods of complementing FM diagnoses have reached high accuracy values: 72.9% accuracy of FM symptomatology questionnaires [66], 78.9% accuracy of neurophysiological reflex exploration of the spinal nociceptive flexion reflex, indicative of central sensitization [20], 95% accuracy of qEEG during polysomnography [67], 85.1% accuracy with different alternative criteria for FM (Salaffi et al., 2020), and 64.8%–71.3% accuracy based on physical examination and laboratory tests to identify FM patients [68]. Another study using an fMRI combination of neurologic pain signature, pain-related response, and multisensory nonpainful sensory stimulation showed 93% discrimination accuracy [29].

To our knowledge, EEG functional connectivity has not been used, so far, to discriminate between chronic pain syndromes. One future line of research should study the discriminative power of brain activity between different pain syndromes using functional connectivity, a line of research that needs further optimization. It is theoretically possible that chronic pain syndromes share common brain signatures, but discriminative methods could also be optimized to increase the accuracy of the results. For example, more specific examination with fMRI has been used to discriminate between pain syndromes with non-significant results, although 78.8% discriminative accuracies were achieved between FM and rheumatoid arthritis [69]. Overall, due to the consistently higher accuracy results of brain parameters over other methods of FM discrimination, neuroscientific methods could help improve FM diagnosis. In particular, EEG seems to be a promising tool with which to improve the early identification of patients at risk of developing a chronic pain condition.

Some possible limitations result from using the reference database, which is a relatively new (albeit increasingly adopted) procedure [70,71]. It is arguable that the FM sample could not be completely comparable with the nonclinical subjects extracted from the standard database because of incompatibilities between different acquisition methods. The use of several methodological techniques can, however, ensure the validity of the comparisons made in the present study, by reducing acquisition noise and sources of confusion [72]. These methods include the use of averaging mounts, band-pass frequency filters that exclude frequencies above 100 Hz [73], and relative power calculations to reduce differences individual measurements in skull thickness or amplifier calibration [74]. These techniques show similar results between acquisition devices when calculating the FFT bands [75], and similar signal-to-noise ratios between devices (up to 12 different ones). Even the comparison between modern low-cost EEG devices with medical-grade instruments shows comparable results for calculating frequency [76]. These techniques and new research opportunities are opening up new avenues for the use of open repositories in neuroscience research and collaboration.

To confirm the validity of the control sample, other studies used the same database [10,77–82], including with FM population [83]. Alterations in functional connectivity are frequent in patients with FM (Hargrove et al., 2010), in particular alterations in frontotemporal connectivity [62,65,84], and are often associated with a lower white matter volume than in controls in frontal regions [28]. Our results replicate these previous findings. However, since we have specifically studied frontotemporal functional connectivity as a region of associations of interest (due to sample size limitations), these results should be viewed with caution. In summary, the comparison with normative samples constitutes a valid method if certain requirements are met (i.e., age-appropriate values, selection of artifact-free segments, and similar registry conditions, among others). Healthy control databases have been demonstrated to be reliable and to lack ethnic bias, making the comparison with clinical samples adequate, cost-effective, culture-fair, and highly sensitive to abnormalities in brain function both to spectra [15] and LORETA comparisons [85].

About the sample size, it would have been interesting to compare patients with FM with depressed individuals to see whether our algorithm correctly differentiates from other comorbid psychiatric pathologies. Another limitation is that there may be different origins of FM which end in the same syndrome. Therefore, we may be facing a particular type of FM pattern that presents specific connectivity abnormalities. However, the syndromic subgroups of FM remain an unsolved problem. We have not been able to measure pain levels or precise psychopathological characteristics through questionnaires or cognitive tests, which may be an interesting line of work in the future, as suggested by some studies [86,87]. Triñanes et al. suggested that types I and II of FM differ by psychopathological profile [87].

This study shows potential distinctive neurophysiological features in patients with FM that put in connection function and structure. In the future, data could be the basis of a reproducible and safe diagnostic method for FM, as previously suggested by other studies [88].

Author Contributions: Conceptualization, R.M.-B. and M.N.G.; methodology, R.M.-B. and M.N.G.; software, R.M.-B.; validation, R.M.-B., L.S.-S.-R., and C.N.; formal analysis, R.M.-B.; investigation, C.N.; resources, M.N.G.; data curation, R.M.-B. and L.S.-S.-R.; writing—original draft preparation, R.M.-B. and C.N.; writing—review and editing, L.S.-S.-R. and C.N.; visualization, M.N.G. and C.N.; supervision, C.N.; project administration, M.N.G.; funding acquisition, C.N. All authors have read and agreed to the published version of the manuscript.

Funding: CN was funded through a Francisco Tomás y Valiente research fellowship (MIAS—UAM). This work is framed in the research project entitled "Criminal Law and Human Behaviour" (RTI2018-097838-B-I00) granted by the Spain Ministry for Science, Innovation, and Universities of Spain (PI: Prof. Eduardo Demetrio Crespo). LSSR was funded by Boston Scientific.

Institutional Review Board Statement: The study was conducted according to the guidelines of the Declaration of Helsinki and approved by the Institutional Ethics Committee of the University of Murcia (2017).

Informed Consent Statement: Informed consent was obtained from all subjects involved in the study. Written informed consent w obtained from the patients to publish this paper.

Data Availability Statement: Data from healthy controls were randomly collected from a public standard database available on the Internet under the auspices of the National Center for Research Resources of the National Institutes of Health.

Acknowledgments: We are deeply thankful to the Fibromyalgia Association in Murcia for its interest and support, particularly to the volunteers and their families. We would also like to thank the Research Support Service of the University of Murcia for their help with the study.

Conflicts of Interest: The authors declare that they have no conflict of interest.

References

1. Queiroz, L.P. Worldwide Epidemiology of Fibromyalgia. *Curr. Pain Headache Rep.* **2013**, *17*, 356. [CrossRef]
2. Goldenberg, D.L. Diagnosing Fibromyalgia as a Disease, an Illness, a State, or a Trait? *Arthritis Care Res.* **2019**, *71*, 334–336. [CrossRef]
3. Ghavidel-Parsa, B.; Bidari, A.; Amir Maafi, A.; Ghalebaghi, B. The Iceberg Nature of Fibromyalgia Burden: The Clinical and Economic Aspects. *Korean J. Pain* **2015**, *28*, 169–176. [CrossRef]
4. Melzack, R. Pain and the Neuromatrix in the Brain. *J. Dent. Educ.* **2001**, *65*, 1378–1382. [CrossRef] [PubMed]
5. Tanasescu, R.; Cottam, W.J.; Condon, L.; Tench, C.R.; Auer, D.P. Functional reorganisation in chronic pain and neural correlates of pain sensitisation: A coordinate based meta-analysis of 266 cutaneous pain fMRI studies. *Neurosci. Biobehav. Rev.* **2016**, *68*, 120–133. [CrossRef]
6. Rainville, P.; Bushnell, M.C.; Duncan, G.H. Representation of Acute and Persistent Pain in the Human CNS: Potential Implications for Chemical Intolerance. *Ann. N. Y. Acad. Sci.* **2006**, *933*, 130–141. [CrossRef] [PubMed]
7. May, A. Chronic pain may change the structure of the brain. *Pain* **2008**, *137*, 7–15. [CrossRef] [PubMed]
8. Apkarian, V.A.; Hashmi, J.A.; Baliki, M.N. Pain and the brain: Specificity and plasticity of the brain in clinical chronic pain. *Pain* **2011**, *152*, S49–S64. [CrossRef]
9. Smallwood, R.F.; Laird, A.R.; Ramage, A.E.; Parkinson, A.L.; Lewis, J.; Clauw, D.J.; Williams, D.A.; Schmidt-Wilcke, T.; Farrell, M.J.; Eickhoff, S.B.; et al. Structural Brain Anomalies and Chronic Pain: A Quantitative Meta-Analysis of Gray Matter Volume. *J. Pain* **2013**, *14*, 663–675. [CrossRef]
10. Fu, M.; Wang, Y.; Chen, Z.; Li, J.; Xu, F.; Liu, X.; Hou, F. Deep Learning in Automatic Sleep Staging With a Single Channel Electroencephalography. *Front. Physiol.* **2021**, *12*, 179. [CrossRef]
11. Baliki, M.N.; Schnitzer, T.J.; Bauer, W.R.; Apkarian, A.V. Brain Morphological Signatures for Chronic Pain. *PLoS ONE* **2011**, *6*, e26010. [CrossRef] [PubMed]
12. Kong, J.; Loggia, M.L.; Zyloney, C.; Tu, P.; LaViolette, P.; Gollub, R.L. Exploring the brain in pain: Activations, deactivations and their relation. *Pain* **2010**, *148*, 257–267. [CrossRef] [PubMed]
13. Ploner, M.; Sorg, C.; Gross, J. Brain Rhythms of Pain. *Trends Cogn. Sci.* **2017**, *21*, 100–110. [CrossRef] [PubMed]
14. Pinheiro, E.S.D.S.; Queirós, F.C.D.; Montoya, P.; Santos, C.L.; Nascimento, M.A.D.; Ito, C.H.; Baptista, A.F. Electroencephalographic Patterns in Chronic Pain: A Systematic Review of the Literature. *PLoS ONE* **2016**, *11*, e0149085. [CrossRef]
15. Prichep, L.S.; John, E.R.; Howard, B.; Merkin, H.; Hiesiger, E.M. Evaluation of the Pain Matrix Using EEG Source Localization: A Feasibility Study. *Pain Med.* **2011**, *12*, 1241–1248. [CrossRef] [PubMed]
16. Jensen, M.P.; Sherlin, L.H.; Gertz, K.J.; Braden, A.L.; Kupper, A.E.; Gianas, A.; Hakimian, S. Brain EEG activity correlates of chronic pain in persons with spinal cord injury: Clinical implications. *Spinal Cord* **2013**, *51*, 55–58. [CrossRef]
17. Vuckovic, A.; Gallardo, V.J.F.; Jarjees, M.; Fraser, M.; Purcell, M. Prediction of central neuropathic pain in spinal cord injury based on EEG classifier. *Clin. Neurophysiol.* **2018**, *129*, 1605–1617. [CrossRef]
18. Sluka, K.A.; Clauw, D.J. Neurobiology of fibromyalgia and chronic widespread. *Pain Neurosci.* **2016**, *338*, 114–129. [CrossRef]
19. Price, D.D.; Staud, R. Neurobiology of fibromyalgia syndrome. *J. Rheumatol. Suppl.* **2005**, *75*, 22–28.
20. Desmeules, J.A.; Cedraschi, C.; Rapiti, E.; Baumgartner, E.; Finckh, A.; Cohen, P.; Vischer, T.L. Neurophysiologic evidence for a central sensitization in patients with fibromyalgia. *Arthritis Rheum.* **2003**, *48*, 1420–1429. [CrossRef]
21. Teng, H.-W.; Tani, J.; Chang, T.-S.; Chen, H.-J.; Lin, Y.-C.; Lin, C.S.-Y.; Sung, J.Y. Altered sensory nerve excitability in fibromyalgia. *J. Formos. Med. Assoc.* **2021**. [CrossRef]
22. Stern, J.; Jeanmonod, D.; Sarnthein, J. Persistent EEG overactivation in the cortical pain matrix of neurogenic pain patients. *Neuroimage* **2006**, *31*, 721–731. [CrossRef]
23. Hubbard, C.S.; Lazaridou, A.; Cahalan, C.M.; Kim, J.; Edwards, R.R.; Napadow, V.; Loggia, M.L. Aberrant Salience? Brain Hyperactivation in Response to Pain Onset and Offset in Fibromyalgia. *Arthritis Rheumatol.* **2020**, *72*, 1203–1213. [CrossRef] [PubMed]

24. Vanneste, S.; Ost, J.; Van Havenbergh, T.; De Ridder, D. Resting state electrical brain activity and connectivity in fibromyalgia. *PLoS ONE* **2017**, *12*, 1–20. [CrossRef] [PubMed]
25. Villafaina, S.; Collado-Mateo, D.; Fuentes-García, J.P.; Cano-Plasencia, R.; Gusi, N. Impact of Fibromyalgia on Alpha-2 EEG Power Spectrum in the Resting Condition: A Descriptive Correlational Study. *BioMed Res. Int.* **2019**, *2019*, 1–6. [CrossRef]
26. Napadow, V.; LaCount, L.; Park, K.; As-Sanie, S.; Clauw, D.J.; Harris, R.E. Intrinsic brain connectivity in fibromyalgia is associated with chronic pain intensity. *Arthritis Rheum.* **2010**, *62*, 2545–2555. [CrossRef] [PubMed]
27. Choe, M.K.; Lim, M.; Kim, J.S.; Lee, D.S.; Chung, C.K. Disrupted Resting State Network of Fibromyalgia in Theta frequency. *Sci. Rep.* **2018**, *8*, 1–9. [CrossRef] [PubMed]
28. Cagnie, B.; Coppieters, I.; Denecker, S.; Six, J.; Danneels, L.; Meeus, M. Central sensitization in fibromyalgia? {A} systematic review on structural and functional brain. *Semin. Arthritis Rheum.* **2014**, *44*, 68–75. [CrossRef]
29. López-Solà, M.; Woo, C.-W.; Pujol, J.; Deus, J.; Harrison, B.J.; Monfort, J.; Wager, T.D. Towards a neurophysiological signature for fibromyalgia. *Pain* **2017**, *158*, 34–47. [CrossRef]
30. Mayer, E.A.; Gupta, A.; Kilpatrick, L.A.; Hong, J.-Y. Imaging brain mechanisms in chronic visceral Pain. *Pain* **2015**, *156* (Suppl. 1), S50–S63. [CrossRef]
31. Bushnell, M.C.; Čeko, M.; Low, L.A. Cognitive and emotional control of pain and its disruption in chronic pain. *Nat. Rev. Neurosci.* **2013**, *14*, 502–511. [CrossRef]
32. González-Roldán, A.M.; Muñoz, M.A.; Cifre, I.; Sitges, C.; Montoya, P. Altered psychophysiological responses to the view of others' pain and anger faces in fibromyalgia patients. *J. Pain. J. Am. Pain Soc.* **2013**, *14*, 709–719. [CrossRef] [PubMed]
33. Napadow, V.; Kim, J.; Clauw, D.J.; Harris, R.E. Decreased intrinsic brain connectivity is associated with reduced clinical pain in fibromyalgia. *Arthritis Rheum.* **2012**, *64*, 2398–2403. [CrossRef] [PubMed]
34. Goldberger, A.L.; Amaral, L.; Glass, L.; Hausdorff Jeffrey, M.; Ivanov Plamen, C.; Mark, R.G.; Stanley, H.E. PhysioBank, PhysioToolkit, and PhysioNet. *Circulation* **2000**, *101*, e215–e220. [CrossRef] [PubMed]
35. Niedermeyer, E. The normal EEG of the waking adult. *Electroencephalogr. Basic. Princ. Clin. Appl. Relat. Fields.* **1999**, *20*, 149–173.
36. Jobert, M.; Wilson, F.J.; Ruigt, G.S.F.; Brunovsky, M.; Prichep, L.S.; Drinkenburg, W.H.I.M. Guidelines for the Recording and Evaluation of Pharmaco-EEG Data in Man: The International Pharmaco-EEG Society (IPEG). *Neuropsychobiology* **2012**, *66*, 201–220. [CrossRef]
37. Tatum, W.O.; Olga, S.; Ochoa, J.G.; Munger Clary, H.; Cheek, J.; Drislane, F.; Tsuchida, T.N. American Clinical Neurophysiology Society Guideline 7. *J. Clin. Neurophysiol.* **2016**, *33*, 328–332. [CrossRef]
38. Feraco, P.; Nigro, S.; Passamonti, L.; Grecucci, A.; Caligiuri, M.E.; Gagliardo, C.; Bacci, A. Neurochemical correlates of brain atrophy in fibromyalgia syndrome: A magnetic resonance spectroscopy and cortical thickness study. *Brain Sci.* **2020**, *10*, 395. [CrossRef] [PubMed]
39. Lin, C.; Lee, S.-H.; Weng, H.-H. Gray Matter Atrophy within the Default Mode Network of Fibromyalgia: A Meta-Analysis of Voxel-Based Morphometry Studies. *BioMed Res. Int.* **2016**, *2016*, 7296125. [CrossRef]
40. McCrae, C.S.; O'Shea, A.M.; Boissoneault, J.; Vatthauer, K.E.; Robinson, M.E.; Staud, R.; Craggs, J.G. Fibromyalgia patients have reduced hippocampal volume compared with healthy controls. *J. Pain Res.* **2015**, *8*, 47–52. [CrossRef]
41. Duschek, S.; Mannhart, T.; Winkelmann, A.; Merzoug, K.; Werner, N.S.; Schuepbach, D.; Montoya, P. Cerebral blood flow dynamics during pain processing in patients with fibromyalgia syndrome. *Psychosom. Med.* **2012**, *74*, 802–809. [CrossRef]
42. Tadel, F.; Baillet, S.; Mosher, J.C.; Pantazis, D.; Leahy, R.M. Brainstorm: A user-friendly application for MEG/EEG analysis. *Comput. Intell. Neurosci.* **2011**, *2011*, 8. [CrossRef]
43. de Oliveira, A.P.S.; de Santana, M.A.; Andrade, M.K.S.; Gomes, J.C.; Rodrigues, M.C.A.; dos Santos, W.P. Early diagnosis of Parkinson's disease using EEG, machine learning and partial directed coherence. *Res. Biomed. Eng.* **2020**, *36*, 311–331. [CrossRef]
44. Gentile, E.; Ricci, K.; Vecchio, E.; Libro, G.; Delussi, M.; Casas-Barragàn, A.; de Tommaso, M. A simple pattern of movement is not able to inhibit experimental pain in fm patients and controls: An sloreta study. *Brain Sci.* **2020**, *10*, 190. [CrossRef]
45. Sullivan, M. *The Statistical Evaluation of Medical Tests for Classification and Prediction*; Oxford University Press: Oxford, UK, 2003.
46. Benbadis, S.R. A spell in the epilepsy clinic and a history of "chronic pain" or "fibromyalgia" independently predict a diagnosis of psychogenic seizures. *Epilepsy Behav.* **2005**, *6*, 264–265. [CrossRef]
47. Dixit, R.; Popescu, A.; Bagić, A.; Ghearing, G.; Hendrickson, R. Medical comorbidities in patients with psychogenic nonepileptic spells (PNES) referred for video-EEG monitoring. *Epilepsy Behav.* **2013**, *28*, 137–140. [CrossRef] [PubMed]
48. Rasker, J.J.; Wolfe, F.; Klaver-Krol, E.G.; Zwarts, M.J.; ten Klooster, P.M. The relation of fibromyalgia and fibromyalgia symptoms to self-reported seizures. *PLoS ONE* **2021**, *16*, e0246051. [CrossRef]
49. Kim, M.; Mawla, I.; Albrecht, D.S.; Admon, R.; Torrado-Carvajal, A.; Bergan, C.; Loggia, M.L. Striatal hypofunction as a neural correlate of mood alterations in chronic pain patients. *Neuroimage* **2020**, *211*, 116656. [CrossRef] [PubMed]
50. Lutz, J.; Jäger, L.; de Quervain, D.; Krauseneck, T.; Padberg, F.; Wichnalek, M.; Schelling, G. White and gray matter abnormalities in the brain of patients with fibromyalgia: A diffusion-tensor and volumetric imaging study. *Arthritis Rheum. J. Am. Coll. Rheumatol.* **2008**, *58*, 3960–3969. [CrossRef]
51. Kuchinad, A.; Schweinhardt, P.; Seminowicz, D.A.; Wood, P.B.; Chizh, B.A.; Bushnell, M.C. Accelerated brain gray matter loss in fibromyalgia patients: Premature aging of the brain? *J. Neurosci.* **2007**, *27*, 4004–4007. [CrossRef]
52. Murga, I.; Guillen, V.; Lafuente, J.V. Cambios en la resonancia magnética cerebral asociados al síndrome de fibromialgia. *Med. Clin.* **2017**, *148*, 511–516. [CrossRef] [PubMed]

53. Amzica, F.; Massimini, M. Glial and Neuronal Interactions during Slow Wave and Paroxysmal Activities in the Neocortex. *Cereb. Cortex.* **2002**, *12*, 1101–1113. [CrossRef]
54. González-Villar, A.J.; Triñanes, Y.; Gómez-Perretta, C.; Carrillo-de-la-Peña, M.T. Patients with fibromyalgia show increased beta connectivity across distant networks and microstates alterations in resting-state electroencephalogram. *Neuroimage* **2020**, *223*, 117266. [CrossRef] [PubMed]
55. Kooi, K.A.; Tucker, R.P.; Marshall, R.E. *Fundamentals of Electroencephalography*; HarperCollins Publishers: New York, NY, USA, 1978.
56. Puiu, T.; Kairys, A.E.; Pauer, L.; Schmidt-Wilcke, T.; Ichesco, E.; Hampson, J.P.; Harris, R.E. Association of Alterations in Gray Matter Volume With Reduced Evoked-Pain Connectivity Following Short-Term Administration of Pregabalin in Patients With Fibromyalgia. *Arthritis Rheumatol.* **2016**, *68*, 1511–1521. [CrossRef] [PubMed]
57. Lee, U.; Kim, M.; Lee, K.; Kaplan, C.M.; Clauw, D.J.; Kim, S.; Harris, R.E. Functional Brain Network Mechanism of Hypersensitivity in Chronic Pain. *Sci. Rep.* **2018**, *8*, 1–11. [CrossRef] [PubMed]
58. Fallon, N.; Chiu, Y.; Nurmikko, T.; Stancak, A. Functional Connectivity with the Default Mode Network Is Altered in Fibromyalgia Patients. *PLoS ONE* **2016**, *11*, e0159198. [CrossRef] [PubMed]
59. Fallon, N.; Chiu, Y.; Nurmikko, T.; Stancak, A. Altered theta oscillations in resting EEG of fibromyalgia syndrome patients. *Eur. J. Pain* **2018**, *22*, 49–57. [CrossRef]
60. van Ettinger-Veenstra, H.; Boehme, R.; Ghafouri, B.; Olausson, H.; Wicksell, R.K.; Gerdle, B. Exploration of Functional Connectivity Changes Previously Reported in Fibromyalgia and Their Relation to Psychological Distress and Pain Measures. *J. Clin. Med.* **2020**, *9*, 3560. [CrossRef]
61. Usui, C.; Kirino, E.; Tanaka, S.; Inami, R.; Nishioka, K.; Hatta, K.; Inoue, R. Music Intervention Reduces Persistent Fibromyalgia Pain and Alters Functional Connectivity Between the Insula and Default Mode Network. *Pain Med.* **2020**, *21*, 1546–1552. [CrossRef]
62. Flodin, P.; Martinsen, S.; Mannerkorpi, K.; Lofgren, M.; Bileviciute-Ljungar, I.; Kosek, E.; Fransson, P. Normalization of aberrant resting state functional connectivity in fibromyalgia patients following a three month physical exercise therapy. *NeuroImage Clin.* **2015**, *9*, 134–139. [CrossRef]
63. Pujol, J.; Macia, D.; Garcia-Fontanals, A.; Blanco-Hinojo, L.; Lopez-Sola, M.; Garcia-Blanco, S.; Deus, J. The contribution of sensory system functional connectivity reduction to clinical pain in fibromyalgia. *Pain* **2014**, *155*, 1492–1503. [CrossRef]
64. Jensen, K.B.; Loitoile, R.; Kosek, E.; Petzke, F.; Carville, S.; Fransson, P.; Kong, J. Patients with fibromyalgia display less functional connectivity in the brain's pain inhibitory network. *Mol. Pain* **2012**, *8*, 32. [CrossRef]
65. Ichesco, E.; Schmidt-Wilcke, T.; Bhavsar, R.; Clauw, D.J.; Peltier, S.J.; Kim, J.; Harris, R.E. Altered resting state connectivity of the insular cortex in individuals with fibromyalgia. *J. Pain* **2014**, *15*, 815–826.e1. [CrossRef]
66. Schmukler, J.; Jamal, S.; Castrejon, I.; Block, J.A.; Pincus, T. Fibromyalgia Assessment Screening Tools (FAST) Based on Only Multidimensional Health Assessment Questionnaire (MDHAQ) Scores as Clues to Fibromyalgia. *ACR Open Rheumatol.* **2019**, *1*, 516–525. [CrossRef] [PubMed]
67. Rosenfeld, V.W.; Rutledge, D.N.; Stern, J.M. Polysomnography with quantitative EEG in patients with and without fibromyalgia. *J. Clin. Neurophysiol.* **2015**, *32*, 164–170. [CrossRef] [PubMed]
68. Elmas, O.; Yildiz, S.; Bilgin, S.; Demirci, S.; Comlekci, S.; Koyuncuoglu, H.R.; Bilgin, G. Physiological parameters as a tool in the diagnosis of fibromyalgia syndrome in females: A preliminary study. *Life Sci.* **2016**, *15*, 51–56. [CrossRef]
69. Sundermann, B.; Burgmer, M.; Pogatzki-Zahn, E.; Gaubitz, M.; Stuber, C.; Wessolleck, E.; Pfleiderer, B. Diagnostic classification based on functional connectivity in chronic pain: Model optimization in fibromyalgia and rheumatoid arthritis. *Acad Radiol.* **2014**, *21*, 369–377. [CrossRef] [PubMed]
70. Johnstone, J.; Gunkelman, J. Use of Databases in QEEG Evaluation. *J. Neurother.* **2003**, *7*, 31–52. [CrossRef]
71. Obeid, I.; Picone, J. The Temple University Hospital EEG Data Corpus. *Front. Neurosci.* **2016**, *10*. [CrossRef] [PubMed]
72. White, J.N. Comparison of QEEG Reference Databases in Basic Signal Analysis and in the Evaluation of Adult ADHD. *J. Neurother.* **2003**, *7*, 123–169. [CrossRef]
73. Scheer, H.J.; Sander, T.; Trahms, L. The influence of amplifier, interface and biological noise on signal quality in high-resolution EEG recordings. *Physiol. Meas.* **2006**, *27*, 109–117. [CrossRef]
74. Thatcher, R.W.; Walker, R.A.; Biver, C.J.; North, D.N.; Curtin, R. Quantitative EEG Normative Databases: Validation and Clinical Correlation. *J. Neurother.* **2003**, *7*, 87–121. [CrossRef]
75. Chavez, M.; Grosselin, F.; Bussalb, A.; De Vico Fallani, F.; Navarro-Sune, X. Surrogate-Based Artifact Removal From Single-Channel EEG. *IEEE Trans. Neural Syst. Rehabil. Eng.* **2018**, *26*, 540–550. [CrossRef] [PubMed]
76. Barham, M.P.; Clark, G.M.; Hayden, M.J.; Enticott, P.G.; Conduit, R.; Lum, J.A.G. Acquiring research-grade ERPs on a shoestring budget: A comparison of a modified Emotiv and commercial SynAmps EEG system. *Psychophysiology* **2017**, *54*, 1393–1404. [CrossRef] [PubMed]
77. Ravan, M.; Begnaud, J. Investigating the Effect of Short Term Responsive VNS Therapy on Sleep Quality Using Automatic Sleep Staging. *IEEE Trans. Biomed. Eng.* **2019**, *66*, 3301–3309. [CrossRef]

78. Jadhav, P.N.; Shanamugan, D.; Chourasia, A.; Ghole, A.R.; Acharyya, A.; Naik, G. Automated detection and correction of eye blink and muscular artefacts in EEG signal for analysis of Autism Spectrum Disorder. In Proceedings of the 2014 36th Annual International Conference of the IEEE Engineering in Medicine and Biology Society, Chicago, IL, USA, 26–30 August 2014; pp. 1881–1884.
79. Piangerelli, M.; Rucco, M.; Tesei, L.; Merelli, E. Topological classifier for detecting the emergence of epileptic seizures. *BMC Res. Notes* **2018**, *11*, 392. [CrossRef] [PubMed]
80. Sharma, M.; Tiwari, J.; Acharya, U.R. Automatic Sleep-Stage Scoring in Healthy and Sleep Disorder Patients Using Optimal Wavelet Filter Bank Technique with EEG Signals. *Int. J. Environ. Res. Public Health* **2021**, *18*, 3087. [CrossRef]
81. Dimitriadis, S.I.; Salis, C.; Linden, D. A novel, fast and efficient single-sensor automatic sleep-stage classification based on complementary cross-frequency coupling estimates. *Clin. Neurophysiol.* **2018**, *129*, 815–828. [CrossRef] [PubMed]
82. Bigdely-Shamlo, N.; Touryan, J.; Ojeda, A.; Kothe, C.; Mullen, T.; Robbins, K. Automated EEG mega-analysis I: Spectral and amplitude characteristics across studies. *NeuroImage* **2020**, *15*, 116361. [CrossRef]
83. Hargrove, J.B.; Bennett, R.M.; Simons, D.G.; Smith, S.J.; Nagpal, S.; Deering, D.E. Quantitative Electroencephalographic Abnormalities in Fibromyalgia Patients. *Clin. EEG Neurosci.* **2010**, *41*, 132–139. [CrossRef] [PubMed]
84. Cifre, I.; Sitges, C.; Fraiman, D.; Muñoz, M.Á.; Balenzuela, P.; González-Roldán, A.; Montoya, P. Disrupted functional connectivity of the pain network in fibromyalgia. *Psychosom. Med.* **2012**, *74*, 55–62. [CrossRef] [PubMed]
85. Thatcher, R.; North, D.; Biver, C. Evaluation and Validity of a LORETA Normative EEG Database. *Clin. EEG Neurosci.* **2005**, *36*, 116–122. [CrossRef] [PubMed]
86. Keller, D.; de Gracia, M.; Cladellas, R. Subtypes of patients with fibromyalgia, psychopathological characteristics and quality of life. *Actas Esp Psiquiatr.* **2011**, *39*, 273–279. [PubMed]
87. Triñanes, Y.; González-Villar, A.; Gómez-Perretta, C.; Carrillo-de-la-Peña, M.T. Profiles in fibromyalgia: Algometry, auditory evoked potentials and clinical characterization of different subtypes. *Rheumatol. Int.* **2014**, *34*, 1571–1580. [CrossRef]
88. Thorp, S.; Healthcare, C.R.; Thorp, S.L.; Suchy, T.; Vadivelu, N.; Helander, E.M.; Kaye, A.D. Functional Connectivity Alterations: Novel Therapy and Future Implications in Chronic Pain Management. *Pain Physician* **2018**, *21*, 207–214. [CrossRef]

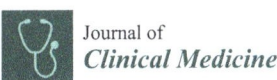

Article

Evaluating Routine Blood Tests According to Clinical Symptoms and Diagnostic Criteria in Individuals with Myalgic Encephalomyelitis/Chronic Fatigue Syndrome

Ingrid H. Baklund [1], Toril Dammen [1], Torbjørn Åge Moum [1], Wenche Kristiansen [2], Daysi Sosa Duarte [2], Jesus Castro-Marrero [3], Ingrid Bergliot Helland [4] and Elin Bolle Strand [4,5,*]

[1] Department of Behavioural Medicine, Faculty of Medicine, University of Oslo, 0315 Oslo, Norway; i.h.m.e.baklund@studmed.uio.no (I.H.B.); Toril.dammen@medisin.uio.no (T.D.); t.a.moum@medisin.uio.no (T.Å.M.)
[2] CFS/ME Center, Division of Medicine, Oslo University Hospital, 0318 Oslo, Norway; wenckr@ous-hf.no (W.K.); daysos@ous-hf.no (D.S.D.)
[3] CFS/ME Unit, Division of Rheumatology, Vall d'Hebron Research Institute, Universitat Autònoma de Barcelona, 08035 Barcelona, Spain; jesus.castro@vhir.org
[4] National Advisory Unit for CFS/ME, Rikshospitalet, Oslo University Hospital, Rikshospitalet OUS, 0372 Oslo, Norway; ihelland@ous-hf.no
[5] Faculty of Health, VID Specialized University, 0370 Oslo, Norway
* Correspondence: elin.bolle.strand@vid.no

Citation: Baklund, I.H.; Dammen, T.; Moum, T.Å.; Kristiansen, W.; Duarte, D.S.; Castro-Marrero, J.; Helland, I.B.; Strand, E.B. Evaluating Routine Blood Tests According to Clinical Symptoms and Diagnostic Criteria in Individuals with Myalgic Encephalomyelitis/Chronic Fatigue Syndrome. *J. Clin. Med.* **2021**, *10*, 3105. https://doi.org/10.3390/jcm10143105

Academic Editors: Giovanni Ricevuti and Lorenzo Lorusso

Received: 14 April 2021
Accepted: 9 July 2021
Published: 14 July 2021

Publisher's Note: MDPI stays neutral with regard to jurisdictional claims in published maps and institutional affiliations.

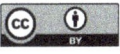

Copyright: © 2021 by the authors. Licensee MDPI, Basel, Switzerland. This article is an open access article distributed under the terms and conditions of the Creative Commons Attribution (CC BY) license (https://creativecommons.org/licenses/by/4.0/).

Abstract: There is a lack of research regarding blood tests within individuals with Myalgic Encephalomyelitis/Chronic Fatigue Syndrome (ME/CFS) and between patients and healthy controls. We aimed to compare results of routine blood tests between patients and healthy controls. Data from 149 patients diagnosed with ME/CFS based on clinical and psychiatric evaluation as well as on the DePaul Symptom Questionnaire, and data from 264 healthy controls recruited from blood donors were compared. One-way ANCOVA was conducted to examine differences between ME/CFS patients and healthy controls, adjusting for age and gender. Patients had higher sedimentation rate (mean difference: 1.38, 95% CI: 0.045 to 2.714), leukocytes (mean difference: 0.59, 95% CI: 0.248 to 0.932), lymphocytes (mean difference: 0.27, 95% CI: 0.145 to 0.395), neutrophils (mean difference: 0.34, 95% CI: 0.0 89 to 0.591), monocytes (mean difference: 0.34, 95% CI: 0.309 to 0.371), ferritin (mean difference: 28.13, 95% CI: −1.41 to 57.672), vitamin B12 (mean difference: 83.43, 95% CI: 62.89 to 124.211), calcium (mean difference: 0.02, 95% CI: −0.02 to 0.06), alanine transaminase (mean difference: 3.30, 95% CI: −1.37 to -7.971), low-density lipoproteins (mean difference: 0.45, 95% CI: 0.104 to 0.796), and total proteins (mean difference: 1.53, 95% CI: −0.945 to 4.005) than control subjects. The patients had lower potassium levels (mean difference: 0.11, 95% CI: 0.056 to 0.164), creatinine (mean difference: 2.60, 95% CI: 0.126 to 5.074) and creatine kinase (CK) (mean difference: 37.57, 95% CI: −0.282 to 75.422) compared to the healthy controls. Lower CK and creatinine levels may suggest muscle damage and metabolic abnormalities in ME/CFS patients.

Keywords: myalgic encephalomyelitis/chronic fatigue syndrome; routine blood tests; diagnostic criteria; functional status; creatinine; creatine kinase

1. Introduction

Myalgic encephalomyelitis, also known as chronic fatigue syndrome (ME/CFS) is a debilitating disease and common symptoms are post-exertional malaise (PEM), headaches, muscle- and joint pain, dyspnoea, nausea, and flu-like symptoms [1,2]. It is affecting all social and racial/ethnic groups, although possibly women more frequently than men [3,4]. The severity of the illness ranges, from ambulant to housebound [5]. A 2020 EUROMENE review found that prevalence ranged from 0.1–2.2% [6]. An American report from 2015, summarizing more than 9000 papers about illness, concluded that "ME/CFS is a serious, chronic, complex, and multisystem disease that frequently and dramatically limits the daily activities of affected patients" [7]. Twenty-five percent of patients become house- or bedbound at some point of their illness course [8].

The illness burden also involves a great personal and societal economic loss. ME/CFS is estimated to affect over 2.5 million across Europe. The condition often results in diminished functionality and increased economic impact. Despite high prevalence rates and disabling nature of the illness, few studies have examined the economic impact at the individual level and the societal cost across Europe [9].

Despite the severe nature of the disease, the pathophysiology is still largely unknown. No cure or specific treatment exists, nor are there any specific biomarkers [10,11].

Most studies on different haematological and biochemical tests reveal that in most cases, no difference is found between ME/CFS patients and healthy controls [11–30]. However, one study reported reduced creatine kinase (CK) levels and a higher sedimentation rate (SR) and thrombocytes in patients compared to normal controls [11]. Furthermore, an elevated neutrophil count has been reported [13,31], and elevated white blood cells [32], monocytes [32], ferritin [15], triglycerides [18,31], mean corpuscular hemoglobin concentration (MCV) [12], albumin [31], C-reactive protein (CRP) [11,33,34], thyroid stimulating hormone (TSH) [21,31], alkaline phosphatase (ALP) [32], antinuclear Antibodies IIF [32], and the complement factors C3 and C4 [35] have also been found in patients compared to controls. A reduced glucose [36], phosphate [31], iron and transferrin saturation [14], vitamin B9 [37], high-density lipoprotein-cholesterol (HDL-cholesterol) [15,18,31], and lower cortisol have also been reported [38–43]. Free T4 has been found to be both elevated [44] and reduced [15], which is also the case for immunoglobulin G (IgG subclass 1 and 2) [24,26,30,32,45,46]. IgG subclasses 3 and 4, however, were reduced [24,45–47], while Immunoglobulin M (IgM) and Immunoglobulin A (IgA) were found to be elevated [32]. Some of these studies have included routine blood tests, or the equivalent [11,13,17,18,32], with various routine test panels, whereas other studies have investigated more specific hypotheses with a limited number of specific blood tests tailored to the hypothesis or in order to exclude fatigue-related conditions.

Several different diagnostic criteria are in clinical use, ranging from the strict International Consensus Criteria (ICC) that capture a condition with more severe symptoms than the other criteria [1], the more lenient Canadian Consensus Criteria (CCC) [3], and the most liberal Fukuda definition [2]. Most patients that fulfil the CCC will also fulfil the Fukuda definition, but the patients fulfilling the CCC may have a higher frequency and severity of functional impairment and physical and cognitive symptoms than those fulfilling the Fukuda criteria [7]. The CCC, and in particular ICC, claim to achieve a more narrow selection of patients, conforming to a hypothesis-specific pathophysiology [48]. It is considered likely that all ME/CFS case definitions capture conditions with different or multifactorial pathogenesis [48], but to the best of our knowledge there is no previous study that has explored differences in blood tests according to various diagnostic criteria for ME/CFS.

Although guidelines for blood sample tests in the diagnostic assessments of ME/CFS do exist, research is sparse regarding how the results of these tests differ from those of healthy controls and across patient characteristics. To address this knowledge gap, we aim to (1) compare the results of routine blood samples from patients and healthy controls (blood volunteer donors); (2) explore the correlation between the blood tests results, illness severity and duration within the patient group; and (3) compare results of routine blood tests between those who fulfill the ICC [1] vs. those only fulfilling the CCC [3] and/or the Fukuda case definition [2].

2. Materials and Methods
2.1. Participants

In this prospective observational cohort study, a total of 149 ME/CFS patients were consecutively referred to a tertiary care center for evaluation (Oslo University Hospital,

Aker, Norway), and 264 healthy volunteer donors, between March 2013 and June 2019, were asked to participate in a thematic register and Biobank for research purposes. Patients had to fulfill the Canadian Consensus criteria (CCC) [3] as applied by a clinician, as well as the following inclusion criteria: aged 18–65 years old and able to understand and speak the Norwegian language. They were evaluated for eligibility and asked to participate during their second consultation by a physician.

From March 2013 to August 2015, 34 patients were included in the study. Unfortunately, relevant data for estimating a participation rate was not collected during this period. From August 2015 to 2019, a total of 288 patients were evaluated for study participation. Two-hundred-and thirteen were considered eligible for study participation at this time. One hundred and seventy-one (80%) agreed to participate, while 42 (20%) declined the request for participation. None were excluded because of age or language, but eight patients were excluded from the current dataset because they did not fulfill any ME/CFS criteria according to their DSQ responses. Of the 171 patients that consented to participation, 48 (28%) did not show up for further assessment and were thus excluded from the study. Most of them reported orally that they felt too ill or fatigued to attend. Thus, 115 patients were included during this period with an estimated participation rate of 40% (115/288). The number of included patients were 149 for the whole period from 2013–2019.

The patients gave a blood sample to the ME/CFS research Biobank and filled out questionnaires with information for the ME/CFS thematic research register. This included clinical and demographic information on patient history and treatment, epidemiology, work/social status, and occupation and DSQ.

The healthy control group consisted of 264 first-time blood volunteer donors at the blood bank at Oslo University Hospital. They were evaluated and no sign of any medical illness was found. They filled out similar questionnaires as the patients and were recruited and assessed during the same time period as the inclusion period for the ME/CFS patients. Both patients and controls were recruited from the area: south-eastern Norway (Helse Sør-Øst).

2.2. ME/CFS Assessment and Diagnosis

The Canadian Consensus Criteria (CCC) [3] as applied by clinicians were used as inclusion criteria. This was assessed during a clinical interview by physicians highly experienced in ME/CFS diagnostics and all patients obtained their diagnosis after a thorough evaluation in interdisciplinary expert groups. In order to exclude somatic and/or psychiatric conditions that could explain the symptoms, several blood tests were taken, and a clinical psychological interview covering diagnostic assessment was carried out.

2.3. Measures

The DePaul Symptom Questionnaire (DSQ) is a 99 items self-report symptom questionnaire originally developed in order to meet the need for more reliable diagnostic categorization of ME/CFS for research purposes [49]. The DSQ can classify patients according to three diagnostic criteria sets: the Fukuda, the CCC and the ICC criteria. For participation in the current study the patients had to fulfil at least one of the diagnostic criteria according to the DSQ, in addition to the Canadian Consensus criteria (CCC) used in the clinical interview. The DSQ assesses information on frequency, severity, onset and duration of symptoms and contains questions on self-reported functioning level classified as very severely or severely impaired, as moderately or as mild degree of impairment. The DSQ is developed from a CFS questionnaire with good inter-rater and test–retest reliability and able to distinguish between CFS, Major Depressive Disorders, and healthy controls [50]. The DSQ has acceptable convergent and discriminant validity [51], test–retest reliability [52], sound psychometric properties to correctly classify ME/CFS within the CCC [53], excellent internal reliability and is able to differentiate between patients and controls [54]. It was translated into Norwegian and retranslated by a professional translator, with permission from the developer (Prof. Leonard A. Jason, DePaul University, Chicago,

IL, USA), and reviewed by researchers and pre-tested in smaller groups of patients [53]. This version has been found useful for detecting and screening symptoms consistent with a CCC diagnosis showing a sensitivity of 98% and a specificity of 38% [53].

The questionnaires were completed by pen and paper at home before being delivered at the hospital at the appointment for blood sampling. To prevent missing data, a research nurse reviewed the questionnaires and the patients were requested to fill in missing data. Data were collected from the self-report questionnaire DSQ and blood tests. Questions from DSQ were applied for categorization of the patient groups that were included in the statistical analyses.

2.4. Patient Groupings: Functional Status, Illness Duration, and Diagnostic Criteria

Function status: The DSQ question 79 was used to categorize patients according to function impairment level (severe, moderate, and mild). The function level categorized as 'severe' was defined as responding positively to either "I am not able to work or do anything, and I am bedridden" or "I can walk around the house, but I cannot do light housework" whereas 'moderate' was defined as responding positively to "I can do light housework, but I cannot work part-time". The final three statements, "I can only work part-time at work or on some family responsibilities", "I can work full time and finish some family responsibilities but I have no energy left for anything else", and "I can do all work or family responsibilities without any problems with my energy" were all categorized as 'mild'. The 'severe' category comprised 43 patients (28.9%), the 'moderate' 75 patients (50.3%), while 31 patients (20.8%) were included in the 'mild' category.

Illness duration: Illness duration was assessed by the DSQ question 69 ("How long ago did your problem with fatigue/energy begin?") and categorized according to the following responses; 1–2 years (9.4%), >2 years (79.2%) and problems starting in childhood (11.4%).

Case criteria applied: The CCC were used as inclusion criteria when the patients initially were diagnosed by the clinicians. In the current study DSQ was applied for diagnostic classification based on different diagnostic criteria and this revealed that all the 149 patients fulfilled the Fukuda case definition, and 93.3% ($n = 139$) fulfilled the CCC, and 63.1% ($n = 94$) patients fulfilled the ICC criteria.

Case criteria groupings: Patients were divided into one of two following case criteria groups: "Non-ICC" that comprised those 55 patients (36.9%) who did not fulfill ICC, but only Fukuda and CCC whereas the "ICC" group consisted of the 94 patients (63.1%) fulfilling all three criteria included the ICC.

2.5. Blood Collection and Processing

Blood samples were collected by experienced nurse at the ME/CFS outpatient clinic in Oslo, or bedside for the most severely ill. The samples were delivered to the central laboratory at Aker Hospital within 30 min from collection and analyzed consecutively. Some serum samples were transported refrigerated to other hospitals for further processing. Standard OUS laboratory protocols were used for all collection, tests, and transport.

2.6. Ethics

All participants were informed about the purposes of the study and they signed a written informed consent form. The study and all data collection, including Biobank sampling and thematic register were approved by the Institutional Review Board at Oslo University Hospital (ref: 2011/8355) and the local Regional Committee for Medical and Health Research Ethics (REC) (REC 2011/473, and REC South-East, 2017/375).

2.7. Statistical Analysis

SPSS (SPSS Inc. Released 2009, PASW Statistics for Windows, Version 25.0. SPSS Inc., Chicago, IL, USA) was used for all statistical analyses. Descriptive statistics were conducted for demographics—i.e., age, gender, body mass index (BMI) and level of education. Analyses of covariance (ANCOVAs) were performed to estimate controlled mean differences between patients and controls for the various biological variables (treated as dependent variables). Gender and age showed significant associations with the patient-control dichotomy as well as with duration and level of functioning among patients and thus were routinely controlled for in the ANCOVAs (procedure UNIANOVA in SPSS) and in linear regressions.

Data plots were inspected for outliers and outliers or extreme values and—when present—these were routinely removed from all dependent variables, in concrete terms by eliminating scores more than three standard deviations above or below the overall mean. Such a trimming of extreme values on average reduced the number of subjects with valid scores by less than 1%. In addition, closer inspection revealed that p-values for the patient versus controls tests were hardly affected at all by the trimming of extreme scores. Mean differences between groups in continuous variables when tested by t-tests (as in the present paper) typically require normally distributed variables within groups, but there is considerable robustness to deviations from normality overall. Log-transformed versions of dependents were visually inspected and yielded almost identical p-values (for t-tests) and within-group means (also when adjusted by ANCOVAs) are reported using the untransformed metric. Units of measurement for the dependent variables are shown as means and standard deviations in all tables. For illustrative purposes confidence intervals (CI) have been added after controlled means for patients and controls in Table 2.

Effect sizes for dichotomous and trichotomous independents in Tables 2 and 3 are cited as "eta", i.e., the square of root of the variance explained by the groups comprising an independent, controlling for possible covariates. Effect sizes for linear trends in ordered trichotomous independents (function status, illness duration), are cited as standardized betas obtained by OLS. Levels of significance for effect sizes are cited as exact p-values (Table 2) and routinely categorized (Table 3).

3. Results

3.1. Study Population Characteristics

Demographic and clinical characteristics of the patients and controls are presented in Table 1. A significant difference in age ($p < 0.001$) and gender ($p = 0.02$) between patients and controls were found and therefore corrected for in ANOVAs. The patients were older and more likely to be female than controls. There was no significant difference in body mass index (BMI) between patients and controls ($p = 0.91$).

Table 1. Mean ± standard deviation, and T-tests conducted on demographic and clinical characteristics for ME/CFS patients and healthy controls.

Variables	ME/CFS Patients ($n = 149$)	Healthy Controls ($n = 264$)	p-Values (Patients vs. Controls)
Age (years) 28 missing	37.7±11.4	31.1±8.4	<0.001
Gender,			
Male n (%)	28 (19)	78 (30)	0.02
Female n (%)	121 (81)	186 (70)	
Education (years completed), 59 missing			
1–10 years (%)	16 (12)	2 (1)	<0.001
10–14 years (%)	52 (35)	59 (29)	
14–16 (%)	59 (40)	87 (42)	
>16 (%)	21 (13)	58 (27)	
BMI (kg/m^2) (26 missing)	24.5 (4.7)	24.5 (4.2)	0.91

3.2. Comparing Patients and Healthy Controls

A higher sedimentation rate (SR) ($p = 0.003$), leukocytes ($p < 0.001$), lymphocytes ($p < 0.001$), neutrophils ($p = 0.003$), monocytes ($p = 0.005$), ferritin ($p = 0.008$), vitamin B12 ($p < 0.001$), P-calcium $p = 0.005$), alanine aminotransferase (ALAT) ($p = 0.002$), alkaline phosphatase (ALP) ($p = 0.033$), low-density lipoprotein cholesterol (LDL-cholesterol) ($p = 0.001$), and free T4 (thyroxine) ($p < 0.001$) were found among patients compared to controls. Lower potassium ($p < 0.001$), creatinine ($p = 0.016$), and CK ($p < 0.001$) were found in patients than in controls. The results are shown in Table 2.

Table 2. Mean scores for routine blood tests in patients with ME/CFS and healthy controls.

Variables	ME/CFS Patients Mean ± SD (95% CI)	n	Healthy Controls Mean ± SD (95% CI)	n	Patients vs. Controls Mean Difference (95% CI)	Eta *	p-Values
Sedimentation rate (5.88/4.13)	6.28 ± 7.47 (5.558;7.0003)	123	4.90 ± 5.29 (4.274;5.525)	215	1.38 (0.045;2.714)	0.161	0.003
Hemoglobin (1.08/13.38)	13.85 ± 1.16 (13.704;13.997)	142	13.85 ± 1.02 (13.723;13.976)	228	0.001 (0.819;1.941)	0.001	0.99
Erythrocytes (4.50/0.42)	4.65 ± 0.43 (4.591;4.71)	142	4.66 ± 0.41 (4.605;4.707)	228	0.01 (1.291;1.469)	0.001	0.89
Hematocrit (0.40/0.03)	0.41 ± 2.81 (0.408;0.417)	141	0.41 ± 0.03 (0.41;0.418)	228	0 (−0.252;0.252)	0.031	0.50
MCHC (33.43/0.93)	33.65 ± 0.96 (33.48;33.81)	142	33.51 ± 0.91 (33.37;33.656)	228	0.14 (−1.765;2.045)	0.063	0.20
MCV (89.19/3.63)	88.85 ± 5.29 (88.219;89.481)	141	89.20 ± 4.72 (88.656;89.746)	227	0.35 (−1.799;2.499)	0.045	0.38
Thrombocytes (242.91/53.84)	241.82 ± 74.41 (232.16;251.487)	140	236.84 ± 50.99 (228.512;245.17)	228	4.98 (−9.153;19.113)	0.045	0.41
Leukocytes (5.42/1.46)	5.76 ± 1.74 (5.504;6.024)	139	5.17 ± 1.37 (4.946;5.393)	228	0.59 (0.248;0.932)	0.187	<0.001
Lymphocytes (1.91/0.59)	2.03 ± 0.65 (1.925;2.133)	142	1.76 ± 0.53 (1.672;1.852)	227	0.27 (0.145;0.395)	0.210	<0.001
Neutrophils (2.92/1.02)	3.11 ± 1.24 (2.928;3.292)	139	2.77 ± 1.06 (2.618;2.931)	226	0.34 (0.089;0.591)	0.105	0.003
Monocytes (0.42/0.13)	0.46 ± 0.16 (0.439;0.484)	140	0.42 ± 0.12 (0.401;0.4441)	226	0.39 (0.309;0.371)	0.148	0.005
Eosinophils (0.17/0.12)	0.18 ± 0.11 (0.154;0.199)	142	0.18 ± 0.11 (0.155;0.195)	228	0.04 (0.017;0.063)	0.001	0.912
Basophils (0.02/0.04)	0.03 ± 0.05 (0.023;0.038)	141	0.02 ± 0.13 (0.016;0.029)	227	0.002 (0.017;0.021)	0.110	0.072
hsCRP (2.50/2.48)	2.7 ± 4.61 (2.093;3.319)	87	2.10 ± 4.88 (1.551;2.629)	129	0.61 (−0.668;1.888)	0.110	0.112
TIBC (63.51/10.27)	60.57 ± 6.84 (56.799;64.332)	38	63.50 ± 9.91 (60.601;66.392)	64	2.93 (−1.43;7.29)	0.138	0.171
Ferritin (70.59/56.67)	110.45 ± 80.81 (91.389;129.509)	37	82.32 ± 54.33 (68.036;96.609)	64	28.13 (−1.41;−57.67)	0.265	0.009
Vitamin B12 (351.17/135.23)	409.7 ± 222.61 (385.366;434.060)	135	326.24 ± 113.6 (305.516;346.954)	229	83.43 (62.89;124.21)	0.281	<0.001
Vitamin B9 (19.19/7.72)	18.36 ± 9.53 (16.909;19.816)	131	18.72 ± 7.22 (17.486;19.949)	226	0.36 (−1.544;−2.264)	0.001	0.693
Sodium (104.15/1.85)	140.34 ± 2.13 (140.013;140.667)	144	140.28 ± 1.68 (139.999;140.566)	230	0.06 (−0.16;−0.27)	0.001	0.779
Potassium (3.82/0.22)	3.81 ± 0.26 (3.77;3.845)	143	3.92 ± 0.25 (3.884;3.949)	229	0.11 (0.056;0.164)	0.235	<0.001
P-calcium (2.30/0.075)	2.3 ± 0.08 (2.307;2.33)	143	2.30 ± 0.25 (2.286;2.308)	230	0.02 (−0.02;0.06)	0.145	0.005
S-calcium (1.22/0.034)	1.22 ± 0.03 (1.217;1.229)	143	1.22 ± 0.08 (1.212;1.223)	228	0 (−0.02;−0.06)	0.077	0.138
Phosphate (1.03/0.17)	1.03 ± 0.17 (1.002;1.061)	144	1.01 ± 0.17 (0.984;1.035)	230	0.02 (0;0.038)	0.020	0.240

Table 2. Cont.

Variables	ME/CFS Patients Mean ± SD (95% CI)	n	Healthy Controls Mean ± SD (95% CI)	n	Patients vs. Controls Mean Difference (95% CI)	Eta *	p-Values
ASAT (21.63/5.68)	22.03 ± 15.3 (21.044;23.008)	142	22.79 ± 8.64 (21.944;23.643)	227	0.76 (−2.035;3.545)	0.063	0.211
ALAT (19.32/9.77)	23.24 ± 26.06 (21.511;24.960)	142	19.94 ± 13.35 (19.444;21.426)	228	3.3 (−1.37;7.971)	0.158	0.002
CK (94.06/66.91)	84.33 ± 34.43 (73.708;95.061)	144	121.90 ± 282.88 (112.559;131.231)	224	37.57 (0.282;75.422)	0.281	<0.001
Creatinine (68.46/11.03)	70.16 ± 11.59 (68.435;71.886)	143	72.76 ± 11.88 (71.263;74.259)	227	2.6 (0.126;5.074)	0.126	0.016
HDL-cholesterol (1.54/0.38)	1.37 ± 0.4 (1.227;1.502)	38	1.50 ± 0.4 (1.395;1.608)	63	0.13 (−0.303;0.043)	0.176	0.082
LDL-cholesterol (2.77/0.42)	3.16 ± 0.88 (2.921;3.393)	37	2.71 ± 0.7 (2.530;2.894)	63	0.45 (0.104;0.796)	0.324	0.001
Triglycerides (1.03/0.53)	1.29 ± 1.44 (1.096;1.474)	36	1.10 ± 0.43 (0.953;1.247)	63	0.19 (−0.312;0.692)	0.176	0.084
Albumin (43.38/2.56)	43.91 ± 2.95 (43.055;44.757)	38	44.23 ± 2.25 (43.577;44.885)	64	0.32 (2.154;2.795)	0.071	0.500
Total protein (70.80/3.51)	72.53 ± 3.6 (71.277;73.784)	38	71.00 ± 8.57 (70.032;71.962)	63	1.53 (−0.945;4.005)	0.214	0.033
TSH (1.92/0.94)	1.93 ± 0.98 (1.756;2.101)	143	1.89 ± 1.34 (1.739;2.040)	220	0.04 (−0.081;0.279)	0.001	0.721
IgG4 (0.49/0.45)	0.64 ± 0.38 (0.471;0.809)	36	0.54 ± 0.29 (0.413;0.669)	62	0.1 (−0.082;0.282)	0.110	0.296
IgA (2.03/0.77)	2.22 ± 0.82 (1.929;2.515)	37	2.13 ± 0.96 (1.903;2.348)	62	0.1 (−0.182;0.475)	0.063	0.559
IgM (1.08/0.41)	1.06 ± 0.62 (0.904;1.218)	35	0.96 ± 0.47 (0.841;1.074)	62	0.1 (−0.142;0.342)	0.122	0.241
Rheumatoid factor IgA (2.55/2.68)	2.89 ± 12.99 (2.412;3.368)	133	2.61 ± 0.96 (2.205;3.017)	221	0.28 (−2.021;2.305)	0.055	0.348
Rheumatoid factor IgM (5.51/4.74)	6.02 ± 13.87 (5.155;6.883)	137	5.26 ± 4.73 (4.521;5.996)	227	0.76 (−1.743;3.263)	0.077	0.156
Anti-CCP (0.85/0.77)	0.94 ± 0.48 (0.641;1.239)	37	0.88 ± 0.6 (0.655;1.104)	63	0.06 (−0.159;0.279)	0.032	0.717

* Values are presented as means ± standard deviation (SD) including confidence interval (95% CI) controlled for gender and age differences by ANCOVA. Effect sizes (Eta) by OLS.

3.3. Comparing Subgroups of Patients between Blood Tests, Clinical Characteristics, and Case Criteria for ME/CFS

Comparing blood results across function impairment status among patients revealed a significant difference in potassium levels ($p = 0.048$), CK ($p < 0.001$) and creatinine ($p = 0.018$), all variables increasing with decreasing function level while ASAT ($p = 0.042$) and ALAT ($p = 0.023$) decreased with more severely impaired function level. Longer illness duration was only significantly associated with potassium levels ($p = 0.007$) that decreased with longer duration. The only difference between different diagnostic criteria was a higher creatinine ($p = 0.015$) among the "non-ICC" group. The results are shown in Table 3.

Table 3. Comparison of baseline mean scores for routine blood tests among ME/CFS patients based on functional status assessment, illness duration, and case criteria for ME/CFS among participants.

Variables (Mean ± SD)	Function Status				Illness Duration				Case Criteria		
	Severe (n = 43)	Moderate (n = 75)	Mild (n = 31)	Beta Eta	1–2 Years (n = 14)	>2 Years (n = 118)	Since Childhood (n = 17)	Beta Eta	Non-ICC (n = 55)	ICC (n = 94)	Beta
Sedimentation rate (7.24 ± 4.46)	6.09	5.88	6.38	0.017 0.045 (ns)	6.70	6.30	3.92	−0.129 0.184 (ns)	5.86	6.16	0.039 (ns)
Hemoglobin (13.3 ± 1.17)	13.85	13.89	14.00	0.043 0.055 (ns)	13.58	13.91	14.09	0.085 0.13 (ns)	13.90	13.91	−0.002 (ns)
Erythrocytes (4.46 ± 0.43)	4.65	4.63	4.70	0.042 0.084 (ns)	4.56	4.65	4.67	0.037 0.077 (ns)	4.65	4.64	−0.011 (ns)
Hematocrit (0.40 ± 0.034)	0.41	0.41	0.42	0.059 0.089 (ns)	0.40	0.41	0.42	0.076 0.015 (ns)	0.41	0.41	0.029 (ns)
MCHC (33.45 ± 0.96)	33.65	33.77	33.54	−0.035 0.10 (ns)	33.81	33.67	33.76	0.009 0.055 (ns)	33.80	33.61	−0.088 (ns)
MCV (89.47 ± 3.41)	88.90	89.09	89.40	0.050 0.055 (ns)	88.44	89.11	89.58	0.078 0.077 (ns)	88.74	89.41	0.098 (ns)
Thrombocytes (242.45 ± 58.26)	248.99	244.11	238.64	−0.057 0.063 (ns)	230.13	245.27	247.14	0.048 0.077 (ns)	238.38	248.60	0.08 (ns)
Leukocytes (5.87 ± 1.55)	5.78	5.75	5.52	−0.055 0.063 (ns)	5.27	5.79	5.56	0.022 0.10 (ns)	5.62	5.78	0.043 (ns)
Lymphocytes (2.05 ± 0.66)	2.09	1.98	1.99	−0.058 0.071 (ns)	1.72	2.05	1.98	0.081 0.14 (ns)	1.99	2.02	0.027 (ns)
Neutrophils (3.20 ± 1.11)	3.02	3.15	2.87	−0.034 0.10 (ns)	2.89	3.11	2.86	−0.035 0.089 (ns)	3.02	3.09	0.023 (ns)
Monocytes (0.45 ± 0.15)	0.47	0.45	0.44	−0.052 0.063 (ns)	0.41	0.46	0.45	0.042 0.089 (ns)	0.43	0.47	0.14 (ns)
Eosinophils (0.17 ± 0.11)	0.18	0.18	0.18	−0.021 0.032 (ns)	0.21	0.17	0.20	−0.024 0.122 (ns)	0.19	0.17	−0.10 (ns)
Basophils (0.029 ± 0.045)	0.034	0.032	0.029	−0.041 0.044 (ns)	0.028	0.033	0.031	0.004 0.032 (ns)	0.028	0.035	0.071 (ns)
hsCRP (1.39 ± 1.86)	0.82	1.15	1.62	0.15 0.15 (ns)	1.05	1.27	0.67	−0.045 0.11 (ns)	1.33	1.032	−0.076 (ns)
Vitamin-B12 (407.74 ± 163)	440.31	386.16	415.44	−0.058 0.14 (ns)	428.75	405.09	382.37	−0.074 0.063 (ns)	406.79	402.31	−0.021 (ns)
Vitamin-B9 (19.21 ± 8.89)	20.72	16.94	18.55	−0.10 0.18 (ns)	19.23	18.53	15.54	−0.12 0.12 (ns)	18.89	7.64	−0.070 (ns)
Sodium (140.03 ± 2.13)	104.20	140.70	139.95	−0.025 0.15 (ns)	140.99	140.49	139.63	−0.13 0.15 (ns)	140.66	140.23	−0.093 (ns)
Potassium (3.77 ± 0.24)	3.76	3.82	3.87	0.16 * 0.17	4.01	3.80	3.77	−0.21 ** 0.27 **	3.82	3.81	−0.019 (ns)
P-calcium (2.30 ± 0.075)	2.33	2.32	2.32	−0.087 0.11 (ns)	2.35	2.32	2.30	−0.14 0.16 (ns)	2.33	2.31	−0.12 (ns)
S-calcium (1.22 ± 0.034)	1.23	1.22	1.22	−0.060 0.063 (ns)	1.23	1.22	1.23	0.046 0.11 (ns)	1.22	1.23	0.076 (ns)
Phosphate (1.03 ± 0.17)	1.042	1.022	1.021	−0.046 0.055 (ns)	1.078	1.019	1.034	−0.024 0.095 (ns)	1.019	1.033	0.048 (ns)
ASAT (20.92 ± 5.24)	23.092	22.13	20.51	−0.17 * 0.17	22.11	22.24	20.67	−0.068 0.095 (ns)	21.61	22.31	0.065 (ns)
ALAT (21.063 ± 11.67)	26.83	23.031	20.58	−0.19 * 0.20	21.93	24.17	20.26	−0.067 0.12 (ns)	22.53	25.097	0.056 (ns)
CK (67.66 ± 34.50)	64.85	87.091	88.34	0.25 *** 0.34 ***	68.41	82.55	88.032	0.11 0.15 (ns)	87.32	77.75	−0.14 (ns)
Creatinine (65.79 ± 10.75)	68.089	70.81	73.38	0.17 * 0.2	65.53	71.34	71.14	0.097 * 0.18	72.90	68.99	−0.18 *
TSH (1.94 ± 0.98)	1.82	1.99	2.16	0.12 0.12 (ns)	1.66	2.040	1.87	0.041 0.12 (ns)	2.034	1.94	−0.043 (ns)

Table 3. Cont.

Variables (Mean ± SD)	Function Status				Illness Duration				Case Criteria		
	Severe (n = 43)	Moderate (n = 75)	Mild (n = 31)	Beta Eta	1–2 Years (n = 14)	>2 Years (n = 118)	Since Childhood (n = 17)	Beta Eta	Non-ICC (n = 55)	ICC (n = 94)	Beta
Rheumatoid factor-IgA (2.76 ± 2.64)	2.55	2.95	2.41	−0.0090 0.089 (ns)	2.94	2.58	3.63	0.063 0.12 (ns)	3.24	2.42	−0.15 (ns)
Rheumatoid factor-IgM (6.12 ± 4.56)	6.12	5.47	6.62	0.028 0.1 (ns)	5.98	5.79	6.095	0.016 0 (ns)	6.47	5.42	−0.11 (ns)

Means and t-tests controlled for age, gender, and BMI among the participants. Values are presented as mean ± SD. A significance threshold was set at * $p < 0.05$, ** $p < 0.01$, and *** $p < 0.001$.

4. Discussion

Our main findings include a lower creatin kinase (±CK) value in routine blood samples among patients than among controls, and lower in those with severe function impairment ME/CFS compared to moderate and mild function impairment. This is in line with the results by Nacul et al. [11]. No differences in blood results were found when comparing categories of illness duration, which could have potentially explained these CK result, because inactivity is known to cause muscle loss and therefore could potentially have influenced the CK level. CK is an enzyme important for energy production, especially in tissues with high and fluctuating energy demands, such as the brain, skeletal muscle, and heart. One of the functions is to maintain constant levels of ATP, acting as a transport mechanism [55]. Measures of CK in the blood might indicate the availability of cellular energy [56]. While an elevated CK is more thoroughly studied, a low CK has been reported less frequently [11], but might be associated with muscle weakness in rheumatoid arthritis [57]. In studies of Huntington's disease, it has been suggested that the loss of CK in the brain may be an important factor for reduced brain energy [11]. As Nacul et al. have suggested, the low concentration in CK among ME/CFS patients, could reflect abnormalities in energy metabolism, which could explain the exertion intolerances that are often reported by patients. Alternatively, it could result from physical inactivity [11]. Our results may indicate that CK could be a possible candidate as a potential marker for ME/CFS. However, the level was within the reference range and there are many factors that can influence CK to be used as a biomarker. It should also be emphasized that CK measured in plasma represents CK from skeletal muscles. Thus, the role of CK in ME/CFS patients should be further explored in future studies.

The creatinine level was also significantly lower among patients than controls and related to severity of impairment with lower levels in those with more severe impairment. This is also found by Nacul et al. that suggested a possible explanation of a low creatinine being the result of poor conversion of creatinine phosphate to creatinine in muscle by CK that could explain the low levels of creatinine [11]. The creatinine level was also lower among the ICC group those fulfilling all case criteria including the most stringent ICC-criteria compared to the non-ICC group those fulfilling only Fukuda definition and CCC, similarly to what we see comparing patients to healthy controls. In the absence of a similar correlation for CK, this difference in diagnosis is harder to explain by such a mechanism.

We also found results somewhat in line with a potentially increased inflammation, with sedimentation rate, leukocytes, lymphocytes, monocytes, and ferritin being higher among patients. The difference, although being highly significant, is small throughout and within the normal range—i.e., 0.53-point difference for leukocytes—and might not be clinically relevant. These findings are similar to those of previous studies, e.g., Bates et al. [32] and may possibly support the idea of a low-grade inflammation in ME/CFS patients. Furthermore, other inflammation parameters, such as CRP, were not significantly different between groups.

Vitamin B12 was higher among patients than controls, but among patients there was no correlation with severity, duration or diagnostic criteria. A possible explanation for this may be that ME/CFS patients frequently take dietary supplements [19]. Unfortunately, we did not register intake of dietary supplements and/or concomitant medications and thus lack such data. It has been suggested that a B12 supplement could be beneficial for ME/CFS patients [58].

An unfavorable lipid profile has been described among ME/CFS patients [18]. We discovered an increase in low density lipoproteins-cholesterol (LDL-cholesterol). However, these values are still within normal ranges.

Other results that are more difficult to explain are moderately lower potassium among patients, which decreased with severity and illness duration, and increased calcium and protein. ALAT was also higher among patients, and both ALAT and ASAT increased with severity. The differences are small, however, and may not be clinically significant, although statistically so. No comparable research that could explain these differences with any certainty is known to the authors. Furthermore, we conducted a large number of analyses and thus some of our results may have occurred by random (we did not apply Bonferroni tests).

Strengths and Limitations

The patients were older and more likely to be female than the controls, but this was controlled for in the statistical analyses. Female gender is more common in the ME/CFS population, and this is therefore representative for this population. There was also a difference in level of education between patients and controls, but education was not related to any of the dependent variables and thus not corrected for. We did not collect information about potential differences in muscle mass and physical activity from study participants. This could potentially be relevant for the observed difference in circulating CK and creatinine levels in study patients. A significant difference in BMI was not found. BMI is not an indicator of body composition.

We did not include patients younger than 18 or older than 65 years or those using another language than Norwegian. Generalization to recent immigration groups and other age groups, for example, should therefore be made with caution.

Furthermore, Aker Hospital is a tertiary care center to which patients with complex symptoms, co-morbid somatic or psychiatric conditions and patients who are difficult to manage in routine clinical contexts are mostly referred. Therefore, generalizing to ME/CFS patients as a group should be done with caution. The interdisciplinary diagnostic evaluation procedures were extensive however, so we regard it as most/extremely likely that our patients are correctly diagnosed, and this is a strength of this study. Other strengths are a relatively high number of ME/CFS patients and healthy donors, and a large variety of variables.

Our participation rate is estimated to be around 40%, but we unfortunately lack data allowing us to compare participants with non-participants (e.g., with respect to demographic and clinical characteristics). We are aware that many listed patients are feeling too ill/fatigued to participate, and this could imply that we have a selection bias against those who are most severely affected. On the other hand, ME/CFS is characterized by symptom fluctuations and it may also have been the case that those who eventually could not participate as agreed in the data collection experienced a bad period with a transient symptom increase without necessarily having a permanently low level of function. In this regard, around 28% of the patients are in the group with the lowest level of function. This is about what we find it in the general ME/CFS population [8].

5. Conclusions

Results of several routine blood tests of ME/CFS patients differed from those healthy controls. Our findings particularly highlight that decreased creatinine and CK levels may indicate greater muscle damage and metabolic disturbances in ME/CFS patients and is worthy of future studies. This is also true of results that may indicate a possible low-grade inflammation in ME/CFS patients.

Author Contributions: All authors were involved in planning and design of the study. E.B.S., W.K. and D.S.D. were responsible for data collection. T.Å.M., I.H.B., T.D. and E.B.S. were responsible for data analysis and writing of the paper. All authors were involved in interpretation of results, drafting, and revising of the manuscript. All authors have read and agreed to the published version of the manuscript.

Funding: This research did not receive any specific grant from funding agencies in the public, commercial, or not-for-profit sectors.

Institutional Review Board Statement: The study was conducted according to the guidelines of the Declaration of Helsinki, and approved by the IRB of Oslo University Hospital (reference number: 2011/8355) and the local Regional Committee for Medical and Health Research Ethics Committee (REC 2011/473 and REC 2017/375).

Informed Consent Statement: All participants in this study received information about the study and gave their consent to attend.

Data Availability Statement: Data and material are available from the corresponding author.

Acknowledgments: We want to thank research nurse Hilde Haukeland from the CFS/ME thematic register/Biobank for her contribution in the data sampling of this project and the participants who provided us with valuable data.

Conflicts of Interest: The authors declare that there is no conflict of interest.

Abbreviations

CFS	Chronic fatigue syndrome
ME	Myalgic encephalomyelitis
ICC	The International Consensus Criteria for ME/CFS
CCC	Canadian Consensus Criteria
CK	Creatine kinase
ESR	Erythrocyte sedimentation rate
DSQ	DePaul Symptom Questionnaires
OUS	Oslo Universitetssykehus (Oslo University Hospital)
BMI	Body mass index
MCHC	Mean corpuscular hemoglobin concentration
MCV	Mean corpuscular volume
hsCRP	High-sensitivity C-reactive protein
TIBC	Total iron binding capacity
ALAT	Alanine transaminase
ASAT	Aspartate aminotransferase
GGT/GT	Gamma-glutamyl transferase
GFR	Glomerular filtration rate
TSH	Thyroid stimulating hormone
HCY	Homocysteine
IgG	Immunoglobulin G
IgG1	Immunoglobulin G subclass 1
IgG2	Immunoglobulin G subclass 2
IgG3	Immunoglobulin G subclass 3
IgG4	Immunoglobulin G subclass 4
IgA	Immunoglobulin A
IgM	Immunoglobulin M
RF	Rheumatoid Factor
Anti-CCP	Anti-cyclic citrullinated peptide
TTGA	Tissue transglutaminase antibody
ALP	Alkaline phosphatase
LDL	Low-density lipoprotein
HDL	High-density lipoprotein
ATP	Adenosine triphosphate
ANCOVA	Analysis of covariance

References

1. Carruthers, B.M.; Van De Sande, M.I.; De Meirleir, K.L.; Klimas, N.G.; Broderick, G.; Mitchell, T.; Staines, D.; Powles, A.C.P.; Speight, N.; Vallings, R.; et al. Myalgic encephalomyelitis: International consensus criteria. *J. Intern. Med.* **2011**, *270*, 327–338. [CrossRef]
2. Fukuda, K. The chronic fatigue syndrome: A comprehensive approach to its definition and study. *Ann. Intern. Med.* **1994**, *121*, 953. [CrossRef]
3. Carruthers, B.M.; Jain, A.K.; De Meirleir, K.L.; Peterson, D.L.; Klimas, N.G.; Lerner, A.M.; Bested, A.C.; Henry, P.F.; Joshi, P.; Powles, A.C.P.; et al. Myalgic encephalomyelitis/chronic fatigue syndrome. *J. Chronic Fatigue Syndr.* **2003**, *11*, 7–115. [CrossRef]
4. Jason, L.A.; Richman, J.A.; Rademaker, A.W.; Jordan, K.M.; Plioplys, A.V.; Taylor, R.R.; McCready, W.; Huang, C.-F.; Plioplys, S. A community-based study of chronic fatigue syndrome. *Arch. Intern. Med.* **1999**, *159*, 2129–2137. [CrossRef]
5. Pendergrast, T.; Brown, A.; Sunnquist, M.; Jantke, R.; Newton, J.L.; Strand, E.B.; Jason, L.A. Housebound versus non-housebound patients with myalgic encephalomyelitis and chronic fatigue syndrome. *Chronic Illn.* **2016**, *12*, 292–307. [CrossRef] [PubMed]
6. Estévez-López, F.; Mudie, K.; Wang-Steverding, X.; Bakken, I.J.; Ivanovs, A.; Castro-Marrero, J.; Nacul, L.; Alegre, J.; Zalewski, P.; Slomko, J.; et al. Systematic review of the epidemiological burden of myalgic encephalomyelitis/chronic fatigue syndrome across europe: Current evidence and EUROMENE research recommendations for epidemiology. *J. Clin. Med.* **2020**, *9*, 1557. [CrossRef] [PubMed]
7. Committee on the Diagnostic Criteria for Myalgic Encephalomyelitis/Chronic Fatigue S, Board on the Health of Select P, Institute of M. *The National Academies Collection: Reports funded by National Institutes of Health. Beyond Myalgic Encephalomyelitis/Chronic Fatigue Syndrome: Redefining an Illness*; Copyright 2015 by the National Academy of Sciences. All rights reserved; National Academies Press: Washington, DC, USA, 2015.
8. Marshall, R.; Paul, L.; Wood, L. The search for pain relief in people with chronic fatigue syndrome: A descriptive study. *Physiother. Theory Pract.* **2011**, *27*, 373–383. [CrossRef] [PubMed]
9. Pheby, D.F.H.; Araja, D.; Berkis, U.; Brenna, B.; Cullinan, J.; De Korwin, J.D.; Gitto, L.; Hughes, D.A.; Hunter, R.M.; Trepel, D.; et al. The development of a consistent Europe-wide approach to investigating the economic impact of ME/CFS: A report from the EUROMENE. *Healthcare* **2020**, *8*, 88. [CrossRef]
10. Smith, M.E.; Haney, E.; McDonagh, M.; Pappas, M.; Daeges, M.; Wasson, N.; Fu, R.; Nelson, H.D. Treatment of myalgic encephalomyelitis/chronic fatigue syndrome: A systematic review for a national institutes of health pathways to prevention workshop. *Ann. Intern. Med.* **2015**, *162*, 841–850. [CrossRef]
11. Nacul, L.D.B.; Kingdon, C.; Clark, M.; De Baros, B.; Cliff, J.M.; Mudie, K.; Dockrell, H.M.; Laceda, E.M. Evidence of clinical pathology abnormalities in people with myalgic encephalomyelitis/chronic fatigue syndrome (me/cfs) from an analytic cross-sectional study. *Diagnostics* **2019**, *9*, 41. [CrossRef]
12. Richards, R.S.; Roberts, T.K.; McGregor, N.R.; Dunstan, R.H.; Butt, H.L. Blood parameters indicative of oxidative stress are associated with symptom expression in chronic fatigue syndrome. *Redox Rep.* **2000**, *5*, 35–41. [CrossRef]
13. Niblett, S.H.; King, K.E.; Dunstan, R.H.; Clifton-Bligh, P.; Hoskin, L.A.; Roberts, T.K.; Fulchert, G.R.; Mcgregor, N.R.; Dunsmore, J.C.; Butt, H.L. Hematologic and urinary excretion anomalies in patients with chronic fatigue syndrome. *Exp. Biol. Med.* **2007**, *232*, 1041–1049. [CrossRef]
14. Van Rensburg, S.J.; Potocnik, F.C.V.; Kiss, T.; Hugo, F.; Van Zijl, P.; Mansvelt, E.; Carstens, M.E.; TheodoroU, P.; Huely, P.R.; Emsley, R.A. Serum concentrations of some metals and steroids in patients with chronic fatigue syndrome with reference to neurological and cognitive abnormalities. *Brain Res. Bull.* **2001**, *55*, 319–325. [CrossRef]
15. Ruiz-Núñez, B.; Tarasse, R.; Vogelaar, E.F.; Janneke Dijck-Brouwer, D.A.; Muskiet, F.A.J. Higher Prevalence of "Low T3 Syndrome" in patients with chronic fatigue syndrome: A case–control study. *Front. Endocrinol.* **2018**, *9*, 97. [CrossRef] [PubMed]
16. Mawle, A.C.; Nisenbaum, R.; Dobbins, J.G.; Gary, H.E.; Stewart, J.A.; Reyes, M.; Steele, L.; Schmid, D.S.; Reeves, W.C. Immune responses associated with chronic fatigue syndrome: A case-control study. *J. Infect. Dis.* **1997**, *175*, 136–141. [CrossRef] [PubMed]
17. Swanink, C.M.A.; Vercoulen, J.H.M.M.; Bleijenberg, G.; Fennis, J.F.M.; Galama, J.M.D.; Meer, J.W.M. Chronic fatigue syndrome: A clinical and laboratory study with a well matched control group. *J. Intern. Med.* **1995**, *237*, 499–506. [CrossRef] [PubMed]
18. Tomic, S.; Brkic, S.; Maric, D.; Mikic, A.N. Lipid and protein oxidation in female patients with chronic fatigue syndrome. *Arch. Med. Sci.* **2012**, *5*, 886–891. [CrossRef]
19. Grant, J.E.; Veldee, M.S.; Buchwald, D. Analysis of dietary intake and selected nutrient concentrations in patients with chronic fatigue syndrome. *J. Am. Diet. Assoc.* **1996**, *96*, 383–386. [CrossRef]
20. Smirnova, I.V.; Pall, M.L. Elevated levels of protein carbonyls in sera of chronic fatigue syndrome patients. *Mol. Cell Biochem.* **2003**, *248*, 93–95. [CrossRef]
21. Moorkens, G.; Berwaerts, J.; Wynants, H.; Abs, R. Characterization of pituitary function with emphasis on GH secretion in the chronic fatigue syndrome. *Clin. Endocrinol.* **2000**, *53*, 99–106. [CrossRef]
22. Ottenweller, J.E.; Sisto, S.A.; McCarty, R.C.; Natelson, B.H. Hormonal responses to exercise in chronic fatigue syndrome. *Neuropsychobiology* **2001**, *43*, 34–41. [CrossRef] [PubMed]
23. Gupta, S.; Vayuvegula, B. A comprehensive immunological analysis in chronic fatigue syndrome. *Scand. J. Immunol.* **1991**, *33*, 319–327. [CrossRef]
24. Natelson, B.H.; LaManca, J.J.; Denny, T.N.; Vladutiu, A.; Oleske, J.; Hill, N.; Bergen, M.T.; Korn, L.; Hay, J. Immunologic parameters in chronic fatigue syndrome, major depression, and multiple sclerosis. *Am. J. Med.* **1998**, *105*, 43s–49s. [CrossRef]

25. Milton, J.D.; Clements, G.B.; Edwards, R.H. Immune responsiveness in chronic fatigue syndrome. *Postgrad Med. J.* **1991**, *67*, 532–537. [CrossRef] [PubMed]
26. Bennett, A.L.; Fagioli, L.R.; Schur, P.H.; Schacterle, R.S.; Komaroff, A.L. Immunoglobulin subclass levels in chronic fatigue syndrome. *J. Clin. Immunol.* **1996**, *16*, 315–320. [CrossRef]
27. Skowera, A.; Stewart, E.; Davis, E.T.; Cleare, A.J.; Unwin, C.; Hull, L.; Ismail, K.; Hossain, G.; Wessely, S.C.; Peakman, M. Antinuclear autoantibodies (±ANA) in Gulf War-related illness and chronic fatigue syndrome (±CFS) patients. *Clin. Exp. Immunol.* **2002**, *129*, 354–358. [CrossRef] [PubMed]
28. Rahman, K.; Burton, A.; Galbraith, S.; Lloyd, A.; Vollmer-Conna, U. Sleep-wake behavior in chronic fatigue syndrome. *Sleep* **2011**, *34*, 671–678. [CrossRef]
29. Wood, B.; Wessely, S.; Papadopoulos, A.; Poon, L.; Checkley, S. Salivary cortisol profiles in chronic fatigue syndrome. *Neuropsychobiology* **1998**, *37*, 1–4. [CrossRef]
30. Lloyd, A.R.; Wakefield, D.; Boughton, C.R.; Dwyer, J.M. Immunological abnormalities in the chronic fatigue syndrome. *Med. J. Aust.* **1989**, *151*, 122–124. [CrossRef] [PubMed]
31. De Lorenzo, F. Chronic fatigue syndrome: Physical and cardiovascular deconditioning. *QJM* **1998**, *91*, 475–481. [CrossRef] [PubMed]
32. Bates, D.W.; Buchwald, D.; Lee, J.; Kith, P.; Doolittle, T.; Rutherford, C.; Churchill, W.H.; Scher, P.H.; Wenert, M.; Wybenga, D. Clinical laboratory test findings in patients with chronic fatigue syndrome. *Arch. Intern. Med.* **1995**, *155*, 97–103. [CrossRef]
33. Groven, N.; Fors, E.A.; Reitan, S.K. Patients with Fibromyalgia and Chronic Fatigue Syndrome show increased hsCRP compared to healthy controls. *Brain Behav. Immun.* **2019**, *81*, 172–177. [CrossRef] [PubMed]
34. Strawbridge, R.; Sartor, M.L.; Scott, F.; Cleare, A.J. Inflammatory proteins are altered in chronic fatigue syndrome-A systematic review and meta-analysis. *Neurosci. Biobehav. Rev.* **2019**, *107*, 69–83. [CrossRef]
35. Sorensen, B.; Streib, J.E.; Strand, M.; Make, B.; Giclas, P.C.; Fleshner, M.; Jones, J.F. Complement activation in a model of chronic fatigue syndrome. *J. Allergy Clin. Immunol.* **2003**, *112*, 397–403. [CrossRef] [PubMed]
36. Germain, A.; Ruppert, D.; Levine, S.M.; Hanson, M.R. Metabolic profiling of a myalgic encephalomyelitis/chronic fatigue syndrome discovery cohort reveals disturbances in fatty acid and lipid metabolism. *Mol. Biosyst.* **2017**, *13*, 371–379. [CrossRef]
37. Jacobson, W.; Saich, T.; Borysiewicz, L.K.; Behan, W.M.; Behan, P.O.; Wreghitt, T.G. Serum folate and chronic fatigue syndrome. *Neurology* **1993**, *43*, 2645–2647. [CrossRef]
38. Roerink, M.E.; Roerink, S.; Skoluda, N.; Van der Schaaf, M.E.; Hermus, A.; Van der Meer, J.W.M.; Knoop, H.; Nater, U.M. Hair and salivary cortisol in a cohort of women with chronic fatigue syndrome. *Horm. Behav.* **2018**, *103*, 1–6. [CrossRef] [PubMed]
39. Nijhof, S.L.; Rutten, J.M.T.M.; Uiterwaal, C.S.P.M.; Bleijenberg, G.; Kimpen, J.L.L.; Putte, E.M.V.D. The role of hypocortisolism in chronic fatigue syndrome. *Psychoneuroendocrinology* **2014**, *42*, 199–206. [CrossRef]
40. Strickland, P.; Morriss, R.; Wearden, A.; Deakin, B. A comparison of salivary cortisol in chronic fatigue syndrome, community depression and healthy controls. *J. Affect. Disord.* **1998**, *47*, 191–194. [CrossRef]
41. Rimes, K.A.; Papadopoulos, A.S.; Cleare, A.J.; Chalder, T. Cortisol output in adolescents with chronic fatigue syndrome: Pilot study on the comparison with healthy adolescents and change after cognitive behavioural guided self-help treatment. *J. Psychosom. Res.* **2014**, *77*, 409–414. [CrossRef]
42. Jerjes, W.K.; Peters, T.J.; Taylor, N.F.; Wood, P.J.; Wessely, S.; Cleare, A.J. Diurnal excretion of urinary cortisol, cortisone, and cortisol metabolites in chronic fatigue syndrome. *J. Psychosom. Res.* **2006**, *60*, 145–153. [CrossRef]
43. Roberts, A.D.; Wessely, S.; Chalder, T.; Papadopoulos, A.; Cleare, A.J. Salivary cortisol response to awakening in chronic fatigue syndrome. *Br. J. Psychiatry* **2004**, *184*, 136–141. [CrossRef] [PubMed]
44. Wyller, V.B.; Vitelli, V.; Sulheim, D.; Fagermoen, E.; Winger, A.; Godang, K.; Bollerslev, J. Altered neuroendocrine control and association to clinical symptoms in adolescent chronic fatigue syndrome: A cross-sectional study. *J. Transl. Med.* **2016**, *14*, 1–12. [CrossRef]
45. Wakefield, D.; Lloyd, A.; Brockman, A. Immunoglobulin subclass abnormalities in patients with chronic fatigue syndrome. *Pediatr. Infect. Dis. J.* **1990**, *9*, 550–553. [CrossRef]
46. Guenther, S.; Loebel, M.; Mooslechner, A.A.; Knops, M.; Hanitsch, L.G.; Grabowski, P.; Wittke, K.; Meisel, C.; Unterwalder, N.; Volk, H.-D.; et al. Frequent IgG subclass and mannose binding lectin deficiency in patients with chronic fatigue syndrome. *Hum. Immunol.* **2015**, *76*, 729–735. [CrossRef] [PubMed]
47. Natelson, B.H.; Lin, J.S.; Lange, G.; Khan, S.; Stegner, A.; Unger, E.R. The effect of comorbid medical and psychiatric diagnoses on chronic fatigue syndrome. *Ann. Med.* **2019**, *51*, 371–378. [CrossRef] [PubMed]
48. Brurberg, K.G.; Fønhus, M.S.; Larun, L.; Flottorp, S.; Malterud, K. Case definitions for chronic fatigue syndrome/myalgic encephalomyelitis (±CFS/ME): A systematic review. *BMJ Open* **2014**, *4*, e003973. [CrossRef] [PubMed]
49. Brown, A.; Molly, B.; Porter, N.; Meredyth, E.; Jason, L.; Jessica, H.; Anderson, V.; Lerch, A.; De Meirleir, K.; Friedberg, F. The development of a revised canadian myalgic encephalomyelitis chronic fatigue syndrome case definition. *Am. J. Biochem. Biotechnol.* **2010**, *6*, 120–135.
50. Hawk, C.; Jason, L.A.; Torres-Harding, S. Differential diagnosis of chronic fatigue syndrome and major depressive disorder. *Int. J. Behav. Med.* **2006**, *13*, 244–251. [CrossRef]
51. Brown, A.A.; Jason, L.A. Validating a measure of myalgic encephalomyelitis/chronic fatigue syndrome symptomatology. *Fatigue* **2014**, *2*, 132–152. [CrossRef]

52. Jason, L.A.; So, S.; Brown, A.A.; Sunnquist, M.; Evans, M. Test-Retest Reliability of the DePaul Symptom Questionnaire. *Fatigue* **2015**, *3*, 16–32. [CrossRef] [PubMed]
53. Strand, E.; Lillestøl, K.; Jason, L.; Tveito, K.; Diep, L.; Valla, S.; Sunnquist, M.; Helland, I.B.; Herder, I.; Dammen, T. Comparing the DePaul Symptom Questionnaire with physician assessments: A preliminary study. *Routledge Fr. Taylor Group* **2016**, *4*, 52–62. [CrossRef]
54. Murdock, K.W.; Wang, X.S.; Shi, Q.; Cleeland, C.S.; Fagundes, C.P.; Vernon, S.D. The utility of patient-reported outcome measures among patients with myalgic encephalomyelitis/chronic fatigue syndrome. *Qual. Life Res.* **2017**, *26*, 913–921. [CrossRef] [PubMed]
55. Teixeira, A.; Borges, G. Creatine Kinase: Structure and function. *Braz. J. Biomotricity* **2012**, *6*, 53–65.
56. Baird, M.F.; Graham, S.M.; Baker, J.S.; Bickerstaff, G.F. Creatine-kinase- and exercise-related muscle damage implications for muscle performance and recovery. *J. Nutr. Metab.* **2012**, *2012*, 960363. [CrossRef]
57. Stucki, G.; Brühlmann, P.; Stoll, T.; Stucki, S.; Willer, B.; Michel, B.A. Low serum creatine kinase activity is associated with muscle weakness in patients with rheumatoid arthritis. *J. Rheumatol.* **1996**, *23*, 603–608. [PubMed]
58. Van Campen, C.L.M.; Riepma, K.; Visser, F.C. Open trial of vitamin b12 nasal drops in adults with myalgic encephalomyelitis/chronic fatigue syndrome: Comparison of responders and non-responders. *Front. Pharmacol.* **2019**, *10*, 1102. [CrossRef] [PubMed]

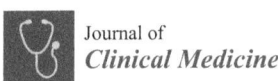

Article

Shadow Burden of Undiagnosed Myalgic Encephalomyelitis/Chronic Fatigue Syndrome (ME/CFS) on Society: Retrospective and Prospective—In Light of COVID-19

Diana Araja [1,2,*], Uldis Berkis [2,3], Asja Lunga [3] and Modra Murovska [2]

1. Department of Dosage Form Technology, Faculty of Pharmacy, Riga Stradins University, 16 Dzirciema Str, LV-1007 Riga, Latvia
2. Institute of Microbiology and Virology, Riga Stradins University, 5 Ratsupites Str, LV-1067 Riga, Latvia; Uldis.Berkis@rsu.lv (U.B.); Modra.Murovska@rsu.lv (M.M.)
3. Development and Project Department, Riga Stradins University, 16 Dzirciema Str, LV-1007 Riga, Latvia; Asja.Lunga@rsu.lv
* Correspondence: Diana.Araja@rsu.lv

Abstract: Background: Myalgic encephalomyelitis/chronic fatigue syndrome (ME/CFS) is a poorly understood, complex, multisystem disorder, with severe fatigue not alleviated by rest, and other symptoms, which lead to substantial reductions in functional activity and quality of life. Due to the unclear aetiology, treatment of patients is complicated, but one of the initial problems is the insufficient diagnostic process. The increase in the number of undiagnosed ME/CFS patients became specifically relevant in the light of the COVID-19 pandemic. The aim of this research was to investigate the issues of undiagnosed potential ME/CFS patients, with a hypothetical forecast of the expansion of post-viral CFS as a consequence of COVID-19 and its burden on society. Methods: The theoretical research was founded on the estimation of classic factors presumably affecting the diagnostic scope of ME/CFS and their ascription to Latvian circumstances, as well as a literature review to assess the potential interaction between ME/CFS and COVID-19 as a new contributing agent. The empirical study design consisted of two parts: The first part was dedicated to a comparison of the self-reported data of ME/CFS patients with those of persons experiencing symptoms similar to ME/CFS, but without a diagnosis. This part envisaged the creation of an assumption of the ME/CFS shadow burden "status quo", not addressing the impact of COVID-19. The second part aimed to investigate data from former COVID-19 patients' surveys on the presence of ME/CFS symptoms, 6 months after being affected by COVID-19. Descriptive and analytical statistical methods were used to analyse the obtained data. Results: The received data assumed that the previously obtained data on the ME/CFS prevalence of 0.8% in the Latvian population are appropriate, and the literature review reports a prevalence of 0.2–1.0% in developed countries. Regarding the reciprocity of ME/CFS and COVID-19, the literature review showed a lack of research in this field. The empirical results show quite similar self-esteem among ME/CFS patients and undiagnosed patients with longstanding disease experience, while former COVID-19 patients show a significantly lower severity of these problems. Notably, "psychological distress (anxiety)" and "episodic fatigue" are significantly predominant symptoms reported by former COVID-19 patients in comparison with ME/CFS patients and undiagnosed patients prior to the COVID-19 pandemic. The results of our analysis predict that the total amount of direct medical costs for undiagnosed patients (out-of-pocket payments) is more than EUR 15 million p.a. (in Latvia), and this may increase by at least 15% due to the consequences of COVID-19. Conclusions: ME/CFS creates a significant shadow burden on society, even considering only the direct medical costs of undiagnosed patients—the number of whom in Latvia is probably at least five times higher than the number of discerned patients. Simultaneously, COVID-19 can induce long-lasting complications and chronic conditions, such as post-viral CFS, and increase this burden. The Latvian research data assume that ME/CFS patients are not a high-risk group for COVID-19; however, COVID-19 causes ME/CFS-relevant symptoms in patients. This increases the need for monitoring of patients for even longer after recovering from COVID-19's symptoms, in order to prevent complications and the progression of chronic diseases. In the

Citation: Araja, D.; Berkis, U.; Lunga, A.; Murovska, M. Shadow Burden of Undiagnosed Myalgic Encephalomyelitis/Chronic Fatigue Syndrome (ME/CFS) on Society: Retrospective and Prospective—In Light of COVID-19. *J. Clin. Med.* **2021**, *10*, 3017. https://doi.org/10.3390/jcm10143017

Academic Editors: Giovanni Ricevuti, Lorenzo Lorusso and Lindsay A. Farrer

Received: 8 June 2021
Accepted: 1 July 2021
Published: 6 July 2021

Publisher's Note: MDPI stays neutral with regard to jurisdictional claims in published maps and institutional affiliations.

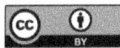

Copyright: © 2021 by the authors. Licensee MDPI, Basel, Switzerland. This article is an open access article distributed under the terms and conditions of the Creative Commons Attribution (CC BY) license (https://creativecommons.org/licenses/by/4.0/).

context of further epidemiological uncertainty, and the possibility of severe post-viral consequences, preventive measures are becoming significantly more important; an integrated diagnostic approach and appropriate treatment could reduce this burden in the future.

Keywords: myalgic encephalomyelitis; chronic fatigue syndrome; ME/CFS; COVID-19; diagnostic; impact on society

1. Introduction

In recent years, the preconditions for an increase in the number of myalgic encephalomyelitis/chronic fatigue syndrome (ME/CFS) patients have emerged, and the growth rate might be contributed to by the COVID-19 pandemic. COVID-19 can induce long-lasting complications and chronic conditions such as post-viral CFS, which is a poorly understood, serious, complex, multisystem disorder, characterised by symptoms lasting at least six months, with severe incapacitating fatigue not alleviated by rest, and other symptoms—many autonomic or cognitive in nature—including profound fatigue, cognitive dysfunction, sleep disturbances, muscle pain, and post-exertional malaise, which lead to substantial reductions in functional activity and quality of life [1].

The prevalence of this disease in developed countries appears to be within the range of 0.2–1%, but this is highly dependent on case definition, geographical area, gender, and age [2]. This disease most commonly occurs between the ages of 20 and 50 years [1], thus causing a significant burden on people of working age and society as a whole. Systematic review and meta-analysis of the prevalence of (ME/CFS), performed in 2020, comprehensively estimated the prevalence of ME/CFS at 0.89%, with women approximately 1.5–2-fold higher than men in all categories. However, the prevalence rates varied widely—particularly by case definitions and diagnostic methods [3].

In Latvia, the number of patients diagnosed with ME/CFS is significantly lower than suggested by the data available in scientific literature on the prevalence of this disease. Therefore, within the framework of this study, it was planned to compare the self-reported data on observed symptoms in ME/CFS patients with those in persons experiencing symptoms similar to those of ME/CFS, but without a diagnosis. This was necessary in order to assess the likelihood and extent of latent ME/CFS in Latvia. Simultaneously, it has been hypothesised that COVID-19 might contribute to the number of undiagnosed patients with ME/CFS, and the obtained results are expected to be relevant to other countries as well.

In Latvia, the first confirmed COVID-19 cases were discerned in March 2020 (Figure 1). Consequently, in the autumn of 2020, circumstances allowed for the analysis of 6 months of ME/CFS-specific exposure data for patients affected by COVID-19 in March 2020.

The number of patients affected by COVID-19 was relatively small in March 2020, and this allowed us to develop a high-coverage cohort to conduct the study. Additionally, a literature review was performed to compare the data obtained in this empirical study with data from other studies. The literature review was devoted to the classic factors assumedly affecting the diagnostic scope of ME/CFS, and the causal interaction between ME/CFS and COVID-19 as a new contributing factor.

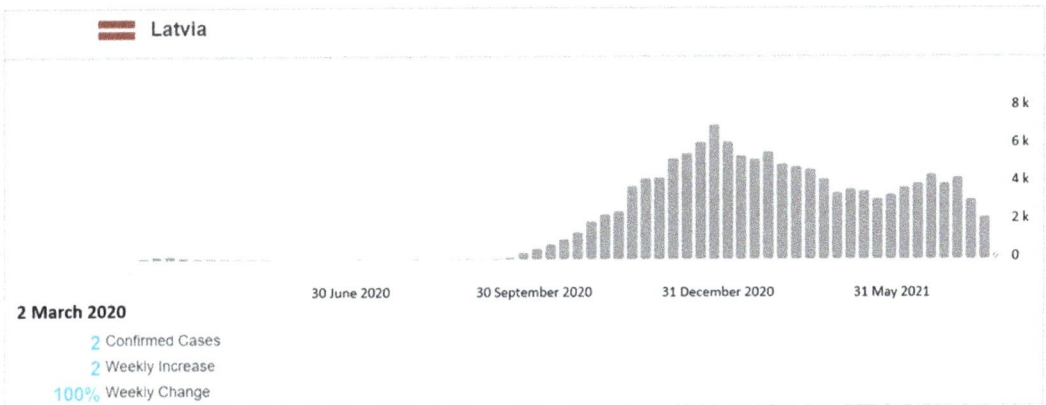

Figure 1. World Health Organisation Coronavirus (COVID-19) Dashboard, confirmed cases in Latvia, March 2020–May 2021 [4].

Consequently, the aim of this research was to investigate the issues of potential undiagnosed ME/CFS patients in Latvia, with a hypothetical forecast of the expansion of a post-viral CFS as a consequence of COVID-19 and its burden on society. The burden of undiagnosed ME/CFS can be described as a shadow burden. To achieve the aim of this research, the following tasks were defined:

- Estimate the literature on classic factors presumably affecting the diagnostic scope of ME/CFS, and their ascription to Latvian circumstances, as well as conducting a literature review to assess the potential relationship between ME/CFS and COVID-19 as a new contributing agent, and its reflection in scientific literature;
- Analyse data from the survey performed both for ME/CFS patients and for persons experiencing symptoms similar to those of ME/CFS, but without a diagnosis (prior to the COVID-19 pandemic), in order to compare the certain socioeconomic and disease management aspects for patients and potential undiagnosed patients. Data from the ME/CFS patients' survey were previously analysed in a comparative study with Italy and the UK. Conversely, the data from undiagnosed patients were not analysed previously; nevertheless, these data create significant potential for assessing the shadow impact of ME/CFS;
- Test the possible interaction between COVID-19 and ME/CFS in Latvian circumstances, by conducting a survey of former COVID-19 patients on the presence of ME/CFS symptoms;
- Make preliminary predictions on the potential shadow impact of ME/CFS on society, limiting this study to direct costs for patients.

The first section of this article is devoted to theoretical aspects and literature review, followed by the description of the methods and materials used in the empirical research, and the presentation of the results. The discussion section draws attention to the potential impact of ME/CFS on society in the light of COVID-19. The publication is finalised by conclusions and recommendations for further research.

2. Theoretical Background and Literature Review

Theoretical contemplations are elaborated in this section, with the initial focus on classic factors assumably affecting the diagnostic scope of ME/CFS, and their ascription to Latvian circumstances. The classification of diagnoses is one of these factors, and the World Health Organisation's approach is used for these purposes in Latvia. To classify ME/CFS by the World Health Organisation's International Statistical Classification of Diseases and Related Health Problems (ICD-10), mainly, two ICD-10 codes—code G93.3 (post-viral fatigue syndrome/myalgic encephalomyelitis (ME)) and code 52.82 (chronic fatigue syndrome (CFS))—are used [5]. Myalgic encephalomyelitis (ME), identified as a new clinical entity with distinctive features in 1956, was originally considered to be a neuromuscular disease [6]. In turn, several case definitions were developed in order to improve the comparability and reproducibility of clinical research and epidemiologic studies. Since the first "ME" case definition was developed in 1986, 25 case definitions/diagnostic criteria were created based on three conceptual factors (aetiology, pathophysiology, and exclusionary disorders). These factors can be categorized into four categories (ME, ME/CFS, CFS, and SEID (systemic exertion intolerance disorder)) [7].

There are eight most prominently cited case definitions and diagnostic criteria, which can be applied for each of the following categories:

- CFS (Fukuda et al. (US Centre for Disease Control (CDC, 1994)) [8], Holmes et al. (1988) [9], Australian (1990) [10], Oxford (1991) [11]);
- ME (Ramsay et al. (1992) [12] and International Consensus Criteria (ICC, 2011) [13]);
- ME/CFS (Canadian Consensus Criteria (CCC, 2003) [14]), and;
- SEID (IOM, 2015) [15], according to the focus of the primary disorder [7].

SEID was proposed by the Institute of Medicine (IOM, now the National Academies of Medicine (NAM), Washington, DC, USA) to resolve diagnostic confusion, as a new clinical entity to replace "ME/CFS". SEID is defined by chronic fatigue, post-exertional "malaise", and unrefreshing sleep, as well as orthostatic intolerance and/or cognitive impairment [16]. However, SEID case criteria do not do justice to either ME or CFS, nor to their definitions. Furthermore, in addition to the theoretical impossibility of replacing two different definitions with a new definition, the SEID case criteria are also applicable to subsets of people with other diseases—for example, multiple sclerosis (MS) and lupus—and psychological conditions—for example, major depression—while only a subset of people with the diagnosis of CFS meet the diagnosis of SEID.

The introduction of SEID did not resolve the impasse, but highlighted the uncertainties of the diagnoses and the need to seek new approaches to improve the diagnostic process.

The authors of this article assume that the discovery of biomarkers and the use of machine learning capacities are the most state-of-the-art approaches to improve the diagnostic process. Several original studies and literature reviews demonstrate the potential of biomarkers in the diagnosis of ME/CFS, and the contribution of precision medicine and personalised healthcare [17–19]. The European ME/CFS Research Network (EUROMENE) (in which Latvia is represented by the Riga Stradins University) has established a database for active biomarker research in Europe, called the EUROMENE ME/CFS Biomarker Landscape project [20]. In Latvia, the investigation of ME/CFS biomarkers is also encouraged and supported by the Latvian Science Council's Fundamental and Applied Research project No lzp-2019/1-0380 "selection of biomarkers in ME/CFS for patient stratification and treatment surveillance/optimisation".

In turn, artificial intelligence and machine learning can greatly support the diagnostic process; however, problems with the initial identification of patients remain topical. In this process, general practitioners (GPs) have an important role, and EUROMENE participants performed a literature review of GPs' knowledge and understanding of ME/CFS (papers were mostly from the United Kingdom), concluding that disbelief and lack of knowledge and understanding of ME/CFS among GPs is widespread, and the resultant diagnostic delays constitute a risk factor for severe and prolonged disease. Failure to diagnose ME/CFS renders attempts to determine its prevalence and, hence, its economic impact, problematic [21]. In addition, a survey of academic and clinical experts who are participants in EUROMENE was conducted to elicit perceptions of GPs knowledge and understanding of ME/CFS, and the results of this survey reported that lack of knowledge and understanding of ME/CFS among GPs is a major cause of missed and delayed diagnoses, which renders attempts to determine the incidence and prevalence of the disease, and to measure its economic impact, problematic. It also contributes to the burden of disease through mismanagement in its early stages [22]. A comparative survey of people with ME/CFS in Italy,

Latvia, and the United Kingdom, performed on behalf of the Socioeconomics Working Group of the EUROMENE, indicated that GPs more frequently had principal responsibility for medical care in Latvia than in Italy or the UK, and this probably reflects the fact that in Latvia GPs perform the gatekeeper role for patients in the diagnostic and treatment process [23].

An additional determining factor is the patients' engagement in outcome measurement and disease management. A literature review performed 10 years ago drew conclusions that the quality and acceptability of reviewed patient-reported outcome measures (PROMs) were limited, and recommendations for patient-reported assessment were difficult [24]. Clear discrepancies existed between what was measured in research and how patients defined their experience of ME/CFS. It was recommended that future PROM development/evaluation must seek to involve patients more collaboratively, in order to measure outcomes of importance using relevant and credible methods of assessment [24]. 10 years later, the situation is more comprehensive, and one literature review defines in total 15 patient-reported outcome (PRO)-derived tools (used in 50 randomised clinical trials (RCTs)) along with two behavioural measurements for adolescents (4 RCTs). The review comprehensively provides the choice pattern of the assessment tools for interventions in RCTs for ME/CFS [25]. However, the environment of RCTs is different from the environment in which patients live daily.

Taking into account the identified challenges that accompanied the process of collecting PROs in the daily lives of ME/CFS patients, EUROMENE member countries' representatives have defined a view on the creation of an app and a web platform for ME/CFS patients' self-empowerment and disease management, where the target users are people suffering from ME/CFS, and the practical challenge is diagnosis, stratification, and monitoring of ME/CFS at the level of the GP, supported by the virtual doctors' consortium, as well as patient self-awareness and proper practical navigation in the healthcare system [26]. This project is currently in the process of seeking funding.

At the same time, the COVID-19 pandemic, resulting from severe acute respiratory syndrome coronavirus 2 (SARS-CoV-2), has severely impacted the population worldwide, with a great mortality rate. According to the lessons from past epidemics, previous research on post-epidemic and post-infection recovery has suggested that the complications include the development of severe fatigue. Certain factors, such as the severity of infection, in addition to the "cytokine storm" experienced by many COVID-19 patients, may contribute to the development of later health problems [27].

In the light of COVID-19's epidemiological uncertainty, the issues of the causes and consequences of the disease remain topical, and CFS is a possible predictor and consequence of COVID-19. A literature review, which included 1161 primary studies published between January 1979 and June 2019, concluded that the four most common causal factors of ME/CFS were: immunological (297 studies), psychological (243), infections (198), and neuroendocrine (198) [28]. The causes can be broadly characterized according to primary disorder (ME—viral, CFS—unknown, ME/CFS—inflammatory, SEID—multisystemic), compulsory symptoms (ME and ME/ CFS—neuroinflammatory, CFS and SEID—fatigue and/or malaise), and required conditions (ME—infective agent, ME/CFS, CFS, SEID—symptoms associated with fatigue, e.g., duration of illness) [7].

Therefore, the increase in the number of undiagnosed ME/CFS patients is becoming specifically relevant in the light of the COVID-19 pandemic. Theoretically, the economic impact assessment of this disease could be based on the current level of costs (direct, indirect, and intangible) to society, by modelling and forecasting techniques. However, data on the prevalence of ME/CFS are widely dispersed, and data on financial impact are even more uncertain. In the framework of EUROMENE, representatives of Ireland in the Socioeconomic Working Group have performed a qualitative study on understanding the economic impact of ME/CFS in Ireland [29]. The identified healthcare barriers and costs are described in Figure 2.

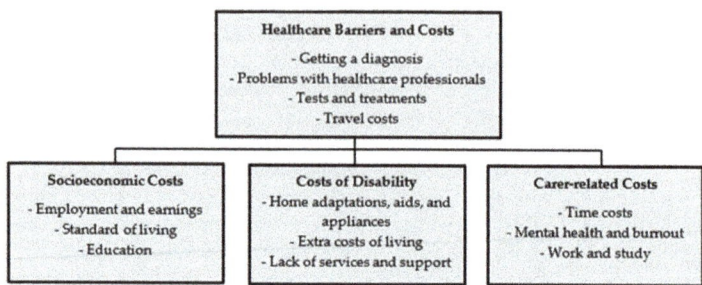

Figure 2. Economic impact of myalgic encephalomyelitis/chronic fatigue syndrome (ME/CFS) [29].

Participants in the mentioned study described a range of problems and costs that related to getting a diagnosis of ME/CFS. As described in the study, for some it took years, with numerous visits to GPs, consultants, and other healthcare professionals, for their illness to be identified or even acknowledged. Participants highlighted how they were often passed from one healthcare professional to another. In many cases, consultations to get a diagnosis were paid for out-of-pocket, at significant personal cost [29].

In the theoretical research on the causal interaction between ME/CFS and COVID-19, the purpose was to identify the main findings regarding the reciprocity of ME/CFS and COVID-19. The search was performed on Medline (via PubMed) and other relevant scientific databases (without restriction for publishing period). The following search key words were used: ("COVID-19") OR ("coronavirus") OR ("SARS-COV-2") AND ("chronic fatigue syndrome") OR ("myalgic encephalomyelitis") OR ("CFS") OR ("ME/CFS"). The flow diagram of the selection process is shown in Figure 3.

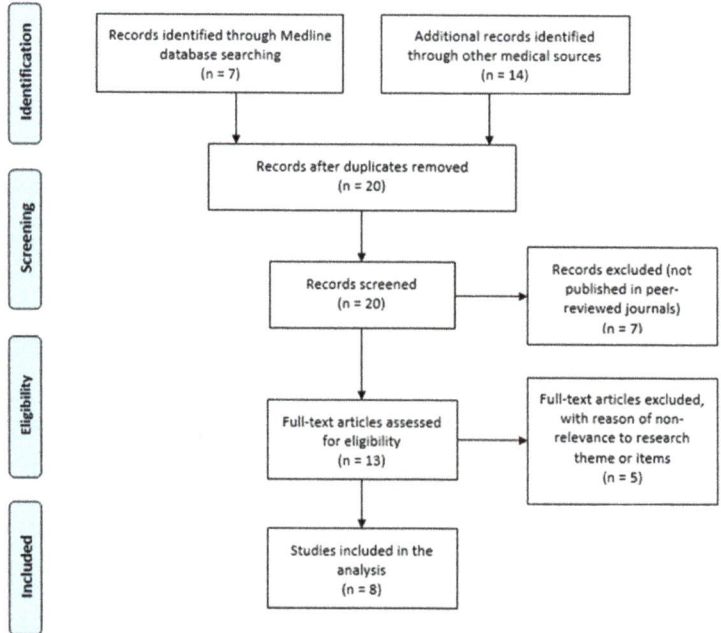

Figure 3. Flow diagram of the selection process for the literature review on the possible interaction between ME/CFS and COVID-19.

A total of 21 articles were identified using the aforementioned search strategy (Figure 3). After the removal of duplicates using reference management software (EndNote, Clarivate Analytics), 20 articles were screened for title and abstract, and 7 articles were excluded due to not being published in peer-reviewed journals. The remaining 13 articles were screened against eligibility criteria; 5 full-text articles were excluded for non-relevance to the research theme or items, and therefore 8 articles were included in the analysis.

The main findings of the literature review are presented in a summary of findings table (Table 1); this table provides key information concerning the research's authors, type of research, and the sum of available data on the main outcomes.

Table 1. Characteristics of the scientific articles included in our analysis to assess the possible interaction between ME/CFS and COVID-19.

Authors	Type of Research	Main Results and Conclusions
Strayer et al. (Oct 2020) [30]	Research Article	The results may have direct relevance to the cognitive impairment and fatigue being experienced by patients clinically recovered from COVID-19 and free of detectable SARS-CoV-2.
Gaber (Jan 2021) [31]	Review	Post-viral fatigue is the most common long-term health issue facing survivors of COVID-19, according to initial reports. The author discusses the risk, diagnosis, and principles of management of post-viral fatigue and its chronic variant—ME/CFS—within the context of the pandemic, and highlights that further research is urgently needed to guide clinical practice. Several symptoms are classically associated with post-viral fatigue and ME/CFS, including physical pain, recurrent headaches, malaise, cognitive impairment, unrefreshing sleep, recurrent sore throats, and lymphadenopathy. These symptoms are strongly associated with the post-exertional phase of the boom-and-bust cycle. Identification of the post-COVID patients needing support and treatment should be a part of the overall COVID-19 response globally.
Friedman et al. (Feb 2021) [32]	Opinion	The similarity and overlap of ME/CFS and long-haul COVID-19 symptoms suggest similar pathological processes. A unifying hypothesis explains the precipitating events, such as viral triggers and other documented exposures; for their overlap in symptoms, ME/CFS and long-haul COVID-19 should be described as post-active-phase-of-infection syndromes (PAPISs). The authors further propose that the underlying biochemical pathways and pathophysiological processes of similar symptoms are similar regardless of the initiating trigger. The authors caution that failure to meet the now combined challenges of ME/CFS and long-haul COVID-19 will impose serious socioeconomic as well as clinical consequences for patients, the families of patients, and society as a whole.
Halpin et al. (Feb 2021) [33]	Research Article	There is currently very limited information on the nature and prevalence of post-COVID-19 symptoms after hospital discharge. In this research, a purposive sample of 100 survivors discharged from a large university hospital was assessed 4–8 weeks after discharge by a multidisciplinary team of rehabilitation professionals. Participants were between 29 and 71 days (mean 48 days) post-discharge from hospital; 32 participants required treatment in an intensive care unit (ICU group), and 68 were managed in hospital wards without needing ICU care (ward group). New illness-related fatigue was the most commonly reported symptom—by 72% of participants in the ICU group and 60.3% in the ward group. There was a clinically significant drop in EQ5D, of 68.8% in the ICU group and 45.6% in the ward group. The authors recommend planning rehabilitation services to manage post-discharge symptoms appropriately and maximize the functional return of COVID-19 survivors.
Simani et al. (Feb 2021) [34]	Research Article	The obtained data revealed the prevalence of CFS among patients with COVID-19, which is almost similar to CFS prevalence in the general population. Moreover, post-traumatic stress disorder (PTSD) in patients with COVID-19 is not associated with an increased risk of CFS. This study suggests that medical institutions should pay attention to the psychological consequences of the COVID-19 outbreak.
Townsend et al. (Feb 2021) [35]	Research Article	The results demonstrate the significant burden of fatigue, symptoms of autonomic dysfunction, and anxiety in the aftermath of COVID-19 infection but, reassuringly, do not demonstrate pathological findings on autonomic testing.
Graham et al. (Mar 2021) [36]	Research Article	A prospective study of the first 100 consecutive patients (50 SARS-CoV-2 laboratory-positive (SARS-CoV-2$^+$) and 50 laboratory-negative (SARS-CoV-2$^-$) individuals) presenting to the Neuro-Covid-19 clinic between May and November 2020 concluded that non-hospitalized COVID-19 "long-haulers" experience prominent and persistent "brain fog" and fatigue that affect their cognition and quality of life.
Toogood et al. (Mar 2021) [37]	Review	Viral infection is an established trigger for the onset of ME/CFS symptoms, raising the possibility of an increase in ME/CFS prevalence resulting from the ongoing COVID-19 pandemic.

The publication period for identified scientific literature was not defined, but the first relevant publication was dated to October 2020, and more research articles were published in 2021. Table 1 shows the main research outcomes of published scientific literature in peer-reviewed journals. Note that the authors pay attention not only to the symptoms, but also to changes in quality-of-life indicators.

3. Materials and Methods of Empirical Research

This section is devoted to the empirical research conducted by the authors to investigate the shadow burden of ME/CFS and its causal interaction with COVID-19 in the context of Latvia. To achieve the aim and objectives of the empirical research, the study design consisted of two parts (Figure 4):

(1) The first part was dedicated to comparison of self-reported data from ME/CFS patients with those from persons experiencing symptoms similar to those of ME/CFS, but without a diagnosis, obtained by the survey performed prior to the COVID-19 pandemic. This part envisaged the creation of an assumption on the ME/CFS shadow burden "status quo"—not addressing the impact of COVID-19—in Latvia.

(2) The second part aimed to investigate the data from COVID-19 patients' surveyed on the presence of ME/CFS symptoms, 6 months after being affected by COVID-19, in Latvia.

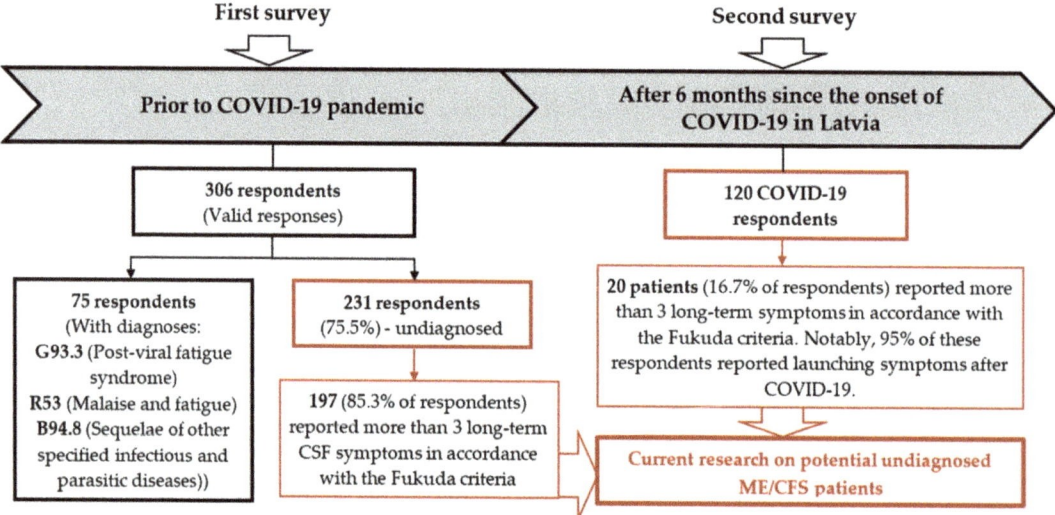

Figure 4. The empirical study design and outcomes.

The first patients' survey (Data S1) was designed mostly to obtain general information (e.g., age, gender, education, etc.) and information on their symptoms, clinical history, and the socio-economic consequences of the disease—including restrictions on daily life, sources of assistance, and understanding and awareness of the disease. The purpose of the survey was indicated in the introductory part of the questionnaire—to evaluate patients' knowledge about ME/CFS, health care received, and problems related to the impact of ME/CFS on quality of life. The questionnaire was addressed to persons who experienced chronic fatigue for at least six months that could not be reduced by rest, headache, muscle aches, enlarged lymph nodes, joint pain, neck pain, memory problems, sleep problems, and other typical symptoms. The survey was approved by the Research Ethics Committee of the Riga Stradins University (Decision No. 6-3/3, 25 October 2018, Riga), launched in February 2019, and lasted for two months. The survey was distributed through GPs, as well as on the social networking platform Mammamuntetiem.lv (accessed on 18 February 2019; a portal for families and parents) that was most relevant to the structure of potential patients (mostly used by persons between the ages of 20 and 50 years). A total of 306 valid responses were received, of which 75 were from patients with G93.3, R53, and B94.8 diagnoses, while 231 respondents had reported CFS-like symptoms but had not been diagnosed (Figure 2). The results of diagnosed ME/CFS patients' surveys were investigated in the scope of Brenna et al.'s Comparative Survey of People with ME/CFS in Italy, Latvia, and the UK [23]. At the same time, the data of undiagnosed patients were not properly analysed, and in this study the authors emphasise the issues of undiagnosed patients, and the possible increase in their number due to the COVID-19 pandemic.

Therefore, the second survey was dedicated to potential ME/CFS patients in the post-COVID-19 phase. This survey's data were obtained from a cohort of former COVID-19 patients established at the Genome Database of Latvian Population national biobank [38], in accordance with the Central Medical Ethics Committee's (Latvia) approval No 01-29.1/5034 (23 September 2020, Riga). ME/CFS was a secondary objective of this questionnaire; therefore, data for the present study were limited to questions about the presence of ME/CFS-like symptoms and quality of life. In Latvia, the first confirmed COVID-19 cases were discerned in March 2020, and consequently, the former COVID-19 patients affected in March 2020 were surveyed in October and November 2020, to establish a 6-month ME/CFS-specific exposure period.

Both questionnaires (inter alia) contained questions about CFS-relevant symptoms, in accordance with the CDC-1994 (Fukuda) criteria. The CDS-1994 case definition and criteria were chosen, as EUROMENE suggests mostly using the Fukuda definition and CCC definition, which identify a more severely affected group of patients. The CDC-1994 definition appeared more robust and less likely to be affected by variations in data collection methods [1]. The threshold was defined as four required accompanying symptoms, in accordance with Fukuda et al. [8,39]. Additionally, quality-of-life measurement was performed. Patients were asked to rate their quality of life (QoL) on a scale from 0 to 100 (where 100 represents the best possible QoL, and 0 the worst) for the year prior to onset of illness, and for the year immediately preceding completion of the survey. The current level of health-related quality of life was assessed using the EuroQol-5D-5L measure (certified translation: EQ-5D-5L Latvian for Latvia). Descriptive and analytical statistical methods were utilised for analysis of the obtained data.

In the Discussion section, the statistical data provided by the national competent authorities of Latvia were also used to make preliminary predictions about the potential shadow impact of ME/CFS on society.

4. Results

This section presents the outcomes of two surveys according to the research methodology: The first—a "status quo" survey—compares data from two groups of respondents prior to the COVID-19 pandemic: self-reported data from ME/CFS patients, and from persons experiencing symptoms similar to those of ME/CFS, but without a diagnosis. The second survey presents former COVID-19 patients' data in order to analyse the presence of ME/CFS-like symptoms and predict ME/CFS expansion.

The main data of descriptive statistics of the first survey are shown in Table 2; There were 75 valid responses from ME/CFS patients, consisting of 62 women and 13 men (20 patients with G93.3 disease code, 46 patients with R53 disease code, and 11 patients with B94.8 disease code; two patients had double diagnoses). Concerning the potentially undiagnosed patients, there were 231 completed responses (with different participation in completing certain questions) but, in both groups, the proportion of females was the same—82.7%. The patients' average age was 50 years (the respondents ranged in age from 17 to 81), while for undiagnosed persons it was 45 years. Other sociodemographic information shows that 60% of patients were married; in both groups, around of a third of respondents lived alone. In addition, 43% of patients were graduates, but a higher proportion (more than half) of undiagnosed persons with higher education degrees was observed. Additionally, comparative results are presented in Table 2 under the following items—household income (by household member), out-of-pocket payments to mitigate the consequences of illness and syndrome, number and variability of symptoms, number of investigations, difficulty explaining the illness and syndrome, and quality of life.

Table 2. Main results of the survey of ME/CFS patients and undiagnosed persons.

Item	Persons' Group	No. of Respondents	Mean	Standard Deviation (SD)	No. Responding "Yes"	%	95% Confidence Interval (%)
Age (Years)	Diagnosed	75	50.0	14.7			46.6–53.3
	Undiagnosed	222	45.1	12.9			43.4–46.8
Gender (No. Females)	Diagnosed	75			62	82.7	74.1–91.2
	Undiagnosed	226			187	82.7	77.8–87.7
Education (No. with Higher Education)	Diagnosed	74			32	43.2	32.0–54.5
	Undiagnosed	225			115	51.1	44.6–57.6
No. Living Alone	Diagnosed	74			25	33.8	23.0–44.6
	Undiagnosed	224			69	30.8	24.8–36.9
Household Income, per Member (EUR, p.a.)	Diagnosed	65	5364.4	2991.1			4637.3–6091.55
	Undiagnosed	213	6365.5	3819.7			5852.5–6878.5
No. Symptoms	Diagnosed	75	7.5	2.5			6.9–8.1
	Undiagnosed	231	6.3	2.8			5.9–6.7
Variability of Symptoms	Diagnosed	75			53	70.7	60.4–81.0
	Undiagnosed	231			178	77.1	71.6–82.5
No. Investigations	Diagnosed	75	5.7	3.2			5.0–6.4
	Undiagnosed	124	4.7	2.5			4.3–5.1
Out-of-Pocket Spending, to Mitigate Symptoms (EUR, p.a.)	Diagnosed	75	1143.0	125.1			1114.7–1171.3
	Undiagnosed	209	979.2	156.1			958.0–1000.4
Difficulty Explaining Illness to Physicians	Diagnosed	75			20	26.7	16.7–36.7
	Undiagnosed	231			76	32.9	26.8–39.0
Family	Diagnosed	75			35	46.7	35.4–58.0
	Undiagnosed	231			100	43.3	36.9–49.7
Friends	Diagnosed	75			20	26.7	16.7–36.7
	Undiagnosed	231			70	30.3	24.4–36.2
Employers	Diagnosed	75			30	40.0	28.9–51.1
	Undiagnosed	231			81	35.1	28.9–41.2
Quality of Life: Prior to Illness	Diagnosed	74	74.6	24.0			69.0–80.2
	Undiagnosed	212	74.1	22.0			71.1–77.1
In Past Year	Diagnosed	74	57.3	16.3			53.5–61.1
	Undiagnosed	219	58.1	16.8			55.9–60.3

It is assumed that this disease has significant impacts on personal income, because patients are frequently unable to work, and spend out-of-pocket resources for treatment. In order to assess the financial situation of patients in Latvia, the data of the Central Statistical Bureau on the mean disposable (net) income per household member were used for comparison. In Latvia, the mean disposable (net) income per household member in 2019 was EUR 6994 [40]. In accordance with the survey data, 48 of the ME/CFS patients (73.9%) reported lower than mean net income per household member, but still, on average, spent more than EUR 1140 p.a. on symptom relief. In the group of undiagnosed persons, 141 respondents (66.2%) reported lower than mean net income per household member, with a slightly lower out-of-pocket payment of EUR 979 p.a. for the mitigation of symptoms and their consequences.

Patients presented on average 7–8 different symptoms, and 9% of patients presented more than 10 symptoms. Significantly, undiagnosed persons reported more than 6 symptoms on average, and 197 (85.3%) of 231 respondents reported more than 3 long-term symptoms similar to ME/CFS symptoms, which is the threshold for the Fukuda criteria. The number of investigations prior to reaching a diagnosis on average was 6, and 43% of patients indicated that more than 12 months passed from their first symptoms to reaching a diagnosis. There was no significant difference in the number of investigations between patients and undiagnosed persons, but for the last group, it had not resulted in reaching a diagnosis. Both groups indicated high variability in symptoms (more than 70%), and undiagnosed persons were more likely to describe their symptoms as variable. The difficulty in explaining the symptoms can be one of the major difficulties for ME/CFS patients (almost 27% of patients reported difficulties in explaining their symptoms to physicians, 47% to family members, 27% to friends, and 40% to employers). The most critical point for both groups is explanation of their symptoms to family and employers.

Concerning the effectiveness of therapies, 64% patients noted the effectiveness of medication (prescription and OTC medicines), and 52% patients reported the effectiveness of non-medication methods (physiotherapy, psychotherapy, osteopathy, homeopathy, nutrition, and food supplements) and complex methods. The complex approach probably provides additional benefits of treatment, taking into account the multisymptom nature and aetiology of the condition. No caregivers other than family were reported; patients mostly took care of themselves.

In the empirical part of the research on investigation of the interaction between ME/CFS and COVID-19, the former COVID-19 patients' survey (the second survey) was performed as a part of the project on the evaluation of the data of the cohort of former COVID-19 patients established at the Genome Database of Latvian Population national biobank. Taking into account that the first confirmed cases of COVID-19 were discerned in March 2020, a 6-month period was required to obtain ME/CFS data, and former COVID-19 patients—affected by COVID-19 in March 2020—were surveyed in October and November 2020. In March 2020, there were 204 confirmed cases of COVID-19 in Latvia [4]. Subsequently, the patients who were affected by COVID-19 in March 2020 were invited to volunteer for a telephone survey in October–November 2020. Respectfully, 120 people agreed, and responded to questions on ME/CFS symptoms and health-related quality of life. Consequently, the sample covers more than half of the patients infected in March 2020, and the data obtained are statistically significant.

The data of the survey showed that 53 patients (44.2%) out of 120 respondents who had not been diagnosed with ME/CFS prior to the COVID-19 pandemic reported at least one of the symptoms characteristic of CFS, in accordance with the Fukuda criteria; 20 respondents (16.7%) reported 4 or more CFS-specific symptoms simultaneously. In order to compare the dominance of symptoms occurring in former COVID-19 patients with data from ME/CFS patients and undiagnosed patients prior to COVID-19, the relevant data are summarised in Figure 5.

The data show (Figure 5) that the predominant symptom in ME/CFS patients is "difficulty concentrating", while in undiagnosed patients "depressed mood" predominates, and "sleep disorders" puts an equally hard burden on all groups of patients. Significantly, non-diagnosed patients and former COVID-19 patients have noticeably higher levels of "psychological distress (anxiety)" compared to ME/CFS patients. "Muscular pain" and "headache" are vastly less common in former COVID-19 patients, but "sore throat" is substantial. "Memory disorders" occur more in undiagnosed patients. "Fluctuating blood pressure", "general malaise, as from flu", "urinary disorders", and "enlarged lymph nodes" are more common in ME/CFS patients. Regarding the different manifestations of fatigue, it should be noted that "persistent fatigue" is more common in former COVID-19 patients and ME/CFS patients, whereas "fluctuating fatigue" is more common in undiagnosed patients. "Episodic fatigue" is relatively less common in ME/CFS patients, but is predominant in former COVID-19 patients and undiagnosed patients. Former COVID-19 patients are also characterised by "fluctuating temperature" and slightly greater dominance of "gastrointestinal disorders" compared to ME/CFS patients and undiagnosed patients.

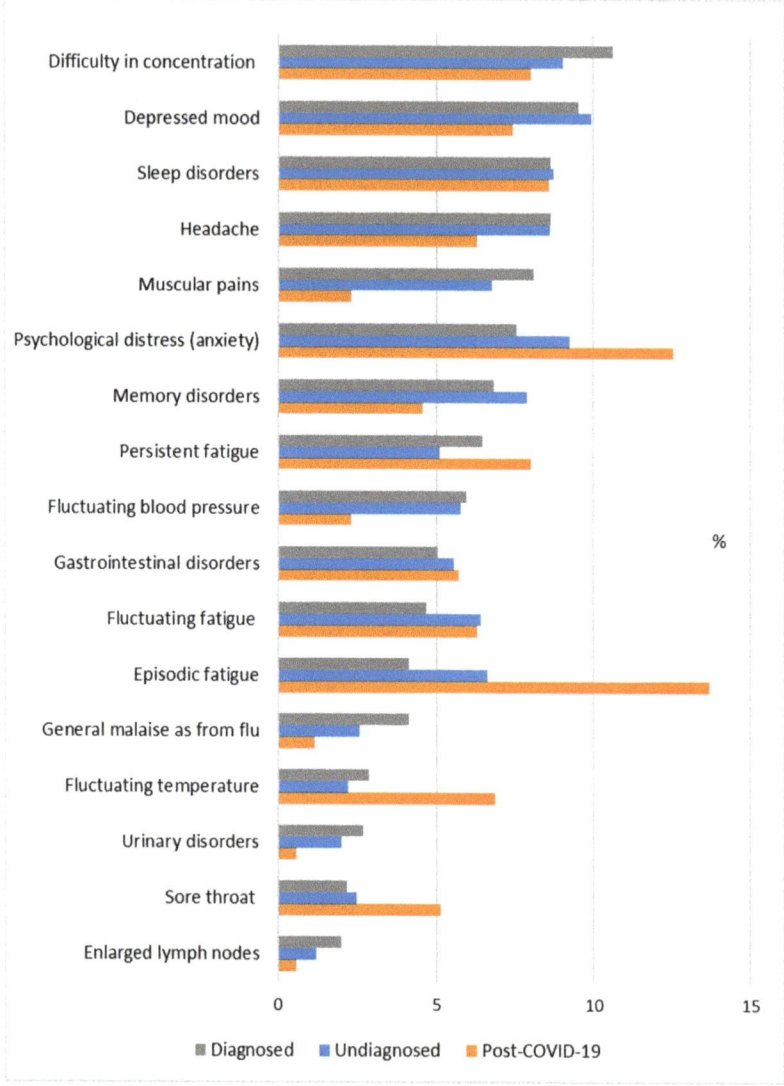

Figure 5. The prevalence of symptoms reported by ME/CFS patients and undiagnosed patients prior to COVID-19 (the first survey), and by former COVID-19 patients 6 months after infection (the second survey), as a percentage of the total number of reported cases of symptoms in each group.

Noticeably, 95% of the post-COVID-19 respondents reported onset of symptoms after being affected by COVID-19. This allows the assumption of COVID-19 as a causative agent of CFS, and probably of ME/CFS.

Concerning to the health-related quality of life measurements, the EuroQol-5D-5L was used to analyse the patients' self-esteem in the following fields: mobility (no/problems in walking about), self-care (no/problems washing or dressing myself), usual activities (e.g., work, study, housework, family or leisure activities—no/problems doing usual activities), pain/discomfort (no/pain or discomfort), and anxiety/depression (not/anxious or depressed). The results are summarised in Figure 6.

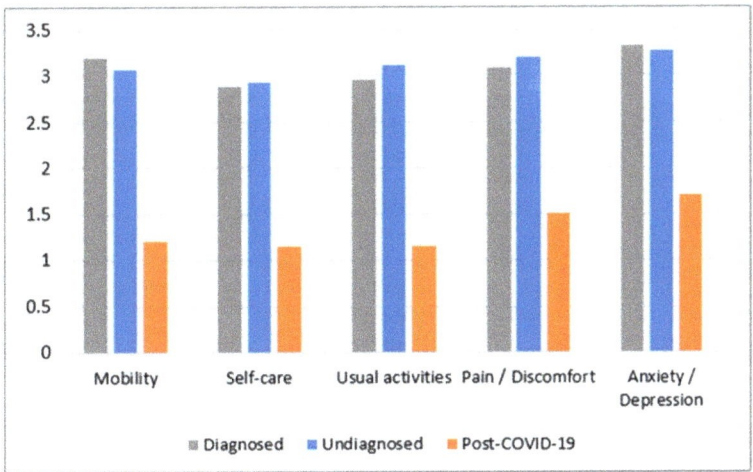

Figure 6. Patient-reported health-related quality of life, as measured by the EuroQol-5D-5L framework (1—the best possible option, and 5—the worst), in ME/CFS patients and undiagnosed persons prior to COVID-19, and former COVID-19 patients (6 months after being affected).

Data on ME/CFS patients (74 respondents), as well as undiagnosed patients (196 respondents) and former COVID-19 patients (20 respondents) who reported four or more ME/CFS-like symptoms, were used to obtain comparable data. The results show (Figure 6) quite similar self-esteem among ME/CFS patients and undiagnosed patients with long-standing disease experience, while former COVID-19 patients show a significantly lower severity of these problems.

It is important to note that there is no considerable difference in self-reported quality of life (using the VAS) between the ME/CFS patients group and the undiagnosed persons group (Table 2) prior to illness and in the past year. Significantly, the quality of life prior to illness was relatively low (scoring less than 75 out of 100), considering the average age of the target groups, and this encourages deeper research in the context of the overall quality of life of the Latvian population.

5. Discussion

As mentioned in the Materials and Methods section, this section is complimented with statistical data provided by the national competent authorities of Latvia, so as to contribute preliminary predictions about the potential shadow impact of ME/CFS on society.

The previously analysed data from the Latvian Centre for Disease Prevention and Control (CDPC) and the National Health Service (NHS) of Latvia tentatively indicated high prevalence of ME/CFS in Latvia. CDCP data from primary care indicated that approximately 700 patients had ICD-10 code G93.3 assigned, while there were approximately 15,000 with ICD-10 code R53, and about 70 with code B94.8. In total, these constitute about 0.8% of the Latvian population, which is considerably higher than the prevalence found in other comparable populations [1]. When discussing these data within the EUROMENE network, the prevalence seemed too high. However, an analysis of the literature shows that there are still no clear definitions of the exact classification of related diseases and case definitions. In addition, new approaches, new disease designations, and a nomenclature of syndrome sets are emerging. GPs, on the other hand, point to problems in making a precise diagnosis [21–23]. In these circumstances, it is possible that the obtained data on the prevalence of 0.8% in Latvia are appropriate, taking into account the fact that the literature review reports a prevalence of 0.2–1.0% in developed countries [2].

In accordance with the data from the Central Statistical Bureau of Latvia, at the beginning of 2020 the population of Latvia was approximately 1,908,000 people [41]. Accordingly, the prevalence of the disease may vary from 3816 to 19,080 patients in Latvia. In 2019, the NHS data show that 3142 patients of diagnosis codes G93.3 (post-viral fatigue syndrome), R53 (malaise and fatigue), and B94.8 (sequelae of other specified infectious and parasitic diseases) received the treatment from the state budget. The survey of potential ME/CFS patients performed in the scope of this research shows that undiagnosed persons reported more than 6 symptoms on average, and 197 (85.3%) of 231 respondents reported more than 3 long-term CFS-like symptoms, which is the threshold for the Fukuda criteria. At the same time, there was no significant difference in self-reported quality of life between the patients group and the undiagnosed persons group. These data confirm a high level of undiagnosed patients in Latvia.

Regarding the correlation with COVID-19, it could be generally assumed that post-viral fatigue syndrome (myalgic encephalomyelitis (ME)) is a logical consequence of viral infection. However, concerning CFS there are currently insufficient data to statistically confirm or reject this interaction. The literature review revealed a lack of research in this field. The present research indicates that the number of undiagnosed ME/CFS patients might increase by at least 15% due to the COVID-19 pandemic. In these circumstances, the COVID-19 pandemic presents a new potential challenge to increase the shadow burden of ME/CFS. The survey data of Latvian COVID-19 patients report alarming results for CFS-like symptoms after COVID-19 infection. Particular attention should be paid to the fact that "psychological distress (anxiety)" and "episodic fatigue" are significantly prevalent symptoms reported by former COVID-19 patients, in comparison with ME/CFS patients and undiagnosed patients prior to the COVID-19 pandemic. Health-related quality-of-life measurements according to EuroQol-5D-5L show better results in former COVID-19 patients compared to ME/CFS patients and undiagnosed patients prior to the COVID-19 period, but this may be explained by the relatively short time period in which persistent symptoms could be observed in former COVID-19 patients.

Concerning the shadow financial burden of ME/CFS on society, with respect to the direct costs faced by potential patients, the survey's data can be useful to predict the approximate out-of-pocket treatment cost per patient. In accordance with the survey data, 73.9% of the ME/CFS patients reported lower than mean net income per household member, but still, on average, spent more than EUR 1140 p.a. on symptom relief. In the group of undiagnosed persons, 66.2% of respondents reported lower than mean net income per household member, with a slightly lower out-of-pocket payment of EUR 979 p.a. for the mitigation of disease consequences.

Assuming that the actual number of patients in Latvia is—for instance—15,770 patients, as forecasted by the CDPC, and each of them spend EUR 979 p.a. to reduce the consequences of the disease, the total direct medical cost for undiagnosed patients is more than EUR 15 million p.a., and may increase by at least 15% in response to the influence of COVID-19.

In these circumstances, prevention programmes can play a significant role, and provide economic benefits as primary prevention and secondary prevention to minimise the diagnostic delays associated with prolonged illness, increased severity, and increased costs [42]. Data on quality of life are also noteworthy, as quality of life prior to illness, as reported by the survey, was relatively low (scoring less than 75 out of 100) considering the average age of the target groups (45–50 years old), and this encourages deeper research in the context of the overall quality of life of the Latvian population.

The present research creates the foundation for determining the "status quo" of undiagnosed patients with ME/CFS in Latvia, and propounds a vision for the further development of the scenario in the light of COVID-19. Simultaneously, the study has several limitations, the most substantial of which is related to the cohort formation of former COVID-19 patients, taking into account that a 6-month period is required to assess the presence of ME/CFS symptoms. The most significant number of confirmed COVID-19 cases in Latvia was observed in December 2020 (Figure 1); thus, in the second half of 2021 it would be valuable to continue this study, with a larger coverage of patients.

6. Conclusions

We came to the realisation that ME/CFS creates a significant shadow burden on society, even taking into account only the direct medical costs of undiagnosed patients—the number of whom in Latvia is probably at least five times higher than the number of discerned patients. A similar situation can be observed in other countries. Simultaneously, the hypothesis tends to be confirmed that COVID-19 might contribute to the number of undiagnosed patients with ME/CFS, and COVID-19 can induce long-lasting complications and chronic conditions—such as post-viral CFS—and increase this burden. The Latvian research data assume that ME/CFS patients are not part of the high-risk group for COVID-19; however, COVID-19 causes ME/CFS-relevant symptoms in patients. This increases the need for monitoring of patients for even longer after recovering from COVID-19's symptoms, in order to prevent complications and the progression of chronic diseases, including ME/CFS. In the context of further epidemiological uncertainty and the possibility of severe post-viral consequences, preventive measures are becoming significantly important, as well as an integrated use of the criteria, identification of biomarkers, and the aid of artificial intelligence for diagnostic purposes and appropriate treatment, all of which could help to reduce this burden in the future. The increased risk of worse outcomes from COVID-19 should be taken into account in decision-making with regard to individual and population-wide risks, prevention, and detection measures.

Supplementary Materials: The following are available online at https://www.mdpi.com/article/10.3390/jcm10143017/s1, Data S1: The patients' survey on ME/CFS symptoms.

Author Contributions: Conceptualization, D.A., U.B., A.L. and M.M.; methodology, D.A., U.B., A.L. and M.M.; validation, D.A., U.B., A.L. and M.M.; formal analysis, D.A., U.B., A.L. and M.M.; investigation, D.A., U.B., A.L. and M.M.; writing—original draft preparation, D.A.; writing—review and editing, D.A., U.B., A.L. and M.M.; visualization, D.A.; project administration, M.M. All authors have read and agreed to the published version of the manuscript.

Funding: This research received no external funding. EUROMENE received funding for networking activities from the COST programme (COST Action 15111), via the COST Association.

Institutional Review Board Statement: This study, as an "in-depth study of chronic fatigue syndrome (ME/CFS), and encouraging of a common approach in international scientific cooperation", was approved by the Research Ethics Committee of the Riga Stradins University (Decision No. 6-3/3 (25 October 2018, Riga) and Decision No. 6-1/05/33 (30 April 2020, Riga)) in the framework of the Latvian Science Council's Fundamental and Applied Research project No. lzp-2019/1-0380 "selection of biomarkers in ME/CFS for patient stratification and treatment surveillance/optimisation". Data from the Genome Database of Latvian Population was used in accordance with the Central Medical Ethics Committee's approval No. 01-29.1/5034 (23 September 2020, Riga).

Informed Consent Statement: Prospective respondents with ME/CFS read a detailed statement, which was accepted by the Research Ethics Committee of the Riga Stradins University (Decision No. 6-3/3, 25 October 2018, Riga), and response therefore indicates informed consent. The former COVID-19 patients' informed consent was obtained in accordance with the Central Medical Ethics Committee's (Latvia) approval No. 01-29.1/5034 (23 September 2020, Riga).

Data Availability Statement: The aggregated data of the ME/CFS survey are available on request from the Riga Stradins University. The former COVID-19 patients' survey data are available at the Latvian Biomedical Research and Study Centre.

Acknowledgments: The study was supported by the Latvian Science Council's Fundamental and Applied Research project No. lzp-2019/1-0380 "selection of biomarkers in ME/CFS for patient stratification and treatment surveillance/optimisation" and by the National Research Program's "COVID-19 consequences mitigation" project No. VPP-COVID-2020/1-0023 "clinical, biochemical, immunogenetic paradigms of COVID-19 infection, and their correlation with socio-demographic, aetiological, pathogenetic, diagnostic, therapeutically and prognostically relevant factors to be included in the guidelines". The Genome Database of Latvian Population, the Latvian Biomedical Research and Study Centre, is acknowledged for providing the former COVID-19 patients' survey data.

Conflicts of Interest: The authors declare no conflict of interest.

References

1. Pheby, D.F.H.; Araja, D.; Berkis, U.; Brenna, E.; Cullinan, J.; de Korwin, J.-D.; Gitto, L.; Hughes, D.A.; Hunter, R.M.; Trepel, D.; et al. The development of a consistent Europe-wide approach to investigating the economic impact of myalgic encephalomyelitis (ME/CFS): A report from the European Network on ME/CFS (EUROMENE). *Healthcare* **2020**, *8*, 88. [CrossRef]
2. Brenna, E.; Gitto, L. The economic burden of Chronic Fatigue Syndrome/Myalgic Encephalomyelitis (CFS/ME): An initial summary of the existing evidence and recommendations for further research. *Eur. J. Pers. Cent. Healthc.* **2017**, *5*, 413–420. [CrossRef]
3. Lim, E.-J.; Ahn, Y.-C.; Jang, E.-S.; Lee, S.-W.; Lee, S.-H.; Son, C.-G. Systematic review and meta-analysis of the prevalence of chronic fatigue syndrome/ myalgic encephalomyelitis (CFS/ME). *J. Transl. Med.* **2020**, *18*, 100. [CrossRef] [PubMed]
4. World Health Organisation Coronavirus (COVID-19) Dashboard with Vaccination Data, Confirmed Cases in Latvia, March 2020–May 2021. Available online: https://covid19.who.int/region/euro/country/lv (accessed on 2 June 2021).
5. World Health Organization. International Statistical Classification of Diseases and Related Health Problems 10th Revision. Available online: https://icd.who.int/browse10/2019/en (accessed on 16 March 2021).
6. Twisk, F. Myalgic Encephalomyelitis (ME) or What? An Operational Definition. *Diagnostics* **2018**, *8*, 64. [CrossRef]
7. Lim, E.-J.; Son, C.-G. Review of case definitions for myalgic encephalomyelitis/ chronic fatigue syndrome (ME/CFS). *J. Transl. Med.* **2020**, *18*, 289. [CrossRef]
8. Fukuda, K.; Straus, S.E.; Hickie, I.; Sharpe, M.; Dobbins, J.G.; Komaroff, A.L. The chronic fatigue syndrome: A comprehensive approach to its definition and study. *Ann. Intern. Med.* **1994**, *121*, 953–959. [CrossRef] [PubMed]
9. Holmes, G.P.; Kaplan, J.E.; Gantz, N.M.; Komaroff, A.L.; Schonberger, L.B.; Straus, S.E.; Jones, J.F.; Dubois, R.E.; Cunningham-Rundles, C.; Pahwa, S.; et al. Chronic fatigue syndrome: A working case definition. *Ann. Intern Med.* **1988**, *108*, 387–389. [CrossRef]
10. Lloyd, A.R.; Hickie, I.; Boughton, C.R.; Spencer, O.; Wakefield, D. Prevalence of chronic fatigue syndrome in an Australian population. *Med. J. Aust.* **1990**, *153*, 522–528. [CrossRef]
11. Sharpe, M.C.; Archard, L.C.; Banatvala, J.E.; Borysiewicz, L.K.; Clare, A.W.; David, A.; Edwards, R.H.; Hawlon, K.E.; Lambert, H.P.; Lane, R.J. A report–chronic fatigue syndrome: Guidelines for research. *J. R. Soc. Med.* **1991**, *84*, 118–121. [CrossRef] [PubMed]
12. Ramsay, A.M.; Dowsett, E.G. Myalgic Encephalomyelitis: Then and Now. In *Clinical and Scientific Basis of Myalgic Encephalomyelitis/Chronic Fatigue Syndrome*, 1st ed.; Hyde, B.M., Goldstein, J., Levine, P., Eds.; The Nightingale Research Foundation: Ottawa, ON, Canada, 1992; pp. 569–595. ISBN 978-0969566205.
13. Carruthers, B.M.; Van de Sande, M.I.; De Meirleir, K.L.; Klimas, N.G.; Broderick, G.; Mitchell, T.; Staines, D.; Powles, A.C.P.; Speight, N.; Vallings, R.; et al. Myalgic encephalomyelitis: International Consensus Criteria. *J. Intern. Med.* **2011**, *270*, 327–338. [CrossRef]
14. Carruthers, B.M.; Van de Sande, M.I. Myalgic Encephalomyelitis/Chronic Fatigue Syndrome: A Clinical Case Definition and Guidelines for Medical Practitioners. An Overview of the Canadian Consensus Document. The National Library of Canada, 2005. Available online: https://www.investinme.org/Documents/PDFdocuments/Canadian_ME_Overview_A4.pdf (accessed on 4 March 2021).
15. Institute of Medicine. Beyond Myalgic Encephalomyelitis/Chronic Fatigue Syndrome; Redefining an Illness. The National Academies Press, 2015. Available online: www.nap.edu (accessed on 12 February 2021).
16. Twisk, F.N.M. Myalgic Encephalomyelitis, Chronic Fatigue Syndrome, and Systemic Exertion Intolerance Disease: Three Distinct Clinical Entities. *Challenges* **2018**, *9*, 19. [CrossRef]
17. Germain, A.; Ruppert, D.; Levine, S.M.; Hanson, M.R. Prospective Biomarkers from Plasma Metabolomics of Myalgic Encephalomyelitis/Chronic Fatigue Syndrome Implicate Redox Imbalance in Disease Symptomatology. *Metabolites* **2018**, *8*, 90. [CrossRef]
18. Almenar-Pérez, E.; Sánchez-Fito, T.; Ovejero, T.; Nathanson, L.; Oltra, E. Impact of Polypharmacy on Candidate Biomarker miRNomes for the Diagnosis of Fibromyalgia and Myalgic Encephalomyelitis/Chronic Fatigue Syndrome: Striking Back on Treatments. *Pharmaceutics* **2019**, *11*, 126. [CrossRef]
19. Sweetman, E.; Noble, A.; Edgar, C.; Mackay, A.; Helliwell, A.; Vallings, R.; Ryan, M.; Tale, W. Current Research Provides Insight into the Biological Basis and Diagnostic Potential for Myalgic Encephalomyelitis/Chronic Fatigue Syndrome (ME/CFS). *Diagnostics* **2019**, *9*, 73. [CrossRef]
20. Scheibenbogen, C.; Freitag, H.; Blanco, J.; Capelli, E.; Lacerda, E.; Authier, J.; Meeus, M.; Castro Marrero, J.; Nora-Krukle, Z.; Oltra, E.; et al. The European ME/CFS Biomarker Landscape project: An initiative of the European network EUROMENE. *J. Transl. Med.* **2017**, *15*, 162. [CrossRef]
21. Pheby, D.F.H.; Araja, D.; Berkis, U.; Brenna, E.; Cullinan, J.; de Korwin, J.-D.; Gitto, L.; Hughes, D.A.; Hunter, R.M.; Trepel, D.; et al. A Literature Review of GP Knowledge and Understanding of ME/CFS: From the Socioeconomic Working Group of the European Network on ME/CFS (EUROMENE). *Medicina* **2021**, *57*, 7. [CrossRef]

22. Cullinan, J.; Pheby, D.; Araja, D.; Berkis, U.; Brenna, E.; de Korwin, J.-D.; Gitto, L.; Hughes, D.; Hunter, R.; Trepel, D.; et al. Perceptions of European ME/CFS Experts Concerning Knowledge and Understanding of ME/CFS among Primary Care Physicians in Europe: A Report from the European ME/CFS Research Network (EUROMENE). *Medicina* **2021**, *57*, 208. [CrossRef] [PubMed]
23. Brenna, E.; Araja, D.; Pheby, D.F.H. Comparative Survey of People with ME/CFS in Italy, Latvia, and the UK: A Report on behalf of the Socioeconomics Working Group of the European ME/CFS Research Network (EUROMENE). *Medicina* **2021**, *57*, 300. [CrossRef] [PubMed]
24. Haywood, K.L.; Staniszewska, S.; Sarah Chapman, S. Quality and acceptability of patient-reported outcome measures used in chronic fatigue syndrome/myalgic encephalomyelitis (CFS/ME): A systematic review. *Qual. Life. Res.* **2012**, *21*, 35–52. [CrossRef] [PubMed]
25. Kim, D.-Y.; Lee, J.-S.; Son, C.-G. Systematic Review of Primary Outcome Measurements for Chronic Fatigue Syndrome/Myalgic Encephalomyelitis (CFS/ME) in Randomized Controlled Trials. *J. Clin. Med.* **2020**, *9*, 3463. [CrossRef] [PubMed]
26. Araja, D.; Berkis, U.; Castro Marrero, J.; Ivanovs, A.; Krumina, A.; Lunga, A.; Murovska, M.; Svirskis, S.; Zalewski, P. Myalgic Encephalomyelitis/Chronic Fatigue Syndrome (ME/CFS) patients' engagement in outcome measuring and disease management through Information Technology. *ICHOM Congr. (Present.)* **2020**. [CrossRef]
27. Islam, M.F.; Cotler, J.; Jason, L.A. Post-viral fatigue and COVID-19: Lessons from past epidemics. *Fatigue Biomed. Health Behav.* **2020**, *8*, 61–69. [CrossRef]
28. Muller, A.E.; Tveito, K.; Bakken, I.J.; Flottorp, S.A.; Mjaaland, S.; Larun, L. Potential causal factors of CFS/ME: A concise and systematic scoping review of factors researched. *J. Transl. Med.* **2020**, *18*, 484. [CrossRef] [PubMed]
29. Cullinan, J.; Ní Chomhraí, O.; Kindlon, T.; Black, L.; Casey, B. Understanding the economic impact of myalgic encephalomyelitis/chronic fatigue syndrome in Ireland: A qualitative study [version 1; peer review: 2 approved]. *HRB Open Res.* **2020**, *3*, 88. [CrossRef]
30. Strayer, D.R.; Young, D.; Mitchell, W.M. Effect of disease duration in a randomized Phase III trial of rintatolimod, an immune modulator for Myalgic Encephalomyelitis/ Chronic Fatigue Syndrome. *PLoS ONE* **2020**, *15*, e0240403. [CrossRef]
31. Gaber, T. Assessment and management of post-COVID fatigue. *Prog. Neurol. Psychiatry* **2021**, *25*, 36–39. [CrossRef]
32. Friedman, K.J.; Murovska, M.; Pheby, D.F.H.; Zalewski, P. Our Evolving Understanding of ME/CFS. *Medicina* **2021**, *57*, 200. [CrossRef]
33. Halpin, S.J.; McIvor, C.; Whyatt, G.; Adams, A.; Harvey, O.; McLean, L.; Walshaw, C.; Kemp, S.; Corrado, J.; Singh, R.; et al. Postdischarge symptoms and rehabilitation needs in survivors of COVID-19 infection: A cross-sectional evaluation. *J. Med. Virol.* **2021**, *93*, 1013–1022. [CrossRef]
34. Simani, L.; Ramezani, M.; Darazam, I.A.; Sagharichi, M.; Aalipour, M.A.; Ghorbani, F.; Pakdaman, H. Prevalence and correlates of chronic fatigue syndrome and post-traumatic stress disorder after the outbreak of the COVID-19. *J. Neuro Virol.* **2021**. [CrossRef]
35. Townsend, L.; Moloney, D.; Finucane, C.; McCarthy, K.; Bergin, C.; Bannan, C.; Kenny, R.-A. Fatigue following COVID-19 infection is not associated with autonomic dysfunction. *PLoS ONE* **2021**, *16*, e0247280. [CrossRef]
36. Graham, E.L.; Clark, J.R.; Orban, Z.S.; Lim, P.H.; Szymanski, A.L.; Taylor, C.; DiBiase, R.M.; Jia, D.T.; Balabanov, R.; Ho, S.U.; et al. Persistent neurologic symptoms and cognitive dysfunction in non-hospitalized Covid-19 'long haulers'. *Ann. Clin. Transl. Neurol.* **2021**, *8*, 1073–1085. [CrossRef] [PubMed]
37. Toogood, P.L.; Clauw, D.J.; Phadke, S.; Hoffman, D. Myalgic encephalomyelitis/ chronic fatigue syndrome (ME/CFS): Where will the drugs come from? *Pharmacol. Res.* **2021**, *165*, 105465. [CrossRef] [PubMed]
38. Rovite, V.; Wolff-Sagi, Y.; Zaharenko, L.; Nikitina-Zake, L.; Grens, E.; Klovins, J. Genome Database of the Latvian Population (LGDB): Design, Goals, and Primary Results. *J. Epidemiol.* **2018**, *28*, 353–360.b. [CrossRef] [PubMed]
39. Close, S.; Marshall-Gradisnik, S.; Byrnes, J.; Smith, P.; Nghiem, S.; Staines, D. The Economic Impacts of Myalgic Encephalomyelitis/Chronic Fatigue Syndrome in an Australian Cohort. *Front. Public Health* **2020**, *8*, 420. [CrossRef] [PubMed]
40. Households' Disposable Income per Household Member, in 2019. Central Statistical Bureau (Republic of Latvia), 2020. Available online: https://www.csb.gov.lv/en/statistics/statistics-by-theme/social-conditions/household-budget/tables/iig040/households-disposable-income-euro-month (accessed on 12 February 2021).
41. Central Statistical Bureau of Latvia. Population in Latvia, at the Beginning of 2020. Available online: https://www.csb.gov.lv/en/statistics/statistics-by-theme/population/number-and-change/search-in-theme/2694 (accessed on 12 April 2021).
42. Pheby, D.F.H.; Araja, D.; Berkis, U.; Brenna, E.; Cullinan, J.; de Korwin, J.; Gitto, L.; Hughes, D.A.; Hunter, R.M.; Trepel, D.; et al. The Role of Prevention in Reducing the Economic Impact of ME/CFS in Europe: A Report from the Socioeconomics Working Group of the European Network on ME/CFS (EUROMENE). *Medicina* **2021**, *57*, 388. [CrossRef] [PubMed]

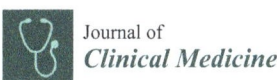

Article

Tolerability and Efficacy of s.c. IgG Self-Treatment in ME/CFS Patients with IgG/IgG Subclass Deficiency: A Proof-of-Concept Study

Carmen Scheibenbogen [1,2,*], Franziska Sotzny [1], Jelka Hartwig [1], Sandra Bauer [1], Helma Freitag [1], Kirsten Wittke [1], Wolfram Doehner [2,3], Nadja Scherbakov [2,3], Madlen Loebel [4] and Patricia Grabowski [1]

[1] Institute of Medical Immunology, Charité–Universitätsmedizin Berlin, Corporate Member of Freie Universität Berlin and Humboldt-Universität zu Berlin, Augustenburger Platz 1, 13353 Berlin, Germany; franziska.sotzny@charite.de (F.S.); jelka.hartwig@gmail.com (J.H.); sandra.bauer@charite.de (S.B.); helma.freitag@charite.de (H.F.); kirsten.wittke@charite.de (K.W.); patricia.grabowski@charite.de (P.G.)

[2] Berlin Institute of Health Center for Regenerative Therapies (BCRT), Charité–Universitätsmedizin Berlin, Corporate Member of Freie Universität Berlin and Humboldt-Universität zu Berlin, Augustenburger Platz 1, 13353 Berlin, Germany; wolfram.doehner@charite.de (W.D.); nadja.scherbakov@charite.de (N.S.)

[3] Center for Stroke Research Berlin, Charité–Universitätsmedizin Berlin, Corporate Member of Freie Universität Berlin and Humboldt-Universität zu Berlin, Augustenburger Platz 1, 13353 Berlin, Germany

[4] Research Center, Carl-Thiem-Klinikum Cottbus gGmbH, Thiemstraße 111, 03048 Cottbus, Germany; M.Loebel@ctk.de

* Correspondence: carmen.scheibenbogen@charite.de

Abstract: Background: Chronic fatigue syndrome (ME/CFS) is a complex disease frequently triggered by infections. IgG substitution may have therapeutic effect both by ameliorating susceptibility to infections and due to immunomodulatory effects. Methods: We conducted a proof of concept open trial with s.c. IgG in 17 ME/CFS patients suffering from recurrent infections and mild IgG or IgG subclass deficiency to assess tolerability and efficacy. Patients received s.c. IgG therapy of 0.8 g/kg/month for 12 months with an initial 2 months dose escalation phase of 0.2 g and 0.4 g/kg/month. Results: Primary outcome was improvement of fatigue assessed by Chalder Fatigue Scale (CFQ; decrease ≥ 6 points) and of physical functioning assessed by SF-36 (increase ≥ 25 points) at month 12. Of 12 patients receiving treatment per protocol 5 had a clinical response at month 12. Two additional patients had an improvement according to this definition at months 6 and 9. In four patients treatment was ceased due to adverse events and in one patient due to disease worsening. We identified LDH and soluble IL-2 receptor as potential biomarker for response. Conclusion: Our data indicate that self-administered s.c. IgG treatment is feasible and led to clinical improvement in a subset of ME/CFS patients.

Keywords: chronic fatigue syndrome; myalgic encephalomyelitis; autoimmunity; immunology; IgG replacement; IgG deficiency; biomarker

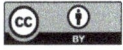

1. Introduction

Chronic Fatigue Syndrome (ME/CFS) is a frequent, severe and complex disease with an estimated prevalence of around 0.5% [1]. Patients suffer from sustained exhaustion accompanied by numerous physical and mental symptoms. ME/CFS onset is typically with an infection and many patients undergo frequently recurrent infections. The underlying pathological mechanism in ME/CFS is not known so far. However, there is ample evidence of dysregulation of the immune system, and both immune activation and deficiency can be found [2,3]. There is increasing evidence, that at least in a subset of ME/CFS patients, autoimmunity contributes to disease etiology [2,4]. Autoantibodies against various antigens including neurotransmitter receptors were reported by several groups (reviewed in [2]). First clinical trials showed that immunomodulatory treatments targeting autoantibodies are effective in a subset of ME/CFS patients [5–7].

Immunoglobulin G (IgG) treatment is effective in autoantibody-mediated autoimmune diseases [8]. Four randomized controlled clinical trials of intravenous (IV) IgG therapy with monthly doses ranging from 0.5 to 2 g/kg body weight were performed more than three decades ago in ME/CFS showing inconsistent results with two positive and two negative studies [9–13]. IgG substitution may have therapeutic effect in ME/CFS both by ameliorating susceptibility to infections and due to immunomodulatory effects.

ME/CFS patients frequently suffer from susceptibility to both viral and bacterial infections. Studies in our own and other patient cohorts show that IgG1 and IgG3 deficiency occurs frequently in ME/CFS patients [3,11,14]. Patients with immunoglobulin deficiency had more frequently an increased rate of infections, mostly of the respiratory tract [3,15].

Thus far, there has been little interest of pharmaceutical companies into clinical trials in ME/CFS presumably due to the complexity of the disease and paucity of knowledge. We thus performed an investigator-initiated trial to study the feasibility and efficacy of an intermediate dose self-administered s.c. IgG treatment in ME/CFS patients. An s.c. IgG treatment regimen was chosen due to better tolerability and possibility of self-administration. The IgG dose of 0.8 g/kg body weight/month was chosen which is the maximum dose recommended by European Medicines Agency (EMA) for IgG treatment of immunodeficient patients but is expected to be effective in autoimmunity as well [8]. Further, we decided to include ME/CFS patients with mild IgG or IgG subclass deficiency and frequent infections as this group of patients may benefit from both immunomodulatory and infection-preventing effect of IgG treatment [10].

Our study provides evidence that self-administered s.c. IgG treatment is feasible and tolerable and can lead to clinical improvement in a subset of ME/CFS patients.

2. Materials and Methods

2.1. Study Design

This was an investigator-initiated one arm trial with support from Baxalta, a member of the Takeda group of companies. HyQvia consists of human normal IgG (10%, Kiovig®, Takeda, Konstanz, Germany) and recombinant human hyaluronidase (rHuPH20, Hylenex®, Takeda, Konstanz, Germany). The clinical study protocol is provided in the supplement section (S1). HyQvia was given as s.c. infusion via the Freedom pump (RMS Medical Products, Chester, NY, USA). Following pretreatment with hyaluronidase up to 300 mL of HyQvia were infused s.c. The first infusion was given at our outpatient clinic and patients were trained for self-therapy. Further infusions were given as home therapy under supervision of a home care nurse. The following doses were given:

Month 1, day 0: total 0.2 g/kg body weight per month (one infusion).
Month 2: total 0.4 g/kg body weight per month (given as one or bi-weekly infusion).
Months 3–12: total 0.8 g/kg body weight per month (given as bi-weekly infusion).

The primary objective of this study was to determine the effect of an intermediate dose of s.c. IgG on patient fatigue and physical functioning as assessed by the Chalder Fatigue Scale (CFQ) and SF-36, physical function domain, respectively. A clinical meaningful response was defined by an improvement of at least 50% of symptoms in the Chalder Fatigue Scale between the first visit and the 12-month follow-up visit. For this an improvement in at least 6 of the 11 items for minimum of one point improvement is required. It means that the composite score decreases by at least 6 points between enrollment and 12-months follow-up. For the SF-36 physical functioning, a clinically meaningful response is defined by an improvement of at least 50% of symptoms, thus the patient scores better in at least 5 of the 10 items between study enrollment and the 12-month follow-up. It means that the composite score increases by at least 25 points between enrollment and 12-months follow-up. The response analysis included only patients receiving the complete 12-months treatment.

Secondary study objectives were to assess the tolerability of HyQvia in patients with ME/CFS, to assess the frequency and severity of infections, to identify markers for response, to assess additional symptoms by scoring the symptoms of Canadian Consensus Criteria

(CCC) and COMPASS-31 and the suitability of step tracking and endothelial function as objective response parameters. Our study was designed in such a way that we wanted to obtain first evidence for efficacy as a prerequisite for a consecutive randomized placebo-controlled trial. Efficacy was defined as seeing a response in at least 5 of 15 patients included in the study. Patients receiving less than 3 months of treatment had to be replaced. Regular site monitoring visits were performed by the Clinical Research Organization GWT, Dresden. The trial was registered at www.clinicaltrialsregister.eu. EudraCT 2016-002370-12.

2.2. Patients

ME/CFS patients were selected who were diagnosed at the outpatient clinic for immunodeficiencies at the Institute of Medical Immunology at the Charité Universitätsmedizin Berlin (Berlin, Germany) and fulfilled the inclusion criteria. In order to obtain an unselected patient sample, all consecutive patients who are eligible for participation and willing to participate were included. The flow chart of participant disposition is shown as Figure 1. Diagnosis of ME/CFS was based on CCC [16] and exclusion of other medical or neurological diseases, which may cause fatigue. Further inclusion criteria were IgG or IgG subclass deficiency with a history of a serious bacterial or recurrent infections (≥ 4 infections during the last year prior to inclusion), and a disease severity according to the Bell scale of ≤ 50 of 100 [17]. However, in none of the patients IgG deficiency and infection history were severe enough for having an indication for IgG substitution (IgG > 5 g/l and none had IgA or IgM deficiency). It was planned to include 15 patients in the trial and replace patients receiving less than 3 months of treatment. All 17 patients who were approached agreed to participate in the trial.

2.3. Assessment of Symptoms and Physical Functioning by Scores

Questionnaires were filled in by the patients at home and validated by the treating physicians together with the patients. Disease severity was determined before and after the 12 months IgG treatment by Bell scale with a score of 0 being equivalent to severest ME/CFS and a score of 100 being healthy. ME/CFS symptoms and physical functioning were further assessed by questionnaires: CFQ, SF-36 physical functioning, COMPASS-31 and CCC symptom scoring, at baseline, then monthly and up to 3 months after the IgG treatment. CFQ evaluates the extent and severity of fatigue assessing fatigue with 0 (healthy) to 33 (severe) [18]. SF-36 (Medical Outcome Study 36-Item Short Form Health Survey) measures health-related quality of life, with a score of 0 being equivalent to maximal disability and a score of 100 being healthy. COMPASS-31 questionnaire assesses autonomic symptoms with a score from 0 (healthy) to 100 (severe) [19]. The severity of symptoms was assessed based on quantification of CCC symptoms using a questionnaire developed by Fluge et al. [20]. Symptoms were classified according to a scale from 1 (no symptoms) to 10 (severe symptoms). The fatigue score was calculated as the mean of fatigue, malaise after exertion, need for rest and daily functioning, cognitive score as mean of memory disturbance, concentration ability and mental tiredness and immune score as mean of painful lymph nodes, sore throat and flu-like symptoms.

2.4. Laboratory Values

Standard laboratory parameters were assessed at the Charité diagnostics laboratory Labor Berlin GmbH (Berlin, Germany). Antibodies against ß2 adrenergic and M3 muscarinic acetylcholine receptors were determined by CellTrend GmbH (Luckenwalde, Germany) using ELISA technology.

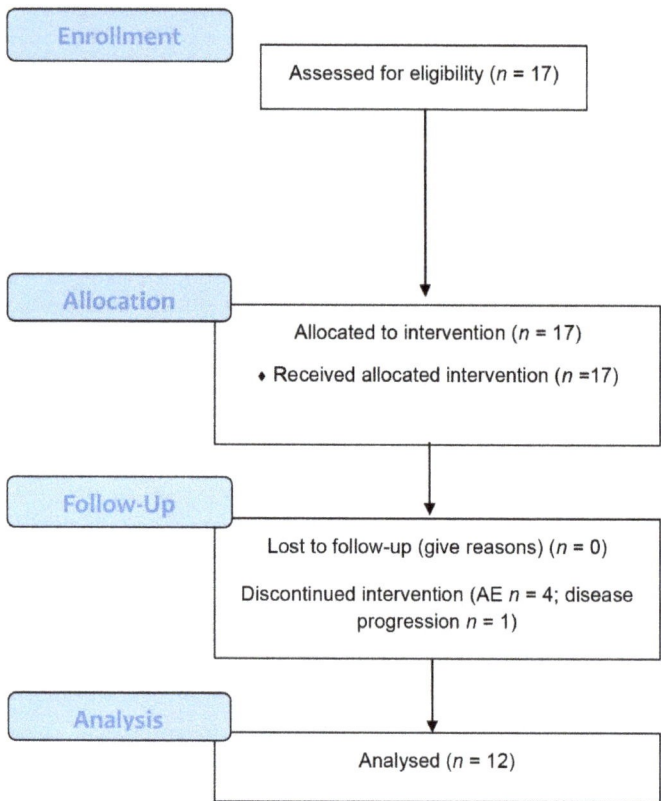

Figure 1. Flow chart of participant disposition. AE = adverse events.

2.5. Functional Assessment

Peripheral endothelial function was evaluated by a pulse arterial tonometry (PAT) device (EndoPAT-2000, Itamar, Israel). Measurement was performed under standardized conditions after at least 15 min of supine rest in a quiet, air-conditioned room. Endothelial dysfunction was defined by reactive hyperemia index (RHI) ≤1.8 as described previously [21]. Steps were counted by a Vivofit® activity tracker (Garmin, Germany). Mean daily number of steps was counted during one week before and after every 3 months for 15 months. Staff members performing these assessments were not involved in implementing any aspect of the intervention.

2.6. Statistical Analysis

Statistical data analyses were done using the software GraphPad Prism 6.0 for Windows, GraphPad Software, La Jolla California USA, www.graphpad.com. Continuous variables were expressed as median and interquartile range (IQR). Univariate comparison of two independent groups was performed using the Mann–Whitney-U test, comparison of two dependent groups was done using the Wilcoxon matched-pairs signed-rank test. A two-tailed *p*-value of <0.05 was considered statistically significant.

3. Results

3.1. Patients and Treatment

A total of 17 ME/CFS patients with a mild IgG or IgG subclass deficiency, but no indication for IgG substitution, were included in this trial (Figure 1). Patient characteristics are summarized in Table 1 (for details see Table S1). The mean age was 46 years, 9 patients were female and 12 patients had an infection-triggered onset. We retrospectively collected the data of the types of infection from the patients records (Table S1). Most patients reported a respiratory tract infection or primary EBV as trigger of disease. At baseline all patients had a Bell score ≤ 50. In 4 of 17 patients physicians decided to cease treatment due to adverse events as described below. In one patient treatment was discontinued at month 3 due to disease worsening (P12). A total of 12 patients received the scheduled 12-months treatment.

Table 1. Patient characteristics.

	Study Cohort (n = 17)
sex (f/m)	9/8
age in years (median (range))	46 (18–70)
age at disease onset in years (median (range))	36 (15–61)
Bell score (median (range))	30 (20–50)
infection-triggered onset	n = 12

3.2. Tolerability

Patients' adverse events are listed in Table S2. Two patients (P1, P14) received only one or two injections and were replaced (Tables S1 and S2). Patient 1 had injection-related grade 3 headache and received only two IgG injections. Patient 14 had a grade 2 injection site reaction with an erythema of approx. 10 cm after the first IgG injection. Treatment was not continued as the patient refused to come into the outpatient clinic for the next injection due to multiple chemical sensitivity. In two patients treatment was ceased at months 3 and 6 due to adverse events (P3, P15). In patient 15 treatment was stopped at month 3 due to elevation grade 3 of the liver enzymes ALT/AST. Pretreatment ALT/AST were normal. A total of 4 weeks after cessation values had returned to grade 1. In patient P3 treatment was not continued at month 6 due to recurrent grade 2 local reaction, flu-like symptoms, headache, and abdominal pain.

In the 12 patients receiving the 12 months treatment 4 patients reported recurrent grade 2 and 2 patients grade 1 headache after injections. In three patients we observed a transient grade 1 increase in the ALT (at month 3, 6 and 9, respectively). P11 had recurrent grade 2 erythematous injection site reaction from month 9 on. All patients had mostly grade 1 flu-like symptoms and injection-site reaction.

3.3. Clinical Treatment Response

A total of 12 patients received IgG treatment per protocol for 12 months. The overall response in all 12 patients showed significantly decreased fatigue (measured by CFQ) and increased physical functioning (measured by SF-36) at months 6, 9 and 12, but not after the dose escalation phase at month 3 (Figure 2a,b). According to the primary response definition five of these patients (P2, 9, 11, 13, 16) had a clinical response with a decrease of at least six points in the CFQ and/or an increase of 25 points in the SF-36 physical functioning at month 12 compared to pretreatment (Figure 2c,d). Two additional patients did fulfill the primary response definition at months 6 and 9 but not at month 12 (P4, 8) (Figure 2c,d). 3 months following cessation of IgG treatment (month 15) physical functioning decreased and fatigue increased again (Figure 2a,b). As expected, we observed a close correlation between fatigue assessed by CFQ and physical functioning assessed by SF-36 ($r = -0.64$; $p = 0.02$). CFQ and SF36 of the three patients ceasing treatment at months 3 (P12, P15) and month 6 (P3) are shown in Figure S1.

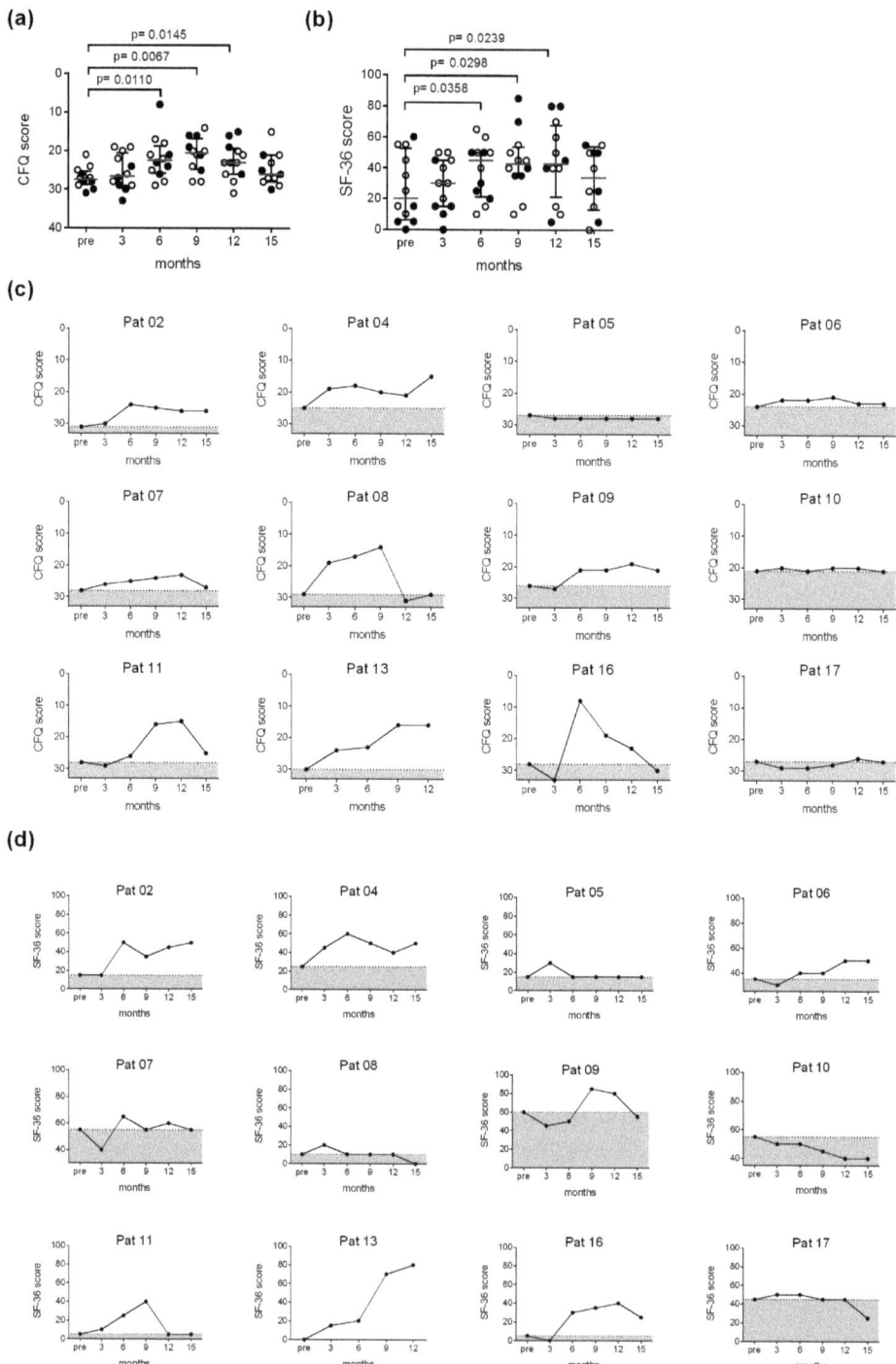

Figure 2. (a) The Chalder Fatigue Scale (CFQ) and the (b) SF-36 physical functioning of all patients receiving 12 months of treatment before (pre), during (months 3–12) and 3 months after the treatment (month 15) is shown. An overall significant

improvement of the fatigue (CFQ) and physical functioning (SF-36) during the IgG treatment was observed (responder indicated as filled circles). A two-tailed Wilcoxon matched-pairs signed-rank test was performed for statistical analysis. The course of individual patients is shown in (**c**) for CFQ and (**d**) for SF-36. (CFQ Score, healthy: 0; SF-36 Score, healthy: 100).

As a secondary outcome parameter, severity of various symptoms was assessed. In the 12 patients receiving the 12 months IgG treatment an overall significant improvement in the severity of cognitive symptoms and immune symptoms could be observed at months 6, 9 and 12 (Figure S2a,b). Improvement of the immune symptoms was already evident at month 3 and remained post IgG treatment at month 15. Muscle pain showed no overall improvement (Figure S2c). The course of symptoms in the individual patients is shown in Figure S2e.

All patients reported moderate to severe symptoms of autonomic dysfunction assessed by the COMPASS-31 questionnaire at baseline (median 50.9, range 12.9–73.8). Again an overall significant improvement of autonomic nervous system function from baseline to months 6 (median 37.14, range 6.99–60.06) and 9 (median 36.05, range 20.16–54.72) was observed (Figure S2d,f).

3.4. Functional Assessment

We tried to objectively assess symptoms by measuring endothelial cell function and daily steps as secondary outcome parameter. The numbers of steps were assessed for a week each month by a Vivofit® activity tracker (Garmin, Germany). Patient 9 could not be evaluated because the tracker of the pretreatment evaluation was lost. All responding patients at month 12 (patients 2, 11, 13 and 16) and also patients 4 and 8 with a response at month 6 and 9 walked more steps during IgG treatment (steps/day pretreatment: median 4565, range 1062–7756; at months 6: median 6067, range 3017–10411; $p = 0.0313$, Figure S3). The number of steps in the five non-responder patients (patients 5, 6, 7, 10, 17) did not increase. There was no seasonal variation in numbers of steps.

A subset of patients with ME/CFS has endothelial dysfunction [22,23]. Endothelial dysfunction defined as a diminished RHI < 1.8 was found pretreatment in 6 of 11 patients receiving 12 months of treatment. At month 15 we observed improvement of endothelial function in six of eight patients (Figure S4). No correlation of pre- or posttreatment endothelial function with clinical response was observed.

3.5. Infections

In the 12 months before initiation of IgG treatment a median of six (range 4–12) mostly respiratory tract infections were reported by the patients. During the 12 months IgG treatment period 11 of 12 patients documented infections to occur less frequently and/or milder with a median of 3.5 (range 0–6) infections (Figure 3, $p = 0.002$).

3.6. Assessment of Potential Biomarkers for Response and Tolerability

In the 12 patients receiving IgG treatment for 12 months we compared demographic and clinical data and laboratory values between the five responders and seven non-responders. There was no obvious difference in age, sex, Bell score and disease duration (Table S1) nor in SF-36, CFQ, COMPASS-31 and symptom scores regarding treatment response (Figure S5). There was also no difference in these parameters when patients 4 and 8 with response at months 6 and 9 were included into the responder group. All responder had an infection-triggered onset. The five patients with a non-infectious disease onset included two patients (P1 and P3) not tolerating treatment, two non-responders and P12 in whom treatment was discontinued due to disease worsening at month 6 (Table S1).

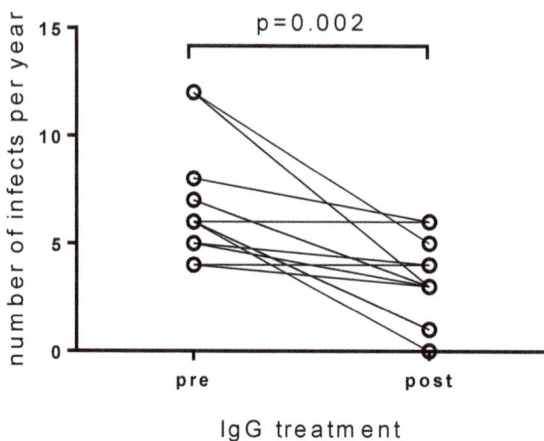

Figure 3. Numbers of infections per year in the 12 months before (pre) and 12 months after (post) initiation of IgG treatment are shown. Numbers of infections significantly decreased during the IgG treatment. A two-tailed Wilcoxon matched-pairs signed-rank test was performed for statistical analysis.

We compared number of leukocytes, lymphocytes, erythrocytes, IgG and IgG subclass levels, CRP level, ANA and levels of several potential disease biomarkers (LDH, CK, soluble IL-2 receptor, IL-8, β2 AdR and M3 AchR AAB and soluble CD26) pretreatment but observed no significant differences between responders and non-responders (Table S3). We observed, however, a trend of a higher pretreatment LDH level and lower soluble IL-2 receptor sCD25 in responders. When we included patients 4 and 8 with a response at months 6 and 9 in the responder group, responders had a significantly higher baseline serum LDH level compared to non-responders (Figure 4a). LDH levels did not decrease in the total patient cohort at month 3 during the dose escalation phase but from month 6 on (at month 9 p = 0.0137, Figure 4b). Further pretreatment values of the soluble IL-2 receptor were significantly lower in responder patients including patients 4 and 8 than in non-responders (Figure 4c). LDH and soluble IL-2 receptor did neither correlate with each other nor with disease severity or symptoms. IgG levels during treatment increased from median 8.5 g/L to maximum median 15.4 g/L at month 9 (Figure 4d). IgG and IgG subclass levels pretreatment did not correlate with response to treatment (Table S3). In the study by Lloyd et al. higher lymphocyte count pretreatment was associated with response to IgG treatment. Here, we could not confirm this observation (Table S3) [10].

When comparing patients not tolerating treatment to those receiving 12 months of treatment we observed no differences in clinical parameters. Interestingly, we observed a lower level of the biomarker sCD26 in the five patients who did not tolerate treatment or had early disease worsening compared to patients who completed IgG treatment (Figure 4e).

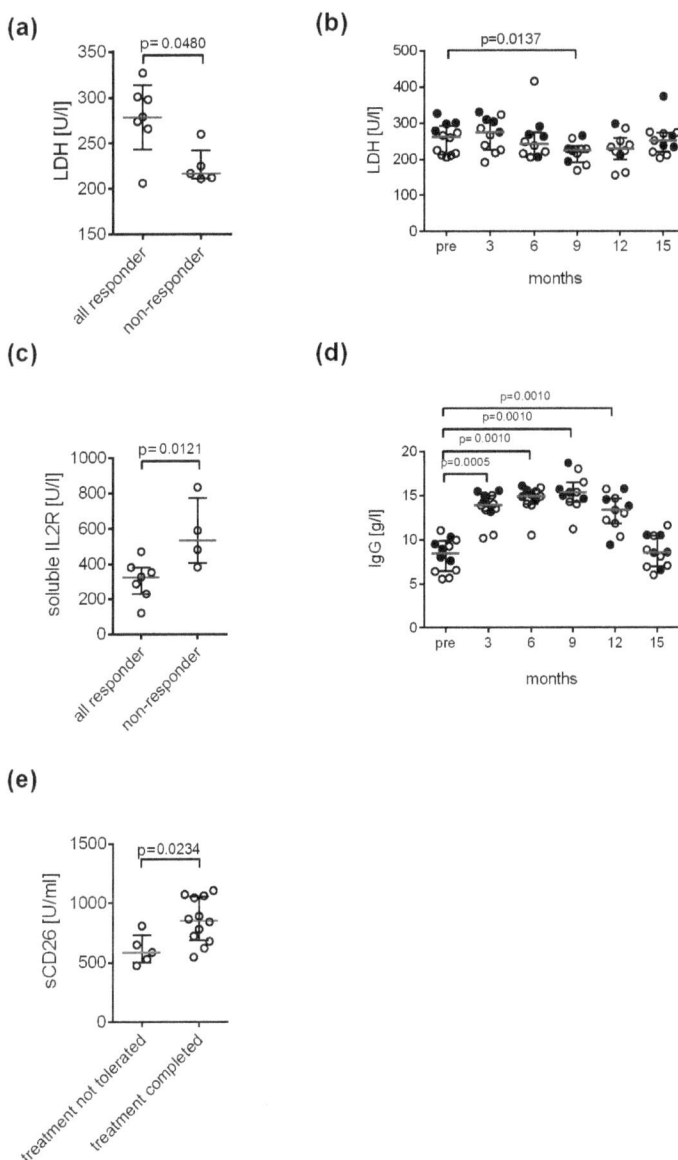

Figure 4. Association of biomarker with response and tolerability. Median and interquartile range pretreatment level of (**a**) LDH and (**c**) the soluble IL-2 receptor of responding patients including patients with a response at month 6 and 9 ($n = 7$) compared to non-responders ($n = 5$) are shown. Responder had significant higher LDH and lower soluble IL-2 receptor pretreatment level. Two tailed Mann–Whitney-U test was performed for statistical analysis. Median and interquartile range (**b**) LDH level and (**d**) IgG level of the patients before (pre), during (months 3–12) and 3 months after the treatment (month 15) are shown (responder indicated as filled circles). A two-tailed Wilcoxon matched-pairs signed-rank test was performed for statistical analysis. (**e**) Median and interquartile range of sCD26 level of patients not tolerating treatment ($n = 5$) compared to those receiving 12 months of treatment ($n = 12$) are plotted. Participants who did not tolerate the treatment had significant lower sCD26 levels. Two tailed Mann–Whitney-U test was performed for statistical analysis.

4. Discussion

In this study we provide evidence that self-administered s.c. IgG treatment is feasible and improved symptoms and physical functioning in a subset of ME/CFS patients with a mild IgG or IgG subclass deficiency. Our results are in line with previous randomized controlled clinical trials (RCT) studies.

Four RCTs of IV immunoglobulin replacement therapy with monthly doses ranging from 0.5–2 g/kg body weight were performed more than three decades ago with two positive and two negative studies [9–13]. In the positive Australian study by Lloyd et al. 10 of 23 (43%) patients receiving IV IgG 2 g/kg on a monthly basis for 3 months but only three of the 26 (12%) placebo recipients responded with a substantial reduction in their symptoms and recommencement of work and activities [10]. In the negative follow-up four-arm study with 99 patients receiving one of three doses of immunoglobulin (0.5, 1, or 2 g/kg) or a placebo solution (1% albumin), all patients showed a similar improvement in their functional capacity [12]. In the other positive study by Rowe et al. in which 71 adolescents received either three infusions of 1 g/kg given one month apart or 1% albumin, both groups had an improved functional score, which was significantly higher in the IgG treated patients at 6 months [13]. In the negative US study Peterson et al. had treated 28 patients in a RCT with IV IgG 1 g/kg or placebo [11]. Both patient groups reported improved health perception. Taken together, improvement of IgG treated patients was reported in all four trials, but also in the placebo group in two of these four trials. This is in line with the results of the recently published multicenter RCT Rituximab study performed in Norway in which around a third of patients reported improvement in both the rituximab and the placebo infusion group [24]. Response definition was, however, less strict, with fatigue improvement for 8 consecutive weeks over a period of 24 months.

How should these findings be translated into a future clinical IgG study in ME/CFS? Our study was designed to observe efficacy in at least 5 of 15 patients as a prerequisite for a consecutive randomized placebo-controlled trial. According to the primary response definition we reached this aim with 5 of 15 patients receiving at least 3 months of treatment having a clinical response. A dose-escalation phase can help in a consecutive randomized placebo-controlled trial to control for placebo effects. In the 12 patients receiving 12 months of treatment we observed overall significantly improved CFQ and SF-36 scores at months 6, 9 and 12, but not after the dose escalation phase at month 3. Objective parameters of response would be desirable in a consecutive randomized placebo-controlled trial. We evaluated the suitability of step counting in our response assessment and observed an increase in number of steps in responder but not non-responder patients.

Further, it is important to implement biomarker for response. IgG deficiency and higher lymphocyte counts were associated with response to treatment in the study by Lloyd et al. [10]. In our study, IgG or IgG subclass deficiency was an inclusion criterion and lymphocyte counts were similar between responders and non-responders. We studied several immune and metabolic biomarkers which were shown to be altered in a subgroup of ME/CFS patients in previous studies [25–28]. Evidence from our study suggests that pretreatment elevated LDH and lower soluble IL-2 receptor levels are a potential response marker. Further we observed a significant decrease in LDH during IgG treatment. How could this be explained? The LDH is an enzyme catalyzing the conversion of pyruvate to lactate and may indicate a preferential energy production via glycolysis rather than the more efficient oxidative phosphorylation as described in ME/CFS [29]. This may result in impaired function of immune cells and lower soluble IL-2 receptor levels, too. Thus, the elevated LDH and lower soluble IL-2 receptor levels may be biomarkers for an impaired metabolism in ME/CFS.

What are the potential mechanisms of IgG treatment in ME/CFS? The infection control by IgG is one possibility as many ME/CFS patients suffer from frequent and long-lasting infections which frequently result in disease aggravation [3]. IgG deficiency is associated with more infections and is frequent in ME/CFS and was reported also in approximately half of the patients in the studies by Lloyd and Peterson [11,12]. IgG deficiency was associated with response to treatment in the study by Lloyd. Therefore, we included in our study only patients with mild IgG or IgG subclass deficiency and recurrent infections. Patients reported less frequent and milder infections during IgG treatment, which may have an effect on amelioration of disease severity. IgG in a dose of 0.8 g/kg body weight s.c. can, however, have immunomodulatory effects as well and it is well known that IgG treatment is effective in autoantibody-mediated autoimmune diseases. There is evidence that infection-triggered ME/CFS is an autoimmune disease [2]. In line with this notion all responder in our study had an infection-triggered onset. In three of the previous RCT studies information on the type of onset is provided with the majority of patients reporting an infection-triggered onset (76–97%) [10–12]; however, the authors did not provide information if this had an impact on response. There is evidence of clinical efficacy of other immunomodulatory treatments targeting autoantibodies in ME/CFS including previous rituximab trials with a dose of 500 mg/m^2, immunoadsorption, and endoxan [5–7]. A total of 3 months following cessation of IgG treatment physical functioning assessed by SF-36 decreased again. Remission times of IgG treatment in autoimmune diseases can be short [8]. Thus, it would be desirable to treat ME/CFS patients for more than 12 months with IgG in a consecutive study.

Treatment with s.c. IgG is usually well tolerated in primary immunodeficiency (PID) [30]. Compared to PID patients we observed side-effects to occur frequently in patients with ME/CFS including headaches and liver enzyme elevations. This is in line with the study by Lloyd et al. who reported that constitutional symptoms occurred with 53 of the 65 IgG (82%) but only 19 of the 78 placebo infusions (24%) [10]. Transient elevation of ALT levels developed in eight IgG recipients but only one placebo recipient [10]. Similarly, in the study by Peterson et al. headaches were reported more frequently in the IgG group [11]. Thus, a higher frequency of adverse events should be taken into account when treating patients with ME/CFS with IgG.

We observed diminished sCD26 to be associated with intolerability of IgG treatment and early disease deterioration. sCD26 was reported in two previous studies to be diminished in a subset of ME/CF patients [25,31]. sCD26 or sDPP4 is well known as an enzyme cleaving glucagon, but also various immune mediators including chemokines and bradykinin [32,33]. It may well be that diminished levels of sCD26 are associated with elevated levels of such immune mediators which may result in more side effects of IgG therapy. Several patients reported better tolerability of the infusions with improvement of their ME/CFS symptoms during treatment. Similarly, more than the expected number of side-effects were observed in the rituximab trial [24].

5. Conclusions

Taken together, our study has several limitations, including a small patient number and a lack of a control arm. The strength of this study is to show the feasibility of a dose escalation s.c. IgG home treatment in ME/CFS patients. Furthermore, it provides first evidence for efficacy of an intermediate dose s.c. IgG treatment and potential biomarkers for response. This warrants an RCT study.

Supplementary Materials: The following are available online at https://www.mdpi.com/article/10.3390/jcm10112420/s1. S1: Clinical study protocol, Table S1: Patient characteristics and treatment response, Table S2: Adverse events, Table S3: Laboratory values pretreatment, Figure S1: CFQ and the SF-36 data of patients 3 and 6, Figure S2: Symptoms of patients during s.c. IgG therapy, Figure S3: Daily steps assessed by Activity tracking, Figure S4: The reactive hyperemia index (RHI) assessed by Endopat, Figure S5: Comparative analysis of pretreatment symptoms of responder vs. non-responder.

Author Contributions: Conceptualization, C.S., K.W., M.L. and P.G.; methodology, C.S.; software, N.S.; validation, H.F., P.G. and C.S., formal analysis, F.S. and J.H.; investigation, C.S., P.G., S.B., N.S., F.S. and H.F.; resources N.S.; data curation, F.S., S.B. and J.H.; writing—original draft preparation, F.S. and C.S.; writing—review and editing, F.S., W.D. and KW; visualization, C.S. and F.S.; supervision,

C.S.; project administration, C.S., K.W. and P.G.; funding acquisition, C.S. All authors have read and agreed to the published version of the manuscript.

Funding: This investigator-initiated trial was supported by a grant from Baxalta, US Inc a member of the Takeda group of companies (grant ID number BT13-21454). The Weidenhammer Zöbele foundation provided personal support.

Institutional Review Board Statement: The study was conducted according to the guidelines of the Declaration of Helsinki, and approved by the Local Ethics Committee (Landesamt für Gesundheit und Soziales, Berlin) and PEI (Paul-Ehrlich Institute) (protocol code IMI2016-2, date of approval 25.1.2017).

Informed Consent Statement: Informed consent was obtained from all subjects involved in the study.

Data Availability Statement: The data presented in this study are available on reasonable request from the corresponding author.

Acknowledgments: The authors thank RMS Medical Products for generously providing the infusion pumps.

Conflicts of Interest: C.S. and K.W. received speaker honoraria from Baxalta/Takeda. P.G., M.A., F.S., J.H., H.F., M.L., S.B., N.S. and W.D. have no conflicts of interest to declare. The funders had no role in the design of the study; in the collection, analyses, or interpretation of data; in the writing of the manuscript, or in the decision to publish the results. M.L. is an employee of "Carl-Thiem-Klinikum Cottbus gGmbH". None of the authors has a conflict of interest with 'Carl-Thiem-Klinikum Cottbus gGmbH'.

References

1. Valdez, A.R.; Hancock, E.E.; Adebayo, S.; Kiernicki, D.J.; Proskauer, D.; Attewell, J.R.; Bateman, L.; DeMaria, A., Jr.; Lapp, C.W.; Rowe, P.C.; et al. Estimating Prevalence, Demographics, and Costs of ME/CFS Using Large Scale Medical Claims Data and Machine Learning. *Front. Pediatr.* **2018**, *6*, 412. [CrossRef] [PubMed]
2. Sotzny, F.; Blanco, J.; Capelli, E.; Castro-Marrero, J.; Steiner, S.; Murovska, M.; Scheibenbogen, C.; European Network on ME/CFS (EUROMENE). Myalgic Encephalomyelitis/Chronic Fatigue Syndrome—Evidence for an autoimmune disease. *Autoimmun. Rev.* **2018**, *17*, 601–609. [CrossRef] [PubMed]
3. Guenther, S.; Loebel, M.; Mooslechner, A.A.; Knops, M.; Hanitsch, L.G.; Grabowski, P.; Wittke, K.; Meisel, C.; Unterwalder, N.; Volk, H.D.; et al. Frequent IgG subclass and mannose binding lectin deficiency in patients with chronic fatigue syndrome. *Hum. Immunol.* **2015**, *76*, 729–735. [CrossRef] [PubMed]
4. Steiner, S.; Becker, S.C.; Hartwig, J.; Sotzny, F.; Lorenz, S.; Bauer, S.; Lobel, M.; Stittrich, A.B.; Grabowski, P.; Scheibenbogen, C. Autoimmunity-Related Risk Variants in PTPN22 and CTLA4 Are Associated With ME/CFS With Infectious Onset. *Front. Immunol.* **2020**, *11*, 578. [CrossRef]
5. Fluge, O.; Bruland, O.; Risa, K.; Storstein, A.; Kristoffersen, E.K.; Sapkota, D.; Naess, H.; Dahl, O.; Nyland, H.; Mella, O. Benefit from B-lymphocyte depletion using the anti-CD20 antibody rituximab in chronic fatigue syndrome. A double-blind and placebo-controlled study. *PLoS ONE* **2011**, *6*, e26358. [CrossRef]
6. Scheibenbogen, C.; Loebel, M.; Freitag, H.; Krueger, A.; Bauer, S.; Antelmann, M.; Doehner, W.; Scherbakov, N.; Heidecke, H.; Reinke, P.; et al. Immunoadsorption to remove ss2 adrenergic receptor antibodies in Chronic Fatigue Syndrome CFS/ME. *PLoS ONE* **2018**, *13*, e0193672. [CrossRef]
7. Rekeland, I.G.; Fossa, A.; Lande, A.; Ktoridou-Valen, I.; Sorland, K.; Holsen, M.; Tronstad, K.J.; Risa, K.; Alme, K.; Viken, M.K.; et al. Intravenous Cyclophosphamide in Myalgic Encephalomyelitis/Chronic Fatigue Syndrome. An Open-Label Phase II Study. *Front. Med.* **2020**, *7*, 162. [CrossRef]
8. Perez, E.E.; Orange, J.S.; Bonilla, F.; Chinen, J.; Chinn, I.K.; Dorsey, M.; El-Gamal, Y.; Harville, T.O.; Hossny, E.; Mazer, B.; et al. Update on the use of immunoglobulin in human disease: A review of evidence. *J. Allergy Clin. Immunol.* **2017**, *139*, S1–S46. [CrossRef]
9. Whiting, P.; Bagnall, A.M.; Sowden, A.J.; Cornell, J.E.; Mulrow, C.D.; Ramirez, G. Interventions for the treatment and management of chronic fatigue syndrome: A systematic review. *JAMA* **2001**, *286*, 1360–1368. [CrossRef]
10. Lloyd, A.; Hickie, I.; Wakefield, D.; Boughton, C.; Dwyer, J. A double-blind, placebo-controlled trial of intravenous immunoglobulin therapy in patients with chronic fatigue syndrome. *Am. J. Med.* **1990**, *89*, 561–568. [CrossRef]
11. Peterson, P.K.; Shepard, J.; Macres, M.; Schenck, C.; Crosson, J.; Rechtman, D.; Lurie, N. A controlled trial of intravenous immunoglobulin G in chronic fatigue syndrome. *Am. J. Med.* **1990**, *89*, 554–560. [CrossRef]
12. Vollmer-Conna, U.; Hickie, I.; Hadzi-Pavlovic, D.; Tymms, K.; Wakefield, D.; Dwyer, J.; Lloyd, A. Intravenous immunoglobulin is ineffective in the treatment of patients with chronic fatigue syndrome. *Am. J. Med.* **1997**, *103*, 38–43. [CrossRef]
13. Rowe, K.S. Double-blind randomized controlled trial to assess the efficacy of intravenous gammaglobulin for the management of chronic fatigue syndrome in adolescents. *J. Psychiatr. Res.* **1997**, *31*, 133–147. [CrossRef]

14. Wakefield, D.; Lloyd, A.; Brockman, A. Immunoglobulin subclass abnormalities in patients with chronic fatigue syndrome. *Pediatr. Infect. Dis. J.* **1990**, *9*, S50–S53. [CrossRef]
15. Lobel, M.; Mooslechner, A.A.; Bauer, S.; Gunther, S.; Letsch, A.; Hanitsch, L.G.; Grabowski, P.; Meisel, C.; Volk, H.D.; Scheibenbogen, C. Polymorphism in COMT is associated with IgG3 subclass level and susceptibility to infection in patients with chronic fatigue syndrome. *J. Transl. Med.* **2015**, *13*, 264. [CrossRef]
16. Carruthers, B.M.; Jain, A.K.; De Meirleir, K.L. Myalgic encephalomyelitis/chronic fatigue syndrome: Clinical working case definition, diagnostic and treatment protocols. *J. Chronic Fatigue Syndr.* **2003**, *11*, 7–115. [CrossRef]
17. Bell, D.S. *The Doctor's Guide to Chronic Fatigue Syndrome: Understanding, Treating, and Living with Cfids*; Da Capo Press: Cambridge, MA, USA, 1995.
18. Chalder, T.; Berelowitz, G.; Pawlikowska, T.; Watts, L.; Wessely, S.; Wright, D.; Wallace, E.P. Development of a fatigue scale. *J. Psychosom. Res.* **1993**, *37*, 147–153. [CrossRef]
19. Sletten, D.M.; Suarez, G.A.; Low, P.A.; Mandrekar, J.; Singer, W. COMPASS 31: A refined and abbreviated Composite Autonomic Symptom Score. *Mayo Clin. Proc.* **2012**, *87*, 1196–1201. [CrossRef]
20. Fluge, O.; Risa, K.; Lunde, S.; Alme, K.; Rekeland, I.G.; Sapkota, D.; Kristoffersen, E.K.; Sorland, K.; Bruland, O.; Dahl, O.; et al. B-Lymphocyte Depletion in Myalgic Encephalopathy/Chronic Fatigue Syndrome. An Open-Label Phase II Study with Rituximab Maintenance Treatment. *PLoS ONE* **2015**, *10*, e0129898. [CrossRef]
21. Scherbakov, N.; Sandek, A.; Martens-Lobenhoffer, J.; Kung, T.; Turhan, G.; Liman, T.; Ebinger, M.; von Haehling, S.; Bode-Boger, S.M.; Endres, M.; et al. Endothelial dysfunction of the peripheral vascular bed in the acute phase after ischemic stroke. *Cerebrovasc. Dis.* **2012**, *33*, 37–46. [CrossRef]
22. Newton, J.L.; Okonkwo, O.; Sutcliffe, K.; Seth, A.; Shin, J.; Jones, D.E. Symptoms of autonomic dysfunction in chronic fatigue syndrome. *QJM Mon. J. Assoc. Physicians* **2007**, *100*, 519–526. [CrossRef] [PubMed]
23. Scherbakov, N.; Szklarski, M.; Hartwig, J.; Sotzny, F.; Lorenz, S.; Meyer, A.; Grabowski, P.; Doehner, W.; Scheibenbogen, C. Peripheral endothelial dysfunction in myalgic encephalomyelitis/chronic fatigue syndrome. *ESC Heart Fail* **2020**. [CrossRef] [PubMed]
24. Fluge, O.; Rekeland, I.G.; Lien, K.; Thurmer, H.; Borchgrevink, P.C.; Schafer, C.; Sorland, K.; Assmus, J.; Ktoridou-Valen, I.; Herder, I.; et al. B-Lymphocyte Depletion in Patients With Myalgic Encephalomyelitis/Chronic Fatigue Syndrome: A Randomized, Double-Blind, Placebo-Controlled Trial. *Ann. Intern. Med.* **2019**. [CrossRef] [PubMed]
25. Fletcher, M.A.; Zeng, X.R.; Maher, K.; Levis, S.; Hurwitz, B.; Antoni, M.; Broderick, G.; Klimas, N.G. Biomarkers in chronic fatigue syndrome: Evaluation of natural killer cell function and dipeptidyl peptidase IV/CD26. *PLoS ONE* **2010**, *5*, e10817. [CrossRef]
26. Loebel, M.; Grabowski, P.; Heidecke, H.; Bauer, S.; Hanitsch, L.G.; Wittke, K.; Meisel, C.; Reinke, P.; Volk, H.D.; Fluge, O.; et al. Antibodies to beta adrenergic and muscarinic cholinergic receptors in patients with Chronic Fatigue Syndrome. *Brain Behav. Immun.* **2016**, *52*, 32–39. [CrossRef]
27. Hilgers, A.; Frank, J. Chronic fatigue syndrome: Immune dysfunction, role of pathogens and toxic agents and neurological and cardial changes. *Wien. Med. Wochenschr.* **1994**, *144*, 399–406.
28. Nacul, L.; de Barros, B.; Kingdon, C.C.; Cliff, J.M.; Clark, T.G.; Mudie, K.; Dockrell, H.M.; Lacerda, E.M. Evidence of Clinical Pathology Abnormalities in People with Myalgic Encephalomyelitis/Chronic Fatigue Syndrome (ME/CFS) from an Analytic Cross-Sectional Study. *Diagnostics* **2019**, *9*, 41. [CrossRef]
29. Fluge, O.; Mella, O.; Bruland, O.; Risa, K.; Dyrstad, S.E.; Alme, K.; Rekeland, I.G.; Sapkota, D.; Rosland, G.V.; Fossa, A.; et al. Metabolic profiling indicates impaired pyruvate dehydrogenase function in myalgic encephalopathy/chronic fatigue syndrome. *JCI Insight* **2016**, *1*, e89376. [CrossRef]
30. Wasserman, R.L.; Church, J.A.; Stein, M.; Moy, J.; White, M.; Strausbaugh, S.; Schroeder, H.; Ballow, M.; Harris, J.; Melamed, I.; et al. Safety, efficacy and pharmacokinetics of a new 10% liquid intravenous immunoglobulin (IVIG) in patients with primary immunodeficiency. *J. Clin. Immunol.* **2012**, *32*, 663–669. [CrossRef]
31. Porter, N.; Lerch, A.; Jason, L.A.; Sorenson, M.; Fletcher, M.A.; Herrington, J. A Comparison of Immune Functionality in Viral versus Non-Viral CFS Subtypes. *J. Behav. Neurosci. Res.* **2010**, *8*, 1–8.
32. Metzemaekers, M.; Van Damme, J.; Mortier, A.; Proost, P. Regulation of Chemokine Activity—A Focus on the Role of Dipeptidyl Peptidase IV/CD26. *Front. Immunol.* **2016**, *7*, 483. [CrossRef]
33. Brown, N.J.; Byiers, S.; Carr, D.; Maldonado, M.; Warner, B.A. Dipeptidyl peptidase-IV inhibitor use associated with increased risk of ACE inhibitor-associated angioedema. *Hypertension* **2009**, *54*, 516–523. [CrossRef]

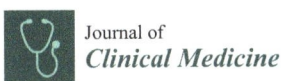

Article

Post-Exertional Malaise May Be Related to Central Blood Pressure, Sympathetic Activity and Mental Fatigue in Chronic Fatigue Syndrome Patients

Sławomir Kujawski [1,*], Joanna Słomko [1], Lynette Hodges [2], Derek F. H. Pheby [3], Modra Murovska [4], Julia L. Newton [5] and Paweł Zalewski [1]

1. Department of Hygiene, Epidemiology, Ergonomics and Postgraduate Education, Division of Ergonomics and Exercise Physiology, Collegium Medicum in Bydgoszcz, Nicolaus Copernicus University in Torun, 85-094 Bydgoszcz, Poland; jslomko@cm.umk.pl (J.S.); p.zalewski@cm.umk.pl (P.Z.)
2. School of Sport, Exercise and Nutrition, Massey University, Palmerston North 4442, New Zealand; l.d.hodges@massey.ac.nz
3. Society and Health, Buckinghamshire New University (Retired), High Wycombe HP11 2JZ, UK; derekpheby@btinternet.com
4. Institute of Microbiology and Virology, Riga Stradiņš University, LV-1067 Riga, Latvia; Modra.Murovska@rsu.lv
5. Population Health Sciences Institute, The Medical School, Newcastle University, Newcastle-upon-Tyne NE2 4AX, UK; julia.newton@ncl.ac.uk
* Correspondence: skujawski@cm.umk.pl; Tel.: +48-52-585-36-15

Abstract: Post-exertional malaise (PEM) is regarded as the hallmark symptom in chronic fatigue syndrome (CFS). The aim of the current study is to explore differences in CFS patients with and without PEM in indicators of aortic stiffness, autonomic nervous system function, and severity of fatigue. One-hundred and one patients met the Fukuda criteria. A Chronic Fatigue Questionnaire (CFQ) and Fatigue Impact Scale (FIS) were used to assess the level of mental and physical fatigue. Aortic systolic blood pressure (sBPaortic) and the autonomic nervous system were measured with the arteriograph and Task Force Monitor, respectively. Eighty-two patients suffered prolonged PEM according to the Fukuda criteria, while 19 did not. Patients with PEM had higher FIS scores ($p = 0.02$), lower central systolic blood pressure ($p = 0.02$) and higher mental fatigue ($p = 0.03$). For a one-point increase in the mental fatigue component of the CFQ scale, the risk of PEM increases by 34%. For an sBPaortic increase of 1 mmHg, the risk of PEM decreases by 5%. For a one unit increase in sympathovagal balance, the risk of PEM increases by 330%. Higher mental fatigue and sympathetic activity in rest are related to an increased risk of PEM, while higher central systolic blood pressure is related to a reduced risk of PEM. However, none of the between group differences were significant after FDR correction, and therefore conclusions should be treated with caution and replicated in further studies.

Keywords: PEM; myalgic encephalomyelitis; brain fog; vascular stiffness

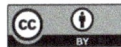

1. Introduction

Chronic Fatigue Syndrome (CFS) is characterized by a substantial deterioration of symptoms that could be provoked in response to physical exercise in patients with post-exertional malaise (PEM) [1]. The National Academy of Medicine reports the prevalence of PEM among CFS patients as being from 69 to 100% [2]. PEM is regarded as a hallmark symptom of CFS [3]. However, some criteria, such as the Fukuda case definition [4], do not require PEM to be present for a CFS diagnosis. The majority of patients, i.e., 73.4%, reported the duration of PEM as being equal to or longer than 24 h [5].

The exact mechanism that underlies PEM is as yet unknown. However, it has been reported that patients with CFS experience shortness of breath [6]. Disruption of the resting respiratory rate induced by PEM has been observed [7].

In addition, an attenuated adrenaline response to physical exercise has been observed in CFS, compared to healthy controls [8], along with more pronounced increases of nitric oxide metabolites after a physical exercise test [9]. The decreased response of adrenaline to physical exercise and a disturbance of nitric oxide metabolites are in line with the observations of Bond et al. [10], who recently proposed that a disturbance in the functioning of the vascular system was a key factor in PEM pathogenesis.

A decrease in the ability of large arteries to adapt readily to an increase in the amount of blood ejected during heart muscle contraction has been reported. Aortic pulse wave, or pulse wave propagation velocity (PWV), and an indirect parameter, the augmentation index (Aix), constitute a relatively simple, non-invasive, and reproducible method to determine arterial stiffness [11]. Arterial stiffness has been found to be associated with cardiovascular events in older cohorts, and, when measured, PWV is considered to be a significant risk factor for cognitive decline. Furthermore, a less elastic arterial system occurs together with impaired autoregulation of cerebral perfusion. In consequence, episodes of hypotension might lead to an increase in the risk of brain hypoperfusion. High arterial stiffness might occur in CFS patients [12] and could serve as a marker of increased cardiovascular risk in this population. Słomko et al. show that CFS patients with sympathetic autonomic dominance had the highest value of arterial stiffness, compared to patients with autonomic balance [13]. Hunter et al. suggest that a higher elasticity of large arteries was correlated with lower subjective fatigue in older women with CFS [14].

The Fukuda criteria can distinguish between CFS and chronic fatigue. However, a further subclassification of the former group into PEM positive and PEM negative subgroups has been suggested [15]. In contrast to the Fukuda criteria, the Canadian Consensus Criteria (CCC) require PEM for a diagnosis of CFS [16]. Therefore, it has been suggested that patients diagnosed on the basis of the Fukuda criteria are a heterogeneous group [17]. However, unlike generalized fatigue, PEM can be associated with extreme disruption of daily life functioning [18]. However, the Fukuda definition, which has been in use for twenty-seven years, has, until recently, been the most widely used case definition for ME/CFS, and is still very widely used in research and clinical practice. The CCC case definition identifies a more severely affected subgroup of those patients identified by the Fukuda definition. The main feature which serves to distinguish those Fukuda-positive patients who are also CCC-positive from those who are not is the presence of PEM. We decided to rely on the Fukuda criteria for CFS to examine the differences between the CFS subgroups of patients with and without PEM. The underlying mechanism of PEM is still not fully understood; therefore we conducted a cross-sectional study to explore the differences in selected physiological parameters and symptoms severity in CFS patients with PEM, compared with those without. The aim of the current study is to examine differences in CFS patients with and without PEM in indicators of aortic stiffness, autonomic nervous system function, and severity of physical and mental fatigue.

2. Materials and Methods

The current study took place from January 2013 to July 2018. The Ethics Committee, of the Ludwik Rydygier Collegium Medicum in Bydgoszcz, Nicolaus Copernicus University, Torun approved the study (KB 332/2013, date of approval: 25 June 2013). Written, informed consent was obtained from all the participants.

2.1. Enrolment

A group of 131 patients with CFS between 25 and 65 years of age were recruited via telephone, e-mail, and mass-media advertisements. The main enrolment criteria included: (1) Fukuda criteria (2) Fatigue Severity Scale score higher than 36 points and persistent fatigue for more than 6 months (3) had suffered from one or more of four additional symptoms: post-exertional malaise, impaired memory and/or concentration, unrefreshing sleep, headache, sore throat, tender lymph nodes (axillary or axillary), muscle or joint pain, (4) perceived fatigue could not be explained by an underlying condition. On inclusion, all

CFS patients received a pre-test health state assessment: basic neurological, psychiatric, clinical examination, and had been referred by a general practitioner and by the neurology and psychiatry departments. The exclusion criteria included: (1) any indication of underlying illness, (2) medical condition explaining fatigue, (3) psychiatric disorders. Hospital Anxiety and Depression Scale (HADS) has been performed to assess anxiety (HADS_A) and depression (HADS_D) symptoms intensity [19]. Beck Depression Inventory (BDI-II) was used to examine depression symptoms intensity [20].

30 participants were excluded as they did not meet the Fukuda criteria ($n = 10$), had an underlying psychiatric illness ($n = 13$), or had another diagnosis, or fatigue was not the primary complain ($n = 7$).

On the day of investigation all subjects were instructed to eat a light breakfast, and refrain from smoking, caffeine, alcohol consumption and vigorous physical activity. All tests were carried out in a chronobiology laboratory (soundproofed room without windows, temperature 22 °C, humidity 60%) and were performed at approximately the same time of day.

2.2. Measurement

Scales

The Chalder Fatigue Questionnaire (CFQ) [21], Fatigue Severity Score (FSS) [22] and the Fatigue Impact Scale (FIS) [23] were administered to provide a comprehensive assessment of fatigue severity. The CFQ assessed physical and psychological fatigue. It consists of 11 items that could be divided to mental (4 items) and physical fatigue (7 items) dimensions. Scoring was made in "Likert" style (in a range from 0 to 3) therefore the total score could be 0 at minimum and 33 at maximum and from 0 to 12 in mental and from 0 to 21 points in physical dimension. Moreover, binary scoring of the total score (0 for absence ad 1 for presence) was done. FSS assessed fatigue in the past week. It consists of nine items that are statements. Patients could choose an option from strongly disagreeing with a statement (1 point) to strongly agreeing with a particular statement (7 points). Total scores ranged from 9 to 63 points. FIS assessed cognitive, physical, and psychosocial fatigue. Higher scores indicate higher severity in all domains. Likert-like scoring with a range of 0–4 points per item was applied to 40 items in total. Therefore the total score could range from 0 to 160 points. In all fatigue questionnaires, the higher the results in points, the more severe fatigue.

The Hospital Anxiety and Depression Scale (HADS) was performed to assess anxiety (HADS_A) and depression (HADS_D) symptoms intensity [19]. The Beck Depression Inventory (BDI-II) was used to examine depression symptoms intensity [20]. Both scales were used only at the baseline to exclude patients with depression.

The Epworth sleepiness scale (ESS) [24] was used to assess patients' general daytime sleepiness.

2.3. Autonomic Symptom Assessment

We used subjective and objective tools to measure the function of the autonomic nervous system. The Autonomic Symptom Profile served to measure presence, frequency, and dynamics of autonomic symptoms severity [25]. Scoring was done based on the Composite Autonomic Symptom Score 31 (COMPASS 31) [26]. Questionnaire contains 31 items assessing six dimensions of autonomic nervous system function, namely response to orthostatic stress, vasomotor and secretomotor reactions, function of, bladder and gastrointestinal tract, as well as pupillomotor reflex. Scores from individual domains were weighted. The total score is 100 points, the higher the score the higher the symptom load. In addition, Orthostatic Grading scale (OGS) was used to assess response to orthostatic stress [27].

Second, ANS functioning was automatically measured with a Task Force Monitor—TFM (CNS Systems, Gratz, Austria). Signals from a three-channel ECG were analyzed using the adaptive autoregressive model [28]. Low frequency (LFnu-RRI) (0.04–0.15 Hz) and high frequency (HFnu-RRI) (0.15–0.4 Hz) components of R-to-R intervals in normalized units, as well as its ratio (LF/HR-RRI), were recorded and analyzed in rest. Assessments were performed after a 5 min waiting period in a supine position, which allowed for signals to stabilize. Then, an assessment at rest was performed in supine position for a further 5 min.

2.4. Arterial Stiffness

Arterial stiffness was measured using an oscillometric non-invasive Arteriograph (TensioMed Kft, Budapest, Hungary, www.tensiomed.com, accessed on 18 March 2021). This is a device that uses a simple upper arm cuff as a sensor, with the cuff pressurized to at least 35 mmHg over the actual systolic pressure. The device determines the PWVaortic and augmentation index according to the manufacturer's instructions. Arteriograph measurement has been described extensively in previous papers [29–31]. The Arteriograph, simultaneously with the arterial stiffness parameters, also records the actual systolic and diastolic blood pressure (BPs) and heart rate.

The difference between the central and peripheral systolic blood pressure was calculated based on measurement from arteriography and TFM, respectively.

2.5. Statistical Analysis

Histogram visual inspection and the Shapiro–Wilk test were applied to test the normality assumption. To examine between-group differences (patients with PEM vs. those without) Mann–Whitney U or independent T-tests were used, depending on assumptions met. To predict presence of PEM in examined patients, a logistic regression model using the GLM function was applied in R. In addition, 95% confidence intervals for log-likelihoods and odds ratios were calculated (confit function using bootstrap). The DescTools package was used to calculate pseudo R2 for the model [32]. Dotwhisker plots were used to visualize odds ratios and confidence intervals [33]. Violin graphs were created using R [34] with a ggstatsplot library [35]. Effect sizes from the ggstatsplot library are reported for between group comparisons. The false discovery rate (FDR) was controlled using a Benjamini–Hochberg adjusted p-value, applying an online calculator available at (https://tools.carbocation.com/FDR, accessed on 18 March 2021). The results contain p-values before as well as after correction.

3. Results

One hundred and one patients met the Fukuda criteria for CFS and were included in the analysis (Table 1). The patients were divided into groups with PEM or without PEM. Eighty-two patients reported prolonged PEM, whilst nineteen patients were free of prolonged PEM. Both groups consisted predominantly of women, comprising fifty-one patients from PEM group (62.2%), and fourteen (73.7%) in the group without PEM. Table 1 describes detailed characteristics about the total group and group differences between the patients with PEM and those without.

Table 2 presents differences in arteriography results between patients with PEM and those without PEM. Table 3 indicates differences between patients with PEM and those without PEM, in respect of autonomic nervous system function indicators.

Patients with PEM had higher overall fatigue, as measured by FIS (81.61 ± 30.3 vs. 63.05 ± 33.9, $t = -2.19$, $p = 0.02$, Hedges' $g = -0.57$ (−1.07, −0.03), and higher mental fatigue (9.13 ± 1.8 vs. 7.95 ± 2.2, $Z = 2.18$, $p = 0.03$, $r = -0.22$ (−0.39, −0.03) (Table 1). Mean fatigue scores in the total sample were 23.68 points (range 0–33 points) in the CFQ scale, 47.03 points (range 9–63 points) in FSS, and 78.12 points (range 0–160 points) in FIS.

Patients with PEM had lower central systolic blood pressure than those without PEM (127.49 ± 15 vs. 141.05 ± 21.1, $Z = -2.37$, $p = 0.02$, $r = 0.24$ (0.06, 0.44) (Table 2). No significant differences in blood pressure measured peripherally were observed (Table 2).

Patients with PEM had higher LFnu-RRI (56.61 ± 16.7 vs. 46.64 ± 13.9, $Z = 2.58$, $p = 0.01$, $r = -0.26$ (−0.45, −0.06), lower HFnu-RRI (43.39 ± 16.7 vs. 53.36 ± 13.9, $Z = -2.58$, $p =

0.01, r = 0.26 (0.07, 0.44) and higher LF/HF-RRI (1.96 ± 2.2 vs. 1.13 ± 0.9, Z = 2.37, p = 0.02, r = −0.24 (−0.42, −0.06). Also, LF/HF was higher in patients with PEM (1.66 ± 1.5 vs. 0.94 ± 0.5, Z = 2.96, p = 0.003, r = −0.29, (−0.45, −0.14). In addition, patients with PEM had higher LFnu-dBP (53.88 ± 14.4 vs. 43.45 ± 13.8, Z = 2.69, p = 0.01, r = −0.27 (−0.47, −0.11) and higher LF/HF-dBP (7.27 ± 6.0 vs. 4.32 ± 3.6, Z = 2.36, p = 0.02, r = −0.23, (−0.45, −0.04) (Table 3).

Table 1. Demographic data of total examined sample (n = 101) and comparison of demographic data and questionnaires results of patients with PEM and without PEM, respectively.

Variable	Total Sample	PEM Mean ± SD	Without PEM Mean ± SD	p-Value	FDR p-Value
Age [years]	38.15 ± 8.0	38.23 ± 8.1	37.79 ± 8.0	0.83	0.88
Height [cm]	171.55 ± 8.4	172.07 ± 8.7	169.32 ± 6.6	0.20	0.15
Weight [kg]	72.22 ± 12.6	72.77 ± 12.6	69.84 ± 12.5	0.36	0.61
BMI	24.47 ± 3.6	24.51 ± 3.5	24.31 ± 3.8	0.83	0.85
Symptoms duration [years]	4.54 ± 4.1	4.75 ± 4.2	3.64 ± 3.7	0.20	0.44
CFQ [points]	23.68 ± 4.6	24.07 ± 4.6	22.00 ± 4.4	0.08	0.21
CFQ_BINARY [points]	14.06 ± 4.8	14.49 ± 4.6	12.21 ± 5.1	0.07	0.22
CFQ_PHYSICAL [points]	10.47 ± 3.9	10.39 ± 4.0	10.79 ± 3.7	0.50	0.69
CFQ_MENTAL [points]	8.91 ± 2.0	9.13 ± 1.8	7.95 ± 2.2	0.03	0.11
FSS [points]	47.03 ± 10.1	47.57 ± 9.4	44.68 ± 12.8	0.46	0.68
FIS [points]	78.12 ± 31.6	81.61 ± 30.3	63.05 ± 33.9	0.02	0.09
HADS_A [points]	9.27 ± 3.5	9.22 ± 3.4	9.47 ± 4.2	0.78	0.87
HADS_D [points]	7.85 ± 3.4	8.00 ± 3.5	7.21 ± 2.9	0.36	0.63
BDI [points]	15.83 ± 7.9	16.15 ± 8.1	14.39 ± 6.9	0.57	0.75
ESS [points]	10.86 ± 5.6	11.01 ± 5.5	10.21 ± 6.3	0.65	0.78
OGS [points]	3.64 ± 3.2	3.71 ± 3.4	3.37 ± 2.5	0.98	0.98
Orthostatic intolerance [points]	11.96 ± 11.0	12.24 ± 11.3	10.74 ± 10.0	0.67	0.77
Vasomotor [points]	0.83 ± 1.4	0.86 ± 1.4	0.70 ± 1.4	0.57	0.73
Secretomotor [points]	5.52 ± 3.9	5.64 ± 3.9	4.96 ± 3.9	0.49	0.70
Gastrointestinal [points]	5.09 ± 4.2	4.89 ± 4.1	5.97 ± 4.7	0.37	0.60
Bladder [points]	0.54 ± 0.9	0.57 ± 1.0	0.41 ± 0.8	0.60	0.74
Pupillomotor [points]	1.15 ± 1.2	1.22 ± 1.2	0.86 ± 0.9	0.38	0.59
Compass-31 Total [points]	25.09 ± 14.7	25.43 ± 15.0	23.64 ± 13.4	0.81	0.88

BMI—body mass index, CFQ—Chalder Fatigue Questionnaire, FSS—Fatigue Severity Scale, FIS—Fatigue Impact Scale, HADS_A—Hospital Anxiety and Depression Scale anxiety, HADS_D—Hospital Anxiety and Depression Scale depression; BDI—Beck Depression Inventory, ESS—*Epworth Sleepiness Scale*, OGS—Orthostatic Grading Scale, Compass-31—Composite Autonomic Symptom Score 31.

Table 2. Comparison of arteriography results of patients with PEM and without PEM.

Variable	PEM Mean ± SD	Without PEM Mean ± SD	p-Value	FDR p-Value
PWVaortic [m/s]	8.33 ± 1.7	8.65 ± 1.8	0.21	0.41
Aixaortic [%]	28.11 ± 14.4	32.95 ± 15.5	0.20	0.41
sBPaortic [mmHg]	127.49 ± 15	141.05 ± 21.1	0.02	0.12
central-peripheral sBP [mmHg]	9.56 ± 21.7	23.41 ± 25.7	0.06	0.20

PWVaortic—Pulse Wave Velocity aortic, sBPaortic—aortic systolic blood pressure, central-peripheral sBP—difference between central and peripheral systolic blood pressure levels.

Table 3. Comparison of autonomic parameters in patients with PEM and without PEM.

Variable	PEM Mean ± SD	Without PEM Mean ± SD	p-Value	FDR p-Value
Spectral analysis of HR variability				
LFnu-RRI	56.61 ± 16.7	46.64 ± 13.9	0.01	0.12
HFnu-RRI	43.39 ± 16.7	53.36 ± 13.9	0.01	0.19
LF/HF-RRI	1.96 ± 2.2	1.13 ± 0.9	0.02	0.08
LF/HF	1.66 ± 1.5	0.94 ± 0.5	0.003	0.11
Spectral analysis of BP variability				
LFnu-dBP	53.88 ± 14.4	43.45 ± 13.8	0.01	0.09
HFnu-dBP	11.67 ± 7.3	18.20 ± 16.0	0.07	0.20
LF/HF-dBP	7.27 ± 6.0	4.32 ± 3.6	0.02	0.11
LFnu-sBP	42.86 ± 14.0	38.14 ± 13.7	0.19	0.44
HFnu-sBP	14.86 ± 9.3	18.74 ± 14.0	0.31	0.57
LF/HF-sBP	4.10 ± 2.8	3.02 ± 1.8	0.17	0.42

LFnu—low frequency normalized units, HFnu—high frequency normalized units, LF/HF—ratio of low frequency to high frequency, RRR—R to R interval, sBP—systolic blood pressure, dBP—diastolic blood pressure.

Figure 1 presents differences between patients without PEM and patients with PEM in the level of the CFQ mental fatigue sub-score (Figure 1a), aortic sBP (Figure 1b) and sympathovagal balance (Figure 1c). This set of variables was then included in logistic regression models as PEM presence predictors.

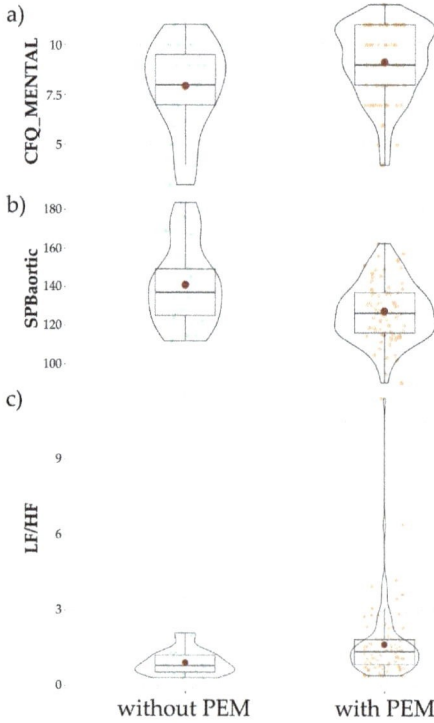

Figure 1. Comparison of patients with PEM vs. without PEM in the CFQ mental fatigue sub-score (a), aortic sBP (b) and sympathovagal balance (c). Red dots indicate mean value, horizontal black line inside the box denotes median value. Green dots before and orange dots after denote results of individual patients. Shape of violin graph indicates distribution of results.

Figure 2 shows the estimate of parameters and their confidence interval (−95%, 95%) in logistic regression analysis. In terms of odds ratios, the results were as follows: for a one point more increase in the mental fatigue component of the CFQ scale, the risk of PEM increases by 34% (CI = 2%, 80%). For an aortic systolic blood pressure increase of 1 mmHg, the risk of PEM decreases by 5% (CI = 9%, 2%). For a one unit more increase in sympathovagal balance, the risk of PEM increases by 330% (CI = 50%, 1516%). (AIC = 81.18, BIC = 91.6, Tjur's R^2 = 0.26) (Table A1 in Appendix A).

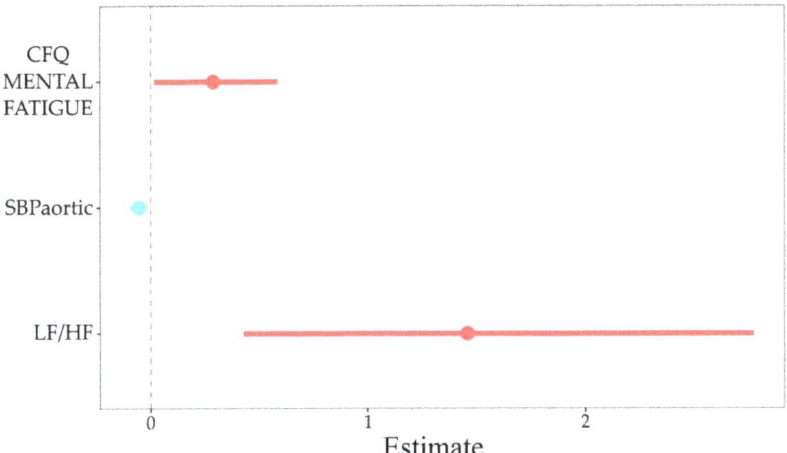

Figure 2. Logistic regression estimates predicting PEM presence. The horizontal axis refers to the odds ratio. Dots denote parameter estimates, while the horizontal lines through the dots denote 95% confidence intervals of the estimates.

4. Discussion

The results of the present study have shown that CFS patients with PEM had significantly higher mental fatigue, overall fatigue being measured by FIS, which was one of the three fatigue scales used in the above research. Moreover, patients with PEM had lower central systolic blood pressure. However, no difference in levels of peripheral blood pressure was observed. Higher mental fatigue is related to a higher risk of PEM, while higher central systolic blood pressure is related to lower risk of PEM. However, none of the between group differences were significant after FDR correction, and therefore conclusions should be treated with caution and replicated in further studies.

As has been noted in the introduction, 73.4% assessed PEM duration as equal to or longer than 24 h [5]. As a result of the dramatic decline in patients' physical and/or cognitive functioning, some patients might have to adjust their lifestyle and activity levels to avoid inducing PEM [2]. Some 25–29% of patients are reported to be bedbound or housebound [2]. The annual cost of CFS in the USA is estimated to be around $18 to $24 billion [2]. PEM was proposed as a prognostic indicator of CFS course [2], so studies of PEM have high clinical significance. Exploration of the PEM mechanism could lead to more effective therapeutic approaches, and thus to improvement of overall patient function.

The above findings are in line with previous research, which suggests that chronic vascular damage might cause a lack of exercise-induced vasodilation and be a potential cause of PEM [10]. In CFS, reduced blood pressure is frequently reported [36,37]. Additionally, an inverse relationship between increasing fatigue and diurnal blood pressure variation has been observed [38]. In our sample, despite a lack of difference in peripheral systolic blood pressure (with a mean lower than 120 mmHg in both groups), increased central systolic blood pressure was observed in patients with PEM. In certain conditions, such as during physical activity, the correlation between peripheral and central systolic blood pressure may decrease [38]. It is tempting to speculate that an increase in central systolic blood pressure in some CFS patients might occur before other pathological changes. Conversely, increased arterial stiffness was observed in healthy young adults in response to acute sleep deprivation. Arterial stiffness might therefore be secondary to comorbidities, such as sleep disturbance [39]. Further studies should examine the exact mechanism underlying the relationship between central systolic blood pressure, PEM fatigue, and factors responsible for blood pressure regulation in CFS. As a result of the rich symptomatology, an attempt should be made to classify different subgroups of CFS patients according to comorbidities. Further studies could possibly focus on the vascular system in all CFS patients, or perhaps just in a specific sub-group. Further exploration of this field would be helpful to establish possible personalized therapeutic approaches in CFS. In the present study, PEM presence was related to a higher mental fatigue component. Moreover, our previous study has shown that arterial stiffness parameters are related to fatigue severity; higher FIS and lower FSS scores were related to lower aortic stiffness [13]. Presumably, some of the mechanisms underlying this relationship could similarly link central blood pressure to PEM. Thus, mental fatigue might be related to dysfunction in ß2 adrenergic receptor and vascular or endothelial function, which in turn could lead to reduced cerebral blood flow (CBF) [40]. A decrease in CBF has been observed in CFS patients [41] and CBF has been shown to be correlated with fatigue severity [42]. Significantly, a negative correlation was seen between CBF and skeletal muscle pH at rest, which might explain why mental fatigue could be related to muscular fatigue [43]. However, the mechanisms described above are purely speculative and need to be examined in further studies.

In the current study, sympathetic nervous system function was more active during rest in the group with PEM, compared with the group without PEM. Moreover, indicators of parasympathetic nervous system activity were lower during rest. Findings in the PEM group are in line with the previous study by Frith et al. [36], where LF-dBP at rest was higher in a CFS group compared to controls. Parasympathetic activity was reduced in the CFS patients after inducing PEM [44]. During physical exercise, cardiac output distribution is governed by the sympathetic nervous system [45]. Surprisingly, in the PEM group, increased sympathetic drive coexisted with lower central systolic blood pressure. It is noteworthy that numerous factors can have an impact on the control of the ANS in the constriction of vascular beds, individual vessels, and even different parts of the same vessel [45]. Those factors include density and subtypes of adrenergic receptors and action of contransmitters, norepinephrine kinetics, density of sympathetic innervations, and degree of basal tone [45]. Additionally, local factors, such as the concentrations of vasoactive tissue metabolites, vessel size, and structure may also play a part in changes in vessel diameter and therefore in cardiac output distribution [45]. The disturbance in some of those factors could play an important role in PEM pathogenesis. Similar mechanisms for PEM have been proposed [40]. However, based on our findings, it is not possible to delineate the exact mechanism underlying the observed disturbances in ANS and whether it is related to PEM. Further studies should examine vascular function in response to stressors and its role in PEM. Understanding PEM mechanisms could contribute to the development of specific PEM therapy.

What is surprising is that the current results, corrected for multiple comparisons, showed no significant differences between the subgroup with PEM and that without PEM, in terms of fatigue as measured by scales. This is in contrast to a previous study, where higher PEM intensity was related to higher frequency and intensity of symptoms, and greater problems with emotional regulation [17]. However, discrepancies in the results observed might be related to a difference in methodology. In the current study, the division of CFS patients into PEM present or PEM absent subgroups was based on a binary variables (presence of prolonged post-exertional malaise), while May et al. divided patients into a group with no to moderate intensity of PEM (loPEM), and a group with severe to very severe PEM (hiPEM) [17]. Future studies should further examine if PEM is a distinct characteristic feature, on which basis a subgroup of CFS patients might be distinguished, or whether PEM is related directionally or non-directionally to other symptoms from which

CFS patients suffer. In addition, it was suggested that further multi-center studies on CFS should apply the same protocols [46]. Therefore, it is necessary to make a decision as to whether PEM should be a symptom required for CFS diagnosis, which would have an impact on the types of criteria of CFS used in research.

Study Limitations

In the above study, PEM was measured subjectively. Further studies should incorporate a protocol based on repeated Cardiopulmonary Exercise Tests, to confirm objectively the presence of PEM in CFS patients. A difference in sample size between the subgroup with PEM and that without PEM was observed, which seems to reflect PEM prevalence in the general population. By increasing the sample size, a higher number of patients without PEM could be included as a control group. Sample size should therefore be increased in further studies on PEM in CFS. Meta-analysis showed that PEM occurs 10.4 times more frequently in CFS patients in comparison with other groups [47]. Comparison between patients with CFS might potentially reduce potentially confounding factors. The present study design is cross sectional, so no conclusions about causality can be drawn based on the current results. Further studies should explore the PEM mechanism applying intervention-based protocols. In addition, to reveal potential biological mechanisms, a deep phenotyping approach could be chosen, using a repeated CPET protocol to elicit PEM and to examine changes in biomarkers related to changes in PEM.

5. Conclusions

Patients with PEM had significantly higher mental fatigue and overall fatigue than those without PEM, as measured by FIS, one of the three fatigue scales used in the above research. They also had higher mental fatigue and sympathetic activity compared with parasympathetic activity during rest and lower central systolic blood pressure. However, none of these differences remained statistically significant after correction for multiple comparisons. Further studies should be conducted to confirm if higher mental fatigue and higher sympathetic activity, compared with parasympathetic activity at rest and lower central systolic blood pressure, are related to a higher risk of PEM.

Author Contributions: Conceptualization, S.K., J.S., L.H. and P.Z.; Formal analysis, S.K. and J.S.; Investigation, J.S. and P.Z.; Methodology, J.S. and P.Z.; Project administration, J.S. and P.Z.; Software, J.S. and S.K.; Supervision, P.Z., J.L.N.; Writing—original draft, S.K. and J.S.; Writing—review and editing, L.H., D.F.H.P., M.M., P.Z., J.L.N. All authors have read and agreed to the published version of the manuscript.

Funding: This research received no external funding.

Institutional Review Board Statement: The study was approved by the Ethics Committee, Ludwik Rydygier Collegium Medicum in Bydgoszcz, Nicolaus Copernicus University, Torun (KB 332/2013, date of approval: 25 June 2013).

Informed Consent Statement: Written informed consent was obtained from all participants.

Data Availability Statement: Individual data is available from the corresponding author S.K. on request.

Acknowledgments: This article/publication is based upon work from COST Action CA15111 "European Network on Myalgic Encephalomyelitis/Chronic Fatigue Syndrome, EUROMENE," supported by COST (European Cooperation in Science and Technology, weblink: www.cost.eu, accessed on 18 March 2021.

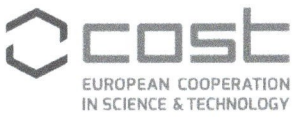
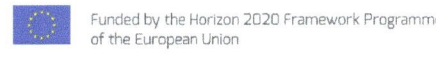

Conflicts of Interest: The authors declare no conflict of interest.

Appendix A

Table A1. Logistic regression predicting PEM presence.

Term	Estimate	−95% CI	95% CI	z Value	p-Value
CFQ_MENTAL_FATIGUE	0.29	0.02	0.59	2.02	0.04
SBPaortic	−0.05	−0.09	−0.02	−2.66	0.01
LF/HF	1.46	0.43	2.78	2.45	0.01

References

1. Oosterwijck, J.V.; Marusic, U.; De Wandele, I.; Paul, L.; Meeus, M.; Moorkens, G.; Lambrecht, L.; Danneels, L.; Nijs, J. The Role of Autonomic Function in Exercise-induced Endogenous Analgesia: A Case-control Study in Myalgic Encephalomyeli-tis/Chronic Fatigue Syndrome and Healthy People. *Pain Physician* **2017**, *20*, E389–E399.
2. Committee on the Diagnostic Criteria for Myalgic Encephalomyelitis/Chronic Fatigue Syndrome; Board on the Health of Select Populations; Institute of Medicine. Beyond Myalgic Encephalomyelitis/Chronic Fatigue Syndrome: Redefining an Illness. In *The National Academies Collection: Reports Funded by National Institutes of Health*; National Academies Press: Washington, DC, USA, 2015; ISBN 9780309316897.
3. Carruthers, B.M.; Van De Sande, M.I.; De Meirleir, K.L.; Klimas, N.G.; Broderick, G.; Mitchell, T.; Staines, D.; Powles, A.C.P.; Speight, N.; Vallings, R.; et al. Myalgic encephalomyelitis: International Consensus Criteria. *J. Intern. Med.* **2011**, *270*, 327–338. [CrossRef]
4. Fukuda, K.; Straus, S.E.; Hickie, I.; Sharpe, M.C.; Dobbins, J.G.; Komaroff, A.; Schluederberg, A.; Jones, J.F.; Lloyd, A.R.; Wessely, S.; et al. The Chronic Fatigue Syndrome: A Comprehensive Approach to Its Definition and Study. *Ann. Int. Med.* **1994**, *121*, 953–959. [CrossRef] [PubMed]
5. Cotler, J.; Holtzman, C.; Dudun, C.; Jason, L.A. A Brief Questionnaire to Assess Post-Exertional Malaise. *Diagnostics* **2018**, *8*, 66. [CrossRef]
6. Hawk, C.; Jason, L.A.; Torres-Harding, S. Differential diagnosis of chronic fatigue syndrome and major depressive disorder. *Int. J. Behav. Med.* **2006**, *13*, 244–251. [CrossRef]
7. Cotler, J.; Katz, B.Z.; Reurts-Post, C.; Vermeulen, R.; Jason, L.A. A hierarchical logistic regression predicting rapid respiratory rates from post-exertional malaise. *Fatigue Biomed. Health Behav.* **2020**, *17*, 1–9. [CrossRef]
8. Strahler, J.; Fischer, S.; Nater, U.M.; Ehlert, U.; Gaab, J. Norepinephrine and epinephrine responses to physiological and pharmacological stimulation in chronic fatigue syndrome. *Biol. Psychol.* **2013**, *94*, 160–166. [CrossRef]
9. Suárez, A.; Guillamó, E.; Roig, T.; Blázquez, A.; Alegre, J.; Bermúdez, J.; Ventura, J.L.; García-Quintana, A.M.; Comella, A.; Segura, R.; et al. Nitric Oxide Metabolite Production During Exercise in Chronic Fatigue Syndrome: A Case-Control Study. *J. Womens Health* **2010**, *19*, 1073–1077. [CrossRef] [PubMed]
10. Bond, J.; Nielsen, T.; Hodges, L. Effects of Post-Exertional Malaise on Markers of Arterial Stiffness in Individuals with Myalgic Encephalomyelitis/Chronic Fatigue Syndrome. *Int. J. Environ. Res. Public Health* **2021**, *18*, 2366. [CrossRef]
11. Sutton-Tyrrell, K.; Najjar, S.S.; Boudreau, R.M.; Venkitachalam, L.; Kupelian, V.; Simonsick, E.M.; Havlik, R.; Lakatta, E.G.; Spurgeon, H.; Kritchevsky, S.; et al. Elevated Aortic Pulse Wave Velocity, a Marker of Arterial Stiffness, Predicts Cardiovascular Events in Well-Functioning Older Adults. *Circulation* **2005**, *111*, 3384–3390. [CrossRef] [PubMed]
12. Allen, J.; Murray, A.; Di Maria, C.; Newton, J.L. Chronic fatigue syndrome and impaired peripheral pulse characteristics on orthostasis–A new potential diagnostic biomarker. *Physiol. Meas.* **2012**, *33*, 231–241. [CrossRef] [PubMed]
13. Słomko, J.; Estévez-López, F.; Kujawski, S.; Zawadka-Kunikowska, M.; Tafil-Klawe, M.; Klawe, J.J.; Morten, K.J.; Szrajda, J.; Murovska, M.; Newton, J.L.; et al. Autonomic Phenotypes in Chronic Fatigue Syndrome (CFS) are Associated with Illness Severity: A Cluster Analysis. *J. Clin. Med.* **2020**, *9*, 2531. [CrossRef] [PubMed]
14. Hunter, G.R.; Neumeier, W.H.; Bickel, C.S.; McCarthy, J.P.; Fisher, G.; Chandler-Laney, P.C.; Glasser, S.P. Arterial Elasticity, Strength, Fatigue, and Endurance in Older Women. *BioMed. Res. Int.* **2014**, *2014*, 1–8. [CrossRef] [PubMed]
15. Maes, M.; Twisk, F.N.M.; Johnson, C. Myalgic Encephalomyelitis (ME), Chronic Fatigue Syndrome (CFS), and Chronic Fatigue (CF) are distinguished accurately: Results of supervised learning techniques applied on clinical and inflammatory data. *Psychiatry Res.* **2012**, *200*, 754–760. [CrossRef] [PubMed]
16. Carruthers, B.M.; Jain, A.K.; De Meirleir, K.L.; Peterson, D.L.; Klimas, N.G.; Lerner, A.M.; van de Sande, M.I. Myalgic encephalomyelitis/chronic fatigue syndrome: Clinical working case definition, diagnostic and treatment protocols. *J. Chronic Fatigue Syndr.* **2003**, *11*, 7–115. [CrossRef]
17. May, M.; Milrad, S.F.; Perdomo, D.M.; Czaja, S.J.; Fletcher, M.A.; Jutagir, D.R.; Hall, D.L.; Klimas, N.; Antoni, M.H. Post-exertional malaise is associated with greater symptom burden and psychological distress in patients diagnosed with Chronic Fatigue Syndrome. *J. Psychosom. Res.* **2020**, *129*, 109893. [CrossRef]

18. Jason, L.A.; Evans, M.; So, S.; Scott, J.; Brown, A. Problems in Defining Post-Exertional Malaise. *J. Prev. Interv. Community* **2015**, *43*, 20–31. [CrossRef]
19. Zigmond, A.S.; Snaith, R.P. The Hospital Anxiety and Depression Scale. *Acta Psychiatr. Scand.* **1983**, *67*, 361–370. [CrossRef] [PubMed]
20. Beck, A.T.; Steer, R.A.; Ball, R.; Ranieri, W.F. Comparison of Beck Depression Inventories-IA and-II in Psychiatric Outpatients. *J. Pers. Assess.* **1996**, *67*, 588–597. [CrossRef]
21. Morriss, R.; Wearden, A.; Mullis, R. Exploring the validity of the chalder fatigue scale in chronic fatigue syndrome. *J. Psychosom. Res.* **1998**, *45*, 411–417. [CrossRef]
22. Valko, P.O.; Bassetti, C.L.; Bloch, K.E.; Held, U.; Baumann, C.R. Validation of the Fatigue Severity Scale in a Swiss Cohort. *Sleep* **2008**, *31*, 1601–1607. [CrossRef] [PubMed]
23. Frith, J.; Newton, J. Fatigue Impact Scale. *Occup. Med.* **2010**, *60*, 159. [CrossRef] [PubMed]
24. Johns, M.W. A New Method for Measuring Daytime Sleepiness: The Epworth Sleepiness Scale. *Sleep* **1991**, *14*, 540–545. [CrossRef] [PubMed]
25. Suarez, G.A.; Opfer-Gehrking, T.L.; Offord, K.P.; Atkinson, E.J.; O'Brien, P.C.; Low, P.A. The Autonomic Symptom Profile: A new instrument to assess autonomic symptoms. *Neurology* **1999**, *52*, 523. [CrossRef] [PubMed]
26. Sletten, D.M.; Suarez, G.A.; Low, P.A.; Mandrekar, J.; Singer, W. COMPASS 31: A Refined and Abbreviated Composite Autonomic Symptom Score. *Mayo Clin. Proc.* **2012**, *87*, 1196–1201. [CrossRef] [PubMed]
27. Kim, H.-A.; Lee, H.; Park, K.-J.; Lim, J.-G. Autonomic dysfunction in patients with orthostatic dizziness: Validation of orthostatic grading scale and comparison of Valsalva maneuver and head-up tilt testing results. *J. Neurol. Sci.* **2013**, *325*, 61–66. [CrossRef]
28. Bianchi, A.M.; Mainardi, L.T.; Meloni, C.; Chierchiu, S.; Cerutti, S. Continuous monitoring of the sympatho-vagal balance through spectral analysis. *IEEE Eng. Med. Biol. Mag.* **1997**, *16*, 64–73. [CrossRef]
29. Németh, Z.; Móczár, K.; Deák, G. Evaluation of the Tensioday ambulatory blood pressure monitor according to the protocols of the British Hypertension Society and the Association for the Advancement of Medical Instrumentation. *Blood Press. Monit.* **2002**, *7*, 191–197. [CrossRef]
30. Ring, M.; Eriksson, M.J.; Zierath, J.R.; Caidahl, K. Arterial stiffness estimation in healthy subjects: A validation of oscillometric (Arteriograph) and tonometric (SphygmoCor) techniques. *Hypertens. Res.* **2014**, *37*, 999–1007. [CrossRef]
31. Horvath, I.G.; Nemeth, A.; Lenkey, Z.; Alessandri, N.; Tufano, F.; Kis, P.; Gaszner, B.; Cziraki, A. Invasive validation of a new oscillometric device (arteriogrph) for measuring augmentation index, central blood pressure and aortic pulse wave velocity. *J. Hypertens.* **2010**, *28*, 2068–2075. [CrossRef]
32. Andri, S.; Ken, A.; Andreas, A.; Nanina, A.; Tomas, A.; Chandima, A.; Antti, A.; Adrian, B.; Kamil, B.; Ben, B.; et al. DescTools: Tools for Descriptive Statistics. R package version 0.99.36. 2020. Available online: https://cran.r-project.org/package=DescTools (accessed on 12 March 2021).
33. Solt, F.; Hu, Y. Dotwhisker: Dot-and-Whisker Plots of Regression Results. The Comprehensive R ArchiveNetwork (CRAN). 2015. Available online: https://cran.r-project.org/web/packages/dotwhisker/vignettes/dotwhisker-vignette.html (accessed on 18 March 2021).
34. R Core Team. *R: A Language and Environment for Statistical Computing*; R Foundation for Statistical Computing: Vienna, Austria, 2013; Available online: http://www.R-project.org/ (accessed on 12 March 2021).
35. Patil, I.; Powell, C. Ggstatsplot: 'ggplot2' Based Plots with Statistical Details. 2018. Available online: https://CRAN.R-project.org/package=ggstatsplot (accessed on 12 March 2021).
36. Frith, J.; Zalewski, P.; Klawe, J.J.; Pairman, J.; Bitner, A.; Tafil-Klawe, M.; Newton, J.L. Impaired blood pressure variability in chronic fatigue syndrome—a potential biomarker. *QJM Int. J. Med.* **2012**, *105*, 831–838. [CrossRef] [PubMed]
37. Newton, J.L.; Sheth, A.; Shin, J.; Pairman, J.; Wilton, K.; Burt, J.A.; Jones, D.E.J. Lower Ambulatory Blood Pressure in Chronic Fatigue Syndrome. *Psychosom. Med.* **2009**, *71*, 361–365. [CrossRef] [PubMed]
38. Wilkinson, I.B.; Maccallum, H.; Flint, L.; Cockcroft, J.R.; Newby, D.E.; Webb, D.J. The influence of heart rate on augmentation index and central arterial pressure in humans. *J. Physiol.* **2000**, *525*, 263–270. [CrossRef]
39. Sunbul, M.; Kanar, B.G.; Durmus, E.; Kivrak, T.; Sari, I. Acute sleep deprivation is associated with increased arterial stiffness in healthy young adults. *Sleep Breath.* **2013**, *18*, 215–220. [CrossRef] [PubMed]
40. Wirth, K.; Scheibenbogen, C. A Unifying Hypothesis of the Pathophysiology of Myalgic Encephalomyelitis/Chronic Fatigue Syndrome (ME/CFS): Recognitions from the finding of autoantibodies against ß2-adrenergic receptors. *Autoimmun. Rev.* **2020**, *19*, 102527. [CrossRef]
41. Yoshiuchi, K.; Farkas, J.; Natelson, B.H. Patients with chronic fatigue syndrome have reduced absolute cortical blood flow. *Clin. Physiol. Funct. Imaging* **2006**, *26*, 83–86. [CrossRef]
42. Boissoneault, J.; Letzen, J.; Robinson, M.; Staud, R. Cerebral blood flow and heart rate variability predict fatigue severity in patients with chronic fatigue syndrome. *Brain Imaging Behav.* **2018**, *13*, 789–797. [CrossRef] [PubMed]
43. He, J.; Hollingsworth, K.G.; Newton, J.L.; Blamire, A.M. Cerebral vascular control is associated with skeletal muscle pH in chronic fatigue syndrome patients both at rest and during dynamic stimulation. *NeuroImage Clin.* **2013**, *2*, 168–173. [CrossRef]
44. Cvejic, E.; Sandler, C.X.; Keech, A.; Barry, B.K.; Lloyd, A.R.; Vollmer-Conna, U. Autonomic nervous system function, activity patterns, and sleep after physical or cognitive challenge in people with chronic fatigue syndrome. *J. Psychosom. Res.* **2017**, *103*, 91–94. [CrossRef]

45. Thomas, G.D. Neural control of the circulation. *Adv. Physiol. Educ.* **2011**, *35*, 28–32. [CrossRef]
46. Estévez-López, F.; Mudie, K.; Wang-Steverding, X.; Bakken, I.J.; Ivanovs, A.; Castro-Marrero, J.; Nacul, L.; Alegre, J.; Zalewski, P.; Słomko, J.; et al. Systematic Review of the Epidemiological Burden of Myalgic Encephalomyelitis/Chronic Fatigue Syndrome Across Europe: Current Evidence and EUROMENE Research Recommendations for Epidemiology. *J. Clin. Med.* **2020**, *9*, 1557. [CrossRef] [PubMed]
47. Brown, A.; Jason, L.A. Meta-analysis investigating post-exertional malaise between patients and controls. *J. Health Psychol.* **2020**, *25*, 2053–2071. [CrossRef] [PubMed]

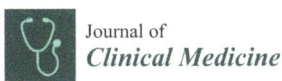

Article

Relationship between Cardiopulmonary, Mitochondrial and Autonomic Nervous System Function Improvement after an Individualised Activity Programme upon Chronic Fatigue Syndrome Patients

Sławomir Kujawski [1,*,†], Jo Cossington [2,†], Joanna Słomko [1], Monika Zawadka-Kunikowska [1], Małgorzata Tafil-Klawe [3], Jacek J. Klawe [1], Katarzyna Buszko [4], Djordje G. Jakovljevic [5], Mariusz Kozakiewicz [6], Karl J. Morten [7], Helen Dawes [2,8], James W. L. Strong [7], Modra Murovska [9], Jessica Van Oosterwijck [10,11], Fernando Estevez-Lopez [12], Julia L. Newton [13], Lynette Hodges [14,‡], Paweł Zalewski [1,‡] and on behalf of the European Network on ME/CFS (EUROMENE)

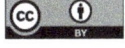

1. Department of Hygiene, Epidemiology, Ergonomy and Postgraduate Education, Ludwik Rydygier Collegium Medicum in Bydgoszcz, Nicolaus Copernicus University in Torun, M. Sklodowskiej-Curie 9, 85-094 Bydgoszcz, Poland; jslomko@cm.umk.pl (J.S.); m.zkunikowska@cm.umk.pl (M.Z.-K.); jklawe@cm.umk.pl (J.J.K.); p.zalewski@cm.umk.pl (P.Z.)
2. Centre for Movement Occupational and Rehabilitation Sciences, Department of Sport, Health Sciences and Social Work, Oxford Brookes University, Headington Rd, Headington, Oxford OX3 0BP, UK; jcossington@brookes.ac.uk (J.C.); hdawes@brookes.ac.uk (H.D.)
3. Department of Human Physiology, Ludwik Rydygier Collegium Medicum in Bydgoszcz, Nicolaus Copernicus University in Torun, Karłowicza 24, 85-092 Bydgoszcz, Poland; malg@cm.umk.pl
4. Department of Biostatistics and Biomedical Systems Theory, Collegium Medicum, Nicolaus Copernicus University, Jagiellonska Street, 85-067 Bydgoszcz, Poland; buszko@cm.umk.pl
5. Institute of Health and Wellbeing, Faculty of Health and Life Sciences, Priory St, Coventry CV1 5FB, UK; djordje.jakovljevic@coventry.ac.uk
6. Department of Geriatrics, Ludwik Rydygier Collegium Medicum in Bydgoszcz, Nicolaus Copernicus University in Torun, M. Sklodowskiej-Curie 9, 85-094 Bydgoszcz, Poland; markoz@cm.umk.pl
7. Nuffield Department of Women's & Reproductive Health, The Women Centre, University of Oxford, Oxford OX3 9DU, UK; karl.morten@wrh.ox.ac.uk (K.J.M.); jamie.strong@kellogg.ox.ac.uk (J.W.L.S.)
8. NIHR Oxford Health Biomedical Research Centre, Oxford OX3 7JX, UK
9. Institute of Microbiology and Virology, Riga Stradiņš University, LV-1067 Riga, Latvia; Modra.Murovska@rsu.lv
10. Department of Rehabilitation Sciences, Ghent University, 9000 Ghent, Belgium; Jessica.VanOosterwijck@UGent.be
11. Research Foundation—Flanders (FWO), 1000 Brussels, Belgium
12. Department of Child and Adolescent Psychiatry/Psychology, Erasmus MC University Medical Center, Postbus 2060, 3000 CB Rotterdam, The Netherlands; fer@estevez-lopez.com
13. Population Health Sciences Institute, The Medical School, Newcastle University, Newcastle-upon-Tyne NE2 4AX, UK; julia.newton@ncl.ac.uk
14. School of Sport, Exercise and Nutrition, Massey University, Palmerston North 4442, New Zealand; L.D.Hodges@massey.ac.nz
* Correspondence: skujawski@cm.umk.pl
† Joint first Authors.
‡ Joint senior Authors.

Abstract: Background: The therapeutic effects of exercise from structured activity programmes have recently been questioned; as a result, this study examines the impact of an Individualised Activity Program (IAP) on the relationship with cardiovascular, mitochondrial and fatigue parameters. Methods: Chronic fatigue syndrome (CFS) patients were assessed using Chalder Fatigue Questionnaire (CFQ), Fatigue Severity Score (FSS) and the Fatigue Impact Scale (FIS). VO$_2$peak, VO$_2$submax and heart rate (HR) were assessed using cardiopulmonary exercise testing. Mfn1 and Mfn2 levels in plasma were assessed. A Task Force Monitor was used to assess ANS functioning in supine rest and in response to the Head-Up Tilt Test (HUTT). Results: Thirty-four patients completed 16 weeks of the IAP. The CFQ, FSS and FIS scores decreased significantly along with a significant increase in Mfn1 and Mfn2 levels ($p = 0.002$ and $p = 0.00005$, respectively). The relationships between VO$_2$ peak and Mfn1 increase in response to IAP (p = 0.03) and between VO$_2$ at anaerobic threshold and ANS response to the HUTT (p = 0.03) were noted. Conclusions: It is concluded that IAP reduces fatigue and improves functional performance along with changes in autonomic and mitochondrial function. However, caution must be applied as exercise was not well tolerated by 51% of patients.

Keywords: myalgic encephalomyelitis; chronic fatigue syndrome; autonomic nervous system; exercise; mitofusin; oxygen consumption

1. Introduction

Chronic Fatigue Syndrome (CFS) is a complex condition characterised by symptoms including chronic fatigue, disturbance in cognitive functions, autonomic dysfunction, pain, ineffective sleep and exercise intolerance [1,2]. Physical or mental exertion might lead to intense debilitating fatigue, musculoskeletal pain, sleep disturbance, headaches, impairments in concentration and short-term memory [3]. Accumulating evidence suggests that the cardiovascular system may be compromised in individuals suffering from CFS, along with reports of autonomic dysfunction [3], impaired heart rate (HR), blood pressure regulation and impaired heart conduction [4].

Autonomic nervous system (ANS) dysfunction is one of the widely described parts of CFS pathomechanism [4]. ANS function can be measured non-invasively using heart rate variability (HRV) [5,6], which differentiates between healthy and diseased states, and is associated with mortality [7]. HRV seems to be a useful biomarker of mental health, stress response and adaptation [8].

Based on HRV, it is proposed that low frequency (LF) variability is an indicator of sympathetic nervous system activity, while high frequency (HF) is an indicator of vagal activity [5,6]. A recent meta-analysis suggests that resting sympathetic hyperactivity, indicated by changes in HRV and blood pressure variability (BPV) might be related to a lower HRmax in CFS patients compared to healthy controls [4]. It is anticipated that chronic sympathetic overactivity might lead to the downregulation of ANS receptors and therefore may suppress HRmax. Moreover, the HR response to a head-up tilt testing (HUTT) was higher in CFS patients compared to healthy controls [4]. The HUTT might serve as a tool in the diagnosis of ANS dysfunction [9,10]. Whilst physical activity programmes might lead to improvement in the ANS in athletes [11], low-volume high-intensity training also improves HRV in sedentary adult men [12]. In addition, the relationship between increased VO2max and increased HRV has also been observed in response to a physical activity program [13].

Although fatigue is multi-dimensional in nature it was recently demonstrated that VO$_2$peak could be an independent predictor of fatigue [14] thus, suggesting the importance of measuring this as a component of health-related fatigue. A recent meta-analysis [15] compared the data of healthy controls and those with CFS from a single exercise test. Franklin et al. [15] demonstrated a pooled mean VO$_2$peak that was 5.2 mL kg^{-1} min^{-1} lower in CFS compared to healthy controls [15]. However, between subject variability was 3.5 (1.5–4.5 mL kg^{-1} min^{-1}) indicating substantial heterogeneity.

In addition to ANS disturbance, mitochondrial dysfunction may also be present in individuals with CFS [16]. The examination of biopsy of muscle tissue using electron microscopy has shown degeneration of mitochondria within this population [17–19]. Healthy mitochondria undergo continual fusion that requires GTPase transmembrane proteins mitofusin 1 (Mfn1) and mitofusin 2 (Mfn2). Deletion of Mfn1 and Mfn2 can lead to a decrease in exercise capacity, which is brought about and worsened by dysfunction in Complex I and IV [20]. Both Mfn1 and 2 are upregulated after physical exercise training in healthy individuals [21]. During starvation or stress, mitochondria form a network structure with mitochondria in a fused state [22]. In this state it is proposed that mitochondria are more efficient at making ATP when substrates are limiting sharing respiratory chain complexes and making the best use of substrates available [23–25]. However, more recently mitochondrial hyperfusion has been linked to various diseases with a negative effect on cell function (reviewed in Rajdeep [26]). Endurance training has the potential to increase mitochondrial functioning, improving biogenesis, mitophagy, and efficiency altering fusion and fission [27]. As already has been mentioned, physical activity programmes might lead to improvement of ANS in healthy participants [12,27]. Therefore, as disturbance in bioenergetics and ANS might be a presumably important parts of CFS pathogenesis, physical exercise program could be applied in patients to improve function of those systems.

Previous studies have documented that a structured activity programme for CFS could be beneficial in some patients in terms of fatigue and disabilities [28–30]. Nevertheless, the therapeutic effectiveness of aerobic physical exercise programmes on CFS seems to be unclear and controversial [31,32]. What seems important is that long-term efficacy of physical exercise programs in CFS patients has been disputed with lack of significant improvement in fatigue and disability compared to patients allocated to receiving standard medical care (SMC) for at least 2 years follow-up [31,32]. Importantly, only four percent of patients from GET group could be considered to be "recovered" when an intention-to-treat approach and protocol-specified definition of recovery is applied [31]. Moreover, long term changes in the examined groups were not statistically significant [31].

This study examines the effects of an Individualised Activity Program (IAP) on self-reported fatigue, respiratory (VO_2submax and VO_2peak), ANS (low frequency to high frequency ratio of R-R interval (LF/HF-RRI) at rest and during HUTT) and mitochondrial (Mfn1 and Mfn2 levels) functioning in CFS patients and the interaction of these outcomes to provide more insight into the disturbance in underlying mechanisms of the exercise effects.

2. Materials and Methods

An activity-based study was performed, which included a homebased exercise intervention and two testing visits, one at baseline, and one post exercise intervention. The patients' progress was supervised during telephone calls which took place every week. The study was approved by the Ethics Committee, Ludwik Rydygier Memorial Collegium Medicum in Bydgoszcz, Nicolaus Copernicus University, Torun, Poland (KB 332/2013, date of approval: 25 June 2013) and written informed consent was obtained from all participants.

2.1. Recruitment and Eligibility

CFS patients were included if they met the diagnostic criteria of the Fukuda case definition for CFS [33]. The patients were recruited based on advertisements in both local and national TV and newspapers. Initially, 1400 volunteers were assessed for eligibility onto the trial with 1308 being excluded. Neurological (myasthenia gravis, traumatic brain injury, stroke, etc.), neurodegenerative (Parkinson's disease, multiple sclerosis, amyotrophic lateral sclerosis, etc.), psychiatric/psychological impairment (atypical depression, generalized anxiety disorder, etc.) and immunologic disorders (systemic lupus erythematosus, type 1 diabetes, celiac disease, rheumatoid arthritis, etc.) which were excluding factors comprised those of which mechanisms might presumably explain primary symptoms of CFS (reasons for exclusion depicted in Figure 1). This left 69 individuals who met the trial inclusion criteria. However, only 53 patients were willing to partake and follow the IAP protocol. Sixteen CFS patients chose not to undertake baseline cardiopulmonary exercise test (CPET). Nineteen patients dropped out due to reported severe post-exertional malaise (PEM) reaction to the IAP [34]. The recruitment and participant flow through the study is shown in Figure 1. A control group was not recruited in the above study.

Anxiety and Depression

A Hospital Anxiety and Depression Scale (HADS) [35] was performed to assess anxiety (HADS_A) and depression (HADS_D) symptoms intensity. Beck Depression Inventory (BDI-II) was used to examine depression symptoms intensity [36]. Both scales were used only at the baseline to exclude patients with depression.

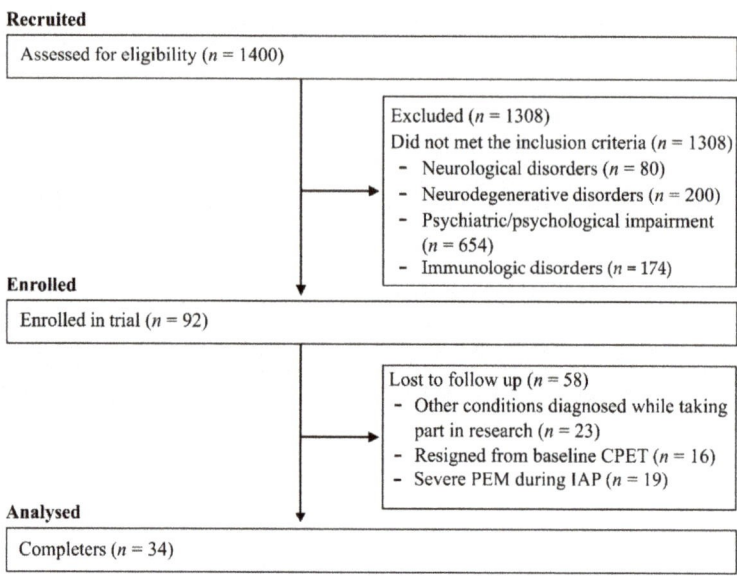

Figure 1. CONSORT-type flow diagram.

2.2. Outcome Measures

2.2.1. Body Composition Analysis

To measure body composition changes a multi frequency bioelectrical impedance analyser (Tanita MC-180MA Body Composition Analyzer, Tanita UK Ltd., Manchester, UK) was applied. All subjects were attributed a 'normal' proprietary algorithm for the impedance measurement. Before measurement, the soles of the feet and the inner part of the hand were cleaned with a sterile dressing to remove any lipid layer. Subjects stood with the ball and heel of each foot in contact with the electrodes on the floor scale. After recording weight in kilograms, the subjects grasped the hand grips with electrode and held them down by their sides with arms extended and away from the body to continue body composition analysis based on bioelectrical impedance signal. Weight kilograms and height in centimetres were measured, and body mass index (BMI) was calculated as well as percent of fat mass and free-fat mass (FFM) in kilograms.

2.2.2. Fatigue

The Chalder Fatigue Questionnaire (CFQ) [37], Fatigue Severity Score (FSS) [38] and the Fatigue Impact Scale (FIS) [39] were administered to provide a comprehensive assessment of fatigue severity. The CFQ assessed physical and psychological fatigue, FSS assessed fatigue in the past week and the FIS assessed cognitive, physical and psychosocial fatigue. Higher scores indicate higher severity in all domains. All questionnaires were administered at baseline and post intervention.

2.2.3. Autonomic Nervous System (ANS) Functioning

ANS functioning was measured with a Task Force Monitor—TFM (CNS Systems, Gratz, Austria). Signals from three-channel ECG were analysed using the adaptive autoregressive model [40]. Low frequency (LFnu-RRI) (0.04–0.15 Hz) and high frequency (HFnu-RRI) (0.15–0.4 Hz) components of R to R intervals in normalized units as well as its ratio (LF/HR-RRI) were recorded and analysed in rest and in response to HUTT. Assessments were performed after 5 min waiting period in supine position which allowed for signals to stabilize. Then, an assessment at rest was performed in supine position which lasted for another 5 min. Heart rate (HR), systolic blood pressure (sBP), diastolic blood pressure (dBP) were measured during rest. Moreover, cardiac index (CI) which is a cardiac output from left ventricle in one minute in relation to body surface area (BSA) was assessed based on cardioimpedance signal. Afterwards, the assessment was performed during a passive HUTT at 70° angle of inclination following the Newcastle protocol [41]. The duration of the HUTT was six minutes which is in line with previous reports [42]. A tilt table with foot support and fastening straps at the knee, hip and chest levels was used to passively change the body position. Differences between mean values of parameters during the third to fourth minute of HUTT along with mean values from the supine position were analysed.

2.2.4. Mitochondrial Function

Blood samples were taken before (baseline) and after IAP (at 16 weeks) to perform biochemical analysis. For plasma, whole blood was collected into commercially available (Vacutainer) anticoagulant EDTA-treated (lavender tops). The cells were removed from plasma by centrifugation for 15 min at $2500\times g$ using a refrigerated ($+4$ °C) centrifuge. The resulting supernatant was designated as plasma. After centrifugation plasma was immediately transferred into a clean sterilized polypropylene tube. The samples were stored at -80 °C until the analysis. Patients started IAP in a sequential manner, therefore some samples of initially recruited patients were frozen longer than the other samples. All samples were defrosted and analysed together. Mfn1 and Mfn2 levels were examined using enzyme-linked immunosorbent assay (ELISA) tests (Cloud-Clone, Katy, TX, USA).

2.2.5. Cardiorespiratory Function

In the presence of a physician, the patients undertook a cardiopulmonary exercise test (CPET) on a treadmill using the Bruce protocol at baseline and at post intervention [43]. A trained technician provided brief instructions and advised the test would end at the moment of full exertion, on the command of the physician, or at any other time point, as stated by the guidelines for safe exercise testing by the American College of Sports Medicine [44]. During exercise there was continuous cardiorespiratory monitoring (Cardiovit CS-200 Ergo-Spiro, Schiller AG, Baar, Switzerland). Heart rate (HR, VO_2, load (watt) and respiratory exchange ratio (RER (VCO_2:VO_2))) were measured to assess cardiopulmonary fitness at baseline and after the intervention. The anaerobic threshold (AT) was determined using the V-slope method [45].

2.3. Intervention

Individualised Activity Programme (IAP)

The IAP has been previously reported [34] and consisted of a prescribed 16-week multimodal home activity programme. The activities were performed 5 days a week, with time (10–40 min) and intensity (30–80% HRpek) increasing gradually across the time period. The HR intensity during activity was individually prescribed based on the actual HRpeak achieved during the CPET. Patients were equipped with HR monitors (Beurer PM 25) to help them in sustaining the recommended HR. Every week, telephone calls were made to resolve potential problems with compliance and to ensure patients were satisfied with the protocol. Patients underwent a minimum of 80 activity sessions, which was the total number of sessions in 16 weeks.

2.4. Statistical Methods

Mitofusins level were not assessed in one patient due to technical difficulties during blood drawing (both before and after physical exercise program) and therefore data on mitofusins level from this patient was not included into analysis. Descriptive statistics include the calculation of means and standard deviations. The Shapiro–Wilk test was used to test the assumption of normality. Variables where values did not meet the normality of distribution assumption, were analysed using Wilcoxon signed-rank test, which was used to compare pre vs. post intervention outcomes. In all other cases t-tests of dependent samples were used. R denotes effect size for Wilcoxon signed-rank test and student t-test provided for statistically significant results [46]. The above tests were performed using statistical package STATISTICA 13.1 (StatSoft, Inc., Tulsa, OK, USA).

Mixed models with random effects were applied to analyse the dependence of CFS, FSS and FIS scales on the CPET and ANS indicators measured at rest and in response to the HUTT. In order to assess the dependence of cardiopulmonary functioning on biochemical parameters and ANS indicators measured at rest and changes in response to tilt mixed models with random effects was performed. In each model, the patients' effects were fitted as random. In the models the maximum likelihood method was applied for estimating variance parameters. Analyses were performed with R version 3.6.2 (R: library lme) [47]. Spearman's correlation was used to analyse relationship between outcomes of the study.

Graphs were created using an R environment [47] with a ggpubr package based on ggplot2 [48]. Benjamini-Hochberg Adjusted P value was chosen to control for False Discovery Rate (FDR). An online calculator for FDR corrections was used (https://www.sdmproject.com/utilities/?show=FDR, accessed on 17 August 2020). *p*-values prior and following FDR correction are reported.

3. Results

Thirty-four CFS patients (20 females, 14 males) completed IAP. Unfortunately, it was not possible for all patients to reach 80% of their HRpeak, and only 1 patient reached this during the last training session. However, 32 patients were able to reach 70% HRmax, and 1 patient achieved 60%HRpeak during the last training sessions. Although patients were encouraged to undertake walking, participants also carried out additional activities including cycling or swimming. All patients chose to perform walking exercises. The mean compliance rate was 80%. Compliance rates for the structured exercise programme were above 60%, which was set as the threshold value. A further examination of the characteristics of IAP completers can be found in Table 1 and Table S1.

Table 1. Patients' characteristics before Individualised Activity Program (IAP).

Variable (Unit)	Mean (SD) before IAP (*n* = 34)
Age (years)	37.06 (7.9)
BMI (kg/m^2)	24.52 (3.2)
FFM (kg)	54.45 (9.7)
Fat (%)	25.04 (6.6)
HADS_A_(points)	10.30 (3.8)
HADS_D_(points)	8.76 (3.2)
BDI_(points)	17.97 (9.1)
HR_(bpm)	69.75 (7.9)
sBP_(mmHg)	116.98 (12)
dBP_(mmHg)	79.45 (10.8)
CI (l/min/m^2)_	3.54 (0.9)

BMI—body mass index, FFM—free-fat mass, HADS_A—Hospital Anxiety and Depression Scale (anxiety score), HADS_D—Hospital Anxiety and Depression Scale (depression score), BDI—Beck Depression Inventory, HR—hear rate, sBP—systolic blood pressure during rest, dBP—diastolic blood pressure during rest, CI—cardiac index.

3.1. Influence of IAP on Fatigue

The influence of the intervention on fatigue was the main area of interest in this study. The structured IAP reduced fatigue levels of the patients in a statistically significant manner on all three scales. The mean scores on the CFQ decreased from 26.12 at baseline to 9.68 post intervention (Z = 5.09, *p* < 0.001, r = 0.62) (Figure 2a). The mean scores on the FSS decreased from 48.91 at baseline to 40.15 post intervention (t = 4.66, *p* < 0.0001, r = 0.63) (Figure 2b). Mean scores on the FIS decreased from 93.59 at baseline to 61.68 post intervention (t = 6.75, *p* < 0.0001, r = 0.76) (Figure 2c) (Table S2).

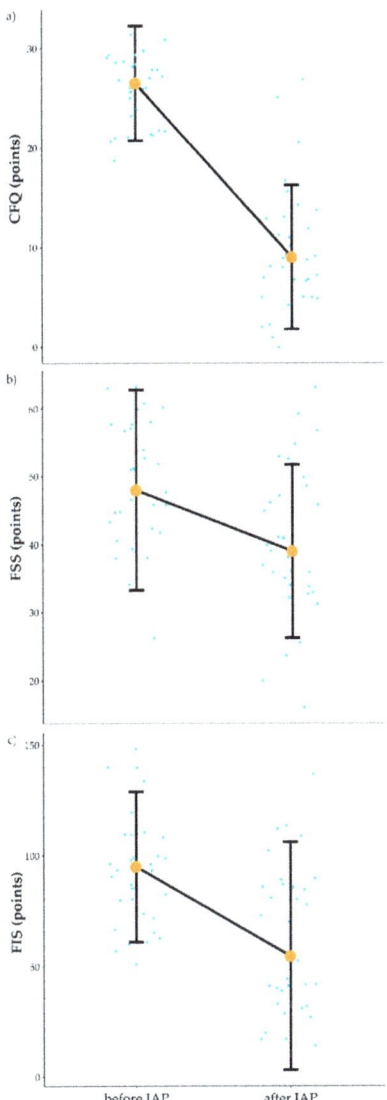

Figure 2. Influence of IAP on fatigue scales. (**a**) influence of IAP on CFS—Chronic Fatigue Scale. (**b**) influence of IAP on FSS—Fatigue Severity Scale. (**c**) influence of IAP on FIS—Fatigue Impact Scale. IAP—Individualised Activity Program, Orange dots connected by black line indicate median value, vertical black lines denote interquartile range. Blue dots before and after denote results of individual patients.

3.2. Influence of IAP on Cardiorespiratory Function

The impact of the intervention on cardiorespiratory function was important in terms of both the occurrence of positive adaptation to the program and indirect evidence of programme compliance. After IAP treadmill workload normalised to body weight at AT was significantly increased (1.31 W/kg before vs. 1.61 W/kg after IAP), $t = -4.53$, $p = 0.00007$, $r = 0.62$ and load/body mass at maximal intensity of physical exercise significantly increased (1.85 W/kg before vs. 2.09 W/kg after), $Z = 2.83$, $p = 0.005$, $r = 0.34$. VT at AT significantly increased (1.66 L vs. 1.81 after), Z = 2.74, p = 0.01, r = 0.33. VO$_2$peak increased significantly (30.3 mL/kg/min before vs. 31.79 after), Z = 1.98, p = 0.047, r = 0.24 (Figure 3) (Table S3). Regarding individual patients, clinically significant improvement defined as improvement of >1.1 mL/kg/min in VO$_2$peak was noted in 19 patients (7 out of 14 males and 12 out of 20 females). The VO$_2$peak improved with 1.66 mL/kg/min when the whole group was considered, and both in males and females. A patient who was able to reach 80% HRmax during the last training session and 18 patients who reached 70% HRmax noted VO$_2$peak clinically significant improvement. A patient who reached 60% and 14 patients who reached 70% HRmax during the last training sessions did not gained clinically significant improvement in VO$_2$peak.

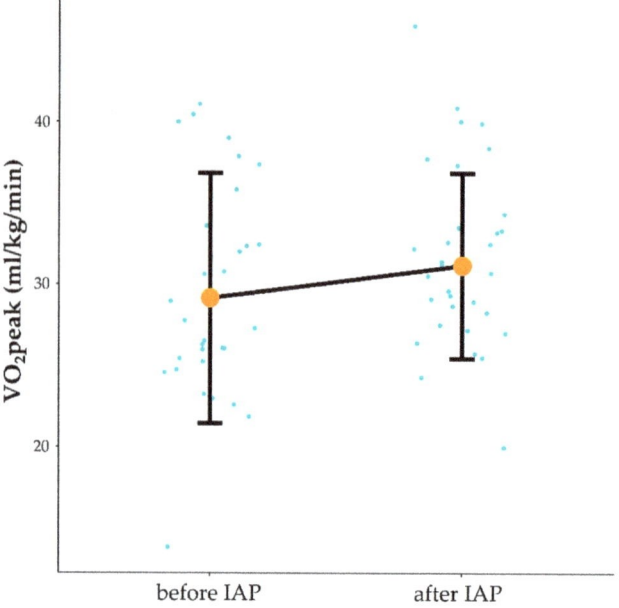

Figure 3. Influence of IAP on VO$_2$peak. VO$_2$peak mL/kg/min—maximal oxygen uptake during physical exercise measured in ml/kg/min, IAP—Individualised Activity Program, Orange dots connected by black line indicate median value, vertical black lines denote interquartile range. Blue dots before and after denote the results of individual patients.

3.3. *Influence of IAP on Mitochondrial Function*

Exploring the effects of IAP on mitochondrial function was one aim of this study. Biochemical analyses showed an increase in both plasma Mfn1 and Mfn2 in response to IAP. Mean value of Mfn1 (increased from 0.22 ng/mL before to 0.33 ng/mL after IAP (Z = 3.07, p = 0.002, r = 0.38)) (Figure 4a). Moreover, Mfn2 mean value (increased from 5.51 ng/mL before vs. to 8.05 ng/mL following the IAP (Z = 4.06, p = 0.00005, r = 0.5) (Figure 4b) (Table S4).

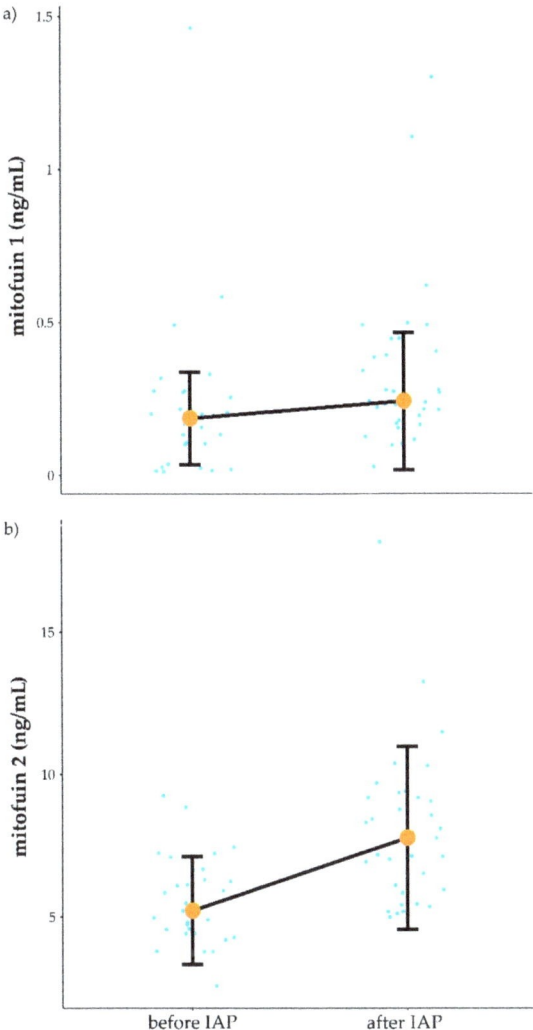

Figure 4. Influence of IAP on Mitofusins. (**a**) influence of IAP on miofusin1 level. (**b**) influence of IAP on mitofusin2 level. IAP—Individualised Activity Program, Orange dots connected by black line indicate median value, vertical black lines denote interquartile range. Blue dots before and after denote the results of individual patients.

3.4. Interaction between VO$_2$peak Improvement, Mitochondrial Plasma Markers and ANS Changes

We explored the role of mitochondria and ANS functions underlying the adaptation to IAP by assessing the indicators of mitochondrial function: MFn1 and MFn2 levels in plasma. The mixed linear model for interaction of VO$_2$peak and Mfn1 was statistically significant (t = 2.5, p = 0.02) (Figure 5).

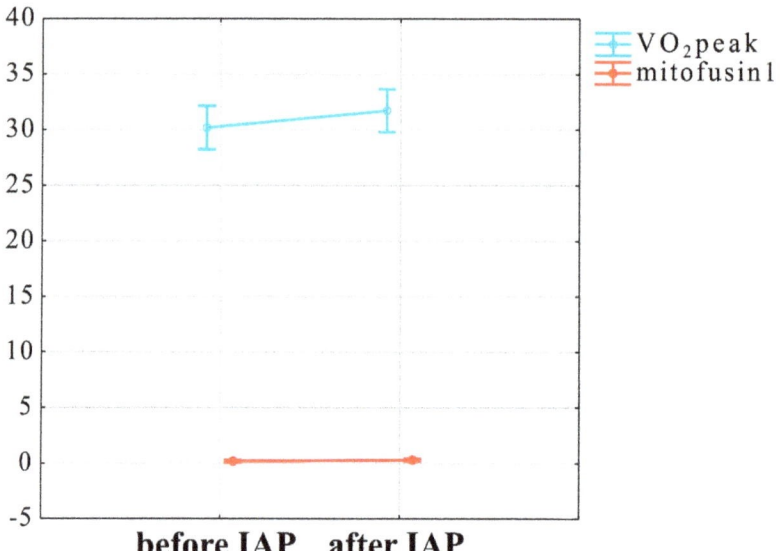

Figure 5. Interaction between influence of IAP on VO$_2$peak and Mfn1. VO$_2$peak—maximal oxygen consumption obtained during physical exercise, mitofusin1—level of mitofusin1, IAP—Individualised Activity Program.

Moreover, the interaction between VO$_2$ at AT (V-slope method) and LF/HF-RRI change in response to HUTT was also significant (t = −2.05, p = 0.048) (Figure 6). Other examined interactions between VO$_2$peak, VO$_2$subpeak, fatigue scale scores and autonomic outcomes or mitofusins were not significant.

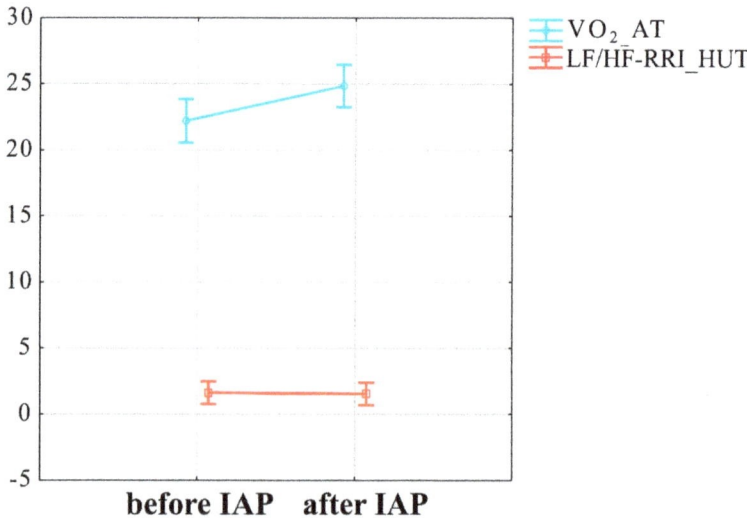

Figure 6. Interaction between influence of IAP on VO$_2$subpeak and sympathovagal balance in response to head-up tilt test. VO$_2$AT—maximal oxygen consumption during anaerobic threshold, LF/HF-RRI_HUTT—low frequency diastolic blood pressure to high frequency R-R interval during head-up tilt test, IAP—Individualised Activity Program.

Influence of IAP on autonomic nervous system function indicators was not significant (Table S5). Heatmap of Spearman's correlation between outcomes of the study is presented on Figure S1.

4. Discussion

This study has noted a statistically significant increase in peak VO_2, alterations in biological factors associated with mitochondria and fatigue in CFS patients who underwent an individualised home-based activity programme. To our knowledge, this is the first study that has associated an increase in maximal aerobic capacity to increased plasma Mfn1 levels. In CFS patients an increase in submax VO_2 related to a decrease in the ratio of sympathetic to parasympathetic activity during HUTT. In a previous study, we noted that CFS patients who completed the IAP showed improved visual attention both in terms of reaction time and correctness of responses and processing speed of simple visual stimuli [34]. It is important to note that there was a significant drop out rate of 51% with IAP [49]. The more sympathetic drive contributes to the control of blood vessels, the longer the reaction time with simple visual stimuli and the lower the HRmax during physical exercise, the chance of a CFS patient completing IAP was reduced [49]. Overall, it could be concluded that an aerobic activity programme characterised by a high frequency of weekly training sessions (5 times/week) and incremental progression of exercise intensity is not well tolerated by a significant number of CFS patients (51% of the patients in the current study). On the other hand, those able to complete the programme noted a reduction in fatigue and improvement in functional performance at the cognitive and cardiovascular level, the latter change being related to changes in autonomic and mitochondrial markers in plasma. It is therefore clear that careful identification of those most likely to benefit and able to participate is needed. Therefore, it would be advisable that any studies seeking to further ascertain the effects of activity programmes in ME/CFS optimally comprise an appropriate control arm, such as a sham intervention or lower intensity exercise regimen with equal assignment of patients classified as more likely to be able to tolerate an aerobic programme comprising high-frequency training sessions. Moreover, benefits and potential harms of training programmes with lower frequency than 5 sessions per week should be examined in further studies.

4.1. Influence of IAP on Self-Reported Fatigue and Peak Oxygen Uptake

The mean CFQ score at baseline was 26.12 in the current study and comparable to 28.2 points scored by the subgroup who received GET in the PACE trial [50]. A 5.4 point decrease in CFQ was previously observed following a 12 week GET trial [51]. The authors of a graded exercise therapy guided self-help trial (GETSET) noted a mean baseline CFQ score of 26.3 for the GET group. After 12-weeks of GET the mean score reduced to 19.1 points, this with a combined effect size of 0.53 [52]. In the current study, the effect size for CFQ scale improvement was 0.62, however, it should be noted that this scale is burdened with many methodological issues which might limit drawing conclusions, especially in longitudinal studies. These issues include problems in the interpretation of the questions when examining the same participants more than once [53]. On the other hand, in our study significant decrease in fatigue were also noted on two other self-reported fatigue measures. The FSS seems to be characterized by high sensitivity and specificity in classification of CFS patients vs. healthy controls [54]. Significant improvement measured by FIS scale was also noted. Hence, these other scales reinforce the observation made using the CFQ assessment. Our study is the first intervention based aerobic activity program in CFS patients that has used three questionnaires to assess the effects on fatigue.

Using CPET testing peak oxygen uptake levels improved by 1.66 mL/kg/min in IAP completers in the whole group regardless of gender. To be considered clinically important in CFS patients peak oxygen uptake needs to increase by 1.1 mL/kg/min [15], therefore, in this study both male and female completers noted improvements higher than the difference between CFS and healthy controls in peak oxygen uptake. Authors of the

PACE trial reported improvement induced by GET in aerobic capacity which was evaluated during a 6-min walk test from 312 m to 379 m at 52-week follow-up. In comparison to the PACE trial, we used CPET, which is the gold standard method to assess physical capacity [51]. In addition, the GETSET study also lacked objective assessments of physical capacity improvement [52].

4.2. Relationship of Peak Oxygen Uptake Improvement and Mitofusin1 Level

The increase in Mfn 1 levels in the plasma of patients who complete the IAP is interesting but difficult to interpret. It is not currently possible to link this increase to what is potentially going on in patients' muscle or other tissues. Mitochondria are constantly being broken down and re-synthesised in energetically active cells including heart, muscle and brain and it has been recently demonstrated that plasma also contains high levels of mitochondria. Some appear to be functional [55] with others are released as a result of cell stress [56]. Mitophagy which drives the break -down of mitochondria and their subsequent recycling is an emerging area of mitochondrial biology with multiple types of mitophagy systems [57]. With most studies carried out in relatively inactive cell lines in vitro it is difficult to know how a highly active tissue like heart and muscle deals with the high demand for mitochondrial turnover. Extracellular vesicles are found at high levels in plasma (reviewed in [58] and contain various cargos including fragments of mitochondria [59] reviewed in [60]. You could speculate that in a very active tissue cells could get rid of larger mitochondrial fragments more rapidly in an extracellular vesicle system than by mitophagy. This could link to the high numbers of mitochondria found in plasma in previous studies and might explain increased levels mitofusin 1 in the plasma of the CFS patients following an IAP. High Mfn1 plasma levels could be linked to either the beneficial or detrimental effects of increased levels of activity in CFS patients. On the positive side, muscle being induced by exercise to form a more network efficient mitochondrial structure could result in an increase in mitochondrial associated Mfn1 debris, expelled to plasma would be linked to enhanced mitochondrial turn over and activity. Detrimentally, high levels of Mfn1 may reflect increased levels of mitochondrial fragmentation linked to induced mitochondrial stress associated with exercise in ME/CFS which may relate to further dysfunction in the future. Without a healthy control group completing the IAP programme it is difficult to know if this increase is just linked to increased exercise or is specific to the CFS group.

Both Mfn1 and Mfn2 play role in the mitochondrial fusion [61]. Mfn1 but not Mfn2 was able to decrease mitochondrial fusion in rodents' skeletal muscle [62]. In a recent rodent-based study, endurance training has been shown to lead to an increase of Mfn1 expression in liver, while a decrease in the sedentary control group with high-fat diet was noted [63].

Exercise training appears to regulate both mitochondrial fusion and fission processes. Seven training sessions of high intensity interval training (HIIT) have been shown to progressively elevate protein content of Mfn1 in human skeletal muscle [64]. In addition, 24 h following a single training session of cycling exercise enhancement of both Mfn1 and Mfn2 mRNA content in human skeletal muscle was observed [21]. However, results of other study contrasts with those discussed above. In a recent study, the effects of a high-intensity interval training (HIIT) program with a progressive increase in intensity on mitochondrial function was assessed. Participants were healthy and recreationally undertaking a physical exercise program before taking part in the study. During the fourth week of the program subjects reached 5 HIIT sessions per week at 8 min intervals with intensity of 90% of VO_2max and 3 min of rest between intervals [65]. After the fourth week disturbances in mitochondria function and impaired glucose homeostasis were observed [65]. It could be speculated that in the case of some of patients in the current study who were unable to complete this was related to the intensity of IAP. Interestingly, both IAP and GET in the PACE trial [51] programmes consisted of five training sessions per week. In contrasts, five HIIT sessions per week has been used to intentionally induce overreaching in healthy participants [65]. We suggest that further studies should consider a personal medicine approach to distinguish whether activity could be considered at all in individual CFS patients. If considered, appropriate the characteristics of a physical activity program need to be considered in terms of frequency, sessions intensity, duration and the type of exercise (interval vs. continuous, endurance vs. strength training, etc.) that are more likely to benefit each particular CFS patient. It seems unlikely that one regime will be appropriate for all those with CFS and for many patients perhaps only pacing would be appropriate at a particular time [66]. Moreover, more studies on predictors of the adverse effects of physical activity/exercise and its underlying pathological mechanism in CFS patients are needed.

4.3. The Relationship between of Submax VO_2 Improvement and ANS Responsiveness

In the current study, improvement in submax VO_2 was related to a decrease in sympathovagal balance in response to the HUTT. Only one patient from 34 was able to reach 80% HRmax intensity during the last training session in a programme. Therefore, the general tendency in our patients was the inability to reach 80% of calculated HRmax even after 15 weeks of training program. Chronotropic intolerance was noted in the current sample and is in line with previous studies on CFS patients [67,68]. A previous study noted that an aerobic exercise training program might lead to improvement in ANS functioning [11]. On the other hand, CFS seems to be an exceptional disorder, in which rapid and dramatic deterioration of symptoms might be induced by physical exercise in patients with post-exertional malaise (PEM) [69]. Poor recovery of diastolic blood pressure and reduced parasympathetic reactivation during recovery from exercise have been previously associated with the pain increases following exercise which are part of the PEM response seen in CFS, evidencing a possible link between ANS dysfunction and PEM [70].

In a study published in 2006, a positive correlation between the measurement of vagal nerve activity and VO_2max was reported for the first time [71]. This positive relationship between HRV and exercise performance is consistent with a large number of previous studies that link variation in heart period [72], total HRV spectral power [73], and HRV triangular index (HRVI) [74] with VO_2max. In addition, cross-sectional studies suggest that higher cardiopulmonary fitness is associated with increased vagal nerve activity [75,76]. The training response was correlated with age (r = 0.39) and with the values of the high-frequency spectral component (HF) of the RR intervals (HF power) analysed during the 24-h recording (r = 0.46), during the day (r = 0.35) and strongest at night (r = 0.52). These data show that the function of the autonomic cardiovascular system is an important determinant of the response to aerobic training in sedentary men. High vagal activity prior to undertaking a training program is associated with an improvement in aerobic capacity as a result of a training program of aerobic exercise in healthy, sedentary individuals [77]. Night-time HF power at baseline was the most effective predictor that explained 27% of the variance in VO_2max improvement with the training program used.

The mechanisms underlying the relationship between ANS and physical training program response remains speculative. Consistent with the high inter-individual and intra-individual variability in training response to exercise, there was also a wide inter-individual variability in the autonomic regulation of the cardiovascular system in healthy subjects, as measured by indices of HR variability [78]. Genetic factors can account for a large proportion (about 20%) of the inter-individual variability in HR [79,80], while demographic and other factors, including blood pressure, blood cholesterol, heart size, body mass index and smoking account, explain only a small part (about 10%) of the variability of the autonomous regulation [80]. It is also possible that there is a mechanistic relationship between the function of the vagus nerve and the response to a training program. In people with optimal vagal function, the cardiovascular system may be better able to adapt to a variety of external stimuli, such as exercise. This adaptive ability can improve overall cardiovascular fitness after regular physical training and thus improve aerobic capacity [77].

4.4. Study Limitations

We have noted a considerable withdrawal rate (35 from 69 patients) from the intervention which was mainly due to the development of PEM. Sixteen patients were unable to complete CPET at baseline and therefore we were unable to incorporate this subgroup in all comparisons. Mitofusins level were analysed using ELISA, which has limits in its precision of measurement level [81]. Moreover, some samples were frozen longer than others, as patients did not start the physical activity program simultaneously. Recently, it has been shown that time of samples being frozen could confound the results [82]. A significant limitation for this study was that PEM was not measured. Moreover, further studies should use questionnaires to examine effects of therapy on potential CFS comorbidities such as anxiety and depression. Due to the relatively small sample size, results on effects of IAP should be replicated in further studies. Additionally, no control group was applied in the above study, limiting the conclusions that can be drown from this study. Future research study should incorporate daily or weekly questionnaires assessing PEM in ME/CFS patients undergoing aerobic exercise program.

Future studies on mechanism underlying PEM should consider a crossover-type trial of a supervised physical activity programme with low load for 12 weeks followed by 12 weeks of high load, to ensure that individuals who take part in the study could be their own controls.

Supplementary Materials: The following are available online at https://www.mdpi.com/article/10.3390/jcm10071542/s1, Table S1: Comparison of results before vs. after IAP in fatigue scales; Table S2: Comparison of results before vs. after IAP in body composition; Table S3: Comparison of results before vs. after IAP in autonomic nervous system functioning; Table S4: Comparison of results before vs. after IAP in mitofusins level; Table S5: Comparison of results before vs. after IAP in CPET results.

Author Contributions: Conceptualization, J.L.N., P.Z., M.T.-K. and J.J.K.; methodology, J.L.N., P.Z., M.T.-K. and J.J.K.; software, S.K.; validation, S.K., J.C., H.D., J.W.L.S., M.M., J.V.O., F.E.-L., J.L.N. and L.H.; formal analysis, S.K. and K.B.; investigation, J.S., M.Z.-K., M.K. and P.Z.; resources, J.S., M.Z.-K., M.T.-K., J.J.K. and P.Z.; data curation, S.K., J.S., M.Z.-K. and P.Z.; writing—original draft preparation, S.K., J.C., H.D. and P.Z.; writing—review and editing, S.K., J.C., J.S., M.Z.-K., M.T.-K., J.J.K., K.B., D.G.J., M.K., K.J.M., H.D., J.W.L.S., M.M., J.V.O., F.E.-L., J.L.N., L.H. and P.Z.; visualization, S.K.; supervision, J.S., M.Z.-K., M.T.-K., J.J.K. and P.Z.; project administration, P.Z.; funding acquisition, P.Z. and K.J.M. All authors have read and agreed to the published version of the manuscript.

Funding: This research received no external funding.

Institutional Review Board Statement: The study was approved by the Ethics Committee, Ludwik Rydygier Memorial Collegium Medicum in Bydgoszcz, Nicolaus Copernicus University, Torun (KB 332/2013, date of approval: 25 June 2013).

Informed Consent Statement: Written informed consent was obtained from all participants.

Data Availability Statement: Individual data is available from the corresponding author S.K. on request.

Acknowledgments: This article/publication is based upon work from COST Action CA15111 "European Network on Myalgic Encephalomyelitis/Chronic Fatigue Syndrome, EUROMENE," supported by COST (European Cooperation in Science and Technology, weblink: www.cost.eu, accessed on 17 August 2020).

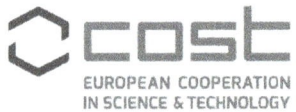
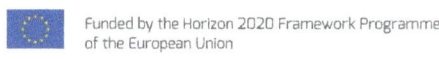

Conflicts of Interest: The authors declare no conflict of interest.

References

1. Prins, J.B.; Bleijenberg, G.; van der Meer, J.W.M. Chronic fatigue syndrome—Authors' reply. *Lancet* **2006**, *367*, 1575. [CrossRef]
2. Jason, L.A.; McManimen, S.; Sunnquist, M.; Brown, A.; Newton, J.L.; Strand, E.B. Examining the Institute of Medicine's Recommendations Regarding Chronic Fatigue Syndrome: Clinical Versus Research Criteria. *J. Neurol. Psychol.* **2015**, *2015*, 441577253.
3. Komaroff, A.L. Advances in understanding the pathophysiology of chronic fatigue syndrome. *JAMA* **2019**, *322*, 499–500. [CrossRef] [PubMed]
4. Nelson, M.J.; Bahl, J.S.; Buckley, J.D.; Thomson, R.L.; Davison, K. Evidence of altered cardiac autonomic regulation in myalgic encephalomyelitis/chronic fatigue syndrome: A systematic review and meta-analysis. *Medicine* **2019**, *98*, e1760. [CrossRef]
5. Fortin, J.; Klinger, T.; Wagner, C.; Sterner, H.; Madritsch, C.; Grullenberger, R. The Task Force Monitor—A Non-invasive Beat-to-beat Monitor for Hemodynamic and Autonomic Function of the Human Body. In *Proceedings of the 20th Annual International Conference of the IEEE*; Engineering in Medicine and Biology Society: Austin, TX, USA, 1988.
6. Fortin, J.; Marte, W.; Grullenberger, R. Continuous non-invasive blood pressure monitoring using concentrically interlocking control loops. *Comput. Biol. Med.* **2006**, *36*, 941–957. [CrossRef] [PubMed]
7. Laborde, S.; Mosley, E.; Thayer, J.F. Heart rate variability and cardiac vagal tone in psychophysiological research–recommendations for experiment planning, data analysis, and data reporting. *Front Psychol.* **2017**, *8*, 213. [CrossRef]
8. Perna, G.; Riva, A.; Defillo, A.; Sangiorgio, E.; Nobile, M.; Caldirola, D. Heart rate variability: Can it serve as a marker of mental health resilience? Special Section on "Translational and Neuroscience Studies in Affective Disorders" Section Editor, Maria Nobile MD, PhD. *J. Affect. Disord.* **2020**, *263*, 754–761. [CrossRef]
9. Naschitz, J.E.; Rosner, I.; Rozenbaum, M.; Gaitini, L.; Bistritzki, I.; Zuckerman, E.; Sabo, E.; Yeshurun, D. The capnography head-up tilt test for evaluation of chronic fatigue syndrome. *Semin. Arthritis Rheum.* **2000**, *30*, 79–86. [CrossRef] [PubMed]
10. Cheshire, W.P.; Goldstein, D.S. Autonomic uprising: The tilt table test in autonomic medicine. *Clin. Auton. Res.* **2019**, *29*, 215–230. [CrossRef]
11. Raczak, G.; Danilowicz-Szymanowicz, L.; Kobuszewska-Chwirot, M.; Ratkowski, W.; Figura-Chmielewska, M.; Szwoch, M. Long-term exercise training improves autonomic nervous system profile in professional runners. *Kardiol. Pol.* **2006**, *64*, 135.
12. Soltani, M.; Baluchi, M.J.; Boullosa, D.; Daraei, A.; Govindasamy, K.; Dehbaghi, K.M.; Mollabashi, S.S.; Doyle–Baker, P.K.; Basati, G.; Saeidi, A.; et al. Endurance training intensity has greater effects than volume on heart rate variability and arterial stiffness adaptations in sedentary adult men: A Randomized Controlled Trial. *Res. Square* **2021**. [CrossRef]
13. Esco, M.R.; Flatt, A.A.; Nakamura, F.Y. Initial weekly HRV response is related to the prospective change in VO2max in female soccer players. *Int. J. Sports Med.* **2016**, *37*, 436–441. [CrossRef]
14. Sebastiao, E.; Hubbard, E.A.; Klaren, E.; Pilutti, L.A.; Motl, R.W. Fitness and its association with fatigue in persons with multiple sclerosis. *Scand. J. Med. Sci. Sports* **2017**, *27*, 1776–1784. [CrossRef]
15. Franklin, J.D.; Atkinson, G.; Atkinson, J.M.; Batterham, A. Peak oxygen uptake in chronic fatigue syndrome/myalgic encephalomyelitis: A meta analysis. *Int. J. Sports Med.* **2019**, *40*, 77–87. [CrossRef]
16. Myhill, S.; Booth, N.E.; McLaren-Howard, J. Chronic fatigue syndrome and mitochondrial dysfunction. *Int. J. Clin. Exp. Med.* **2009**, *2*, 1.
17. Behan, W.M.H.; More, I.A.R.; Behan, P.O. Mitochondrial abnormalities in the postviral fatigue syndrome. *Acta Neuropathol.* **1991**, *83*, 61–65. [CrossRef] [PubMed]
18. Byrne, E.; Trounce, I.; Dennett, X. Chronic relapsing myalgia (postviral): Clinical, histological and biochemical studies. *Aust. N. Z. J. Med.* **1985**, *15*, 305–308. [CrossRef] [PubMed]
19. Vecchiet, L.; Montanari, G.; Pizzigallo, E.; Iezzi, S.; de Bigontina, P.; Dragani, L.; Vecchiet, J.; Giamberardino, M.A. Sensory characterization of somatic parietal tissues in humans with chronic fatigue syndrome. *Neurosci. Lett.* **1996**, *208*, 117–120. [CrossRef]
20. Bell, M.B.; Bush, Z.; McGinnis, G.R.; Rowe, G.C. Adult skeletal muscle deletion of Mitofusin 1 and 2 impedes exercise performance and training capacity. *J. Appl. Physiol.* **2019**, *126*, 341–353. [CrossRef] [PubMed]
21. Cartoni, R.; Léger, B.; Hock, M.B.; Praz, M.; Crettenand, A.; Pich, S.; Ziltener, J.L.; Luthi, F.; Dériaz, O.; Zorzano, A.; et al. Mitofusins 1/2 and ERRalpha expression are increased in human skeletal muscle after physical exercise. *J. Physiol.* **2005**, *567*, 349–358. [CrossRef]
22. Lebeau, J.; Saunders, J.M.; Moraes, V.W.; Madhavan, A.; Madrazo, N.; Anthony, M.C.; Wiseman, R.L. The PERK arm of the unfolded protein response regulates mitochondrial morphology during acute endoplasmic reticulum stress. *Cell Rep.* **2018**, *22*, 2827–2836. [CrossRef]
23. Tondera, D.; Grandemange, S.; Jourdain, A.; Karbowski, M.; Mattenberger, Y.; Herzig, S.; Da Cruz, S.; Clerc, P.; Raschke, I.; Merkwirth, C.; et al. SLP-2 is required for stress-induced mitochondrial hyperfusion. *EMBO J.* **2009**, *28*, 1589–1600. [CrossRef]
24. Sgarbi, G.; Matarrese, P.; Pinti, M.; Lanzarini, C.; Ascione, B.; Gibellini, L.; Dika, E.; Patrizi, A.; Tommasino, C.; Capri, M.; et al. Mitochondria hyperfusion and elevated autophagic activity are key mechanisms for cellular bioenergetic preservation in centenarians. *Aging* **2014**, *6*, 296–310. [CrossRef]
25. Rossignol, R.; Gilkerson, R.; Aggeler, R.; Yamagata, K.; Remington, S.J.; Capaldi, R.A. Energy substrate modulates mitochondrial structure and oxidative capacity in cancer cells. *Cancer Res.* **2004**, *64*, 985–993. [CrossRef] [PubMed]
26. Das, R.; Chakrabarti, O. Mitochondrial hyperfusion: A friend or a foe. *Biochem. Soc. Trans.* **2020**, *48*, 631–644. [CrossRef] [PubMed]

27. Drake, J.C.; Wilson, R.J.; Yan, Z. Molecular mechanisms for mitochondrial adaptation to exercise training in skeletal muscle. *FASEB J.* **2016**, *30*, 13–22. [CrossRef]
28. Cvejic, E.; Lloyd, A.R.; Vollmer-Conna, U. Neurocognitive improvements after best-practice intervention for chronic fatigue syndrome: Preliminary evidence of divergence between objective indices and subjective perceptions. *Compr. Psychiatry* **2016**, *66*, 166–175. [CrossRef] [PubMed]
29. Castell, B.D.; Kazantzis, N.; Moss-Morris, R.E. Cognitive behavioral therapy and graded exercise for chronic fatigue syndrome: A meta-analysis. *Clin. Psychol. Sci. Pract.* **2011**, *18*, 311–324. [CrossRef]
30. Larun, L.; Brurberg, K.G.; Odgaard-Jensen, J.; Price, J.R. Exercise therapy for chronic fatigue syndrome. *Cochrane Database Syst. Rev.* **2016**, *25*, CD003200. [CrossRef]
31. Wilshire, C.E.; Kindlon, T.; Courtney, R.; Matthees, A.; Tuller, D.; Geraghty, K.; Levin, B. Rethinking the treatment of chronic fatigue syndrome—A reanalysis and evaluation of findings from a recent major trial of graded exercise and CBT. *BMC Psychol.* **2018**, *6*, 6. [CrossRef] [PubMed]
32. McPhee, G. Cognitive behaviour therapy and objective assessments in chronic fatigue syndrome. *J. Health Psychol.* **2017**, *22*, 1181–1186. [CrossRef]
33. Fukuda, K.; Straus, S.E.; Hickie, I.; Sharpe, M.C.; Dobbins, J.G.; Komaroff, A. The chronic fatigue syndrome: A comprehensive approach to its definition and study. *Ann. Intern Med.* **1994**, *121*, 953–959. [CrossRef] [PubMed]
34. Zalewski, P.; Kujawski, S.; Tudorowska, M.; Morten, K.; Tafil-Klawe, M.; Klawe, J.J.; Strong, J.; Estévez-López, F.; Murovska, M.; Newton, J.L. The Impact of a Structured Exercise Programme upon Cognitive Function in Chronic Fatigue Syndrome Patients. *Brain Sci.* **2019**, *10*, 4. [CrossRef]
35. Zigmond, A.S.; Snaith, R.P. The hospital anxiety and depression scale. *Acta Psychiatr. Scand.* **1983**, *67*, 361–370. [CrossRef]
36. Beck, A.T.; Steer, R.A.; Ball, R.; Ranieri, W. Comparison of Beck Depression Inventories -IA and -II in psychiatric outpatients. *J. Pers. Assess.* **1996**, *67*, 588–597. [CrossRef] [PubMed]
37. Morriss, R.; Wearden, A.; Mullis, R. Exploring the validity of the Chalder Fatigue scale in chronic fatigue syndrome. *J. Psychosom. Res.* **1998**, *45*, 411–417. [CrossRef]
38. Valko, P.O.; Bassetti, C.L.; Bloch, K.E.; Held, U.; Baumann, C.R. Validation of the fatigue severity scale in a Swiss cohort. *Sleep* **2008**, *31*, 1601–1607. [CrossRef] [PubMed]
39. Frith, J.; Newton, J. Fatigue impact scale. *Occup. Med.* **2010**, *60*, 159. [CrossRef] [PubMed]
40. Bianchi, A.M.; Mainardi, L.T.; Meloni, C.; Chierchiu, S.; Cerutti, S. Continuous monitoring of the sympatho-vagal balance through spectral analysis. *IEEE Eng. Med. Biol. Mag.* **1997**, *16*, 64–73. [CrossRef] [PubMed]
41. Kenny, R.A.; O'Shea, D.; Parry, S.W. The Newcastle protocols for head-up tilt table testing in the diagnosis of vasovagal syncope, carotid sinus hypersensitivity, and related disorders. *Heart* **2000**, *83*, 564–569. [CrossRef] [PubMed]
42. Estévez, M.; Machado, C.; Leisman, G.; Estévez-Hernández, T.; Arias-Morales, A.; Machado, A.; Montes-Brown, J. Spectral analysis of heart rate variability. *Int. J. Disabil. Hum. Dev.* **2016**, *15*, 5–17. [CrossRef]
43. Froelicher, V.F.; Thompson, A.; Noguera, I.; Davis, G.; Stewart, A.J.; Triebwasser, J.H. Prediction of Maximal Oxygen Consumption: Comparison of the Bruce and Balke treadmill protocols. *Chest* **1975**, *68*, 331–336. [CrossRef] [PubMed]
44. Linda, S.; Thompson, W.R.; Gordon, N.F.; Pescatello, L.S. (Eds.) *ACSM's Guidelines for Exercise Testing and Prescription*; Wolters Kluwer Lippincott Williams & Wilkins: Philadelphia, PA, USA, 2010; Volume 8, pp. 35–96.
45. Schneider, D.A.; Phillips, S.E.; Stoffolano, S.H. The simplified V-slope method of detecting the gas exchange threshold. *Med. Sci. Sports Exerc.* **1993**, *25*, 1180–1184. [CrossRef] [PubMed]
46. Field, A. *Discovering Statistics using SPSS*; Sage Publications: London, UK, 2009; 550p.
47. R Core Team. *R: A Language and Environment for Statistical Computing*; R Foundation for Statistical Computing: Vienna, Austria, 2018; Available online: https://ggplot2.tidyverse.org (accessed on 9 October 2019).
48. Wickham, H. *ggplot2: Elegant Graphics for Data Analysis*; Springer: New York, NY, USA, 2016; ISBN 978-3-319-24277-4.
49. Kujawski, S.; Cossington, J.; Słomko, J.; Dawes, H.; Strong, J.W.; Estevez-Lopez, F.; Murovska, M.; Newton, J.L.; Hodges, L.; Zalewski, P. Prediction of Discontinuation of Structured Exercise Programme in Chronic Fatigue Syndrome Patients. *J. Clin. Med.* **2020**, *9*, 3436. [CrossRef] [PubMed]
50. Sharpe, M.; Goldsmith, K.A.; Johnson, A.L.; Chalder, T.; Walker, J.; White, P.D. Rehabilitative treatments for chronic fatigue syndrome: Long-term follow-up from the PACE trial. *Lancet Psychiatry* **2015**, *2*, 1067–1074. [CrossRef]
51. White, P.D.; Goldsmith, K.A.; Johnson, A.L.; Potts, L.; Walwyn, R.; DeCesare, J.C.; Baber, H.L.; Burgess, M.; Clark, L.V.; Cox, D.L.; et al. Comparison of adaptive pacing therapy, cognitive behaviour therapy, graded exercise therapy, and specialist medical care for chronic fatigue syndrome (PACE): A randomised trial. *Lancet* **2011**, *377*, 823–836. [CrossRef]
52. Clark, L.V.; Pesola, F.; Thomas, J.M.; Vergara-Williamson, M.; Beynon, M.; White, P.D. Guided graded exercise self-help plus specialist medical care versus specialist medical care alone for chronic fatigue syndrome (GETSET): A pragmatic randomised controlled trial. *Lancet* **2017**, *390*, 363–373. [CrossRef]
53. Wilshire, C.E.; McPhee, G.; Science for MECFQ. Submission to the public review on common data elements for ME/CFS: Problems with the Chalder Fatigue Questionnaire. Science for ME. 2018. Available online: https://huisartsvink.files.wordpress.com/2018/08/wilshire-mcphee-cfq-cde-critique-for-s4me-final.pdf (accessed on 26 March 2021).
54. Jason, L.A.; Evans, M.; Brown, M.; Porter, N.; Brown, A.; Hunnell, J.; Anderson, V.; Lerch, A. Fatigue scales and chronic fatigue syndrome: Issues of sensitivity and specificity. *Disabil. Stud. Q. Winter* **2011**, *31*, 1375. [CrossRef]

55. Al Amir Dache, Z.A.A.; Otandault, A.; Tanos, R.; Pastor, B.; Meddeb, R.; Sanchez, C.; Arena, G.; Lasorsa, L.; Bennett, A.; Grange, T.; et al. Blood contains circulating cell-free respiratory competent mitochondria. *FASEB J.* **2020**, *34*, 3616–3630. [CrossRef] [PubMed]
56. Puhm, F.; Afonyushkin, T.; Resch, U.; Obermayer, G.; Rohde, M.; Penz, T.; Schuster, M.; Wagner, G.; Rendeiro, A.F.; Melki, I.; et al. Mitochondria Are a Subset of Extracellular Vesicles Released by Activated Monocytes and Induce Type I IFN and TNF Responses in Endothelial Cells. *Circ. Res.* **2019**, *125*, 43–52. [CrossRef]
57. Zachari, M.; Ktistakis, N.T. Mammalian Mitophagosome Formation: A Focus on the Early Signals and Steps. *Front. Cell Dev. Biol.* **2020**, *8*, 171. [CrossRef]
58. Bhattacharyya, K.; Mukherjee, S. Fluorescent Metal Nano-Clusters as Next Generation Fluorescent Probes for Cell Imaging and Drug Delivery. *Bull. Chem. Soc. Jpn.* **2018**, *91*, 447–454. [CrossRef]
59. Bernimoulin, M.; Waters, E.K.; Foy, M.; Steele, B.M.; Sullivan, M.; Falet, H.; Walsh, M.T.; Barteneva, N.; Geng, J.-G.; Hartwig, J.H.; et al. Differential stimulation of monocytic cells results in distinct populations of microparticles. *J. Thromb. Haemost.* **2009**, *7*, 1019–1028. [CrossRef]
60. Sugiura, A.; McLelland, G.; Fon, E.A.; McBride, H.M. A new pathway for mitochondrial quality control: Mitochondrial-derived vesicles. *EMBO J.* **2014**, *33*, 2142–2156. [CrossRef]
61. Westermann, B. Mitochondrial fusion and fission in cell life and death. *Nat. Rev. Mol. Cell Biol.* **2010**, *11*, 872–884. [CrossRef]
62. Eisner, V.; Lenaers, G.; Hajnóczky, G. Mitochondrial fusion is frequent in skeletal muscle and supports excitation–contraction coupling. *J. Cell Biol.* **2014**, *205*, 179–195. [CrossRef]
63. Goncalves, I.O.; Passos, E.; Diogo, C.V.; Rocha-Rodrigues, S.; Santos-Alves, E.; Oliveira, P.J.; Ascensão, A.; Magalhaes, J. Exercise mitigates mitochondrial permeability transition pore and quality control mechanisms alterations in nonalcoholic steatohepatitis. *Appl. Physiol. Nutr. Metab.* **2016**, *41*, 298–306. [CrossRef] [PubMed]
64. Perry, C.G.R.; Lally, J.; Holloway, G.P.; Heigenhauser, G.J.F.; Bonen, A.; Spriet, L.L. Repeated transient mRNA bursts precede increases in transcriptional and mitochondrial proteins during training in human skeletal muscle. *J. Physiol.* **2010**, *588*, 4795–4810. [CrossRef] [PubMed]
65. Flockhart, M.; Nilsson, L.C.; Tais, S.; Ekblom, B.; Apró, W.; Larsen, F.J. Excessive exercise training causes mitochondrial functional impairment and decreases glucose tolerance in healthy volunteers. *Cell Metab.* **2021**. [CrossRef]
66. National Institute for Health and Care Excellence. Myalgic Encephalomyelitis (or Encephalopathy)/Chronic Fatigue Syndrome: Diagnosis and Management. Draft Guidance Consultation. 2020. Available online: https://www.nice.org.uk/guidance/indevelopment/gid-ng10091 (accessed on 26 March 2021).
67. Davenport, T.E.; Lehnen, M.; Stevens, S.R.; Vanness, J.M.; Stevens, J.; Snell, C.R. Chronotropic Intolerance: An Overlooked Determinant of Symptoms and Activity Limitation in Myalgic Encephalomyelitis/Chronic Fatigue Syndrome? *Front. Pediatr.* **2019**, *7*, 82. [CrossRef]
68. Hodges, L.; Nielsen, T.; Cochrane, D.; Baken, D. The physiological time line of post-exertional malaise in Myalgic Encephalomyelitis/Chronic Fatigue Syndrome (ME/CFS). *Transl. Sports Med.* **2020**, *3*, 243–249. [CrossRef]
69. Holtzman, C.S.; Bhatia, S.; Cotler, J.; Jason, L.A. Assessment of Post-Exertional Malaise (PEM) in Patients with Myalgic Encephalomyelitis (ME) and Chronic Fatigue Syndrome (CFS): A Patient-Driven Survey. *Diagnostics* **2019**, *9*, 26. [CrossRef] [PubMed]
70. Van Oosterwijck, J.; Marušič, U.; De Wandele, I.; Paul, L.; Meeus, M.; Moorkens, G.; Lambrecht, L.; Danneels, L.; Nijs, J. The Role of Autonomic Function in Exercise-induced Endogenous Analgesia: A Case-control Study in Myalgic Encephalomyelitis/Chronic Fatigue Syndrome and Healthy People. *Pain Physician* **2017**, *20*, E389–E399.
71. Buchheit, M.; Gindre, C. Cardiac parasympathetic regulation: Respective associations with cardiorespiratory fitness and training load. *Am. J. Physiol. Circ. Physiol.* **2006**, *291*, H451–H458. [CrossRef] [PubMed]
72. Kenney, W.L. Parasympathetic control of resting heart rate: Relationship to aerobic power. *Med. Sci. Sports Exerc.* **1985**, *17*, 451–455. [CrossRef] [PubMed]
73. Pichot, V.; Busso, T.; Roche, F.; Garet, M.; Costes, F.; Duverney, D.; Lacour, J.-R.; Barthélémy, J.-C. Autonomic adaptations to intensive and overload training periods: A laboratory study. *Med. Sci. Sports Exerc.* **2002**, *34*, 1660–1666. [CrossRef]
74. Kouidi, E.; Haritonidis, K.; Koutlianos, N.; Deligiannis, A. Effects of athletic training on heart rate variability triangular index. *Clin. Physiol. Funct. Imaging* **2002**, *22*, 279–284. [CrossRef]
75. Maciel, B.C.; Gallo, L.; Neto, J.A.M.; Filho, E.C.L.; Filho, J.T.; Manço, J.C. Parasympathetic contribution to bradycardia induced by endurance training in man. *Cardiovasc. Res.* **1985**, *19*, 642–648. [CrossRef]
76. Shin, K.; Minamitani, H.; Onishi, S.; Yamazaki, H.; Lee, M. Autonomic differences between athletes and nonathletes: Spectral analysis approach. *Med. Sci. Sports Exerc.* **1997**, *29*, 1482–1490. [CrossRef]
77. Hautala, A.J.; Mäkikallio, T.H.; Kiviniemi, A.; Laukkanen, R.T.; Nissilä, S.; Huikuri, H.V.; Tulppo, M.P. Cardiovascular autonomic function correlates with the response to aerobic training in healthy sedentary subjects. *Am. J. Physiol. Circ. Physiol.* **2003**, *285*, H1747–H1752. [CrossRef]
78. Bouchard, C. Individual differences in the response to regular exercise. *Int. J. Obes. Relat. Metab. Disord.* **1995**, *19* (Suppl. 4), S5–S8.
79. Singh, J.P.; Larson, M.G.; O'Donnell, C.J.; Tsuji, H.; Evans, J.C.; Levy, D. Heritability of Heart Rate Variability: The Framingham Heart Study. *Circulation* **1999**, *99*, 2251–2254. [CrossRef] [PubMed]

80. Singh, J.P.; Larson, M.G.; O'Donnell, C.J.; Tsuji, H.; Corey, D.; Levy, D. Genome scan linkage results for heart rate variability (the Framingham Heart Study). *Am. J. Cardiol.* **2002**, *90*, 1290–1293. [CrossRef]
81. Hosseini, S.; Vázquez-Villegas, P.; Rito-Palomares, M.; Martinez-Chapa, S.O. Advantages, Disadvantages and Modifications of Conventional ELISA. In *Tunable Low-Power Low-Noise Amplifier for Healthcare Applications*; Springer: Singapore, 2018; pp. 67–115.
82. Gómez-Mora, E.; Carrillo, J.; Urrea, V.; Rigau, J.; Alegre, J.; Cabrera, C.; Oltra, E.; Castro-Marrero, J.; Blanco, J. Impact of Long-Term Cryopreservation on Blood Immune Cell Markers in Myalgic Encephalomyelitis/Chronic Fatigue Syndrome: Implications for Biomarker Discovery. *Front. Immunol.* **2020**, *11*, 582330. [CrossRef] [PubMed]

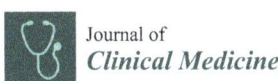

Article

MoCA vs. MMSE of Fibromyalgia Patients: The Possible Role of Dual-Task Tests in Detecting Cognitive Impairment

Alvaro Murillo-Garcia [1], Juan Luis Leon-Llamas [1,*], Santos Villafaina [1], Paloma Rohlfs-Dominguez [1,2] and Narcis Gusi [1]

[1] Physical Activity and Quality of Life Research Group (AFYCAV), Faculty of Sport Science, University of Extremadura, 10003 Cáceres, Spain; alvaromurillo@unex.es (A.M.-G.); svillafaina@unex.es (S.V.); palomaroh@unex.es (P.R.-D.); ngusi@unex.es (N.G.)

[2] Department of Psychology and Anthropology, University of Extremadura, 10003 Caceres, Spain

* Correspondence: leonllamas@unex.es

Abstract: Fibromyalgia is a syndrome that is characterized by widespread pain; fatigue; stiffness; reduced physical fitness; sleep disturbances; psychological symptoms, such as anxiety and depression; and deficits in cognitive functions, such as attention, executive function, and verbal memory deficits. It is important to analyze the potentially different performance on the Mini-Mental State Examination (MMSE) and the Montreal Cognitive Assessment (MoCA) test in patients with fibromyalgia as well as examine the relationship of that performance with physical and cognitive performance. A total of 36 women with fibromyalgia participated in the study. Participants completed the MoCA test, the MMSE, and the TUG physical fitness test under dual-task conditions. The results obtained on cognitive tests were 28.19 (1.74) on the MMSE and 25.17 (2.79) on the MoCA. The participants' performance on cognitive tests was significantly related to the results of the TUG dual-task test. In this way, cognitive performance on a dual-task test can be used to support the diagnosis of cognitive impairment in patients with fibromyalgia. The MoCA test may be a more sensitive cognitive screening tool than the MMSE for patients with fibromyalgia.

Keywords: fibromyalgia; dual task; MMSE; MoCA; TUG; cognitive

Citation: Murillo-Garcia, A.; Leon-Llamas, J.L.; Villafaina, S.; Rohlfs-Dominguez, P.; Gusi, N. MoCA vs. MMSE of Fibromyalgia Patients: The Possible Role of Dual-Task Tests in Detecting Cognitive Impairment. *J. Clin. Med.* **2021**, *10*, 125. https://doi.org/10.3390/jcm10010125

Received: 9 December 2020
Accepted: 29 December 2020
Published: 1 January 2021

Publisher's Note: MDPI stays neutral with regard to jurisdictional clai-ms in published maps and institutio-nal affiliations.

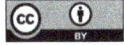

Copyright: © 2021 by the authors. Licensee MDPI, Basel, Switzerland. This article is an open access article distributed under the terms and conditions of the Creative Commons Attribution (CC BY) license (https://creativecommons.org/licenses/by/4.0/).

1. Introduction

Fibromyalgia is a syndrome that is characterized by widespread pain; fatigue; stiffness; reduced physical fitness; sleep disturbances, in particular insomnia [1]; psychological symptoms, such as anxiety and depression [2]; and deficits in cognitive functions, such as attention, executive function, and verbal memory deficits [1,3]. The global prevalence of fibromyalgia is 2.7%, being more prevalent in 50-year-old or older women [4].

A significant body of evidence indicates that cognitive activity is involved in natural motor activities such as walking [5], which is an activity of daily living. When we say cognitive activity, we mean that there is thought. Therefore, when walking, at the same time, we may be thinking of the destination to reach and on what we plan to do there. We may be calculating the distances between obstacles, such as cars or other pedestrians, or even the time we will take to reach the destination. The simultaneously execution of a motor task (such as walking) and a cognitive task (such as thinking) is called a dual task [6]. In this regard, activities of daily living often require the ability to simultaneously perform a cognitive and a motor task, that is, dual-task performance [7]. When an individual faces a dual task in daily life, successful execution of both of these tasks (i.e., the motor task (walking) and the cognitive task (thinking)) decreases because of dual-task interference [6]. This interference occurs because the individual has to divide their attention resources between both of the tasks. "Attention is the cognitive mechanism through which the information that is received by our senses is filtered and/or cognitive resources are assigned to particular elements of that information that are relevant to the observer" [8].

A decrease in the successful execution of a motor task usually leads to accidents, such as falls, especially in older people [5]. In experimental contexts, to replicate the situation in which an individual is walking and cognitive activity occurs, the cognitive motor dual task is usually used [6]. Within this paradigm, participants are asked to perform a cognitive and a motor task at the same time.

Previous studies have found that patients with fibromyalgia usually show reduced dual-task performance in comparison to healthy counterparts [9,10]. Moreover, the ability to perform daily activities is conditioned by physical fitness [11] and the fear of falling [12]. Therefore, physical function is a relevant outcome in patients with fibromyalgia [13]. There are several physical fitness tests that measure subjects' mobility. Among these tests, we emphasize the Timed Up and Go (TUG) test, which is a widely used instrument that evaluates mobility and the risk of falls in older adults [14,15]. In the TUG test, patients have to get up from a chair without using the arm rests. Then, they have to walk 3 m as quickly as possible without running, turn around, walk back to the chair, and sit down without using arm rests [16]. The TUG test provides a valid prognostic assessment to predict falls in elderly people [17], and it has been associated with fall history, indicating that older adults with slower TUG scores report a fall history more often than those in other categories (or compared to other instruments) [18]. TUG scores have been associated with executive function in 70-year-old or older participants, "indicating that a longer time on the TUG is associated with lower executive function performance". These associations have been found specifically using the trail making test (which evaluates the components of executive function that represent complex visual scanning, speed, attention, and the ability to shift sets) and the Stroop word-color test (which evaluates components of executive function representing a person's ability to deal with conflicting stimuli) [19]. In addition, the dual-task TUG test has also been shown to be an effective tool to determine the risk of falls and to better discriminate between fallers and nonfallers, even in a scenario where all standard tests and measures are insufficient to show significant differences [20].

A previous study evaluated the influence of dual-task conditions in patients with fibromyalgia in comparison to healthy people [9]. In this study, both groups performed three physical fitness tests (arm curl, handgrip, and 10-step stair tests) under two conditions: (a) regular condition (single task), that is, without performing any additional cognitive activity, and (b) dual-task condition, that is, while thinking of three words that were given before each test and had to be recalled and verbalized after the execution of each test. As a result, women with fibromyalgia showed lower physical performance (achieving the significance level in the arm curl test and in the 10-step stair test) than healthy people under both single- and dual-task conditions [9]. In addition, Moriarty et al. conducted a review of clinical and preclinical research to establish whether chronic pain negatively affects cognition. The authors concluded that pain is associated with impaired cognitive function and might be a consequence of competing limited neural resources, neuroplasticity, and/or dysregulated brain neurochemistry [21].

The Mini-Mental State Examination (MMSE) [22] is a widely used screening tool for dementia [23], and it is validated for Spanish-speaking communities [24]. A meta-analysis of the accuracy of the MMSE in the detection of dementia and mild cognitive impairment showed that the cut-off of 23/24 was the most used in the 34 analyzed studies [25]. However, the MMSE has a series of limitations, especially regarding its use in more educated patients [26]. To address this problem, the Montreal Cognitive Assessment (MoCA) was developed as a tool to screen patients with mild cognitive impairment whose performance on the MMSE is usually located at the normal range [27]. A meta-analysis compared the diagnostic accuracy of a range of cut-off scores from nine studies that evaluated the validity of the MoCA. The results showed that a cut-off score of 23/30 has a better diagnostic accuracy across parameters than the originally recommended 26/30 cut-off score, reducing the rate of false positives [28].

Previous research has examined which cognitive screening tool (MMSE vs. MoCA) is more effective [28,29]. In this regard, the MoCA seems superior to the MMSE in the detection of cognitive impairment in patients at a higher risk for incident dementia [29]. Another study supported that the MoCA is, as a cognitive screening tool, superior to the MMSE in detecting cognitive decline in its early stages [30]. In addition, the MoCA, but not the MMSE, has adequate psychometric properties as a screening instrument for the detection of mild cognitive impairment or dementia in Parkinson's disease [31]. However, that question has not been studied in patients with fibromyalgia, although cognitive impairment is one of the symptoms [32].

Considering all the above, the aim of the present study was to analyze the differences between the cognitive assessment of both the MMSE and MoCA in patients with fibromyalgia as well as examine the relationship of the cognitive assessment score with physical and cognitive performance under dual-tasks conditions.

2. Experimental Section

2.1. Design

This study was designed as an explorative and descriptive study.

2.2. Participants

A total of 36 women with fibromyalgia participated in the study. The inclusion criteria were: women aged between 30 and 75 years old diagnosed with fibromyalgia by a rheumatologist, according to the criteria that have been established by the American College of Rheumatology [1]. Participants were excluded from the study if they met the following exclusion criteria: (a) being pregnant and (b) not being able to stand and sit on a chair once.

All participants provided signed written consent to participate in the study. All procedures were approved by the university's bioethical committee (approval number: 62/2017) and followed the recommendations of the updated Declaration of Helsinki.

2.3. Procedures

First, anthropometric measurements of the participants were taken to calculate the body mass index (BMI). Subsequently, the participants completed the Spanish version of the Fibromyalgia Impact Questionnaire (FIQ), which evaluates the impact of symptoms of the disease from 0 to 100, indicating the minimum to maximum impact, respectively. The FIQ is an extensively validated fibromyalgia-specific tool that captures the overall effects of fibromyalgia symptomatology (pain, fatigue, feeling rested, stiffness, anxiety, depression, physical impairment, feel good, or work missed) [33–35]. After, trained research staff administered the MoCA and MMSE, both previously used in patients with fibromyalgia [36–38].

The MoCA test is a brief cognitive screening tool with high sensitivity and specificity for detecting mild cognitive impairment, which evaluates the following cognitive abilities: attention, concentration, executive functions (including the capacity for abstraction), memory, language, visuoconstructive abilities, calculation, and orientation [27]. The required administration time is approximately ten minutes. The maximum score is 30 [39]. In the present study, a score of 23 or higher was considered normal. In this sense, a meta-analysis compared the diagnostic accuracy of a range of cut-off scores of nine studies that evaluated the validity of the MoCA test. Its results showed that a cut-off score of 23/30 has a better diagnostic accuracy across parameters than the originally recommended 26/30 cut-off score, reducing the rate of false positives [28].

The MMSE is a widely used test of cognitive function; it includes tests of orientation, attention, memory, language, and visual-spatial skills. A higher score represents a better cognitive state. In the present study, a score of 24 or higher was considered normal. A meta-analysis of the accuracy of the MMSE in the detection of dementia and mild cognitive impairment showed that the cut-off of 23/24 was the most used in the 34 studies that were analyzed [25].

Finally, the participants completed the TUG physical fitness test under single- and dual-task conditions. The order of single- and dual-task conditions was randomized.

Particularly, under the single-task condition, the participants had to get up from a chair without using arm rests; then, they had to walk 3 m as quickly as possible without running, turn around, walk back to the chair, and sit down without using arm rests [16]. The dual-task condition consisted of counting aloud backward two by two while performing the tests, starting from a random number higher than 100 [40].

2.4. Data Analysis

The SPSS statistical package version 24 (IBM Corp., Armonk, NY, USA) was used to analyze the data. Descriptive analyses were conducted to obtain means and standard deviations (SDs) regarding participants' age and anthropometric measurements. Moreover, parametric and nonparametric tests were conducted based on the results of the Shapiro–Wilk test. Thus, Pearson´s and Spearman's rho correlation analyses were conducted to evaluate the relationship between the participants' performance on cognitive tests (MMSE vs. MoCA) and cognitive performance on the TUG test under dual-task conditions. In addition, the dual-task cost (DTC) of the TUG test [41] was calculated as follows:

$$DTC = (\text{Dual-task TUG time} - \text{Single-task TUG time})/\text{Single-task TUG time}$$

The TUG cognitive performance variable was calculated by dividing the number of cognitive hits (correct answers in the subtractions) between the seconds spent on the dual-task test.

3. Results

Table 1 shows the participants' descriptive characteristics in terms of means and SDs, including age 55.11 (8.74) years, BMI 28.30 (3.44) kg/m^2, FIQ-100 53.50 (20.31), and medications: analgesics/relaxants (33.3%), hypotensive drugs (11.1%), antidepressants (41.7%), and others (80.6%).

Table 1. Characteristics of the participants.

Variable (n = 36) (Maximum–Minimum Values)	Mean (SD)
Age (years) (34–70)	55.11 (8.74)
BMI (kg/m^2) (24–39)	28.30 (3.44)
FIQ-100 (9–86)	53.50 (20.31)
Medication	**n (Percentage)**
Analgesics/Relaxants	12 (33.3%)
Hypotensive drugs	4 (11.1%)
Antidepressants	15 (41.7%)
Others	29 (80.6%)

BMI, body mass index; FIQ, Fibromyalgia Impact Questionnaire; SD, standard deviation.

Table 2 shows the results of the participants' performance on the TUG test, in terms of means and SDs, under single-task, 7.55 (1.96) seconds, and dual-task, 8.20 (2.30) seconds, conditions. In addition, this table shows the dual-task cost on the TUG test: −0.08 (1.11) seconds. Table 2 shows the results regarding the participants' performance on the TUG test, which is related to cognitive performance: 0.53 (0.28). The number of cognitive hits, 4.14 (2.09), and misses, 0.11 (0.38), in the subtractions on the dual-task TUG test are also reported in Table 2. Finally, the results obtained on cognitive tests (MMSE: 28.19 (1.74) and MoCA: 25.17 (2.79)) are also reported in Table 2.

Table 2. Performance on the TUG test, dual-task TUG test, and cognitive tests (MMSE and MoCA).

Variable (n = 36) (Maximum–Minimum Values)	Mean	SD
TUG (5.43–15.06)	7.55	1.96
TUG Dual-Task (5.39–15.42)	8.20	2.30
TUG Dual-Task Cost (−0.07–0.45)	0.08	0.11
TUG Cognitive Performance (0–1)	0.53	0.28
TUG Hits (0–7)	4.14	2.09
TUG Misses (0–2)	0.11	0.38
MMSE (23–30)	28.19	1.74
MoCA (19–31)	25.17	2.79

TUG, Timed Up and Go; MMSE, Mini-Mental State Examination; MoCA, Montreal Cognitive Assessment.

Table 3 shows the correlation analyses between the participants' performance on the TUG test under single- and dual-task conditions and the participants' performance on cognitive tests (MMSE and MoCA test) without finding a correlation in any of the tests. In addition, the correlation analyses between cognitive test results and the dual-task cost, cognitive performance, and hits and misses on the TUG test under the dual-task condition are reported in Table 3. As can be observed, the participants' performance on cognitive tests was only significantly related to the results of the TUG dual-task cognitive performance test.

Table 3. Correlations between the TUG test and cognitive tests.

Variable (n = 36)	MMSE		MoCA Test	
TUG	Spearman's CC	−0.206	Spearman's CC	−0.136
	p-value	0.227	p-value	0.082
TUG Dual-Task	Spearman's CC	−0.260	Spearman's CC	−0.105
	p-value	0.126	p-value	0.541
TUG Dual-Task Cost	Spearman's CC	−0.077	Spearman's CC	0.020
	p-value	0.657	p-value	0.906
TUG Dual-Task Cognitive Performance	Spearman's CC	0.355	Pearson's CC	0.348
	p-value	0.034 *	p-value	0.038 *
TUG Hits	Spearman's CC	0.169	Spearman's CC	0.297
	p-value	0.324	p-value	0.078
TUG Misses	Spearman's CC	0.059	Spearman's CC	−0.187
	p-value	0.732	p-value	0.275

* p-value <0.05. CC, correlation coefficient; TUG, Timed Up and Go; MMSE, Mini-Mental State Examination; MoCA, Montreal Cognitive Assessment.

Finally, results of the participants' performance on the MMSE and the MoCA are shown in Tables 4 and 5, respectively, in terms of frequencies. Regarding Table 4 (performance on the MMSE), only 2.8% of the participants had cognitive impairment (with the cut-off point at 24) and 25% of the participants answered all the questions correctly. Regarding Table 5 (on performance on the MoCA), 16.7% of the participants had cognitive impairment (with the cut-off point at 23) and only 5.6% of the participants answered all the questions correctly. Thus, the results showed a ceiling effect, with 25.0% of the participants achieving a perfect score on the MMSE compared to 5.6% on the MoCA.

Table 4. Results regarding the participants' performance on the MMSE.

MMSE (n = 36)	Frequency	Percentage	Accumulated Percentage
0–22	0	0%	0
23	1	2.8%	2.8%
24	0	0%	2.8%
25	3	8.3%	11.1%
26	1	2.8%	13.9%
27	5	13.9%	27.8%
28	7	19.4%	47.2%
29	10	27.8%	75.0%
30	9	25.0%	100%
Total	36	100%	

Table 5. Results regarding the participants' performance on the MoCA test.

MoCA (n = 36)	Frequency	Percentage	Accumulated Percentage
0–19	1	2.8%	2.8%
20	2	5.6%	8.3%
21	1	2.8%	11.1%
22	2	5.6%	16.7%
23	4	11.1%	27.8%
24	2	5.6%	33.3%
25	8	22.2%	55.6%
26	2	5.6%	61.1%
27	7	19.4%	80.6%
28	5	13.9%	94.4%
29	0	0%	94.4%
30	2	5.6%	100%
Total	36	100	

4. Discussion

This is the first study to analyze, compare, and correlate the results of two well-known cognitive assessment tests (MMSE and MoCA) with the physical and cognitive performance on the TUG test under single- and dual-task conditions in people with fibromyalgia. We found positive correlation between the results of the cognitive tests (MMSE and MoCA) and the cognitive performance on the TUG test under dual-task condition. According to the results of the MMSE, only 2.8% of the participants had cognitive impairment. However, according to the results of the MoCA test, 16.7% of the participants had cognitive impairment. In both tests, the strictest cut-off points were used to avoid false positives (23 in the MoCA and 24 in the MMSE). In addition, although less-strict cut-off points were used in each test (26 in the MoCA and 27 in the MMSE), a difference between the results of both tests still existed. Finally, using less strict cut-off points in each test, 13.9% of the population had cognitive impairment on the MMSE and 55.6% on the MoCA.

Despite the experimental results of neuroimaging studies, a diagnosis of cognitive and behavioral impairment in patients with fibromyalgia still relies on the use of validated tests of neuropsychiatric assessment [42]. In addition, several studies have confirmed that a diagnosis of cognitive impairment using a single test is not enough and have recommended relying on other methods to ensure the diagnosis [31,43,44]. Furthermore, in people with fibromyalgia, comorbid symptoms such as depression, anxiety, insomnia, and fatigue may impact cognitive function, but they do not entirely explain the mental impairment. Chronic pain may disrupt attention and induce neuroplasticity in the central nervous system [42]. Thus, it is difficult to find a gold standard for the evaluation of cognitive impairment in fibromyalgia. Therefore, it is important to know which of the cognitive tests used is most adequate to help in the diagnosis of cognitive impairment in fibromyalgia.

The findings of the present study are consistent with most of the research that has been conducted to date: the MMSE does not perform well as a screening instrument (mainly due to the ceiling effect). This may be partially due to a lack of sensitivity to milder cognitive deficits [31,45]. The present results show the instrument ceiling effect, with 25.0% of the participants achieving a perfect score on the MMSE compared to 5.6% on the MoCA. As shown in a previous study, the poorer performance of the MMSE in detecting cognitive impairment may be due to a series of several factors, apart from a lack of sensitivity to milder cognitive deficits. First, the MMSE may be less effective at assessing complex cognitive domains such as visuospatial skills, executive function, and abstract reasoning. In addition, the MMSE includes one test for attention, while the MoCA includes two additional tests (digit span and vigilance). Similarly, the three-item test on delayed recall in the MMSE is less difficult than the five-item test on delayed recall in the MoCA. Thus, the attention and delayed-recall items in the MMSE are easier than in the MoCA [46]. The differences that have been described above between performance on the MMSE and performance on the MoCA are important when assessing cognitive impairment in patients with fibromyalgia because a previous study found memory and vocabulary deficits in patients with fibromyalgia, showing that memory function in patients with fibromyalgia is not age-appropriate [47]. For the above reasons, it is possible to recommend the MoCA test to help in the diagnosis of mild cognitive impairment in fibromyalgia patients.

The results obtained in the TUG test are similar to results of other studies on fibromyalgia patients, both under single-task [40,48,49] and dual-task [40] conditions. Among the measures that were obtained from the dual-task TUG test, we identified cognitive performance. This variable was calculated by dividing the number of cognitive hits between the seconds spent on the dual-task test. In this regard, we found a positive correlation between the results of both cognitive tests (MMSE and MoCA) and the cognitive performance on the TUG test under a dual-task condition. A previous study found significant correlations between performance on the TUG test (under dual-task conditions) and MoCA and MMSE scores [41]. In this study, the cognitive task consisted of reciting the days of the week in reverse order starting from Sunday while performing the TUG test. These findings suggested that the TUG test under the dual-task condition might be used in clinical practice as a functional and practical test for the early screening of cognitive dysfunction among older adults. However, the authors recommended additional studies including more challenging cognitive tasks during the TUG test to obtain stronger correlations with cognitive tests. Therefore, in the current study, we selected a dual-task condition that consisted of counting aloud backward two by two while performing the tests, starting from a random number higher than 100 [40]. This might be the reason we found a correlation only between cognitive performance on the TUG test under the dual-task condition and the results of both cognitive tests (MMSE and MoCA), being even stricter for the assessment of cognitive impairment. Moreover, the cognitive task used under the dual-task condition (counting aloud backward two by two) requires some of the cognitive domains that are assessed on the MMSE or the MoCA, such as working memory, calculation, or attention, among others. This is relevant since when clinicians or researchers conduct evaluations under the dual-task paradigm, physical performance is usually presented, ignoring cognitive performance under the dual-task condition. However, our results suggested that cognitive performance under the dual-task condition provides us with cognitive information in the same line using the MoCA and MMSE. Thus, to complement the patients' cognitive assessments, this variable should be considered rather than physical performance under the dual-task condition or even the DTC.

Previously, it was shown that physical performance on the TUG test under single- and dual-task conditions could predict mild cognitive impairment [19]. However, the results of the current study did not show correlations between physical performance on the TUG (single- and dual-task) test and cognitive performance on cognitive tests. Importantly, we found a positive correlation between the results of cognitive tests (MMSE and MoCA) and cognitive performance on the TUG test under the dual-task condition. This relationship between cognitive performance on cognitive tests and cognitive performance on the TUG test under the dual-task condition may help support the cognitive impairment diagnosis in fibromyalgia patients, highlighting its importance.

The present study had limitations: the small number of participants and all the participants being women. Thus, the results cannot be extrapolated to men with fibromyalgia. Moreover, our data cannot be compared with normative data (for the MoCA and the MMSE) due to both the specificity of the fibromyalgia population and the lack of normative values for this population. Furthermore, since there is no gold standard to measure cognitive impairment in patients with fibromyalgia, the sensitivity and specificity of both cognitive tests could not be calculated in the present study. The main conclusion was based on the ceiling effect of both tests.

5. Conclusions

The MoCA may be a more sensitive cognitive screening tool than the MMSE for patients with fibromyalgia. The results of both cognitive tests correlated with cognitive performance on the dual-task TUG test. As such, cognitive performance on a dual-task test can be used to support the diagnosis of cognitive impairment in patients with fibromyalgia because it provides a functional assessment related to real-life activities, although more research is needed to generalize the present results to populations with fibromyalgia.

Author Contributions: Conceptualization, A.M.-G. and S.V.; methodology, J.L.L.-L.; software, N.G.; validation, S.V., J.L.L.-L., and A.M.-G.; formal analysis, S.V.; investigation, P.R.-D.; resources, N.G.; data curation, S.V.; writing—original draft preparation, A.M.-G.; writing—review and editing, P.R.-D.; visualization, J.L.L.-L.; supervision, S.V.; project administration, N.G.; funding acquisition, N.G. All authors have read and agreed to the published version of the manuscript.

Funding: In the framework of the Spanish National R + D + i Plan, the current study was co-funded by the Spanish Ministry of Sciences and Innovation (reference PID2019-107191RB-I00). This study was also funded by the Research Grant for Groups (GR18155) funded by the Junta de Extremadura (Regional Government of Extremadura) and the European Regional Development Fund (ERDF/FEDER) "a way of doing Europe". This study was supported by the Biomedical Research Networking Center on Frailty and Healthy Aging (CIBERFES) and FEDER funds from the European Union (CB16/10/00477).

Institutional Review Board Statement: All procedures were approved by the university bioethical committee (approval number: 62/2017) and followed the recommendations of the updated Declaration of Helsinki.

Informed Consent Statement: All participants provided signed written consent to participate in the study.

Data Availability Statement: All data are available by the corresponding author (S.G.) upon reasonable request.

Acknowledgments: The author A.M.-G. was supported by a grant from the Spanish Ministry of Education, Culture, and Sport (FPU17/031330). The author J.L.L.-L. was supported by a grant from the Spanish Ministry of Education, Culture, and Sport (FPU18/05655). The author S.V. was supported by a grant from the Regional Department of Economy and Infrastructure of the Government of Extremadura and the European Social Fund (PD16008). The funders played no role in the study design, data collection and analysis, the decision to publish, or the preparation of the manuscript.

Conflicts of Interest: The authors certify that there is no conflict of interest with any financial organization regarding the material discussed in the manuscript.

References

1. Wolfe, F.; Clauw, D.J.; Fitzcharles, M.-A.; Goldenberg, D.L.; Katz, R.S.; Mease, P.; Russell, A.S.; Russell, I.J.; Winfield, J.B.; Yunus, M.B. The American College of Rheumatology preliminary diagnostic criteria for fibromyalgia and measurement of symptom severity. *Arthritis Care Res.* **2010**, *62*, 600–610. [CrossRef]
2. Galvez-Sánchez, C.M.; Montoro, C.I.; Duschek, S.; del Paso, G.A.R. Depression and trait-anxiety mediate the influence of clinical pain on health-related quality of life in fibromyalgia. *J. Affect. Disord.* **2020**, *265*, 486–495. [CrossRef]
3. Kalfon, T.B.-O.; Gal, G.; Shorer, R.; Ablin, J.N. Cognitive functioning in fibromyalgia: The central role of effort. *J. Psychosom. Res.* **2016**, *87*, 30–36. [CrossRef]
4. Queiroz, L.P. Worldwide epidemiology of fibromyalgia. *Curr. Pain Headache Rep.* **2013**, *17*, 356. [CrossRef] [PubMed]
5. Li, K.Z.H.; Bherer, L.; Mirelman, A.; Maidan, I.; Hausdorff, J.M. Cognitive involvement in balance, gait and dual-tasking in aging: A focused review from a neuroscience of aging perspective. *Front. Neurol.* **2018**, *9*, 913. [CrossRef] [PubMed]
6. Kimura, T.; Matsuura, R. Additional effects of a cognitive task on dual-task training to reduce dual-task interference. *Psychol. Sport Exerc.* **2020**, *46*, 101588. [CrossRef]
7. Yuan, J.; Blumen, H.M.; Verghese, J.; Holtzer, R. Functional connectivity associated with gait velocity during walking and walking-while-talking in aging: A resting-state fMRI study. *Hum. Brain Mapp.* **2015**, *36*, 1484–1493. [CrossRef] [PubMed]
8. Sánchez-López, A.; Quinto-Guillen, R.; Pérez-Lucas, J.; Jurado-Barba, R.; Martínez-Grass, I.; Ponce-Alfaro, G.; Rubio-Valladolid, G. Validación de la versión española del Test Stroop de Alcohol. *An. Psicol.* **2015**, *31*, 504–523.
9. Villafaina, S.; Collado-Mateo, D.; Domínguez-Muñoz, F.J.; Fuentes-García, J.P.; Gusi, N. Impact of adding a cognitive task while performing physical fitness tests in women with fibromyalgia: A cross-sectional descriptive study. *Medicine* **2018**, *97*, e13791. [CrossRef]
10. Villafaina, S.; Polero, P.; Collado-Mateo, D.; Fuentes-García, J.P.; Gusi, N. Impact of adding a simultaneous cognitive task in the elbow's range of movement during arm curl test in women with fibromyalgia. *Clin. Biomech.* **2019**, *65*, 110–115. [CrossRef]
11. Panton, L.B.; Kingsley, J.D.; Toole, T.; Cress, M.E.; Abboud, G.; Sirithienthad, P.; Mathis, R.; McMillan, V. A comparison of physical functional performance and strength in women with fibromyalgia, age-and weight-matched controls, and older women who are healthy. *Phys. Ther.* **2006**, *86*, 1479–1488. [CrossRef] [PubMed]
12. Collado-Mateo, D.; Gallego-Diaz, J.M.; Adsuar, J.C.; Domínguez-Muñoz, F.J.; Olivares, P.; Gusi, N. Fear of falling in women with fibromyalgia and its relation with number of falls and balance performance. *BioMed Res. Int.* **2015**, *2015*, 589014. [CrossRef]
13. Da Silva Costa, I.; Gamundí, A.; Miranda, J.G.V.; França, L.G.S.; De Santana, C.N.; Montoya, P. Altered functional performance in patients with fibromyalgia. *Front. Hum. Neurosci.* **2017**, *11*, 14.
14. Herman, T.; Mirelman, A.; Giladi, N.; Schweiger, A.; Hausdorff, J.M. Executive control deficits as a prodrome to falls in healthy older adults: A prospective study linking thinking, walking, and falling. *J. Gerontol. Ser. A Biomed. Sci. Med. Sci.* **2010**, *65*, 1086–1092. [CrossRef] [PubMed]
15. Herman, T.; Giladi, N.; Hausdorff, J.M. Properties of the 'timed up and go'test: More than meets the eye. *Gerontology* **2011**, *57*, 203–210. [CrossRef] [PubMed]
16. Podsiadlo, D.; Richardson, S. The timed "Up & Go": A test of basic functional mobility for frail elderly persons. *J. Am. Geriatr. Soc.* **1991**, *39*, 142–148. [PubMed]
17. Hofheinz, M.; Mibs, M. The prognostic validity of the timed up and go test with a dual task for predicting the risk of falls in the elderly. *Gerontol. Geriatr. Med.* **2016**, *2*, 2333721416637798. [CrossRef]
18. Asai, T.; Oshima, K.; Fukumoto, Y.; Yonezawa, Y.; Matsuo, A.; Misu, S. Association of fall history with the Timed Up and Go test score and the dual task cost: A cross-sectional study among independent community-dwelling older adults. *Geriatr. Gerontol. Int.* **2018**, *18*, 1189–1193. [CrossRef]
19. McGough, E.L.; Kelly, V.E.; Logsdon, R.G.; McCurry, S.M.; Cochrane, B.B.; Engel, J.M.; Teri, L. Associations between physical performance and executive function in older adults with mild cognitive impairment: Gait speed and the timed "up & go" test. *Phys. Ther.* **2011**, *91*, 1198–1207.
20. Ponti, M.; Bet, P.; Oliveira, C.L.; Castro, P.C. Better than counting seconds: Identifying fallers among healthy elderly using fusion of accelerometer features and dual-task Timed Up and Go. *PLoS ONE* **2017**, *12*, e0175559. [CrossRef]
21. Moriarty, O.; McGuire, B.E.; Finn, D.P. The effect of pain on cognitive function: A review of clinical and preclinical research. *Prog. Neurobiol.* **2011**, *93*, 385–404. [CrossRef] [PubMed]
22. Folstein, M.F.; Folstein, S.E.; McHugh, P.R. "Mini-mental state": A practical method for grading the cognitive state of patients for the clinician. *J. Psychiatr. Res.* **1975**, *12*, 189–198. [CrossRef]
23. Tariq, S.H.; Tumosa, N.; Chibnall, J.T.; Perry Iii, M.H.; Morley, J.E. Comparison of the Saint Louis University mental status examination and the mini-mental state examination for detecting dementia and mild neurocognitive disorder—A pilot study. *Am. J. Geriatr. Psychiatry* **2006**, *14*, 900–910. [CrossRef] [PubMed]
24. Blesa, R.; Pujol, M.; Aguilar, M.; Santacruz, P.; Bertran-Serra, I.; Hernández, G.; Sol, J.M.; Peña-Casanova, J.; Group Normacodem. Clinical validity of the 'mini-mental state'for Spanish speaking communities. *Neuropsychologia* **2001**, *39*, 1150–1157. [CrossRef]
25. Mitchell, A.J. A meta-analysis of the accuracy of the mini-mental state examination in the detection of dementia and mild cognitive impairment. *J. Psychiatr. Res.* **2009**, *43*, 411–431. [CrossRef] [PubMed]
26. Anthony, J.C.; LeResche, L.; Niaz, U.; Von Korff, M.R.; Folstein, M.F. Limits of the 'Mini-Mental State'as a screening test for dementia and delirium among hospital patients. *Psychol. Med.* **1982**, *12*, 397–408. [CrossRef]

27. Nasreddine, Z.S.; Phillips, N.A.; Bédirian, V.; Charbonneau, S.; Whitehead, V.; Collin, I.; Cummings, J.L.; Chertkow, H. The Montreal Cognitive Assessment, MoCA: A brief screening tool for mild cognitive impairment. *J. Am. Geriatr. Soc.* **2005**, *53*, 695–699. [CrossRef]
28. Carson, N.; Leach, L.; Murphy, K.J. A re-examination of Montreal Cognitive Assessment (MoCA) cutoff scores. *Int. J. Geriatr. Psychiatry* **2018**, *33*, 379–388. [CrossRef]
29. Dong, Y.; Lee, W.Y.; Basri, N.A.; Collinson, S.L.; Merchant, R.A.; Venketasubramanian, N.; Chen, C.L.-H. The Montreal Cognitive Assessment is superior to the Mini–Mental State Examination in detecting patients at higher risk of dementia. *Int. Psychogeriatr.* **2012**, *24*, 1749–1755. [CrossRef]
30. Roalf, D.R.; Moberg, P.J.; Xie, S.X.; Wolk, D.A.; Moelter, S.T.; Arnold, S.E. Comparative accuracies of two common screening instruments for classification of Alzheimer's disease, mild cognitive impairment, and healthy aging. *Alzheimer's Dement.* **2013**, *9*, 529–537. [CrossRef]
31. Hoops, S.; Nazem, S.; Siderowf, A.D.; Duda, J.E.; Xie, S.X.; Stern, M.B.; Weintraub, D. Validity of the MoCA and MMSE in the detection of MCI and dementia in Parkinson disease. *Neurology* **2009**, *73*, 1738–1745. [CrossRef] [PubMed]
32. Wu, Y.-L.; Huang, C.-J.; Fang, S.-C.; Ko, L.-H.; Tsai, P.-S. Cognitive impairment in fibromyalgia: A meta-analysis of case–control studies. *Psychosom. Med.* **2018**, *80*, 432–438. [CrossRef] [PubMed]
33. Burckhardt, C.S.; Clark, S.; Bennett, R. Fibromyalgia and quality of life: A comparative analysis. *J. Rheumatol.* **1993**, *20*, 475–479. [PubMed]
34. Bennett, R. The Fibromyalgia Impact Questionnaire (FIQ): A review of its development, current version, operating characteristics and uses. *Clin. Exp. Rheumatol.* **2005**, *23*, S154–S162.
35. Esteve-Vives, J.; Redondo, J.R.; Salvat, M.I.S.; de Gracia Blanco, M.; de Miquele, C.A. Proposal for a consensus version of the Fibromyalgia Impact Questionnaire (FIQ) for the Spanish population. *Reumatol. Clínica* **2007**, *3*, 21–24. [CrossRef]
36. Rodríguez-Andreu, J.; Ibáñez-Bosch, R.; Portero-Vázquez, A.; Masramon, X.; Rejas, J.; Gálvez, R. Cognitive impairment in patients with fibromyalgia syndrome as assessed by the mini-mental state examination. *BMC Musculoskelet. Disord.* **2009**, *10*, 162. [CrossRef]
37. Borg, C.; Padovan, C.; Thomas-Antérion, C.; Chanial, C.; Sanchez, A.; Godot, M.; Peyron, R.; De Parisot, O.; Laurent, B. Pain-related mood influences pain perception differently in fibromyalgia and multiple sclerosis. *J. Pain Res.* **2014**, *7*, 81–87. [CrossRef]
38. Aparicio, V.A.; Segura-Jimenez, V.; Alvarez-Gallardo, I.C.; Soriano-Maldonado, A.; Castro-Pinero, J.; Delgado-Fernandez, M.; Carbonell-Baeza, A. Fitness testing in the fibromyalgia diagnosis: The al-Ándalus project. *Med. Sci. Sports Exerc.* **2015**, *47*, 451–459. [CrossRef]
39. Hobson, J. The montreal cognitive assessment (MoCA). *Occup. Med.* **2015**, *65*, 764–765. [CrossRef]
40. Martín-Martínez, J.P.; Villafaina, S.; Collado-Mateo, D.; Pérez-Gómez, J.; Gusi, N. Effects of 24-week exergame intervention on physical function under single-and dual-task conditions in fibromyalgia: A randomized controlled trial. *Scand. J. Med. Sci. Sports* **2019**, *29*, 1610–1617. [CrossRef]
41. Lima, L.C.A.; Ansai, J.H.; Andrade, L.P.; Takahashi, A.C.M. The relationship between dual-task and cognitive performance among elderly participants who exercise regularly. *Braz. J. Phys. Ther.* **2015**, *19*, 159–166. [CrossRef] [PubMed]
42. Bertolucci, P.H.F.; de Oliveira, F.F. Cognitive impairment in fibromyalgia. *Curr. Pain Headache Rep.* **2013**, *17*, 344. [CrossRef] [PubMed]
43. Petersen, R.C. Mild cognitive impairment as a diagnostic entity. *J. Intern. Med.* **2004**, *256*, 183–194. [CrossRef] [PubMed]
44. Flicker, C.; Ferris, S.H.; Reisberg, B. Mild cognitive impairment in the elderly: Predictors of dementia. *Neurology* **1991**, *41*, 1006. [CrossRef]
45. Dong, Y.; Sharma, V.K.; Chan, B.P.-L.; Venketasubramanian, N.; Teoh, H.L.; Seet, R.C.S.; Tanicala, S.; Chan, Y.H.; Chen, C. The Montreal Cognitive Assessment (MoCA) is superior to the Mini-Mental State Examination (MMSE) for the detection of vascular cognitive impairment after acute stroke. *J. Neurol. Sci.* **2010**, *299*, 15–18. [CrossRef]
46. Nys, G.M.S.; Van Zandvoort, M.J.E.; de Kort, P.L.M.; Jansen, B.P.W.; Kappelle, L.J.; de Haan, E.H.F. Restrictions of the Mini-Mental State Examination in acute stroke. *Arch. Clin. Neuropsychol.* **2005**, *20*, 623–629. [CrossRef]
47. Park, D.C.; Glass, J.M.; Minear, M.; Crofford, L.J. Cognitive function in fibromyalgia patients. *Arthritis Rheum. Off. J. Am. Coll. Rheumatol.* **2001**, *44*, 2125–2133. [CrossRef]
48. Collado-Mateo, D.; Domínguez-Muñoz, F.J.; Adsuar, J.C.; Merellano-Navarro, E.; Olivares, P.R.; Gusi, N. Reliability of the timed up and go test in fibromyalgia. *Rehabil. Nurs. J.* **2018**, *43*, 35–39. [CrossRef]
49. Collado-Mateo, D.; Dominguez-Muñoz, F.J.; Adsuar, J.C.; Merellano-Navarro, E.; Gusi, N. Exergames for women with fibromyalgia: A randomised controlled trial to evaluate the effects on mobility skills, balance and fear of falling. *PeerJ* **2017**, *5*, e3211. [CrossRef]

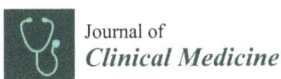

Review

The Emerging Role of Gut Microbiota in Myalgic Encephalomyelitis/Chronic Fatigue Syndrome (ME/CFS): Current Evidence and Potential Therapeutic Applications

Angelica Varesi [1,2,*], Undine-Sophie Deumer [3], Sanjana Ananth [4] and Giovanni Ricevuti [5,*]

1. Department of Biology and Biotechnology, University of Pavia, 27100 Pavia, Italy
2. Almo Collegio Borromeo, 27100 Pavia, Italy
3. Department of Biological Sciences, Faculty of Natural Sciences and Mathematics, University of Cologne, 50674 Cologne, Germany; udeumer@small.Uni-Koeln.de
4. Department of Metabolism, Digestion and Reproduction, Faculty of Medicine, Imperial College London, London SW7 2AZ, UK; s.ananth@imperial.ac.uk
5. Department of Drug Sciences, School of Pharmacy, University of Pavia, 27100 Pavia, Italy
* Correspondence: angelica.varesi@collegioborromeo.eu (A.V.); giovanni.ricevuti@unipv.it (G.R.)

Citation: Varesi, A.; Deumer, U.-S.; Ananth, S.; Ricevuti, G. The Emerging Role of Gut Microbiota in Myalgic Encephalomyelitis/Chronic Fatigue Syndrome (ME/CFS): Current Evidence and Potential Therapeutic Applications. *J. Clin. Med.* **2021**, *10*, 5077. https://doi.org/10.3390/jcm10215077

Academic Editor: Moussa Antoine Chalah

Received: 15 September 2021
Accepted: 28 October 2021
Published: 29 October 2021

Publisher's Note: MDPI stays neutral with regard to jurisdictional claims in published maps and institutional affiliations.

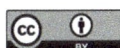

Copyright: © 2021 by the authors. Licensee MDPI, Basel, Switzerland. This article is an open access article distributed under the terms and conditions of the Creative Commons Attribution (CC BY) license (https://creativecommons.org/licenses/by/4.0/).

Abstract: The well-known symptoms of Myalgic Encephalomyelitis/Chronic Fatigue Syndrome (ME/CFS) are chronic pain, cognitive dysfunction, post-exertional malaise and severe fatigue. Another class of symptoms commonly reported in the context of ME/CFS are gastrointestinal (GI) problems. These may occur due to comorbidities such as Crohn's disease or irritable bowel syndrome (IBS), or as a symptom of ME/CFS itself due to an interruption of the complex interplay between the gut microbiota (GM) and the host GI tract. An altered composition and overall decrease in diversity of GM has been observed in ME/CFS cases compared to controls. In this review, we reflect on genetics, infections, and other influences that may factor into the alterations seen in the GM of ME/CFS individuals, we discuss consequences arising from these changes, and we contemplate the therapeutic potential of treating the gut to alleviate ME/CFS symptoms holistically.

Keywords: ME/CFS; dysbiosis; therapy; diagnosis; intestinal permeability; metabolic endotoxemia; LPS

1. Introduction

Since the late 19th century, reasonably reliable medical records have been available which describe a multisystemic and debilitating disease of unknown origin causing chronic and severe fatigue which prevents individuals from carrying out normal levels of day-to-day activities [1]. Today, this disease is known under the terms myalgic encephalomyelitis and chronic fatigue syndrome (ME/CFS) and is diagnosed based on symptoms using established consensus criteria (i.e., Fukuda, Canadian Consensus Criteria, Oxford, International Consensus Criteria, etc.) [2–5]. Besides disabling fatigue, cognitive dysfunction, sleep problems, autonomic dysfunction, and post-exertional malaise are often reported in individuals with ME/CFS [6]. While ME/CFS is clearly accompanied by immunological alterations and inflammatory dysfunctions [7–12], recent findings suggests that a link between microbial dysbiosis and disease pathogenesis is also possible [13–15]. Although the precise etiology of ME/CFS is poorly understood, genetic predisposition, viral infection, and stress have been considered to be linked with disease origin and chronicity [6,16–18]. For example, the finding that relatives of ME/CFS cases report significantly higher rates of ME/CFS or similar fatigue-like symptoms compared to random controls may indicate a genetic contribution to disease onset [19–21]. However, independent studies on different cohorts often lack reproducibility, thus evidencing the need for new larger investigations [22]. Similarly, pathogens such as Epstein-Barr Virus (EBV), Human Herpesvirus (HHV)-6, and Human Parvovirus B19 are suspected of contributing to the development of the disease via antiviral immune activation and systemic inflammation [23–29], but their necessity for ME/CFS development remains debated [30]. Indeed, several studies comparing ME/CFS cases with controls failed to support the hypothesis of involvement of a viral infection in disease pathogenesis [29,31–35]. Moreover, it should be noted that the vast majority of people recover from infections without consequences, therefore making it difficult to establish a clear correlation between infection and ME/CFS. Other infectious diseases such as Lyme disease or COVID-19 have also been suggested to increase the risk of developing ME/CFS [36,37]; yet the mechanism behind this is largely unknown. One hypothesis is that the infection causes inflammation in the body, which dysregulates the immune response and inflammatory cascades in the long term [10,11,18,38]; but how this impacts the onset of ME/CFS has yet to be defined.

The term "gut microbiota" (GM) describes the microbial community in the gastrointestinal (GI) tract, which consists of a plethora of bacteria, archaea, phages, yeasts, protozoa, and fungal species that exist in a symbiotic relationship with the human gut. Owing to advancements in genomic studies and metagenomic analysis, GM composition has been studied regarding development of certain diseases such as neuro-psychological disorders, cancer, cardio-metabolic disorders, and inflammatory bowel disease (IBD) [39,40]. *Firmicutes, Bacteroides, Proteobacteria, Fusobacteria, Verrucomicrobia, Cyanobacteria*, and *Actinobacteria* are the major taxonomic groups typically found in the gut [41,42]. As the GM and their habitat are involved in a complex interplay, host environmental factors such as pH, transit time, bile acids, digestive enzymes, and mucus play an important role in GM composition [42–44]. Non-host factors involved can be nutrients and medications, as well as bacterial properties such as adhesion, metabolic capacity, and enzymes [44,45]. The microbiota produces many chemical mediators that can travel to distant regions, such as the brain, and affect the host's health positively or negatively [46,47]. Indeed, by synthesizing nutrients and vitamins, producing beneficial or toxic metabolites, inhibiting microbial and viral pathogens, detoxifying food, and contributing to the development of a healthy immune system, GM are essential for the host [42–44]. Depending on the GM composition, effects on the immune system can differ. Immune cell priming partly takes place in the gut and signals for the development of T regulatory, T helper (Th-1 and Th-2), and Th-17 cells are generated, which are involved in immune system regulation and cytokine secretion as a defense against foreign antigens [48–51]. Furthermore, the GM has other metabolic functions such as bile acid transformation by microbial enzymes for cholesterol and glucose metabolism, amino acid synthesis and vitamin production [52,53]. Another beneficial function for the host is short-chain fatty acid (SCFAs) production, which includes acetate, butyrate, and propionate required for energy production and cholesterol synthesis [54,55]. As ME/CFS is a systemic disease, GI disturbances are another class of symptoms commonly reported [56–58]. Indeed, comorbidities such as irritable bowel syndrome (IBS) or Crohn's disease may be found in ME/CFS individuals, thus suggesting a possible role of the gut microbiome in disease progression [59,60]. However, whether and how the GM is involved in ME/CFS pathogenesis and development is still unknown. Here, we briefly review the most relevant studies addressing how dysbiosis and intestinal permeability may contribute to disease phenotype, and we discuss the possible therapeutic applications aimed at restoring eubiosis and intestinal barrier integrity in the context of ME/CFS.

2. Main Findings

2.1. Alterations of Human Microbiome in ME/CFS

In the past years, studies have been conducted to investigate the kind of alterations taking place in the gut microbiome in ME/CFS and their implications for those suffering from ME/CFS. Significant dysregulations in the overall composition of microbiota and shifted ratios between several bacterial taxa in comparison to healthy controls have been detected ([61,62], Figure 1, Table 1). For example, a modified microbiome was found in saliva, gut, and feces of ME/CFS cases, linking the GM to the disease [12,63]. Moreover, when 16S ribosomal ribonucleic acid (rRNA) sequencing was used to compare stool samples from 43 ME/CFS individuals and 36 healthy controls, an altered GM composition and imbalance in microbial diversity have been reported ([64] Table 1). Subsequently, similar results were obtained using the same technique [13,14,63,65,66]. Interestingly, a striking decrease in relative abundance and diversity of *Firmicutes* bacteria, and a higher number of *Bacteroidetes* was detected [14]. Often, a lower *Bacteroides/Firmicutes* ratio can be accompanied by an increase in *Enterobacteriaceae*, therefore suggesting a complete reshuffling of the gut microbiota composition [63,64]. Since shifts in microbial ratios have also been identified in autoimmune conditions such as Crohn's disease, Systemic Lupus Erythematosus 2, and Diabetes Type 2, it would be interesting to investigate whether the microbiome may be linked to ME/CFS autoimmune manifestations, if they occur [63,67–70]. While environmental and genetic factors can alter the microbiome [42,44], changes in GM composition according to geographical origin should also be considered in ME/CFS [64]. In this respect, studies involving matched healthy controls are crucial. When accounting for these differences, Nagy-Szakal et al. report a differential microbiota composition in ME/CFS cases with or without IBS comorbidity when compared to the same number of matched controls. Indeed, while an increase in *Alipstes* and a decrease in *Faecalibacterium* seem to characterize ME/CFS individuals who also present IBS, a rise in unclassified *Bacteroides*, but not in *Bacteroides vulgatus*, appears typical of ME/CFS without IBS comorbidity [13]. However, as disturbances may arise due to the high prevalence of IBS comorbidity in individuals with ME/CFS, these results should be confirmed in larger cohorts before drawing any conclusion [13].

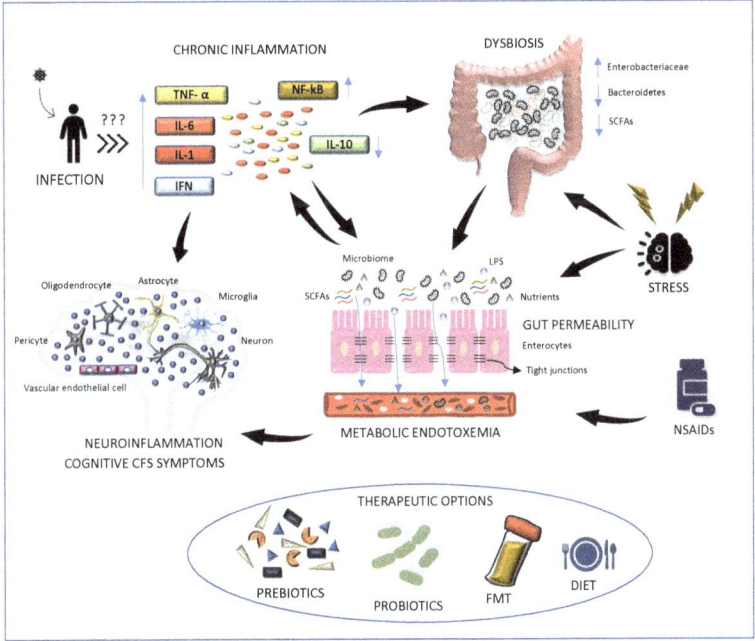

Figure 1. Role of dysbiosis and gut permeability in ME/CFS pathogenesis.

Table 1. Summary of studies concerning dysbiosis in ME/CFS.

Reference	Journal	Participants	Classification Criteria	Analysis Performed	Results
Giloteaux et al., 2016 [71]	Am Jour Case Rep	A pair of 34 year old monozygotic male twins, 1 ME/CFS and 1 control	Fukuda (1994) [4]	Two-day CPET; stool biochemical and molecular analysis; 16S RNA sequencing	↓ Microbial diversity ↓ *Faecalibacterium* and *Bifidobacterium*
Shukla et al., 2015 [66]	PLOS One	10 ME/CFS and 10 matched healthy controls	Fukuda (1994) [4]	Maximal exercise challenge, stool examination before and 15 min, 48 h, 72 h after exercise. PCR and 16S rRNA sequence	↑ Abundance changes of major bacterial phyla (after exercise) ↓ Bacterial clearance (after exercise)
Kitami et al., 2020 [65]	Sci Rep	48 ME/CFS and 52 controls	Fukuda (1994) [4] and International Consensus Criteria (2011) [5]	Stool microbiome analysis by DNA extraction and 16S rRNA sequencing	↑ *Coprobacillus*, *Eggerthella* and *Blautia*
Mandarano et al., 2018 [61]	PeerJ	49 ME/CFS and 39 healthy controls	Fukuda (2004) [4]	18S rRNA sequencing in stool samples	↓ Eukaryotic diversity (nonsignificant) ↑ *Basidiomycota/Ascomycota* ratio (nonsignificant)
Nagy-Szakal et al., 2017 [13]	Microbiome	50 ME/CFS and 50 matched healthy controls	Fukuda (2004) [4] and/or Canadian Criteria (2003) [3]	Fecal bacterial metagenomics (shotgun metagenomic sequences)	↑ Dysbiosis ↑ *Alistipes* (in ME/CFS with IBS), *Bacteroides* (in ME/CFS without IBS) ↓ *Faecalibacterium* (in ME/CFS with IBS), *Bacteroides vulgatus* (in ME/CFS without IBS)
Lupo et al., 2021 [63]	Sci Rep	35 ME/CFS and 70 healthy controls (35 had relatives with ME/CFS and 35 not)	Fukuda (2004) [4]	Fecal bacterial analysis by 16S rRNA Illumina sequencing	↓ *Anaerostipes* (*Lachnospiraceae*) ↑ *Bacteroides* and *Phascolarctobacterium*
Giloteaux et al., 2016 [14]	Microbiome	49 ME/CFS and 39 healthy controls	Fukuda (2004) [4]	16S rRNA sequencing from stool	↓ Diversity ↓ *Firmicutes* phylum ↑ Pro-inflammatory species (*Proteobacteria* species)
Frémont et al., 2013 [64]	Anaerobe	43 ME/CFS and 36 healthy controls	Fukuda (1994) [4]	High-throughput 16S rRNA sequencing from stool samples	↑ *Lactonifactor* and *Alistipes* ↓ Several *Firmicutes* populations
Sheedy et al., 2009 [62]	In Vivo	108 ME/CFS and 177 healthy controls	Holmes (1988) [72]/Fukuda (1994) [4]/Canadian Definition Criteria (2003) [3]	Fecal sample collection and identification of facultative anaerobic organisms using standard criteria [73]	↑ Dlactic acid producing *Enterococcus* and *Streptococcus* spp.

CPET: cardiopulmonary exercise test; ↓ decrease; ↑ increase.

GM dysbiosis may also represent a cause of increased gut permeability [60]. In this respect, a correlation between changes in GM and a higher level of inflammation was observed in some studies [60,64]. Moreover, increased commensal bacterial translocation and enhanced gut inflammation have been found in ME/CFS cases compared to controls, as discussed in more detail in Section 2.2 [60,74,75] (Figure 1). Although the exact mechanism behind this phenomenon largely remains unknown, one hypothesis is that the rise in *Enterobacteriaceae* found in dysbiosis may mediate intestinal inflammation and permeability, as increased levels of lipopolysaccharide derived from these bacteria is detected in ME/CFS [74,76,77] (Figure 1). However, it should be noted that this is far from being proven, and more research is needed to address this point. Another possibility is that bacterial metabolites contribute to the disease by interfering with the estrogen receptor and Vitamin D receptor pathways, as the latter is also involved in development of autoimmune disorders, which often occur as comorbidities of ME/CFS as mentioned previously, but this topic remains to be addressed [64,78,79]. Last, when searching for a possible mechanism for how dysbiosis influences ME/CFS pathogenesis, the gut-brain-axis, and the autonomic and enteric nervous systems should also be considered [60,80].

Although the importance of gut microbiome in health and disease is becoming more and more prominent, several limitations still need to be addressed in respect to ME/CFS. Indeed, if the data cited above report evidence for a dysregulated gut microbiota composition, it is also true that contradictory studies are present in the literature. For example, when 18S rRNA sequencing was used to analyze eukaryotic diversity in ME/CFS cases compared to controls, insignificant differences were reported [61]. Likewise, even though alterations in the human gut microbiome (i.e., the multitude of genes of the gut microbiota), have been observed in multiple studies in ME/CFS cases, results have failed to be reproduced between studies, likely due to study design [12,14,81]. The reason for this discrepancy could be found, at least in part, in the narrowness of the cohort analyzed in each study. In this respect, in order to have reliable and statistically significant results new investigations should be carried out involving more participants, both ME/CFS cases and controls. Similarly, the idea of using rRNA sequencing as a new diagnostic tool in ME/CFS, although attractive, has yet to be validated to avoid misdiagnosis. Altogether, these data point out that gut microbiota alterations seem to characterize ME/CFS in those affected, but the role of dysbiosis in disease pathogenesis and progression should be further investigated.

2.2. Increased Gut Permeability in ME/CFS

The intestinal barrier is a single-cell epithelial layer that allows the selective absorption of nutrients, electrolytes, and water through a mucous membrane. In health, epithelial cells are tightly connected by desmosomes, adherens junctions and tight junctions, which are made up of occludin, claudins, and junctional adhesion molecules respectively. Thus, intraluminal translocation of bacteria and toxins into the bloodstream is prevented [82]. However, when homeostasis is altered, for example due to gut inflammation, dysbiosis, chronic NSAID intake, or stress, the barrier integrity is lost and commensal bacteria can reach the bloodstream (Figure 1) [60,82,83]. The presence of circulating lipopolysaccharide (LPS) derived from gram-negative endobacteria, also known as metabolic endotoxemia, then activates the inflammatory TLR4 pathway and immune cells produce pro-inflammatory cytokines and LPS-directed IgM/IgA, thus enhancing systemic inflammation [74,76,84,85].

Metabolic endotoxemia and gut permeability have already been considered in the pathophysiological mechanism of several diseases such as obesity, diabetes, nonalcoholic fatty liver disease, atherosclerosis, metabolic syndrome, or septic shock, as well as ME/CFS [60,75,84–86]. In this respect, serum IgA and IgM levels against LPS of enterobacteria are significantly higher in ME/CFS cases than controls, and correlate with disease severity [74]. Likewise, raised IgA response to commensal bacteria and enhanced inflammation have been reported in 128 ME/CFS cases when compared to healthy volunteers [76]. Remarkably, significant improvement was obtained if a leaky gut diet was combined with anti-inflammatory and anti-oxidative substances, thus suggesting a new therapeutic approach in ME/CFS treatment [77]. Similar results were also obtained in depressed patients, suggesting that gut permeability and consequently enhanced immune response might explain overlap between major depressive disorder (MDD) and ME/CFS cognitive symptom [87,88]. A growing body of evidence demonstrates the importance of neuroinflammation in the development of neurodegenerative and neuroprogressive diseases [89,90]. Given the ability of bacterial translocation to drive systemic inflammation, blood-brain barrier disruption and neuroinflammation, some authors hypothesize that this mechanism might explain the onset of neurological abnormalities in ME/CFS, but this remains to be proven [83,91,92]. Based on this hypothesis, leaky gut targeting may reduce both gastrointestinal and cognitive symptoms, thus representing a promising approach in ME/CFS therapy but more research is needed before drawing conclusions.

There is evidence that ME/CFS could be classified as an autoimmune disease [93], and gut permeability may also play a role in this context. After a viral trigger, dysbiosis and genetic predisposition favor the generation of immune cell clones prone to autoreactivity, leading to self-antigen immunization and autoimmunity [16]. In addition, a link between fatigue, autoimmunity, and intestinal barrier breakdown has also been established [94]. The fact that dysbiosis and bacterial translocation cause an increase in pro-inflammatory cytokines (i.e., IL-1 and TNF-α) is an additional mechanism that could explain the relationship between gut, ME/CFS and autoimmunity [95]. However, the role and the importance of autoimmunity in ME/CFS pathophysiology are not yet clear, and more studies are needed to confirm these suggestions.

A complex relationship between dysbiosis, intestinal permeability, chronic inflammation, and cognitive symptoms is reported in ME/CFS. A viral infection may represent an important trigger of systemic inflammation, which in turn promotes dysbiosis and neuroinflammation. In these conditions, *Enterobacteriaceae* growth is favored, while *Bacteroidetes* and SCFA production are impaired. This imbalanced gut composition, together with chronic inflammation, stress and NSAIDs prolonged intake, favors tight-junction disruption and leaky gut. While in base-line conditions only nutrients and SCFAs can reach the bloodstream, upon intestinal barrier integrity loss, bacterial and LPS translocation are also possible. Given that the resulting metabolic endotoxemia exacerbates pro-inflammatory cytokine production and release, this chronic-low grade inflammation contributes to neuroinflammation and neurological abnormalities.

Therapeutic options aimed at restoring gut barrier integrity and eubiosis have been proposed. Among those, prebiotics, probiotics, fecal microbiota transplantation (FMT), and diet interventions have all shown promising results, but more studies are needed to determine their efficacy.

2.3. Oxidative Stress and Inflammation in Disease Pathogenesis

Oxidative stress refers to a condition in which high levels of intracellular reactive oxygen species (ROS) accumulate and cause protein, lipid, and DNA damage [96]. Although antioxidants are supposed to counteract the buildup of ROS, their levels in chronic conditions, such as IBD, remain low [97]. In addition, chronic low-grade inflammation and oxidative stress are both associated with ME/CFS [60,98]. For example, an increase in oxidative stress level and a decrease in antioxidant levels in resting conditions have been reported in ME/CFS cases when compared to controls [99]. Moreover, elevated urinary 8-hydroxy-deoxoguanosine (8-OHdG) levels, a well-known marker of oxidative DNA damage, was shown to correlate with malaise and depression in ME/CFS [100]. Similar to IBS, high levels of pro-inflammatory cytokines (i.e., IFN-γ, IL-4, IL-5, TGF-α and IL-1) are also detected in ME/CFS [101,102]. Although it is not yet clear whether inflammation can directly cause fatigue, the enhancement of 92 circulating inflammatory markers in ME/CFS individuals resembles the analysis obtained for Q fever fatigue [103]. Given the lack of defined biomarkers in ME/CFS, the possibility of relying on inflammatory, oxidative/nitrosative stress, and antioxidants markers has been proposed [60,99,104].

Although several factors contribute to the establishment of inflammation and oxidant/antioxidant imbalance (i.e., viral infection, reduced antioxidants, stress, depression [60,75,105]), dysbiosis, and metabolic endotoxemia also play an important role [60,83,91]. In this respect, a model has been established according to which stress, dysbiosis, and systemic inflammation all contribute to reducing the tight-junction protein occludin, thus causing the intestinal lining to lose its barrier function [60,82,83]. Increased gut permeability, in turn, further exacerbates chronic inflammation via endotoxemia and TLR4 pathway activation, leading to neuroinflammation and oxidative/nitrosative stress [83,85]. As evident in Idiopathic Chronic Fatigue (ICF), oxidative stress may finally represent a key pathophysiological mechanism in ME/CFS [83,106,107]. Even though it still requires fundamental validations, if this model turns out to be true, it will certainly constitute a new key target in ME/CFS treatment, thus confirming the central role of gut homeostasis in both gastrointestinal and extra-intestinal disease pathogenesis.

2.4. Therapies Aimed at Microbiota May Alleviate ME/CFS Symptoms

Given the frequent association of ME/CFS with chronic inflammation, dysbiosis and gut permeability [108], it is worth speculating that approaches aimed at replenishing the microbial balance, restoring mucosal barrier integrity, and lowering inflammation may be therapeutically relevant. Prebiotics, probiotics, specific diet, particular molecule intake, and fecal transplantation have been proposed, in this respect (Figure 1) [109]. NADH, probiotics, high cocoa polyphenol rich chocolate and Coenzyme Q10 proved all capable of improving fatigue in ME/CFS-diagnosed cases, but questions remain on whether the results can be replicated on a larger sample size [110].

2.4.1. Probiotics

Probiotics are living microorganisms which normally reside in the human body. *Lactobacilli* spp., *E. coli*-Nisle 1917, *Bifodobacteria* spp., some *Streptococcus* types, and the yeast *Saccharomyces boulardii* are all considered probiotics [60]. Recently, their application as adjuvant therapy in IBS treatment mostly showed positive results [111–124]. In addition, administration of *Akkermansia muciniphila* and *Lactobacillus sakei* OK67 to high-fat diet (HFD) fed mice were independently able to enhance tight-junction function, increasing occludin gene expression and decreasing intestinal permeability [125,126]. Remarkably, during L. sakei OK67 treatment, a significant decrease in the inflammatory markers TNF-α, IL-1β and NF-κB has also been reported [126]. In the context of ME/CFS, the same promising results were replicated applying an 8-week long treatment of four probiotic mixtures [127]. Moreover, the administration of *Bifidobacterium infantis* 35624 to 48 ME/CFS cases confirmed the ability of probiotics to reduce the systemic pro-inflammatory markers CRP, TNF-α and IL-6 [128].

Anxiety, depression, and psychiatric disorders are often found in ME/CFS affected individuals [129] and finding an alternative to the currently employed psychotropic medications is crucial. Results from a 12-week randomized, double-blind, and placebo controlled clinical trial report that a mixture of *Lactobacillus helveticus* R0052 and *Bifidobacterium longum* R0175 could be effective in decreasing inflammation and improving psychiatric manifestations in MDD patients following a gluten-free diet [130]. Since both MDD and ME/CFS show psychiatric symptom overlap [131], it is interesting to see whether probiotic use in chronic fatigue would prove equally beneficial. Preliminary evidence suggests that a significant drop in anxiety, associated with eubiosis reestablishment, can be observed if *Lactobacillus casei* strain Shirota is administered daily for 2 months in ME/CFS cases [132]. In addition, improvements in neurocognitive functions among *L. paracasei* spp. *paracasei* F19, *L. acidophilus* NCFB 1748 and *B. lactis* Bb12 receiving ME/CFS-diagnosed individuals are particularly notable [109]. Overall, these studies show that probiotics, alone or in combination, will probably emerge as a remedy supporting ME/CFS therapy.

2.4.2. Prebiotics

Prebiotics are non-digestible carbohydrate nutrients which are used as food by the GM. Fructo-oligosaccharides and galacto-oligosaccharides are the two main prebiotic classification groups [133]. Upon bacterial degradation, they produce SCFAs that diffuse via systemic circulation, hence influencing both gastrointestinal and extra-intestinal functionality [134]. Given their ability to selectively promote the expansion of only some intestinal microorganisms and revising gut microbiota makeup and function [133], they are proposed as promising adjuvant therapy in many diseases (e.g., IBS, Crohn's disease, bowel motility, autism, obesity and colorectal cancer) [133]. Multiple oligosaccharides have proven effective in reversing microbiota dysbiosis through *Lactobacilli* growth promotion, *Proteobacteria* reduction, and *Firmicutes/Bacteroidetes* ratio decrease in diet-induced obese rats and mice [135–137]. In addition, significant amelioration of gut permeability and systemic inflammation have also been reported. Rats and mice fed with prebiotics, such as bovine milk oligosaccharides, oligofructose-enriched inulin, spirulina platensis, and FOS/GOS, showed lower plasma LPS, decrease in serum pro-inflammatory cytokine levels, reduced gut inflammation and improved tight-junction integrity [135–139]. Altogether, these studies suggest that prebiotics may be helpful for ME/CFS cases presenting dysbiosis, leaky gut and systemic basal inflammation, but clinical trials are needed before drawing further conclusions.

2.4.3. Diet

A change in dietary habit is a rapid, reproducible and direct way of modifying the gut microbiota [140]. Diet, other than being involved in some disease pathophysiology, if adequate and taken at set times, is capable of balancing microbiota composition and mitigating inflammation, similar to prebiotics [141,142]. In the last few years, IBS, obesity, and Crohn's patients have benefited from this therapy, and dietary interventions have also been considered in the neuropsychiatric field [143–149].

Glucose/fructose-based diets and long-term protein-based diets have been correlated with dysbiosis, leaky gut, increased systemic inflammation and increased levels of plasma endotoxins [150,151]. Consequently, gluten-free diets, starch and sucrose-reduced diet, and dietary regimens aimed at lowering caloric intake can decrease C-reactive protein (CRP) and LPS binding protein levels, counteract intestinal permeability, and ameliorate gastrointestinal and extra-intestinal symptoms of IBS and obesity [130,152,153]. Similarly, microbiota diversity and metabolic endotoxemia are improved by polyunsaturated fatty acid omega-3 intake, and polyphenol and fiber consumption are preferred [142,154]. Eicosapentaenoic acid which is found in omega-3 rich fish oil has also been found to alleviate symptoms in ME/CFS cases [155,156]. In diet-induced obese rats and mice, some benefits can also be achieved by specific nutrient integration. In this respect, apple polysaccharides, flos lanicera administration and Bofutsushasan (a Japanese herbal medicine) have proven effective in favoring *Lactobacillus* and *Bacteroidetes* growth, enhancing tight junction function and reducing the pro-inflammatory cytokines TNF-α and IL-6 [157–159]. Additionally, integration of *Sarcodon imbricatus* or intake of a mixture composed of *Angelica gigas*, *Cnidium officinale*, and *Paeonia lactiflora*, proved effective in restoring the oxidant/antioxidant homeostasis and in reducing fatigue in ME/CFS mouse models [160,161].

Although more clinical trials are needed in humans, these results indicate that the ability to act on microbiome makeup, gut permeability, inflammation and neurocognitive symptoms at the same time proposes dietary intervention as a promising additional adjuvant approach in ME/CFS treatment.

2.4.4. Fecal Microbiota Transplantation (FMT)

Fecal microbiota transplantation (FMT), also known as stool transplantation or bacteriotherapy, is the process of transplanting stool from a healthy donor into a patient's intestine [162]. The aim of the therapy is to restore dysbiosis by infusing a balanced and healthy microbiota population into the gut of the recipient. In most cases the transplantation takes place via colonoscopy, but enema or orally administered capsules are also available [163,164]. Although it is only approved for recurrent or refractory *Clostridium difficile* infection treatment [165], FMT is now being tested as an experimental therapeutic option for primary *Clostridium difficile* infection, obesity, insulin resistance, metabolic syndrome, metabolic fatty acid liver disease, fibromyalgia, ulcerative colitis, Crohn's disease, ME/CFS, functional constipation, IBS, and even cancer [164,166–169]. In addition, several neuropsychiatric disorders have been proposed as potentially benefitting from FMT. Studies are being carried out using stool transplantation in autism, Parkinson's Disease, Alzheimer's Disease, and Multiple Sclerosis, but the success of these trials is debatable [170–172]. Recently, promising perspectives came from the use of FMT in immune-checkpoint inhibitor-associated colitis, IBS, and IBD, but larger cohort trials are needed [162,164,173]. FMT ability to decrease inflammation, reduce intestinal permeability via SCFA production and restore immune dysbiosis [174] proposes this nascent therapy as a promising approach also in ME/CFS treatment. In a study of 34 ME/CFS participants who received FMT, 41% showed persistent relief after 11–28 months, while 35% reported only little or late relief [175]. Moreover, a 70% response rate was obtained when 13 non-pathogenic bacteria were administered via colonoscopy in 60 ME/CFS individuals. Additionally, at 15–20 years follow up, 58% of cases reported maintained response without recurrence [176].

Despite the potential of FMT in a wide range of diseases, limitations are still evident. Lack of consistency and shared standard protocols, selection criteria, route of administration, therapy duration, long-term risks, and donor selection are all open questions that have not yet been addressed [162,167,170,177–179]. Moreover, several authors underline that no solid conclusions can be drawn from existing studies, and larger clinical trials are needed in order to clarify FMT efficiency in various human disorders [162,170,174,180,181]. It would also be worthwhile to see if the multiple donor FMT proved more effective than the single donor approach, as already suggested in the literature [182].

While several limitations exist, these data indicate that FMT application in multiple intestinal dysbiosis-associated extra-intestinal diseases may soon represent a novel therapeutic approach for ME/CFS cases.

3. Discussion

Altogether, this short review summarizes the main findings concerning dysbiosis and gut permeability in ME/CFS. While GM homeostasis has proved to be fundamental in many diseases, its role in ME/CFS pathogenesis and disease development is still partially unclear and needs to be fully addressed to enable proper treatment of the disease. Studies on larger cohorts, use of consistent criteria for the diagnosis of ME/CFS, and reduction of confounding variables by controlling factors that influence microbiome composition prior to sample collection are needed in this respect. At the same time, therapeutic applications aimed at eubiosis re-establishment and leaky-gut prevention should be tested further in humans, as current promising insights are often based on data from mice and rats. Similarly, microbiome alterations or metabolic endotoxemia should be considered as potential disease biomarkers, even though GI symptoms overlap with those of other disorders and may represent a concern for precise differential diagnosis. Nevertheless, the importance of the GM in ME/CFS is evident through the links between GM alterations, inflammation, autoimmunity, and the gut-brain axis. Overall, we give an overview of the promising microbiome-based therapeutic applications for the chronic and strongly debilitating disease that is ME/CFS, and encourage deeper research in this field.

Author Contributions: Conceptualization, A.V. and G.R.; methodology, A.V. and G.R.; writing-original draft, A.V., U.-S.D., S.A. and G.R.; writing-review and editing, A.V. and U.-S.D.; supervision, G.R. All authors have read and agreed to the published version of the manuscript.

Funding: This research received no external funding.

Institutional Review Board Statement: Not applicable.

Informed Consent Statement: Not applicable.

Data Availability Statement: Data sharing not applicable.

Conflicts of Interest: The authors declare no conflict of interest.

References

1. Prins, J.B.; van der Meer, J.W.; Bleijenberg, G. Chronic Fatigue Syndrome. *Lancet* **2006**, *367*, S0140–S6736. [CrossRef]
2. Sharpe, M.C.; Archard, L.C.; Banatvala, J.E.; Borysiewicz, L.K.; Clare, A.W.; David, A.; Edwards, R.H.; Hawton, K.E.; Lambert, H.P.; Lane, R.J. A Report—Chronic Fatigue Syndrome: Guidelines for Research. *J. R. Soc. Med.* **1991**, *84*, 118–121. [CrossRef] [PubMed]
3. Carruthers, B.; Jain, A.; de Meirleir, K.; Peterson, D.; Klimas, N.; Lerner, A.; Bested, A.; Pierre, F.; Joshi, P.; Powles, A.; et al. Myalgic Encephalomyelitis/Chronic Fatigue Syndrome: Clinical Working Case Definition, Diagnostic and Treatment Protocols. *J. Chronic Fatigue Syndr.* **2003**, *11*, 7–115. [CrossRef]
4. Fukuda, K. The Chronic Fatigue Syndrome: A Comprehensive Approach to Its Definition and Study. *Ann. Intern. Med.* **1994**, *121*, 953–959. [CrossRef]
5. Carruthers, B.M.; van de Sande, M.I.; de Meirleir, K.L.; Klimas, N.G.; Broderick, G.; Mitchell, T.; Staines, D.; Powles, A.C.P.; Speight, N.; Vallings, R.; et al. Myalgic Encephalomyelitis: International Consensus Criteria. *J. Intern. Med.* **2011**, *270*, 327–338. [CrossRef]
6. Bested, A.; Marshall, L. Review of Myalgic Encephalomyelitis/Chronic Fatigue Syndrome: An Evidence-Based Approach to Diagnosis and Management by Clinicians. *Rev. Environ. Health* **2015**, *30*, 223–249. [CrossRef] [PubMed]
7. Mandarano, A.H.; Maya, J.; Giloteaux, L.; Peterson, D.L.; Maynard, M.; Gottschalk, C.G.; Hanson, M.R. Myalgic Encephalomyelitis/Chronic Fatigue Syndrome Patients Exhibit Altered T Cell Metabolism and Cytokine Associations. *J. Clin. Investig.* **2020**, *130*, 1491–1505. [CrossRef] [PubMed]
8. Lorusso, L.; Mikhaylova, S.V.; Capelli, E.; Ferrari, D.; Ngonga, G.K.; Ricevuti, G. Immunological Aspects of Chronic Fatigue Syndrome. *Autoimmun. Rev.* **2009**, *8*, 287–291. [CrossRef]
9. Wirth, K.; Scheibenbogen, C. A Unifying Hypothesis of the Pathophysiology of Myalgic Encephalomyelitis/Chronic Fatigue Syndrome (ME/CFS): Recognitions from the Finding of Autoantibodies against SS2-Adrenergic Receptors. *Autoimmun. Rev.* **2020**, *19*, 102527. [CrossRef] [PubMed]
10. Maes, M.; Twisk, F.N.M.; Kubera, M.; Ringel, K. Evidence for Inflammation and Activation of Cell-Mediated Immunity in Myalgic Encephalomyelitis/Chronic Fatigue Syndrome (ME/CFS): Increased Interleukin-1, Tumor Necrosis Factor-α, PMN-Elastase, Lysozyme and Neopterin. *J. Affect. Disord.* **2012**, *136*, 933–939. [CrossRef]
11. Cortes Rivera, M.; Mastronardi, C.; Silva-Aldana, C.; Arcos-Burgos, M.; Lidbury, B. Myalgic Encephalomyelitis/Chronic Fatigue Syndrome: A Comprehensive Review. *Diagnostics* **2019**, *9*, 91. [CrossRef]
12. Magnus, P.; Gunnes, N.; Tveito, K.; Bakken, I.J.; Ghaderi, S.; Stoltenberg, C.; Hornig, M.; Lipkin, W.I.; Trogstad, L.; Håberg, S.E. Chronic Fatigue Syndrome/Myalgic Encephalomyelitis (CFS/ME) Is Associated with Pandemic Influenza Infection, but Not with an Adjuvanted Pandemic Influenza Vaccine. *Vaccine* **2015**, *33*, 6173–6177. [CrossRef] [PubMed]
13. Nagy-Szakal, D.; Williams, B.L.; Mishra, N.; Che, X.; Lee, B.; Bateman, L.; Klimas, N.G.; Komaroff, A.L.; Levine, S.; Montoya, J.G.; et al. Fecal Metagenomic Profiles in Subgroups of Patients with Myalgic Encephalomyelitis/Chronic Fatigue Syndrome. *Microbiome* **2017**, *5*, 44. [CrossRef]
14. Giloteaux, L.; Goodrich, J.K.; Walters, W.A.; Levine, S.M.; Ley, R.E.; Hanson, M.R. Reduced Diversity and Altered Composition of the Gut Microbiome in Individuals with Myalgic Encephalomyelitis/Chronic Fatigue Syndrome. *Microbiome* **2016**, *4*, 30. [CrossRef] [PubMed]
15. Navaneetharaja, N.; Griffiths, V.; Wileman, T.; Carding, S. A Role for the Intestinal Microbiota and Virome in Myalgic Encephalomyelitis/Chronic Fatigue Syndrome (ME/CFS)? *J. Clin. Med.* **2016**, *5*, 55. [CrossRef]
16. Blomberg, J.; Gottfries, C.-G.; Elfaitouri, A.; Rizwan, M.; Rosén, A. Infection Elicited Autoimmunity and Myalgic Encephalomyelitis/Chronic Fatigue Syndrome: An Explanatory Model. *Front. Immunol.* **2018**, *9*, 229. [CrossRef]
17. Sullivan, P.F.; Evengard, B.; Jacks, A.; Pedersen, N.L. Twin Analyses of Chronic Fatigue in a Swedish National Sample. *Psychol. Med.* **2005**, *35*, 1327–1336. [CrossRef]
18. Glassford, J.A.G. The Neuroinflammatory Etiopathology of Myalgic Encephalomyelitis/Chronic Fatigue Syndrome (ME/CFS). *Front. Physiol.* **2017**, *8*, 88. [CrossRef]
19. Hickie, I.; Bennett, B.; Lloyd, A.; Heath, A.; Martin, N. Complex Genetic and Environmental Relationships between Psychological Distress, Fatigue and Immune Functioning: A Twin Study. *Psychol. Med.* **1999**, *29*, 269–277. [CrossRef]
20. Van de Putte, E.; van Doornen, L.; Engelbert, R.; Kuis, W.; Kimpen, J.; Uiterwaal, C. Mirrored Symptoms in Mother and Child with Chronic Fatigue Syndrome. *Pediatrics* **2006**, *117*, 2074–2079. [CrossRef] [PubMed]
21. Albright, F.; Light, K.; Light, A.; Bateman, L.; Cannon-Albright, L.A. Evidence for a Heritable Predisposition to Chronic Fatigue Syndrome. *BMC Neurol.* **2011**, *11*, 1–6. [CrossRef]
22. Dibble, J.J.; McGrath, S.J.; Ponting, C.P. Genetic Risk Factors of ME/CFS: A Critical Review. *Hum. Mol. Genet.* **2020**, *29*, R118–R125. [CrossRef] [PubMed]

23. Jacobson, S.K.; Daly, J.S.; Thorne, G.M.; McIntosh, K. Chronic Parvovirus B19 Infection Resulting in Chronic Fatigue Syndrome: Case History and Review. *Clin. Infect. Dis.* **1997**, *24*, 1048–1051. [CrossRef]
24. Aoki, R.; Kobayashi, N.; Suzuki, G.; Kuratsune, H.; Shimada, K.; Oka, N.; Takahashi, M.; Yamadera, W.; Iwashita, M.; Tokuno, S.; et al. Human Herpesvirus 6 and 7 Are Biomarkers for Fatigue, Which Distinguish between Physiological Fatigue and Pathological Fatigue. *Biochem. Biophys. Res. Commun.* **2016**, *478*, 424–430. [CrossRef]
25. Niller, H.H.; Wolf, H.; Ay, E.; Minarovits, J. Epigenetic Dysregulation of Epstein-Barr Virus Latency and Development of Autoimmune Disease. *Adv. Exp. Med. Biol.* **2011**, *711*, 82–102. [CrossRef] [PubMed]
26. Kerr, J.R. The Role of Parvovirus B19 in the Pathogenesis of Autoimmunity and Autoimmune Disease. *J. Clin. Pathol.* **2016**, *69*, 279–291. [CrossRef]
27. Kerr, J.R.; Bracewell, J.; Laing, I.; Mattey, D.L.; Bernstein, R.M.; Bruce, I.N.; Tyrrell, D.A.J. Chronic Fatigue Syndrome and Arthralgia Following Parvovirus B19 Infection. *J. Rheumatol.* **2002**, *29*, 595–602.
28. Seishima, M.; Mizutani, Y.; Shibuya, Y.; Arakawa, C. Chronic Fatigue Syndrome after Human Parvovirus B19 Infection without Persistent Viremia. *Dermatology* **2008**, *216*, 341–346. [CrossRef] [PubMed]
29. Cameron, B.; Flamand, L.; Juwana, H.; Middeldorp, J.; Naing, Z.; Rawlinson, W.; Ablashi, D.; Lloyd, A. Serological and Virological Investigation of the Role of the Herpesviruses EBV, CMV and HHV-6 in Post-Infective Fatigue Syndrome. *J. Med. Virol.* **2010**, *82*, 1684–1688. [CrossRef]
30. Rasa, S.; Nora-Krukle, Z.; Henning, N.; Eliassen, E.; Shikova, E.; Harrer, T.; Scheibenbogen, C.; Murovska, M.; Prusty, B.K. Chronic Viral Infections in Myalgic Encephalomyelitis/Chronic Fatigue Syndrome (ME/CFS). *J. Transl. Med.* **2018**, *16*, 1–25. [CrossRef]
31. Soto, N.E.; Straus, S.E. Chronic Fatigue Syndrome and Herpesviruses: The Fading Evidence. *Herpes J. IHMF* **2000**, *7*, 46–50.
32. Levine, P.H.; Jacobson, S.; Pocinki, A.G.; Cheney, P.; Peterson, D.; Connelly, R.R.; Weil, R.; Robinson, S.M.; Ablashi, D.V.; Salahuddin, S.Z. Clinical, Epidemiologic, and Virologic Studies in Four Clusters of the Chronic Fatigue Syndrome. *Arch. Intern. Med.* **1992**, *152*, 1611–1616. [CrossRef] [PubMed]
33. Blomberg, J.; Rizwan, M.; Böhlin-Wiener, A.; Elfaitouri, A.; Julin, P.; Zachrisson, O.; Rosén, A.; Gottfries, C.-G. Antibodies to Human Herpesviruses in Myalgic Encephalomyelitis/Chronic Fatigue Syndrome Patients. *Front. Immunol.* **2019**, *10*, 1946. [CrossRef]
34. Burbelo, P.D.; Bayat, A.; Wagner, J.; Nutman, T.B.; Baraniuk, J.N.; Iadarola, M.J. No Serological Evidence for a Role of HHV-6 Infection in Chronic Fatigue Syndrome. *Am. J. Transl. Res.* **2012**, *4*, 443.
35. Domingues, T.D.; Grabowska, A.D.; Lee, J.-S.; Ameijeiras-Alonso, J.; Westermeier, F.; Scheibenbogen, C.; Cliff, J.M.; Nacul, L.; Lacerda, E.M.; Mouriño, H.; et al. Herpesviruses Serology Distinguishes Different Subgroups of Patients From the United Kingdom Myalgic Encephalomyelitis/Chronic Fatigue Syndrome Biobank. *Front. Med.* **2021**, *8*, 959. [CrossRef]
36. Clauw, D.J. Perspectives on Fatigue from the Study of Chronic Fatigue Syndrome and Related Conditions. *PM&R* **2010**, *2*, 414–430. [CrossRef]
37. Simani, L.; Ramezani, M.; Darazam, I.A.; Sagharichi, M.; Aalipour, M.A.; Ghorbani, F.; Pakdaman, H. Prevalence and Correlates of Chronic Fatigue Syndrome and Post-Traumatic Stress Disorder after the Outbreak of the COVID-19. *J. Neurovirol.* **2021**, *27*, 154–159. [CrossRef]
38. Kennedy, G.; Khan, F.; Hill, A.; Underwood, C.; Belch, J.J.F. Biochemical and Vascular Aspects of Pediatric Chronic Fatigue Syndrome. *Arch. Pediatr. Adolesc. Med.* **2010**, *164*, 817–823. [CrossRef] [PubMed]
39. Tilg, H.; Adolph, T.E.; Gerner, R.R.; Moschen, A.R. The Intestinal Microbiota in Colorectal Cancer. *Cancer Cell* **2018**, *33*, 954–964. [CrossRef] [PubMed]
40. Ogino, S.; Nowak, J.A.; Hamada, T.; Phipps, A.I.; Peters, U.; Milner, D.A., Jr.; Giovannucci, E.L.; Nishihara, R.; Giannakis, M.; Garrett, W.S.; et al. Integrative Analysis of Exogenous, Endogenous, Tumour and Immune Factors for Precision Medicine. *Gut* **2018**, *67*, 1168–1180. [CrossRef] [PubMed]
41. Rinninella, E.; Raoul, P.; Cintoni, M.; Franceschi, F.; Miggiano, G.; Gasbarrini, A.; Mele, M. What Is the Healthy Gut Microbiota Composition? A Changing Ecosystem across Age, Environment, Diet, and Diseases. *Microorganisms* **2019**, *7*, 14. [CrossRef]
42. Bäckhed, F.; Ley, R.E.; Sonnenburg, J.L.; Peterson, D.A.; Gordon, J.I. Host-Bacterial Mutualism in the Human Intestine. *Science* **2005**, *307*, 1915–1920. [CrossRef] [PubMed]
43. Thursby, E.; Juge, N. Introduction to the Human Gut Microbiota. *Biochem. J.* **2017**, *474*, 1823–1836. [CrossRef] [PubMed]
44. Nicholson, J.K.; Holmes, E.; Kinross, J.; Burcelin, R.; Gibson, G.; Jia, W.; Pettersson, S. Host-Gut Microbiota Metabolic Interactions. *Science* **2012**, *336*, 1262–1267. [CrossRef] [PubMed]
45. Prakash, S.; Rodes, L.; Coussa-Charley, M.; Tomaro-Duchesneau, C.; Tomaro-Duchesneau, C.; Coussa-Charley, M. Rodes Gut Microbiota: Next Frontier in Understanding Human Health and Development of Biotherapeutics. *Biol. Targets Ther.* **2011**, *5*, 71. [CrossRef]
46. Morais, L.H.; Schreiber, H.L.; Mazmanian, S.K. The Gut Microbiota–Brain Axis in Behaviour and Brain Disorders. *Nat. Rev. Microbiol.* **2021**, *19*, 241–255. [CrossRef] [PubMed]
47. Mayer, E.A.; Tillisch, K.; Gupta, A. Gut/Brain Axis and the Microbiota. *J. Clin. Investig.* **2015**, *125*, 926–938. [CrossRef] [PubMed]
48. Atarashi, K.; Tanoue, T.; Shima, T.; Imaoka, A.; Kuwahara, T.; Momose, Y.; Cheng, G.; Yamasaki, S.; Saito, T.; Ohba, Y.; et al. Induction of Colonic Regulatory T Cells by Indigenous Clostridium Species. *Science* **2011**, *331*, 337–341. [CrossRef]
49. Ivanov, I.I.; Atarashi, K.; Manel, N.; Brodie, E.L.; Shima, T.; Karaoz, U.; Wei, D.; Goldfarb, K.C.; Santee, C.A.; Lynch, S.V.; et al. Induction of Intestinal Th17 Cells by Segmented Filamentous Bacteria. *Cell* **2009**, *139*, 485–498. [CrossRef]

50. Khan, R.; Petersen, F.C.; Shekhar, S. Commensal Bacteria: An Emerging Player in Defense against Respiratory Pathogens. *Front. Immunol.* **2019**, *10*, 1203. [CrossRef]
51. Zhang, H.; DiBaise, J.K.; Zuccolo, A.; Kudrna, D.; Braidotti, M.; Yu, Y.; Parameswaran, P.; Crowell, M.D.; Wing, R.; Rittmann, B.E.; et al. Human Gut Microbiota in Obesity and after Gastric Bypass. *Proc. Natl. Acad. Sci. USA* **2009**, *106*, 2365–2370. [CrossRef]
52. Malaguarnera, L. Vitamin D and Microbiota: Two Sides of the Same Coin in the Immunomodulatory Aspects. *Int. Immunopharmacol.* **2020**, *79*, 106112. [CrossRef]
53. Wahlström, A.; Sayin, S.I.; Marschall, H.-U.; Bäckhed, F. Intestinal Crosstalk between Bile Acids and Microbiota and Its Impact on Host Metabolism. *Cell Metab.* **2016**, *24*, 41–50. [CrossRef] [PubMed]
54. Canfora, E.E.; Jocken, J.W.; Blaak, E.E. Short-Chain Fatty Acids in Control of Body Weight and Insulin Sensitivity. *Nat. Rev. Endocrinol.* **2015**, *11*, 577–591. [CrossRef] [PubMed]
55. Morrison, D.J.; Preston, T. Formation of Short Chain Fatty Acids by the Gut Microbiota and Their Impact on Human Metabolism. *Gut Microbes* **2016**, *7*, 189–200. [CrossRef] [PubMed]
56. Johnston, S.; Staines, D.; Marshall-Gradisnik, S. Epidemiological Characteristics of Chronic Fatigue Syndrome/Myalgic Encephalomyelitis in Australian Patients. *Clin. Epidemiol.* **2016**, *8*, 97. [CrossRef]
57. Wallis, A.; Ball, M.; McKechnie, S.; Butt, H.; Lewis, D.P.; Bruck, D. Examining Clinical Similarities between Myalgic Encephalomyelitis/Chronic Fatigue Syndrome and d-Lactic Acidosis: A Systematic Review. *J. Transl. Med.* **2017**, *15*, 1–22. [CrossRef]
58. Corbitt, M.; Campagnolo, N.; Staines, D.; Marshall-Gradisnik, S. A Systematic Review of Probiotic Interventions for Gastrointestinal Symptoms and Irritable Bowel Syndrome in Chronic Fatigue Syndrome/Myalgic Encephalomyelitis (CFS/ME). *Probiotics Antimicrob. Proteins* **2018**, *10*, 466–477. [CrossRef] [PubMed]
59. Riedl, A.; Schmidtmann, M.; Stengel, A.; Goebel, M.; Wisser, A.-S.; Klapp, B.F.; Mönnikes, H. Somatic Comorbidities of Irritable Bowel Syndrome: A Systematic Analysis. *J. Psychosom. Res.* **2008**, *64*, 573–582. [CrossRef]
60. Lakhan, S.E.; Kirchgessner, A. Gut Inflammation in Chronic Fatigue Syndrome. *Nutr. Metab.* **2010**, *7*, 79. [CrossRef]
61. Mandarano, A.H.; Giloteaux, L.; Keller, B.A.; Levine, S.M.; Hanson, M.R. Eukaryotes in the Gut Microbiota in Myalgic Encephalomyelitis/Chronic Fatigue Syndrome. *PeerJ* **2018**, *6*, e4282. [CrossRef]
62. Sheedy, J.R.; Wettenhall, R.E.H.; Scanlon, D.; Gooley, P.R.; Lewis, D.P.; McGregor, N.; Stapleton, D.I.; Butt, H.L.; de Meirleir, K.L. Increased D-Lactic Acid Intestinal Bacteria in Patients with Chronic Fatigue Syndrome. *In Vivo* **2009**, *23*, 621–628. [PubMed]
63. Lupo, G.F.D.; Rocchetti, G.; Lucini, L.; Lorusso, L.; Manara, E.; Bertelli, M.; Puglisi, E.; Capelli, E. Potential Role of Microbiome in Chronic Fatigue Syndrome/Myalgic Encephalomyelits (CFS/ME). *Sci. Rep.* **2021**, *11*, 7043. [CrossRef] [PubMed]
64. Frémont, M.; Coomans, D.; Massart, S.; de Meirleir, K. High-Throughput 16S RRNA Gene Sequencing Reveals Alterations of Intestinal Microbiota in Myalgic Encephalomyelitis/Chronic Fatigue Syndrome Patients. *Anaerobe* **2013**, *22*, 50–56. [CrossRef]
65. Kitami, T.; Fukuda, S.; Kato, T.; Yamaguti, K.; Nakatomi, Y.; Yamano, E.; Kataoka, Y.; Mizuno, K.; Tsuboi, Y.; Kogo, Y.; et al. Deep Phenotyping of Myalgic Encephalomyelitis/Chronic Fatigue Syndrome in Japanese Population. *Sci. Rep.* **2020**, *10*, 19933. [CrossRef] [PubMed]
66. Shukla, S.K.; Cook, D.; Meyer, J.; Vernon, S.D.; Le, T.; Clevidence, D.; Robertson, C.E.; Schrodi, S.J.; Yale, S.; Frank, D.N. Changes in Gut and Plasma Microbiome Following Exercise Challenge in Myalgic Encephalomyelitis/Chronic Fatigue Syndrome (ME/CFS). *PLoS ONE* **2015**, *10*, e0145453. [CrossRef]
67. Manichanh, C. Reduced Diversity of Faecal Microbiota in Crohn's Disease Revealed by a Metagenomic Approach. *Gut* **2006**, *55*, 205–211. [CrossRef]
68. Hevia, A.; Milani, C.; López, P.; Cuervo, A.; Arboleya, S.; Duranti, S.; Turroni, F.; González, S.; Suárez, A.; Gueimonde, M.; et al. Intestinal Dysbiosis Associated with Systemic Lupus Erythematosus. *mBio* **2014**, *5*, e01548-14. [CrossRef]
69. Gianchecchi, E.; Fierabracci, A. Recent Advances on Microbiota Involvement in the Pathogenesis of Autoimmunity. *Int. J. Mol. Sci.* **2019**, *20*, 283. [CrossRef] [PubMed]
70. Larsen, N.; Vogensen, F.K.; van den Berg, F.W.J.; Nielsen, D.S.; Andreasen, A.S.; Pedersen, B.K.; Al-Soud, W.A.; Sørensen, S.J.; Hansen, L.H.; Jakobsen, M. Gut Microbiota in Human Adults with Type 2 Diabetes Differs from Non-Diabetic Adults. *PLoS ONE* **2010**, *5*, e9085. [CrossRef]
71. Giloteaux, L.; Hanson, M.R.; Keller, B.A. A Pair of Identical Twins Discordant for Myalgic Encephalomyelitis/Chronic Fatigue Syndrome Differ in Physiological Parameters and Gut Microbiome Composition. *Am. J. Med. Case Rep.* **2016**, *17*, 720–729. [CrossRef]
72. Holmes, G.P. Chronic Fatigue Syndrome: A Working Case Definition. *Ann. Intern. Med.* **1988**, *108*, 387–389. [CrossRef]
73. Balows, A.; Hausler, W.; Herrmann, K.; Isenberg, H.; Shadomy, H. *Manual of Clinical Microbiology*; ASM Press: Washington, DC, USA, 2007.
74. Maes, M.; Mihaylova, I.; Leunis, J.C. Increased Serum IgA and IgM against LPS of Enterobacteria in Chronic Fatigue Syndrome (CFS): Indication for the Involvement of Gram-Negative Enterobacteria in the Etiology of CFS and for the Presence of an Increased Gut-Intestinal Permeability. *J. Affect. Disord.* **2007**, *99*, 237–240. [CrossRef]
75. Morris, G.; Maes, M. Oxidative and Nitrosative Stress and Immune-Inflammatory Pathways in Patients with Myalgic Encephalomyelitis (ME)/Chronic Fatigue Syndrome (CFS). *Curr. Neuropharmacol.* **2014**, *12*, 168–185. [CrossRef] [PubMed]
76. Maes, M.; Twisk, F.N.M.; Kubera, M.; Ringel, K.; Leunis, J.C.; Geffard, M. Increased IgA Responses to the LPS of Commensal Bacteria Is Associated with Inflammation and Activation of Cell-Mediated Immunity in Chronic Fatigue Syndrome. *J. Affect. Disord.* **2012**, *136*, 909–917. [CrossRef]

77. Maes, M.; Leunis, J.-C. Normalization of Leaky Gut in Chronic Fatigue Syndrome (CFS) Is Accompanied by a Clinical Improvement: Effects of Age, Duration of Illness and the Translocation of LPS from Gram-Negative Bacteria. *Neuro Endocrinol. Lett.* **2008**, *29*, 902–910.
78. Malla, M.A.; Dubey, A.; Kumar, A.; Yadav, S.; Hashem, A.; Abd_Allah, E.F. Exploring the Human Microbiome: The Potential Future Role of Next-Generation Sequencing in Disease Diagnosis and Treatment. *Front. Immunol.* **2019**, *9*, 2868. [CrossRef]
79. Lemke, D.; Klement, R.J.; Schweiger, F.; Schweiger, B.; Spitz, J. Vitamin D Resistance as a Possible Cause of Autoimmune Diseases: A Hypothesis Confirmed by a Therapeutic High-Dose Vitamin D Protocol. *Front. Immunol.* **2021**, *12*, 655739. [CrossRef] [PubMed]
80. Komaroff, M.A.L.; Buchwald, M.D.S. CHRONIC FATIGUE SYNDROME: An Update. *Annu. Rev. Med.* **1998**, *49*, 1–13. [CrossRef]
81. Du Preez, S.; Corbitt, M.; Cabanas, H.; Eaton, N.; Staines, D.; Marshall-Gradisnik, S. A Systematic Review of Enteric Dysbiosis in Chronic Fatigue Syndrome/Myalgic Encephalomyelitis. *Syst. Rev.* **2018**, *7*, 241. [CrossRef] [PubMed]
82. Groschwitz, K.R.; Hogan, S.P. Intestinal Barrier Function: Molecular Regulation and Disease Pathogenesis. *J. Allergy Clin. Immunol.* **2009**, *124*, 3–20. [CrossRef]
83. Alhasson, F.; Das, S.; Seth, R.; Dattaroy, D.; Chandrashekaran, V.; Ryan, C.N.; Chan, L.S.; Testerman, T.; Burch, J.; Hofseth, L.J.; et al. Altered Gut Microbiome in a Mouse Model of Gulf War Illness Causes Neuroinflammation and Intestinal Injury via Leaky Gut and TLR4 Activation. *PLoS ONE* **2017**, *12*, e0172914. [CrossRef] [PubMed]
84. Mohammad, S.; Thiemermann, C. Role of Metabolic Endotoxemia in Systemic Inflammation and Potential Interventions. *Front. Immunol.* **2021**, *11*, 594150. [CrossRef]
85. Lucas, K.; Maes, M. Role of the Toll like Receptor (TLR) Radical Cycle in Chronic Inflammation: Possible Treatments Targeting the TLR4 Pathway. *Mol. Neurobiol.* **2013**, *48*, 190–204. [CrossRef] [PubMed]
86. Munford, R. Endotoxemia-Menace, Marker, or Mistake? *J. Leukoc. Biol.* **2016**, *100*, 687–698. [CrossRef] [PubMed]
87. Maes, M.; Kubera, M.; Leunis, J.C.; Berk, M. Increased IgA and IgM Responses against Gut Commensals in Chronic Depression: Further Evidence for Increased Bacterial Translocation or Leaky Gut. *J. Affect. Disord.* **2012**, *141*, 55–62. [CrossRef] [PubMed]
88. Maes, M.; Mihaylova, I.; Kubera, M.; Leunis, J. An IgM-Mediated Immune Response Directed against Nitro-Bovine Serum Albumin (Nitro-BSA) in Chronic Fatigue Syndrome (CFS) and Major Depression: Evidence That Nitrosative Stress Is Another Factor Underpinning the Comorbidity between Major Depression and CFS. *Neuro Endocrinol. Lett.* **2008**, *29*, 313–319. [PubMed]
89. Sartori, A.C.; Vance, D.E.; Slater, L.Z.; Crowe, M. The Impact of Inflammation on Cognitive Function in Older Adults: Implications for Healthcare Practice and Research. *J. Neurosci. Nurs.* **2012**, *44*, 206–217. [CrossRef] [PubMed]
90. Gorelick, P.B. Role of Inflammation in Cognitive Impairment: Results of Observational Epidemiological Studies and Clinical Trials. *Ann. N.Y. Acad. Sci.* **2010**, *1207*, 155–162. [CrossRef]
91. Slyepchenko, A.; Maes, M.; Jacka, F.N.; Köhler, C.A.; Barichello, T.; McIntyre, R.S.; Berk, M.; Grande, I.; Foster, J.A.; Vieta, E.; et al. Gut Microbiota, Bacterial Translocation, and Interactions with Diet: Pathophysiological Links between Major Depressive Disorder and Non-Communicable Medical Comorbidities. *Psychother. Psychosom.* **2016**, *86*, 31–46. [CrossRef]
92. Morris, G.; Maes, M.; Berk, M.; Puri, B.K. Myalgic Encephalomyelitis or Chronic Fatigue Syndrome: How Could the Illness Develop? *Metab. Brain Dis.* **2019**, *34*, 385–415. [CrossRef]
93. Sotzny, F.; Blanco, J.; Capelli, E.; Castro-Marrero, J.; Steiner, S.; Murovska, M.; Scheibenbogen, C. Myalgic Encephalomyelitis/Chronic Fatigue Syndrome—Evidence for an Autoimmune Disease. *Autoimmun. Rev.* **2018**, *17*, 601–609. [CrossRef]
94. Morris, G.; Berk, M.; Carvalho, A.; Caso, J.; Sanz, Y.; Maes, M. The Role of Microbiota and Intestinal Permeability in the Pathophysiology of Autoimmune and Neuroimmune Processes with an Emphasis on Inflammatory Bowel Disease Type 1 Diabetes and Chronic Fatigue Syndrome. *Curr. Pharm. Des.* **2016**, *22*, 6058–6075. [CrossRef]
95. Morris, G.; Berk, M.; Galecki, P.; Maes, M. The Emerging Role of Autoimmunity in Myalgic Encephalomyelitis/Chronic Fatigue Syndrome (ME/Cfs). *Mol. Neurobiol.* **2014**, *49*, 741–756. [CrossRef]
96. Schieber, M.; Chandel, N.S. ROS Function in Redox Signaling and Oxidative Stress. *Curr. Biol.* **2014**, *24*, R453–R462. [CrossRef] [PubMed]
97. Sido, B.; Hack, V.; Hochlehnert, A.; Lipps, H.; Herfarth, C.; Dröge, W. Impairment of Intestinal Glutathione Synthesis in Patients with Inflammatory Bowel Disease. *Gut* **1998**, *42*, 485–492. [CrossRef]
98. Morris, G.; Puri, B.K.; Walker, A.J.; Maes, M.; Carvalho, A.F.; Walder, K.; Mazza, C.; Berk, M. Myalgic Encephalomyelitis/Chronic Fatigue Syndrome: From Pathophysiological Insights to Novel Therapeutic Opportunities. *Pharmacol. Res.* **2019**, *148*, 104450. [CrossRef] [PubMed]
99. Fukuda, S.; Nojima, J.; Motoki, Y.; Yamaguti, K.; Nakatomi, Y.; Okawa, N.; Fujiwara, K.; Watanabe, Y.; Kuratsune, H. A Potential Biomarker for Fatigue: Oxidative Stress and Anti-Oxidative Activity. *Biol. Psychol.* **2016**, *118*, 88–93. [CrossRef] [PubMed]
100. Maes, M.; Mihaylova, I.; Kubera, M.; Uytterhoeven, M.; Vrydags, N.; Bosmans, E. Increased 8-Hydroxy-Deoxyguanosine, a Marker of Oxidative Damage to DNA, in Major Depression and Myalgic Encephalomyelitis/Chronic Fatigue Syndrome. *Neuro Endocrinol. Lett.* **2009**, *30*, 715–722.
101. Monro, J.A.; Puri, B.K. A Molecular Neurobiological Approach to Understanding the Aetiology of Chronic Fatigue Syndrome (Myalgic Encephalomyelitis or Systemic Exertion Intolerance Disease) with Treatment Implications. *Mol. Neurobiol.* **2018**, *55*, 7377–7388. [CrossRef]

102. Ivashkin, V.; Poluektov, Y.; Kogan, E.; Shifrin, O.; Sheptulin, A.; Kovaleva, A.; Kurbatova, A.; Krasnov, G.; Poluektova, E. Disruption of the Pro-Inflammatory, Anti-Inflammatory Cytokines and Tight Junction Proteins Expression, Associated with Changes of the Composition of the Gut Microbiota in Patients with Irritable Bowel Syndrome. *PLoS ONE* **2021**, *16*, e0252930. [CrossRef]
103. Raijmakers, R.P.H.; Roerink, M.E.; Jansen, A.F.M.; Keijmel, S.P.; Gacesa, R.; Li, Y.; Joosten, L.A.B.; van der Meer, J.W.M.; Netea, M.G.; Bleeker-Rovers, C.P.; et al. Multi-Omics Examination of Q Fever Fatigue Syndrome Identifies Similarities with Chronic Fatigue Syndrome. *J. Transl. Med.* **2020**, *18*, 448. [CrossRef]
104. Maes, M. A New Case Definition of Neuro-Inflammatory and Oxidative Fatigue (NIOF), a Neuroprogressive Disorder, Formerly Known as Chronic Fatigue Syndrome or Myalgic Encephalomyelitis: Results of Multivariate Pattern Recognition Methods and External Validation by Neuro-Immune Biomarkers. *Neuro Endocrinol. Lett.* **2015**, *36*, 320–329.
105. Borton, M.A.; Sabag-Daigle, A.; Wu, J.; Solden, L.M.; O'Banion, B.S.; Daly, R.A.; Wolfe, R.A.; Gonzalez, J.F.; Wysocki, V.H.; Ahmer, B.M.M.; et al. Chemical and Pathogen-Induced Inflammation Disrupt the Murine Intestinal Microbiome. *Microbiome* **2017**, *5*, 47. [CrossRef] [PubMed]
106. Lee, J.S.; Kim, H.G.; Lee, D.S.; Son, C.G. Oxidative Stress Is a Convincing Contributor to Idiopathic Chronic Fatigue. *Sci. Rep.* **2018**, *8*, 12890. [CrossRef]
107. Maes, M.; Twisk, F. Why Myalgic Encephalomyelitis/Chronic Fatigue Syndrome (ME/CFS) May Kill You: Disorders in the Inflammatory and Oxidative and Nitrosative Stress (IO&NS) Pathways May Explain Cardiovascular Disorders in ME/CFS. *Neuro Endocrinol. Lett.* **2009**, *30*, 677–693.
108. Logan, A.C.; Rao, A.V.; Irani, D. Chronic Fatigue Syndrome: Lactic Acid Bacteria May Be of Therapeutic Value. *Med. Hypotheses* **2003**, *60*, 915–923. [CrossRef]
109. Sullivan, Å.; Nord, C.E.; Evengård, B. Effect of Supplement with Lactic-Acid Producing Bacteria on Fatigue and Physical Activity in Patients with Chronic Fatigue Syndrome. *Nutr. J.* **2009**, *8*, 4. [CrossRef] [PubMed]
110. Campagnolo, N.; Johnston, S.; Collatz, A.; Staines, D.; Marshall-Gradisnik, S. Dietary and Nutrition Interventions for the Therapeutic Treatment of Chronic Fatigue Syndrome/Myalgic Encephalomyelitis: A Systematic Review. *J. Hum. Nutr. Diet.* **2017**, *30*, 247–259. [CrossRef]
111. Staudacher, H.M.; Lomer, M.C.E.; Farquharson, F.M.; Louis, P.; Fava, F.; Franciosi, E.; Scholz, M.; Tuohy, K.M.; Lindsay, J.O.; Irving, P.M.; et al. A Diet Low in FODMAPs Reduces Symptoms in Patients With Irritable Bowel Syndrome and A Probiotic Restores Bifidobacterium Species: A Randomized Controlled Trial. *Gastroenterology* **2017**, *153*, 936–947. [CrossRef] [PubMed]
112. Hod, K.; Sperber, A.D.; Ron, Y.; Boaz, M.; Dickman, R.; Berliner, S.; Halpern, Z.; Maharshak, N.; Dekel, R. A Double-Blind, Placebo-Controlled Study to Assess the Effect of a Probiotic Mixture on Symptoms and Inflammatory Markers in Women with Diarrhea-Predominant IBS. *Neurogastroenterol. Motil.* **2017**, *29*, e13037. [CrossRef]
113. Ishaque, S.M.; Khosruzzaman, S.M.; Ahmed, D.S.; Sah, M.P. A Randomized Placebo-Controlled Clinical Trial of a Multi-Strain Probiotic Formulation (Bio-Kult®) in the Management of Diarrhea-Predominant Irritable Bowel Syndrome. *BMC Gastroenterol.* **2018**, *18*, 71. [CrossRef] [PubMed]
114. Francavilla, R.; Piccolo, M.; Francavilla, A.; Polimeno, L.; Semeraro, F.; Cristofori, F.; Castellaneta, S.; Barone, M.; Indrio, F.; Gobbetti, M.; et al. Clinical and Microbiological Effect of a Multispecies Probiotic Supplementation in Celiac Patients with Persistent IBS-Type Symptoms: A Randomized, Double-Blind, Placebo-Controlled, Multicenter Trial. *J. Clin. Gastroenterol.* **2019**, *53*, E117–E125. [CrossRef] [PubMed]
115. Leventogiannis, K.; Gkolfakis, P.; Spithakis, G.; Tsatali, A.; Pistiki, A.; Sioulas, A.; Giamarellos-Bourboulis, E.J.; Triantafyllou, K. Effect of a Preparation of Four Probiotics on Symptoms of Patients with Irritable Bowel Syndrome: Association with Intestinal Bacterial Overgrowth. *Probiotics Antimicrob. Proteins* **2019**, *11*, 627–634. [CrossRef] [PubMed]
116. Oh, J.H.; Jang, Y.S.; Kang, D.; Chang, D.K.; Min, Y.W. Efficacy and Safety of New Lactobacilli Probiotics for Unconstipated Irritable Bowel Syndrome: A Randomized, Double-Blind, Placebo-Controlled Trial. *Nutrients* **2019**, *11*, 2887. [CrossRef] [PubMed]
117. Lewis, E.D.; Antony, J.M.; Crowley, D.C.; Piano, A.; Bhardwaj, R.; Tompkins, T.A.; Evans, M. Efficacy of Lactobacillus Paracasei Ha-196 and Bifidobacterium Longum R0175 in Alleviating Symptoms of Irritable Bowel Syndrome (IBS): A Randomized, Placebo-Controlled Study. *Nutrients* **2020**, *12*, 1159. [CrossRef]
118. Lorenzo-Zúñiga, V.; Llop, E.; Suárez, C.; Álvarez, B.; Abreu, L.; Espadaler, J.; Serra, J. I. 31, a New Combination of Probiotics, Improves Irritable Bowel Syndrome-Related Quality of Life. *World J. Gastroenterol.* **2014**, *20*, 8709–8716. [CrossRef]
119. Skrzydło-Radomańska, B.; Prozorow-Król, B.; Cichoż-Lach, H.; Majsiak, E.; Bierła, J.B.; Kosikowski, W.; Szczerbiński, M.; Gantzel, J.; Cukrowska, B. The Effectiveness of Synbiotic Preparation Containing Lactobacillus and Bifidobacterium Probiotic Strains and Short Chain Fructooligosaccharides in Patients with Diarrhea Predominant Irritable Bowel Syndrome—a Randomized Double-Blind, Placebo-Controlled Study. *Nutrients* **2020**, *12*, 1999. [CrossRef]
120. Pinto-Sanchez, M.; Hall, G.; Ghajar, K.; Nardelli, A.; Bolino, C.; Lau, J.; Martin, F.; Cominetti, O.; Welsh, C.; Rieder, A.; et al. Probiotic Bifidobacterium Longum NCC3001 Reduces Depression Scores and Alters Brain Activity: A Pilot Study in Patients With Irritable Bowel Syndrome. *Gastroenterology* **2017**, *153*, 448–459. [CrossRef]
121. Yuan, F.; Ni, H.; Asche, C.; Kim, M.; Walayat, S.; Ren, J. Efficacy of Bifidobacterium Infantis 35624 in Patients with Irritable Bowel Syndrome: A Meta-Analysis. *Curr. Med. Res. Opin.* **2017**, *33*, 1191–1197. [CrossRef]

122. Andresen, V.; Gschossmann, J.; Layer, P. Heat-Inactivated Bifidobacterium Bifidum MIMBb75 (SYN-HI-001) in the Treatment of Irritable Bowel Syndrome: A Multicentre, Randomised, Double-Blind, Placebo-Controlled Clinical Trial. *Lancet Gastroenterol. Hepatol.* **2020**, *5*, 658–666. [CrossRef]
123. Zhao, Q.; Yang, W.R.; Wang, X.H.; Li, G.Q.; Xu, L.Q.; Cui, X.; Liu, Y.; Zuo, X.L. Clostridium Butyricum Alleviates Intestinal Low-Grade Inflamm TNBS-Induced Irritable Bowel Syndrome in Mice by Regulating Functional Status of Lamina Propria Dendritic Cells. *World J. Gastroenterol.* **2019**, *25*, 5469–5482. [CrossRef]
124. Basturk, A.; Artan, R.; Yilmaz, A. Efficacy of Synbiotic, Probiotic, and Prebiotic Treatments for Irritable Bowel Syndrome in Children: A Randomized Controlled Trial. *Turk. J. Gastroenterol.* **2020**, *27*, 439–443. [CrossRef] [PubMed]
125. Chelakkot, C.; Choi, Y.; Kim, D.K.; Park, H.T.; Ghim, J.; Kwon, Y.; Jeon, J.; Kim, M.S.; Jee, Y.K.; Gho, Y.S.; et al. Akkermansia Muciniphila-Derived Extracellular Vesicles Influence Gut Permeability through the Regulation of Tight Junctions. *Exp. Mol. Med.* **2018**, *50*, e450. [CrossRef] [PubMed]
126. Lim, S.M.; Jeong, J.J.; Woo, K.H.; Han, M.J.; Kim, D.H. Lactobacillus Sakei OK67 Ameliorates High-Fat Diet-Induced Blood Glucose Intolerance and Obesity in Mice by Inhibiting Gut Microbiota Lipopolysaccharide Production and Inducing Colon Tight Junction Protein Expression. *Nutr. Res.* **2016**, *36*, 337–348. [CrossRef]
127. Venturini, L.; Bacchi, S.; Capelli, E.; Lorusso, L.; Ricevuti, G.; Cusa, C. Modification of Immunological Parameters, Oxidative Stress Markers, Mood Symptoms, and Well-Being Status in CFS Patients after Probiotic Intake: Observations from a Pilot Study. *Oxid. Med. Cell. Longev.* **2019**, *2019*, 1684198. [CrossRef]
128. Groeger, D.; O'Mahony, L.; Murphy, E.F.; Bourke, J.F.; Dinan, T.G.; Kiely, B.; Shanahan, F.; Quigley, E.M.M. Bifidobacterium Infantis 35624 Modulates Host Inflammatory Processes beyond the Gut. *Gut Microbes* **2013**, *4*, 325–339. [CrossRef]
129. Caswell, C.; Daniels, J. *Anxiety and Depression in Chronic Fatigue Syndrome: Prevalence and Effect on Treatment. A Systematic Review, Meta-Analysis and Meta-Regression*; British Association of Behavioural and Cognitive Psychotherapy: Glasgow, UK, 2018.
130. Karakula-Juchnowicz, H.; Rog, J.; Juchnowicz, D.; Łoniewski, I.; Skonieczna-Ydecka, K.; Krukow, P.; Futyma-Jedrzejewska, M.; Kaczmarczyk, M. The Study Evaluating the Effect of Probiotic Supplementation on the Mental Status, Inflammation, and Intestinal Barrier in Major Depressive Disorder Patients Using Gluten-Free or Gluten-Containing Diet (SANGUT Study): A 12-Week, Randomized, Double-Blind, and Placebo-Controlled Clinical Study Protocol. *Nutr. J.* **2019**, *18*, 50. [CrossRef]
131. Griffith, J.; Zarrouf, F. A Systematic Review of Chronic Fatigue Syndrome: Don't Assume It's Depression. *Prim. Care Companion J. Clin. Psychiatry* **2008**, *10*, 120–128. [CrossRef]
132. Rao, A.V.; Bested, A.C.; Beaulne, T.M.; Katzman, M.A.; Iorio, C.; Berardi, J.M.; Logan, A.C. A Randomized, Double-Blind, Placebo-Controlled Pilot Study of a Probiotic in Emotional Symptoms of Chronic Fatigue Syndrome. *Gut Pathog.* **2009**, *1*, 6. [CrossRef] [PubMed]
133. Davani-Davari, D.; Negahdaripour, M.; Karimzadeh, I.; Seifan, M.; Mohkam, M.; Masoumi, S.J.; Berenjian, A.; Ghasemi, Y. Prebiotics: Definition, Types, Sources, Mechanisms, and Clinical Applications. *Foods* **2019**, *8*, 92. [CrossRef] [PubMed]
134. Den Besten, G.; van Eunen, K.; Groen, A.K.; Venema, K.; Reijngoud, D.J.; Bakker, B.M. The Role of Short-Chain Fatty Acids in the Interplay between Diet, Gut Microbiota, and Host Energy Metabolism. *J. Lipid Res.* **2013**, *54*, 2325–2340. [CrossRef] [PubMed]
135. Boudry, G.; Hamilton, M.K.; Chichlowski, M.; Wickramasinghe, S.; Barile, D.; Kalanetra, K.M.; Mills, D.A.; Raybould, H.E. Bovine Milk Oligosaccharides Decrease Gut Permeability and Improve Inflammation and Microbial Dysbiosis in Diet-Induced Obese Mice. *J. Dairy Sci.* **2017**, *100*, 2471–2481. [CrossRef] [PubMed]
136. Yu, T.; Wang, Y.; Chen, X.; Xiong, W.; Tang, Y.; Lin, L. Spirulina Platensis Alleviates Chronic Inflammation with Modulation of Gut Microbiota and Intestinal Permeability in Rats Fed a High-Fat Diet. *J. Cell. Mol. Med.* **2020**, *24*, 8603–8613. [CrossRef]
137. Zhang, Z.; Lin, T.; Meng, Y.; Hu, M.; Shu, L.; Jiang, H.; Gao, R.; Ma, J.; Wang, C.; Zhou, X. FOS/GOS Attenuates High-Fat Diet Induced Bone Loss via Reversing Microbiota Dysbiosis, High Intestinal Permeability and Systemic Inflammation in Mice. *Metab. Clin. Exp.* **2021**, *119*, 154767. [CrossRef]
138. Cani, P.; Possemiers, S.; van de Wiele, T.; Guiot, Y.; Everard, A.; Rottier, O.; Geurts, L.; Naslain, D.; Neyrinck, A.; Lambert, L.; et al. Changes in Gut Microbiota Control Inflammation in Obese Mice through a Mechanism Involving GLP-2-Driven Improvement of Gut Permeability. *Gut* **2009**, *58*, 1091–1103. [CrossRef]
139. Nettleton, J.E.; Klancic, T.; Schick, A.; Choo, A.C.; Shearer, J.; Borgland, S.L.; Chleilat, F.; Mayengbam, S.; Reimer, R.A. Low-Dose Stevia (Rebaudioside A) Consumption Perturbs Gut Microbiota and the Mesolimbic Dopamine Reward System. *Nutrients* **2019**, *11*, 1248. [CrossRef]
140. David, L.A.; Maurice, C.F.; Carmody, R.N.; Gootenberg, D.B.; Button, J.E.; Wolfe, B.E.; Ling, A.V.; Devlin, A.S.; Varma, Y.; Fischbach, M.A.; et al. Diet Rapidly and Reproducibly Alters the Human Gut Microbiome. *Nature* **2014**, *505*, 559–563. [CrossRef] [PubMed]
141. Klingbeil, E.; De, C.B.; Serre, L. Microbiota Modulation by Eating Patterns and Diet Composition: Impact on Food Intake. *Am. J. Physiol. Regul. Integr. Comp. Physiol.* **2018**, *315*, R1254–R1260. [CrossRef]
142. Merra, G.; Noce, A.; Marrone, G.; Cintoni, M.; Tarsitano, M.G.; Capacci, A.; de Lorenzo, A. Influence of Mediterranean Diet on Human Gut Microbiota. *Nutrients* **2021**, *13*, 7. [CrossRef]
143. El-Salhy, M.; Hatlebakk, J.G.; Hausken, T. Diet in Irritable Bowel Syndrome (IBS): Interaction with Gut Microbiota and Gut Hormones. *Nutrients* **2019**, *11*, 1824. [CrossRef]
144. Varjú, P.; Farkas, N.; Hegyi, P.; Garami, A.; Szabó, I.; Illés, A.; Solymár, M.; Vincze, Á.; Balaskó, M.; Pár, G.; et al. Low Fermentable Oligosaccharides, Disaccharides, Monosaccharides and Polyols (FODMAP) Diet Improves Symptoms in Adults Suffering from

Irritable Bowel Syndrome (IBS) Compared to Standard IBS Diet: A Meta-Analysis of Clinical Studies. *PLoS ONE* **2017**, *12*, e0182942. [CrossRef] [PubMed]
145. Cuomo, R.; Andreozzi, P.; Zito, F.P.; Passananti, V.; de Carlo, G.; Sarnelli, G. Irritable Bowel Syndrome and Food Interaction. *World J. Gastroenterol.* **2014**, 8837–8845.
146. Singh, R.K.; Chang, H.W.; Yan, D.; Lee, K.M.; Ucmak, D.; Wong, K.; Abrouk, M.; Farahnik, B.; Nakamura, M.; Zhu, T.H.; et al. Influence of Diet on the Gut Microbiome and Implications for Human Health. *J. Transl. Med.* **2017**, *15*, 73. [CrossRef]
147. Liu, R.; Hong, J.; Xu, X.; Feng, Q.; Zhang, D.; Gu, Y.; Shi, J.; Zhao, S.; Liu, W.; Wang, X.; et al. Gut Microbiome and Serum Metabolome Alterations in Obesity and after Weight-Loss Intervention. *Nat. Med.* **2017**, *23*, 859–868. [CrossRef]
148. Suskind, D.L.; Lee, D.; Kim, Y.M.; Wahbeh, G.; Singh, N.; Braly, K.; Nuding, M.; Nicora, C.D.; Purvine, S.O.; Lipton, M.S.; et al. The Specific Carbohydrate Diet and Diet Modification as Induction Therapy for Pediatric Crohn's Disease: A Randomized Diet Controlled Trial. *Nutrients* **2020**, *12*, 3749. [CrossRef] [PubMed]
149. Marx, W.; Moseley, G.; Berk, M.; Jacka, F. Nutritional Psychiatry: The Present State of the Evidence. *Proc. Nutr. Soc.* **2017**, *76*, 427–436. [CrossRef]
150. Snelson, M.; Clarke, R.E.; Nguyen, T.; Penfold, S.A.; Forbes, J.M.; Tan, S.M.; Coughlan, M.T. Long Term High Protein Diet Feeding Alters the Microbiome and Increases Intestinal Permeability, Systemic Inflammation and Kidney Injury in Mice. *Mol. Nutr. Food Res.* **2021**, *65*, e2000851. [CrossRef] [PubMed]
151. Do, M.; Lee, E.; Oh, M.-J.; Kim, Y.; Park, H.-Y. High-Glucose or -Fructose Diet Cause Changes of the Gut Microbiota and Metabolic Disorders in Mice without Body Weight Change. *Nutrients* **2018**, *10*, 761. [CrossRef]
152. Nilholm, C.; Roth, B.; Ohlsson, B. A Dietary Intervention with Reduction of Starch and Sucrose Leads to Reduced Gastrointestinal and Extra-Intestinal Symptoms in IBS Patients. *Nutrients* **2019**, *11*, 1662. [CrossRef]
153. Ott, B.; Skurk, T.; Hastreiter, L.; Lagkouvardos, I.; Fischer, S.; Büttner, J.; Kellerer, T.; Clavel, T.; Rychlik, M.; Haller, D.; et al. Effect of Caloric Restriction on Gut Permeability, Inflammation Markers, and Fecal Microbiota in Obese Women. *Sci. Rep.* **2017**, *7*, 11955. [CrossRef]
154. Kaliannan, K.; Wang, B.; Li, X.Y.; Kim, K.J.; Kang, J.X. A Host-Microbiome Interaction Mediates the Opposing Effects of Omega-6 and Omega-3 Fatty Acids on Metabolic Endotoxemia. *Sci. Rep.* **2015**, *5*, 11276. [CrossRef]
155. Puri, B.K. The Use of Eicosapentaenoic Acid in the Treatment of Chronic Fatigue Syndrome. *Prostaglandins Leukot. Essent. Fat. Acids* **2004**, *70*, 399–401. [CrossRef]
156. Puri, B.K. Long-Chain Polyunsaturated Fatty Acids and the Pathophysiology of Myalgic Encephalomyelitis (Chronic Fatigue Syndrome). *J. Clin. Pathol.* **2007**, *60*, 122–124. [CrossRef]
157. Wang, J.H.; Bose, S.; Kim, G.C.; Hong, S.U.; Kim, J.H.; Kim, J.E.; Kim, H. Flos Lonicera Ameliorates Obesity and Associated Endotoxemia in Rats through Modulation of Gut Permeability and Intestinal Microbiota. *PLoS ONE* **2014**, *9*, e86117. [CrossRef] [PubMed]
158. Wang, S.; Li, Q.; Zang, Y.; Zhao, Y.; Liu, N.; Wang, Y.; Xu, X.; Liu, L.; Mei, Q. Apple Polysaccharide Inhibits Microbial Dysbiosis and Chronic Inflammation and Modulates Gut Permeability in HFD-Fed Rats. *Int. J. Biol. Macromol.* **2017**, *99*, 282–292. [CrossRef] [PubMed]
159. Fujisaka, S.; Usui, I.; Nawaz, A.; Igarashi, Y.; Okabe, K.; Furusawa, Y.; Watanabe, S.; Yamamoto, S.; Sasahara, M.; Watanabe, Y.; et al. Bofutsushosan Improves Gut Barrier Function with a Bloom of Akkermansia Muciniphila and Improves Glucose Metabolism in Mice with Diet-Induced Obesity. *Sci. Rep.* **2020**, *10*, 5544. [CrossRef] [PubMed]
160. Wang, X.; Qu, Y.; Zhang, Y.; Li, S.; Sun, Y.; Chen, Z.; Teng, L.; Wang, D. Antifatigue Potential Activity of Sarcodon Imbricatus in Acute Excise-Treated and Chronic Fatigue Syndrome in Mice via Regulation of Nrf2-Mediated Oxidative Stress. *Oxidative Med. Cell. Longev.* **2018**, *2018*, 9140896. [CrossRef] [PubMed]
161. Kwon, D.A.; Kim, Y.S.; Kim, S.K.; Baek, S.H.; Kim, H.K.; Lee, H.S. Antioxidant and Antifatigue Effect of a Standardized Fraction (HemoHIM) from Angelica Gigas, Cnidium Officinale, and Paeonia Lactiflora. *Pharm. Biol.* **2021**, *59*, 391–400. [CrossRef]
162. Tan, P.; Li, X.; Shen, J.; Feng, Q. Fecal Microbiota Transplantation for the Treatment of Inflammatory Bowel Disease: An Update. *Front. Pharmacol.* **2020**, *11*, 574533. [CrossRef]
163. Gupta, A.; Khanna, S. Fecal Microbiota Transplantation. *JAMA* **2017**, *318*, 102. [CrossRef] [PubMed]
164. Rodiño-Janeiro, B.K.; Vicario, M.; Alonso-Cotoner, C.; Pascua-García, R.; Santos, J. A Review of Microbiota and Irritable Bowel Syndrome: Future in Therapies. *Adv. Ther.* **2018**, *35*, 289–310. [CrossRef] [PubMed]
165. Surawicz, C.M.; Brandt, L.J.; Binion, D.G.; Ananthakrishnan, A.N.; Curry, S.R.; Gilligan, P.H.; McFarland, L.V.; Mellow, M.; Zuckerbraun, B.S. Guidelines for Diagnosis, Treatment, and Prevention of Clostridium Difficile Infections. *Am. J. Gastroenterol.* **2013**, *108*, 478–498. [CrossRef] [PubMed]
166. Malnick, S.D.H.; Fisher, D.; Somin, M.; Neuman, M.G. Treating the Metabolic Syndrome by Fecal Transplantation—Current Status. *Biology* **2021**, *10*, 447. [CrossRef] [PubMed]
167. Choi, H.H.; Cho, Y.S. Fecal Microbiota Transplantation: Current Applications, Effectiveness, and Future Perspectives. *Clin. Endosc.* **2016**, *49*, 257–265. [CrossRef] [PubMed]
168. Juul, F.E.; Garborg, K.; Bretthauer, M.; Skudal, H.; Øines, M.N.; Wiig, H.; Rose, Ø.; Seip, B.; Lamont, J.T.; Midtvedt, T.; et al. Fecal Microbiota Transplantation for Primary Clostridium Difficile Infection. *N. Engl. J. Med.* **2018**, *378*, 2535–2536. [CrossRef]
169. Chen, D.; Wu, J.; Jin, D.; Wang, B.; Cao, H. Fecal Microbiota Transplantation in Cancer Management: Current Status and Perspectives. *Int. J. Cancer* **2019**, *145*, 2021–2031. [CrossRef]

170. Evrensel, A.; Ceylan, M.E. Fecal Microbiota Transplantation and Its Usage in Neuropsychiatric Disorders. *Clin. Psychopharmacol. Neurosci.* **2016**, *14*, 231–237. [CrossRef]
171. Xu, M.Q.; Cao, H.L.; Wang, W.Q.; Wang, S.; Cao, X.C.; Yan, F.; Wang, B.M. Fecal Microbiota Transplantation Broadening Its Application beyond Intestinal Disorders. *World J. Gastroenterol.* **2015**, *21*, 102–111. [CrossRef]
172. Kim, M.; Kim, Y.; Choi, H.; Kim, W.; Park, S.; Lee, D.; Kim, D.; Kim, H.; Choi, H.; Hyun, D.; et al. Transfer of a Healthy Microbiota Reduces Amyloid and Tau Pathology in an Alzheimer's Disease Animal Model. *Gut* **2020**, *69*, 283–294. [CrossRef]
173. Wang, Y.; Wiesnoski, D.H.; Helmink, B.A.; Gopalakrishnan, V.; Choi, K.; DuPont, H.L.; Jiang, Z.D.; Abu-Sbeih, H.; Sanchez, C.A.; Chang, C.C.; et al. Fecal Microbiota Transplantation for Refractory Immune Checkpoint Inhibitor-Associated Colitis. *Nat. Med.* **2018**, *24*, 1804–1808. [CrossRef]
174. Shen, Z.-H.; Zhu, C.-X.; Quan, Y.-S.; Yang, Z.-Y.; Wu, S.; Luo, W.-W.; Tan, B.; Wang, X.-Y. Relationship between Intestinal Microbiota and Ulcerative Colitis: Mechanisms and Clinical Application of Probiotics and Fecal Microbiota Transplantation. *World J. Gastroenterol.* **2018**, *24*, 14. [CrossRef] [PubMed]
175. Borody, T. Bacteriotherapy for Chronic Fatigue Syndrome: A Long-Term Follow up Study. In Proceedings of the 1995 CFS National Consensus Conference; 1995.
176. Borody, T.J.; Nowak, A.; Finlayson, S. The GI Microbiome and Its Role in Chronic Fatigue Syndrome: A Summary of Bacteriotherapy The GI Microbiome and Its Role in Chronic Fatigue Syndrome: A Summary of Bacteriotherapy. *ACNEM J.* **2012**, *31*, 3–8.
177. Schmulson, M.; Bashashati, M. Fecal Microbiota Transfer for Bowel Disorders: Efficacy or Hype? *Curr. Opin. Pharmacol.* **2018**, *43*, 72–80. [CrossRef] [PubMed]
178. Lopetuso, L.; Ianiro, G.; Allegretti, J.; Bibbò, S.; Gasbarrini, A.; Scaldaferri, F.; Cammarota, G. Fecal Transplantation for Ulcerative Colitis: Current Evidence and Future Applications. *Expert Opin. Biol. Ther.* **2020**, *20*, 343–351. [CrossRef] [PubMed]
179. Shanahan, F.; Quigley, E. Manipulation of the Microbiota for Treatment of IBS and IBD-Challenges and Controversies. *Gastroenterology* **2014**, *146*, 1554–1563. [CrossRef]
180. Imdad, A.; Nicholson, M.; Tanner-Smith, E.; Zackular, Z.; Gomez-Duarte, O.; Beaulieu, D.; Acra, S. Fecal Transplantation for Treatment of Inflammatory Bowel Disease. *Cochrane Database Syst. Rev.* **2018**, *11*, CD012774. [CrossRef]
181. Aroniadis, O.C.; Brandt, L.J. Fecal Microbiota Transplantation: Past, Present and Future. *Curr. Opin. Gastroenterol.* **2013**, *29*, 79–84. [CrossRef]
182. Levy, A.N.; Allegretti, J.R. Insights into the Role of Fecal Microbiota Transplantation for the Treatment of Inflammatory Bowel Disease. *Ther. Adv. Gastroenterol.* **2019**, *12*, 1756284819836893. [CrossRef]

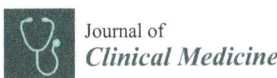

Review

Myalgic Encephalomyelitis/Chronic Fatigue Syndrome (ME/CFS): An Overview

Undine-Sophie Deumer [1,†], Angelica Varesi [2,3,*,†], Valentina Floris [4], Gabriele Savioli [5], Elisa Mantovani [6], Paulina López-Carrasco [7], Gian Marco Rosati [8], Sakshi Prasad [9] and Giovanni Ricevuti [10,*]

1. Department of Biological Sciences, Faculty of Natural Sciences and Mathematics, University of Cologne, 50674 Cologne, Germany; udeumer@smail.uni-koeln.de
2. Department of Biology and Biotechnology, University of Pavia, 27100 Pavia, Italy
3. Almo Collegio Borromeo, 27100 Pavia, Italy
4. Department of Internal Medicine and Therapeutics, University of Pavia, 27100 Pavia, Italy; valentina.floris01@universitadipavia.it
5. Emergency Department, IRCCS Policlinico San Matteo, 27100 Pavia, Italy; gabrielesavioli@gmail.com
6. Department of Neurosciences, Biomedicine and Movement Sciences, Neurology Section, University of Verona, 37129 Verona, Italy; elisa.mantovani@univr.it
7. División de Neurociencias, Instituto de Fisiología Celular, Universidad Nacional Autónoma de México (UNAM), Mexico City 04510, Mexico; pcarrasco@ifc.unam.mx
8. Medicine and Surgery, Humanitas University, 20090 Milano, Italy; gianmarcorosati23@gmail.com
9. National Pirogov Memorial Medical University, 21018 Vinnytsya, Ukraine; sakshiprasad8@gmail.com
10. School of Pharmacy, Department of Drug Sciences, University of Pavia, 27100 Pavia, Italy
* Correspondence: angelica.varesi@collegioborromeo.eu (A.V.); giovanni.ricevuti@unipv.it (G.R.)
† These authors contributed equally.

Abstract: Myalgic encephalomyelitis/chronic fatigue syndrome (ME/CFS) is a chronic systemic disease that manifests via various symptoms such as chronic fatigue, post-exertional malaise, and cognitive impairment described as "brain fog". These symptoms often prevent patients from keeping up their pre-disease onset lifestyle, as extended periods of physical or mental activity become almost impossible. However, the disease presents heterogeneously with varying severity across patients. Therefore, consensus criteria have been designed to provide a diagnosis based on symptoms. To date, no biomarker-based tests or diagnoses are available, since the molecular changes observed also largely differ from patient to patient. In this review, we discuss the infectious, genetic, and hormonal components that may be involved in CFS pathogenesis, we scrutinize the role of gut microbiota in disease progression, we highlight the potential of non-coding RNA (ncRNA) for the development of diagnostic tools and briefly mention the possibility of SARS-CoV-2 infection causing CFS.

Keywords: ME/CFS; immunity; dysbiosis; COVID-19; hormone; depression; genetics; miRNA; therapy; diagnosis

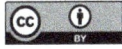

1. Introduction

Myalgic encephalomyelitis/chronic fatigue syndrome (ME/CFS) is a complex chronic disease of unknown origin that affects nearly 0.9% of the population worldwide [1,2]. Disease symptoms are often broad, and they overlap with many other conditions, making ME/CFS hard to diagnose. Excessive fatigue, malaise, muscle pain, unrefreshing sleep, dysbiosis, cognitive dysfunction, neuroendocrine and immune alterations are all reported in ME/CFS patients [3]. While ME/CFS is often a chronic condition, some patients can experience periods of partial recovery in between relapses, and disease progression differs largely between patients [4]. Although viral infections have been considered the main trigger of disease onset for a long time, a clear mechanism of pathogenesis is still undefined [5]. It is now becoming clear that ME/CFS origin could instead be explained by a complex relationship between genetic predisposition and environmental factors, with each component contributing to disease manifestation [6]. In this respect, sex, socio-economic status, and age have been reported to correlate with disease presentation, with females being predominantly diagnosed but not necessarily affected more often [7].

Although several consensus criteria have been established in the literature (i.e., Canadian Consensus Criteria, Fukuda, Oxford, International Criteria, etc.) no blood test or diagnostic tool is commercially available [3]. However, the lack of a single set of defined consensus criteria might lead to misdiagnosis. Similarly, a clear therapeutic approach is still lacking. Although different meta-analysis and clinical trials have shown robust evidence in favor of cognitive-behavioral therapy (CBT) and graded exercise therapy (GET) [8–17], more research should be carried out to find advanced therapeutic approaches [6,18].

Given these limitations, identifying the components which contribute to disease pathogenesis and understanding how they cause disease symptoms may lead to novel diagnostic and therapeutic approaches [6]. Several reviews are available in the literature addressing general and specific topics related to ME/CFS, yet a complete overview of the different aspects leading to disease pathogenesis and progression is still lacking. In this review, we address comprehensively how immune dysfunction, hormonal imbalance, genetics/epigenetics, and cognitive alterations affect ME/CFS patients, providing insights into the emerging role of non-coding RNAs and gut microbiome alterations in disease pathogenesis. Lastly, we also include a brief summary of the potential relationship between the newly coined "long-COVID" and chronic fatigue.

2. Methods

To review the role of inflammation, immunity, genetics, epigenetics, cognitive symptoms, dysbiosis, non-coding RNAs, and hormones in ME/CFS, we carried out an exhaustive search in PubMed (U.S. National Library of Medicine) publication database. The following keywords were used alone or in combination: "chronic fatigue syndrome", "myalgic encephalomyelitis", "ME/CFS", "inflammation", "cognitive symptoms", "dysbiosis", "microbiome", "miRNA", "non-coding RNA", "COVID-19", "long-COVID", "fatigue", "therapy", "diagnosis", "cytokine", "genetic", "polymorphism", "epigenetic", "HPA axis", "depression", "intestinal permeability" and "infection". Recent publications were preferred, but no limiting period was imposed in our screening. Furthermore, books, general newspapers, and Institutional Websites were reviewed for possible integration.

3. Results

3.1. The Role of Inflammation and Immunity in ME/CFS

Like other inter-cellular communication, homeostasis of the immune system is dysregulated in CFS [19]. This means ME/CFS patients will experience symptoms related to immunological changes such as high susceptibility to infections, especially of the upper respiratory tract, long recovery times, chronically swollen and tender lymph nodes, and feeling feverish often [3]. It is not clear yet whether CFS is an inherently low-grade inflammatory disease or whether it is only accompanied by systemic inflammation [5]. The underlying causes for each of the symptoms have not yet been fully elucidated, but the following paragraph aims at summarizing the current state of knowledge in the field.

Multiple changes can be observed concerning the state of inflammation in the body of CFS patients in comparison to healthy people. An inflammatory, cell-mediated immune response is active even when pathogens are absent. This may be an abnormal reaction to common antigens which are harmless [20]. This cell-mediated immune response is generally characterized by a decreased function of natural killer (NK) cells, reduced response of T-cells to antigens [21,22], and persistence of autoreactive cells [23–25]. The activated state of the immune system is also indicated by an increase in the biomarker neopterin, which is released by monocytes and macrophages, and a high concentration of acute-phase reactants [5,26]. With impaired NK cell function, the ability of the organism to fight infections decreases. The more severely the function of these cells is impaired, the worse ME/CFS symptoms the patient suffers from typically are, and patients are more likely to contract recurrent infections due to immune suppression [3,27]. One can also observe an expansion of effector memory cells exhibiting type 2 responsiveness which means there is low-grade, chronic inflammation. A phenotypic shift in T-helper cells from Th1- to Th2-cells was already discovered in the early 1990s [3,28–30]. T-cells also show increased CD26 surface expression, defective regulatory cell functions, fast exhaustion, and dysregulated cell metabolism [5,19,28,31]. Contradictory studies have been published on whether CFS patients show an increase or decrease in T-regulatory cells [32,33]. Furthermore, CFS patients show persistence of autoreactive cells that can generate autoantibodies during common infections, for example, against ß2-adrenergic receptors and M3 acetylcholine receptors [23,24]. Neutrophils and lymphocytes are more prone to apoptosis than in healthy individuals [34].

The finding of low-grade inflammation is also supported by an altered cytokine profile, pro- as well as anti-inflammatory cytokine levels are reported to be elevated in subsets of patients [5,21]. However, contradictory studies have been published on this topic depending on the methods which were used [21,35]. Cytokine levels which are often reported as increased are IL-1β, IL-1, IL-4, IL-5, IL-6, IL-12 [5], and IL-2 [26,36,37], those which appear decreased are IL-8, IL-13, IL-15, and IL-23 [5,38,39]. Furthermore, TNF-α and IFN-γ levels are increased as well as those of NF-κB, a transcription factor regulated by cytokines such as TNF-α and IL-1β [5,27,37,40–42]. As mentioned before, the overall results of these studies are not conclusive, for example for IL-8 and IL-13, increased levels have been reported as well [38]. One of the reasons why these results may differ so much between studies could be the influence of other factors such as sleep, obesity, nutrition, and cognition on the state of inflammation in the body. The time point of measurement during disease progression could also play a role. If changes are observed, they are most pronounced in the first three years of the disease. This is of clinical significance as it enables distinguishing between the early and late stages of ME/CFS [43]. Besides total cytokine levels, the network of cytokine interactions also seems to diverge from the norm [39]. A chronically high level of cytokines may interfere with the stress response to body issues and could partly explain chronic fatigue and flu-like symptoms in many patients' experiences.

It is not clear what exactly causes the onset of symptoms in ME/CFS, but viral infections and stress have been discussed as a possible origin of the disease, while an additional genetic component is also likely [3,44–46]. Infectious pathogens such as viruses could be the original cause of the inflammatory state by activating antiviral immune responses, which then trigger systemic inflammation [5,26,34,45]. The virus infection most widely reported in relation to CFS is Epstein-Barr virus (EBV) since a considerable number of patients report symptom onset after contracting EBV [47–49]. However, it should be noted that an estimate of >90% of the adult population generally test positive for past EBV infection, and most do not develop ME/CFS. Human herpesvirus 6 (HHV-6) and human parvovirus B19 have also been reported as possible causes of CFS [50–54]. The probability of patients developing CFS after severe viral infections or other illnesses such as Lyme disease has consistently been reported as 5% to 10% [55]. Regardless of which virus infection may trigger ME/CFS, specific immunological changes that CFS and viral infections have in common include altered antiviral response elements, for example, the 2-5A synthetase/ribonuclease L (RNase L) antiviral defense pathway in monocytes, which is mediated by interleukins [3,31,56], and elevated cytokine levels. RNase L then destroys cell membranes in CFS patients, including mitochondrial membranes which causes additional oxidative stress [57]. When suffering acutely from a sore throat, patients very often present with a viral reactivation, which may also be accompanied by tender, swollen lymph nodes [3]. Besides viral infections, another possible explanation for dysregulation of the inflammatory cascade is impairment of the hypothalamus–pituitary–adrenal (HPA) axis, since the systemic hypocortisolism which has been reported in this respect is known to impact immunological homeostasis and drive Th2-cell identity [28,58] (see also HPA axis paragraph). Patients who received cognitive behavioral therapy (CBT) showed lower cortisol levels after treatment compared to untreated patients [58].

Multiple studies have reported elevated levels of oxidative stress in CFS patients [5,34,59]. The antioxidant capacity seems to be decreased in subgroups of patients, but even in patients with normal antioxidant capacity, an increase in oxidative stress is observed. The activity of oxidative and nitrosative pathways is enhanced while levels of antioxidants such as zinc and enzymes like coenzyme Q10 are decreased [5,21,60,61]. This may lead to excessive formation of free radicals, which cannot be eliminated and will damage the cells by targeting fatty acids and proteins [5,21]. These are then recognized as abnormal by the immune system and may in part lead to a chronic inflammatory state. An IgM-mediated immune response directed against O&NS-modified epitopes in ME/CFS has been observed [5,61]. In this context, mitochondrial dysfunction, which has been observed as well [5], can also play a role as this organelle is crucial for reactive oxygen species (ROS) regulation. ROS-induced damage to the mitochondria and elevated pro-inflammatory cytokines, which are both also consequences of viral infection, can activate NF-kB transcription.

Since the inflammatory signaling pathways generally seem to be disturbed, one possible explanation for the symptoms of the disease could be a disrupted gut barrier [45]. The leaky gut hypothesis is supported by the finding that IgA levels in CFS patients against lipopolysaccharides (LPS) of gram-negative bacteria are increased, which is accompanied by increased translocation of these bacteria [5] and the fact that CFS and irritable bowel syndrome (IBS) often occur together [62]. Another possible explanation for the pronounced immune response could be autoimmunity. A few factors support this idea, such as a high prevalence in women which is common in autoimmune diseases, the increase in baseline inflammation, and that it often occurs as a comorbidity of other autoimmune diseases [3,47,55,63,64]. As mentioned above, CFS can occur after infection with EBV, which is also a known risk factor for developing autoimmune diseases [65,66]. If patients are treated against autoantibodies, the condition improves [25,64]. What strongly speaks against the idea of CFS being an autoimmune disease, however, is the lack of tissue damage.

Besides these differences in the baseline state of the immune system in CFS patients compared to healthy people, patients also experience post-exertional malaise (PEM) [55,67,68]. One possible explanation for this might be a more pronounced immune response in ME/CFS patients after exercise than in healthy people [69]. Upon exercise, physically but also mentally, symptoms usually worsen within 24 h, however, there is contradictory evidence against an immune response that diverges from the norm, possibly due to differences in study design [68]. Reports have been made of an increase in TLR-4 and IL-10 gene expression after exercise [69]. While the gene expression was increased, the circulating cytokine levels in response to exercise appear to be similar in CFS and control groups in some studies but diverge strongly in others [69,70]. When studying the complement response to exercise in CFS patients, some evidence was found for a stronger response than in controls. This is of interest because an altered complement response might cause PEM [69]. Moreover, patients seem to suffer from increased oxidative stress faster and longer after exercise than healthy controls, and their antioxidant response is delayed and reduced [46,59]. This fits with the higher level of oxidative stress in these patients even without exercise and supports the hypothesis that some of the symptoms are caused by malfunctions in ROS regulation. Further findings point towards decreased ATP levels, increased lactate, hyperactive RNase L activated by IFN, and hyperactive NF-κB relative to healthy controls. Overall, the evidence suggests that the immune response of CFS patients to exercise is more pronounced than that of healthy people [70].

3.2. Genetic and Epigenetic Alterations

Although CFS pathogenesis is still largely unknown, several studies suggest the possibility of a genetic predisposition. First hints came from the observation that mothers and children diagnosed with CFS share very similar symptoms, in contrast to fathers and their children [71]. Moreover, the analysis of data obtained from the Utah health care system highlighted a strong contribution in favor of CFS heritability [72]. Many pathways have then been linked to disease symptoms and severity, such as regulatory pathways of immunity and neurotransmission, inflammation and oxidative stress, the catecholamine pathway, and the serotoninergic system [73] (Table 1). TNF-α, IL-1β, IL-4, IL-6, HLA, IFN-γ, GRIK2, SCL6A4, COMT, and NR3C1 genes have all been found to be correlated with the disease [73]. For a summary of the most significant findings regarding CFS and genetic predisposition please refer to Table 1.

Despite most studies reporting the association between CFS and one or a few polymorphisms, it should be noted that, being a multifactorial disease, a varied genetic contribution is more likely to explain predisposition and heredity than a single variation. In this respect, many variations scarcely contribute by themselves, but when put together they increase the risk. Thus, searching for haplotypes or combined genetic polymorphisms will be helpful in establishing a genetic screening test able to diagnose and/or stratify CFS patients [74]. Possibly, this could also be useful for the administration of personalized and tailored therapy [75].

Genetic predisposition has also been hypothesized to be involved in autoimmunity. Blomberg et al. present a model in which, following infection, certain genetic backgrounds and dysbiosis might favor the generation of B-cell clones prone to react against self-antigens, thus explaining why some patients present signs of autoimmunity [46].

Besides classical genetics, a growing body of evidence suggests that epigenetics is also linked to CFS and can potentially explain the major pathways involved in the disease. In one study, methylation patterns of 10 CFS patients have been compared to 10 controls, and immune, metabolic and neurological pathways have been associated with the disease [4]. Moreover, differential methylation in the PRF1 gene and in several CpG loci of T lymphocytes was also detected in CFS patients in contrast to healthy subjects [76,77]. Perhaps not surprisingly, the genetic and epigenetic alterations found in CFS often reside in the same genes and affect the same functions, thus confirming the importance of the previously mentioned pathways in disease pathophysiology.

Although the new discoveries in CFS and genetics are rising in expectancy in terms of new diagnostic and therapeutic tools, it should be considered that studies with a higher number of participants are needed to achieve true significance. Indeed, independent research is usually conducted on a very limited number of CFS cases and analysis on different patient cohorts often fails to reproduce matching results [74]. Therefore, while the recent data can certainly increase our knowledge of disease mechanisms and has translational potential, more confirming evidence is needed before applying this knowledge in clinical practice.

Table 1. Summary of the most significant genetic alterations found in CFS patients.

Ref.	N° Patients	Gene/Protein	Alteration	Pathway
Smith et al., 2011 [78]	40 CFS + 40 controls	GRIK2 (glutamate receptor, ionotropic, kinase 2)	G allele of rs 2247215 (GRIK2)	Glutamatergic neurotransmission
		NPAS2 (neural PAS domain protein 2)	T allele of rs 356653 (NPAS2)	Circadian rhythm regulation
Schlauch et al., 2016 [79]	42 CFS + 38 controls	CLEC4M (C-Type lectin domain family 4 member M)	C > T missense mutation (CLEC4M)	Signal transduction and kinase reaction
		GRIK3 (glutamate ionotropic receptor kainate type subunit 3)	CT genotype at rs3913434 (GRIK3)	Glutamatergic neurotransmission

Table 1. Cont.

Ref.	N° Patients	Gene/Protein	Alteration	Pathway
Meyer et al., 2015 [80]	120 CFS (12–18 years) + 38 controls	• SCL6A4 (solute carrier family 6 member 4), encodes for 5-HTT	• SNP rs25531 A > G and short (S) vs. long (L) 5-HTTLPR allele	• Serotonin reuptake
Lobel et al., 2015 [81]	74 CFS + 76 controls	• COMT (catechol-O-methyltransferase)	• rs 4680 polymorphism	• Catecholamine inactivation
De Luca et al., 2015 [82]	89 FM/CFS + 196 controls	• NOS2A (nitric oxide synthase 2A)	• NOS2A −2.5 kb $(CCTTT)_{11}$ allele	• Inflammation and oxidative stress
Fukuda et al., 2013 [83]	155 CFS	• GCH (GTP cyclohydrolase I)	• C+243T polymorphism (GCH)	• tetrahydrobiopterin (BH4) biosynthesis
		• TH (tyrosine hydroxylase)	• C-824T polymorphism (TH)	• Catecholamines biosynthesis
Smith et al., 2008 [84]	40 CFS + 55 with insufficient fatigue + 42 controls	• HTR2A (5-hydroxytryptamine receptor 2A)	• -1438G/A, C102T and rs1923884	• Serotoninergic system
Carlo-Stella et al., 2006 [85]	54 CFS	• TNF promoter	• -857 TT and CT genotypes (TNF)	• Inflammation
		• IFN-gamma	• 874 A/A (IFN-gamma)	• Inflammation
Perez et al., 2019 [86]	383 ME/CFS	• GPBAR1 (G protein-coupled bile acid receptor 1)	• rs199986029	• Macrophage functions and regulation of energy homeostasis by bile acids
		• HLA-C (major histocompatibility complex, class I, C)	• rs41560916	• Immune system
		• BCAM (basal cell adhesion molecule)	• rs3810141	• Intracellular signaling mediator
Carlo-Stella et al., 2009 [87]	75 CFS + 141 controls	• RAGE (receptor for advanced glycation end-product)	Haplotypes: • RAGE-374A, HLA-DRB1*1104 allele	• Immunity and inflammation
		• HLA-DRB1 (major histocompatibility complex, class II, DR beta 1)	• RAGE-374A, HLA-DRB1*1301 allele	

Table 1. Cont.

Ref.	N° Patients	Gene/Protein	Alteration	Pathway
Sommerfeldt et al., 2011 [88]	53 CFS (12–18 years)	• COMT (catechol-O-methyltransferase)	• AA genotype of SNP Rs4680 (COMT)	• Catecholamine inactivation
		• β^2-adrenergic receptor	• CG and CC genotype of SNP Rs1042714 (β^2-adrenergic receptor)	• Catecholamine signaling

3.3. Cognitive Symptoms and Depression

It is well known that cognitive symptoms such as sleep disorders, depression, anxiety, and mood swings are often found in and characterize CFS. Indeed, a recent systematic review and meta-analysis reported that around half of the ME/CFS patients present with anxiety and/or depression [89].

Diagnosis of CFS is achieved by using well-established diagnostic criteria (Canadian Consensus Criteria, Fukuda, Oxford, International Criteria, etc.). In this respect, carefully defining the forms of associated chronic fatigue (i.e., in cancer, multiple sclerosis, inflammatory bowel disease, psychiatric conditions) is critical to reaching a conclusive diagnosis. Typically, a detailed medical history of the patient including symptoms, the associated disability, the choice of coping strategies, and the patient's own understanding of their illness are considered. Since CFS and major depression (MD) share very similar characteristics, many CFS patients are initially diagnosed as depressed [80]. Although the diagnosis of MD should be an exclusion criterion for ME/CFS, distinguishing between MD and reactive depression, which can be a comorbidity of CFS, is not always easy. However, while the two conditions show some similar symptoms, they can still be distinguished. For example, in depressed people, fatigue is associated with apathy, whereas in CFS patients it is associated with intense frustration about their condition [90]. In addition, every CFS evaluation should include a mental status examination to identify abnormalities in mood, intellectual function, memory, and personality changes. Particular attention should be directed toward acute depressive, anxious or self-destructive thoughts and observable signs such as psychomotor problems. Moreover, a physical examination may show a frequently sore throat and tender cervical or axillary lymph nodes in CFS, which are not found in depression [90].

As briefly mentioned, not only is there a clear symptom overlap, but several articles also show that ME/CFS and MD can be defined as comorbid [90]. Multiple reasons for this co-occurrence can be discussed. For example, one of the main symptoms of CFS/ME is chronic pain of differing quality and fatigue, and depression is a comorbidity of pain itself [91]. Another possible reason for this comorbidity may be immune system dysregulation, as discussed above. Patients with ME/CFS have poorly functioning NK cells, which is linked to the severity of the illness and disturbed cognitive function, while low NK cytotoxicity has also been found in other diseases including MD disorder [3]. Recent works have also found that, during chronic inflammation, microglia are activated and participate in creating a neuro-inflammatory environment that is similarly found in patients with depression [92]. Leaky gut and metabolic endotoxemia may also explain MD and CFS symptom overlap. Recent studies demonstrated that both diseases show activated immune-inflammatory pathways, including increased Gram-negative bacteria translocation and higher levels of pro-inflammatory cytokines, such as IL-1 [93]. Interestingly, in chronic depression increased levels of IL-1 are associated with higher levels of fatigue and psychosomatic symptoms, including hyperalgesia, insomnia, and neurocognitive deficits [94]. Furthermore, depression sometimes also results from CFS. Poor concentration, groping for words, short-term memory loss, and reading impairment are reported in CFS patients, with severely affected patients experiencing strongly disabling cognitive symptoms [3,95]. This complex psychological condition often prevents patients from continuing their normal lives, leading to severe depression that in turn may worsen the already serious cognitive symptoms.

However, not all CFS patients present with depression. Clinical reports of CFS patients without a history of depression show that antidepressant treatments may even be harmful in these cases [3,90]. Although clinical diagnosis based on symptom manifestation is certainly fundamental, results of some studies suggest that diagnostic tools based on molecular and biological analysis could improve the diagnosis. While further investigation is needed, Table 2 summarizes the proposed biomarkers based on which diagnostic tools could be created to distinguish between CFS and MD (Table 2).

It should be noted that the neuropsychological conditions described in ME/CFS have been hypothesized to originate at least in part from neuroinflammation. Higher levels of proinflammatory cytokines have been found in the cerebral spinal fluid of CFS patients than in healthy controls, and activation of microglia and astrocytes has been verified by positron emission tomography (PET) scan. Over-activity of microglia and astrocytes showed a correlation with symptom severity in patients. However, MD cannot be attributed to neuroinflammation [96–98].

Table 2. Proposed biomarkers for CFS/MD differential diagnosis.

Ref.	Condition	Number of Participants	Markers Analyzed	MD	CFS	Potential Biomarker
Maes at al., 2012 [99]	Plasma pro-inflammatory cytokines	26 controls, 97 ME/CFS, 85 MD	• IL-1	↓	↑	Plasma levels of IL-1 and TNF-α
			• TNF-α	↓	↑	
Robertson et al., 2005 [100]	Lymphocyte subset	25 controls, 24 MD, 23 CFS	• Resting T (CD3+/CD25-)	↓	↑	Resting T cells or CD20+/CD5+ B cells levels
			• CD20+/CD5+ B cells	↑	↓	
Scott et al., 1999 [101]	Cortisol, adrenal androgens, DHEA, DHEA-S, 17-α-hydroxyprogesterone levels	11 controls, 15 MD, 15 CFS	• DHEA	↑	↓	DHEA levels
Iacob et al., 2016 [102]	Exploratory factor analysis and regression analysis on 34 genes	61 controls, 31 medication-responsive MD 42 medication-resistant MD, 33 CFS	• Purinergic and cellular modulators gene groups;	↓	↑	Purinergic, cellular modulators, nociception, and stress mediator gene expression analysis.
			• Nociception and stress mediators group	↓	↑	
Morris et al., 2018 [103]	SPECT imaging	38 controls, 14 MD, 45 CFS	• Mid cerebral uptake index	↑	↓	SPECT imaging abnormalities
Costa et al., 1995 [104]	SPECT imaging	40 controls, 29 MD, 67 CFS	• Global and brainstem hypoperfusion	↓	↑	^{99m}Tc-HMPAO SPECT differences

Table 2. Cont.

Ref.	Condition	Number of Participants	Markers Analyzed	MD	CFS	Potential Biomarker
Goldstein et al., 1995 [105]	SPECT imaging	19 controls, 26 MD, 33 CFS	• Dorsofrontal hypoperfusion	↓	↑	99mTc-HMPAO SPECT imaging patterns of rCBF
			• Right orbitofrontal lobe, left temporal lobe and left anterior frontal lobes hypoperfusion	↑	↓	
MacHale et al., 2000 [106]	SPECT imaging	15 controls, 12 MD, 30 CFS	• Left prefrontal cortex hyperperfusion	↑	↓	99mTc-HMPAO SPECT differences
			• Left thalamus hyperperfusion	↓	↑	

MD: major depression; DHEA: dehydroepiandrosterone; DHEA-S: sulphate derivative of DHEA; SPECT: single-photon emission computerized tomography (also known as single-photon emission tomography (SPET)); CBF: cerebral blood flow; 99mTc-HMPAO: (99m)Tc-hexamethyl-propylenamine-oxime. ↑: increased; ↓: decreased.

To date, there is no standard therapy available that will effectively alleviate symptoms of the disease. There are, however, different approaches that have been tried in the past which appear promising. Classical approaches are exercise treatment to slowly build increased resistance to fatigue, and cognitive behavioral therapy (CBT) to alleviate the psychological strain of the disease [3,55,58]. A major concern in CFS is chronic pain treatment.

In this respect, meditation and relaxation response, warm baths, massages, stretching, acupuncture, hydrotherapy, chiropractic, yoga, Tai Chi, TENS (transcutaneous electrical nerve stimulation), physiotherapy and nerve blocks have all been proposed, but their efficacy is still unclear [3]. Although mild pain killers and non-steroidal anti-inflammatory drugs (NSAIDs), such as ibuprofen and naproxen, can be used in clinical practice to temporally relieve headache, muscle pain, and fever, they often fail to treat chronic pain, thus not providing relief in the long term [107–109]. Moreover, evidence for their efficacy as adjuvant medicine in ME/CFS treatment is still lacking [110], and no large-scale clinical trials support their prescription. A possible explanation for the lack of efficacy in ME/CFS should be sought in the origin of pain in these patients [111]. In this respect, central sensitization, which is pain hypersensitivity due to amplification of neuronal signaling, may play a major role. The nervous system is tuned to high pain reactivity, resulting in hyperalgesia. Neurological changes can be observed in these patients such as the ectopic firing of dorsal root ganglia cells or anatomical changes to neurons and the dorsal horn. Neuroinflammation can possibly contribute to central sensitization. NSAIDs may still be used to modulate the activity of nociceptors, but antidepressants have shown higher efficacy in managing this type of pain while physical therapy and psychotherapy are also helpful [112,113].

Oftentimes, doctors advise CFS patients to rest physically. However, it is important to point out that patients, especially those with a depressive disorder and no contraindications for physical stress, should be recommended to undergo structured and supervised physical training, as exercise therapy has been shown to improve symptoms in some patients [114]. Data from eight randomized clinical trials concluded that physical therapy improves exhaustion, quality of sleep, and health status of the patients in the long term, thus showing beneficial potential [12]. This finding contradicts the widespread opinion that patients always feel uncomfortable after physical exertion, a phenomenon known as PEM [115].

One of the aims of CFS treatment is the prevention of depression and suicidal tendencies by managing the physical and emotional issues resulting from ME/CFS [3]. Short-term studies of CBT in CFS have shown improvement in function and symptom management, especially in conjunction with other treatment modalities and compared to relaxation controls [116]. Symptoms of fatigue decreased mood, and physical fitness have been shown to be significantly ameliorated in patients following CBT [9,11,14,15], even in children and adolescents [10,117,118]. Moreover, the ability of CBT to relieve pain in ME/CFS has also been reported [119]. However, the outcome of CBT for CFS as a psychotherapeutic intervention and CBT effectiveness in improving cognitive function and quality of life still need to be fully addressed, as some gaps remain in the current evidence base [120–124].

Considering the overlap with depression which has already been discussed, it is not surprising that antidepressants might also be useful in treating mental aspects of CFS [124]. A large meta-analysis including 94 studies showed that antidepressants were approximately 3.5 times more effective than placebo in treating chronic pain in CFS patients [125]. Fluoxetine, for example, has shown the ability to improve symptoms and immune function [126] while Bupropion was found effective for the treatment of fatigue and depression in nine fluoxetine resistant CFS patients [127]. However, some authors underline the lack of studies on the efficacy of antidepressants in treating ME/CFS, and more studies on different antidepressant molecules should be carried out before establishing a therapy [128].

3.4. HPA Axis and Hormonal Imbalance

When suffering from ME/CFS, patients can experience dysregulation in the levels of hormones produced by the HPA axis [129]. Indeed, despite the heterogeneity of symptoms affecting CFS patients, and the evidence of multifactorial pathogenesis, a hormonal imbalance has been demonstrated to have a direct link with some of the symptoms present in CFS, such as debilitating fatigue, difficulty with concentration, and disturbed sleep [130]. In this respect, meta-analysis evidence supports the presence of hypocortisolism in CFS patients. Cortisol levels are fundamental to maintaining hormone homeostasis, and when altered they may cause metabolic, inflammatory, and memory alterations, although it is not sure if inflammation is a cause or consequence of a hormonal imbalance. Moreover, a loss of morning peak ACTH (adrenocorticotropic hormone) and decreased responsiveness to pharmacological challenge are also reported in CFS cases compared to controls [130]. Several symptoms of CFS resemble those of hypothyroidism caused by lower thyroid hormone activity that may be due to underlying chronic inflammation. A case-control study demonstrated that chronic fatigue syndrome patients exhibited lower FreeT3 (triiodothyronine), TT3 (total triiodothyronine), decreased peripheral conversion of T4 (thyroxine) to T3, normal/high-normal TT4 (total thyroxine) level, and lower protein binding of thyroid hormones [131].

It is well-known that the prevalence of CFS is substantially higher in females compared to men. Moreover, women with CFS have a significantly greater probability of reporting an earlier onset of menopause due to any gynecological surgeries (hysterectomy and oophorectomy) as well as pelvic pain and associated endometriosis compared to controls. The consequences of a hysterectomy and early onset menopause will bring about a decline in sex hormone levels. Low levels of estrogen can affect the immune system, causing chronic fatigue and sleep disorders. Indeed, as the delicate balance between estrogen and progesterone is lost, an improper inflammation response can arise [132].

It is now clear that proper function of the HPA axis is important for homeostasis. As patients present with changes in the HPA axis, it is reasonable to wonder about possible neuroendocrine implications in CFS etiopathogenesis. However, the main question is whether HPA alterations are implicated in the genesis of the disease or if they are secondary to the development of CFS. In this respect, it would be worth investigating which role is played by hormonal imbalance in disease pathogenesis [133]. One popular hypothesis is the so-called "allostatic load condition", where the neuroendocrine system responds to a stressor (allostatic state) in order to reset the physiological set-point (homeostasis). If this mechanism fails, an allostatic overload takes place, and the way the body deals with the stressor perpetuates stress and the chronicity of the condition [134]. Possibly, this situation may proceed dysfunction of the HPA axis. However, clear evidence in support of this suggestion is still lacking, and more studies need to be carried out to understand the role of neuroendocrinology in CFS pathogenesis [135].

3.5. Dysbiosis and Intestinal Permeability

Several papers have pointed out an alteration in the gut microbiome composition in CFS patients, and involvement of dysbiosis in disease pathogenesis has been hypothesized [136–138]. In particular, a decrease in microbial diversity and a drop in Firmicutes number was found in CFS patients compared to controls [137]. Moreover, other studies confirmed a reduction in Bacteroidetes/Firmicutes ratio and an increase in Enterobacteriaceae, thus providing evidence of a complete reorganization in intestinal microbiome composition and function [139,140]. The use of microbiota alteration as a diagnostic biomarker has also been suggested, but disease overlap with other intestinal disorders may represent a disturbing factor during diagnosis and patient stratification [138]. Although the gut microbiome is crucial in different disorders, the role of dysbiosis in CFS pathogenesis remains to be fully addressed, and its role in this disease is still up to debate [141]. After 18S RNA sequencing in the stool of 49 ME/CFS patients and 39 healthy individuals, Mandrano et al. reported a nonsignificant difference in eukaryotic diversity [142]. Therefore, more studies are needed to fully understand gut microbiome involvement in disease pathogenesis and progression.

Dysbiosis is a well-known cause of increased gut permeability. This phenomenon, also known as leaky gut, allows bacterial translocation into the bloodstream, thus increasing systemic inflammation via an immune response mediated by higher levels of LPS derived from Enterobacteriaceae [26,143–145]. More commensal bacterial translocation and increased gut inflammation have been reported in ME/CFS cases when compared to healthy controls, similar to what has already been found in obesity, diabetes, metabolic syndrome, nonalcoholic fatty liver disease, and septic shock. [143,145–148]. Therapeutic interventions aimed at re-establishing eubiosis and reducing intestinal permeability may be helpful in this respect. It has been demonstrated that a leaky gut diet, together with anti-inflammatory and anti-oxidative substances, is able to significantly improve CFS conditions [149]. Moreover, the use of probiotics and/or prebiotics should also be considered, and preliminary studies in mice and rats show promising results [150–153]. Finally, positive outcomes were reported using fecal microbiota transplantation (FMT) in CFS patients [154], but further evidence is needed. In addition, several concerns about FMT, for example, a lack of consistency, donor problems, long-term safety, etc., still raise doubts about safety and feasibility, limiting its use in the clinical practice [155–159].

Altogether, these data point out that intestinal microbiome involvement in disease pathogenesis and progression should be further analyzed, and that promising novel therapeutic tools targeting leaky gut and dysbiosis could potentially arise for CFS patients.

3.6. Non-Coding RNAs

Non-coding RNAs (ncRNA) control various levels of gene expression, chromatin architecture, epigenetic memory, transcription, RNA splicing, editing, and translation [160]. One specific type of ncRNA, the microRNAs (miRNA), alter and modulate several developmental, physiological, and pathophysiological processes [161]. This modulation can be achieved in different ways: by silencing genes, by initiating the cleavage of their respective target mRNA, or by inhibiting gene translation after complete or partial binding to their target sequence [162].

Altered protein expression characterizes chronic pain and contributes to the development of long-term hyper-excitability of nociceptive neurons in the periphery. Moreover, the central nervous system is characterized by expressional changes of signaling molecules, transmitters, ion channels, or structural proteins [163]. As miRNAs are part of mechanisms of gene expression, they are likely to contribute to these changes.

There is a need for unbiased, specific diagnostic biomarkers for ME/CFS to expedite patient diagnosis and treatment, as some previously proposed biomarkers such as activin B are controversially discussed [164,165]. miRNA profiles represent a promising strategy to discover biomarkers and more recently to diagnose patients. A limitation for the biomarker discovery studies in ME/CFS is the low number of participants that have been recruited. Patients with ME/CFS show differential expression of miRNA coding genes that regulate cytotoxicity, cytokine secretion, and apoptosis [166]. Therefore, miRNAs have the potential to be utilized as biomarkers for disease diagnosis and prognosis, but it is imperative to find a way to make markers as accurate as possible for the patient, considering their gender, age, and lifestyle. Indeed, it has previously been shown that differential expression of miRNAs in ME/CFS depends also on gender, exercise, and disease state. It is extremely important to align assessment and reporting with Common Data Elements (CDE) in human subject research to improve data quality that allows for comparisons across multiple studies [167]. The pathways in which each miRNA exerts its activity are not clear yet, but several miRNAs have been identified as altered in ME/CFS patients.

Most of the miRNAs differentially expressed in patients with CFS are involved in immune response regulation. For example, up-regulation of miR-150-5p is seen in both T-cell and B-cell maturation and differentiation and influences the release of pro-inflammatory cytokines. MiR-199-3p is a negative regulator of NF-κB and IL-8. Low miR-199-3p expression, seen in ME/CFS subjects, is linked with poor survival outcomes in carcinomas, possibly affecting the disease-related physiological burden. Another dysregulated miR-223 modulates the TLR4/TLR2/NF-κB/STAT3 signaling pathway consequently affecting inflammatory cytokine expression [161]. The cytokines released in response to the inflammatory assault, particularly TNF-α, are directly suppressed by miR-130a-3p, reducing inflammation, and associated oxidative stress. MiR-146a regulates the expression of STAT1 and reduces IFN-γ secretion, resulting in the loss of the repressive effect of regulatory T lymphocytes, while miR-374a-5p regulates the expression of ubiquitin ligase, mTOR signaling pathway, and monocyte chemoattractant protein (MCP)-1, critical in inflammatory and immune response. The overexpressed miR-4443 increases pro-inflammatory cytokines by activated the NF-κB pathway via targeting TRAF4. The expression of miR-558, miR-146a, miR-150, miR-124, and miR-143 associates directly with higher expression of immune inflammatory-related genes encoding TNF-α, IL-6, and COX-2 in adolescents with CFS [161]. In addition, NK cells have demonstrated the greatest changes in miRNA expression with upregulation of hsa-miR-99b and hsa-miR-330-3p. This is consistent with the ME/CFS phenotype characterized by NK cells activity alterations [168].

Another important factor in ME/CFS is endothelial function. Silent information regulator 1 (Sirt1) reduces inflammation and oxidative stress and increases the production of nitric oxide by activating the endothelial nitric oxide synthase. MiR-21, miR-34a, miR-92a, miR-126, and miR-200c regulate endothelial function via the Sirt1/eNOS axis but it is necessary to further explore how this regulation occurs and its effectors [169].

In 2020, a new technique consisting of a post-exertional stress challenge that provokes PEM in ME/CFS patients was developed, allowing to obtain measurements of the differential expression of circulating miRNAs in severely affected patients. This study led to the discovery and validation of eleven miRNAs associated with ME/CFS and the creation of a machine learning algorithm that allows the classification of ME/CFS patients into four clusters associated with symptom severity, providing a foundation for the development of a new non-invasive test to diagnose ME/CFS. These miRNA signatures and clusters could potentially be used to predict responses to pharmacological treatments for ME/CFS and may even allow clinicians to identify individuals for whom such treatments could be beneficial [170].

MiRNAs are not the only type of ncRNA with a promising role in CFS diagnosis and prognosis. Emerging roles of long non-coding RNAs (lncRNAs) in immune regulation and disease processes are being discovered. The levels in peripheral blood mononuclear cells (PMBCs) of NTT and EMX2OS (two lncRNA associated with immune response) have been associated with more severe ME/CFS, suggesting a potential diagnostic value of these lncRNAs. For NTT, it has been proposed to exert its function on nearby genes involved in cell proliferation, apoptosis, or inflammation, due to its large size (17 kb). A marked positive correlation between NTT and IFNGR1, another lncRNA, was observed in ME/CFS, suggesting that the NTT/IFNGR1 axis might play role in disease pathogenesis. The expression level of EMX2OS was found to have elevated PBMCs from CFS patients. The role of EMX2OS in PBMC is currently unclear and requires more experiments to be elucidated [171].

Together, the previously mentioned studies provide a basis to develop an integral diagnosis and prognosis program which not only includes metabolic analytes but also molecular ones, such as miRNA or lncRNA, for diagnosing and choosing the best treatment for ME/CFS patients.

3.7. ME/CFS and COVID-19

As of August 2021, the Coronavirus disease 2019 (COVID-19) outbreak caused by the Severe Acute Respiratory Syndrome Coronavirus 2 (SARS-CoV-2) has led to nearly 216 million cumulative cases, with 4.5 million deaths worldwide (WHO, 2021, https://www.who.int/publications/m/item/weekly-epidemiological-update-on-covid-19---31-august-2021, accessed on 31 August 2021).

The clinical interest recently shifted from the acute to the chronic COVID-19 phase which is causing additional disease management issues. Indeed, a proportion of COVID-19 survivors fail to revert to their preexisting condition and report persistent debilitating symptoms likened to CFS several months after COVID-19 acute infection resolution [172–174]. This chronic post-viral syndrome has been termed as "long-COVID" or "post-acute COVID-19 syndrome" and has been reported to affect patients irrespective of the severity of the acute infection [175]. However, it should be noted that the term "long-COVID", although widely used now, is still poorly defined, as multiple entities beyond chronic fatigue are included, thus raising questions about the conclusiveness of studies on long-COVID. In this respect, basic research on the underlying molecular and cellular mechanisms can be of great help in defining more about post-COVID-19 and ME/CFS symptoms relationship. Estimates of long-COVID vary widely based on the timing of follow-up. One study reports that nearly 90% of 143 patients experienced at least one symptom, in particular fatigue and dyspnea, two months after acute infection recovery [176]. The percentage of patients with persistent symptoms at nine months follow-up was reported to have dropped to 30%, according to a longitudinal prospective cohort study also including outpatients with mild acute disease course, with fatigue, loss of smell and taste and, "brain fog" being among the most common referred complaints [177].

With a wide array of symptoms centered around fatigue, brain fog, diffuse myalgia, non-restorative sleep, and depressive symptoms, long-COVID resembles ME/CFS, which is frequently associated with viral infections [178,179]. Interestingly, clusters of ME/CFS-like symptoms have been observed following other coronavirus outbreaks, including SARS in 2001 and MERS in 2012 [180]. Reduced quality of life and persistent pain and fatigue were reported at 6 months after hospital discharge in 30% of SARS and MERS survivors [181]. Besides this, one study reported that 27% of SARS survivors met the criteria for ME/CFS 41 months after infection [182]. Moreover, in a recent meta-analysis of post-infectious symptoms following SARS and MERS, fatigue was the most debilitating symptom in 19.3% of patients up to 39 months after infection resolution [183].

The prevalence and duration of long-COVID symptoms resembling ME/CFS are still under investigation and there are some uncertainties because of heterogeneous patient populations, follow-up duration, and inclusion criteria [184]. Only a few studies so far have applied ME/CFS diagnostic criteria. A retrospective analysis reported that 85.3% of 231 COVID-19 survivors gathered from the Genome Database of Latvian Population national biobank reached the threshold for ME/CFS diagnosis, with three or more long-term ME/CFS-like symptoms persisting at 6 months follow-up [185]. A single-center prospective longitudinal study found that only 13% of 130 patients with moderate-to-severe COVID-19 pneumonia met the criteria for ME/CFS 6 months after discharge [186]. In a small, single-center pilot study, ME/CFS-like features were found in 27% of 37 COVID-19 survivors, six months after recovery, with no difference in clinical inflammation, lung function, serum neurofilament light chain (a biomarker of axonal damage), and objective cognitive testing when comparing patients with versus without ME/CFS-like features [187]. Another study found that 14.2% of 120 COVID-19 survivors met the ME/CFS diagnostic criteria 6 months after infection onset [188]. A case series described ME/CFS-like patterns after COVID-19 infection resolution in three adolescents and young adults 6 months after recovery [189].

Despite the similarities between the symptoms of long-COVID patients and ME/CFS, further evidence is required to list COVID-19 among the infections associated with ME/CFS. Last, additional investigations with longer follow-ups, more uniform criteria for ME/CFS diagnosis, including both in- and outpatients with infections of different severity and a control group of people affected by other infections are required to better characterize risk factors, prevalence, and progression of long-COVID ME/CFS-like features, and to design specific interventions and treatments.

4. Discussion

Altogether, the insights presented show that ME/CFS is a complex systemic disease that affects many organs. By reviewing the most important pathways and systems associated with disease pathogenesis and symptoms, our review encourages to account for ME/CFS as a multifactorial disease that cannot be diagnosed or treated appropriately if it is not considered in its entirety. Consequently, any diagnostic method based on blood tests or biomarkers needs to take into account disease heterogeneity and complexity. Moreover, inter-individual variability in ME/CFS manifestations is striking and should be considered when developing novel therapeutic tools. Personalized and tailored approaches should be preferred to a one-size-fits-all therapy in this respect, but much remains to be elucidated to define specific patient subgroups.

Although more studies are urgently needed, our summary provides a general overview that can be useful to provide a better understanding of ME/CFS pathogenesis and to find new diagnostic/therapeutic opportunities for a disease that, although strongly debilitating, is still largely unexplored.

Author Contributions: Conceptualization, A.V. and G.R.; methodology, A.V. and U.-S.D.; writing-original draft preparation, U.-S.D., A.V., V.F., G.S., E.M., P.L.-C., G.M.R., S.P.; writing-review and editing, U.-S.D., A.V. and G.R.; supervision, U.-S.D., A.V. and G.R. All authors have read and agreed to the published version of the manuscript.

Funding: This research received no external funding.

Institutional Review Board Statement: Not applicable.

Informed Consent Statement: Not applicable.

Data Availability Statement: Data sharing not applicable.

Conflicts of Interest: The authors declare no conflict of interest.

References

1. Lim, E.-J.; Ahn, Y.-C.; Jang, E.-S.; Lee, S.-W.; Lee, S.-H.; Son, C.-G. Systematic Review and Meta-Analysis of the Prevalence of Chronic Fatigue Syndrome/Myalgic Encephalomyelitis (CFS/ME). *J. Transl. Med.* **2020**, *18*, 1–15. [CrossRef] [PubMed]
2. Son, C.-G. Review of the Prevalence of Chronic Fatigue Worldwide. *J. Korean Orient. Med.* **2012**, *33*, 25–33.
3. Bested, A.; Marshall, L. Review of Myalgic Encephalomyelitis/Chronic Fatigue Syndrome: An Evidence-Based Approach to Diagnosis and Management by Clinicians. *Rev. Environ. Health* **2015**, *30*, 223–249. [CrossRef] [PubMed]

4. Helliwell, A.M.; Sweetman, E.C.; Stockwell, P.A.; Edgar, C.D.; Chatterjee, A.; Tate, W.P. Changes in DNA Methylation Profiles of Myalgic Encephalomyelitis/Chronic Fatigue Syndrome Patients Reflect Systemic Dysfunctions. *Clin. Epigenet.* **2020**, *12*, 1–20. [CrossRef]
5. Cortes Rivera, M.; Mastronardi, C.; Silva-Aldana, C.; Arcos-Burgos, M.; Lidbury, B. Myalgic Encephalomyelitis/Chronic Fatigue Syndrome: A Comprehensive Review. *Diagnostics* **2019**, *9*, 91. [CrossRef]
6. Daniels, J.; Parker, H.; Salkovskis, P.M. Prevalence and Treatment of Chronic Fatigue Syndrome/Myalgic Encephalomyelitis and Co-Morbid Severe Health Anxiety. *Int. J. Clin. Health Psychol.* **2020**, *20*, 10–19. [CrossRef]
7. Faro, M.; Sàez-Francàs, N.; Castro-Marrero, J.; Aliste, L.; Fernández de Sevilla, T.; Alegre, J. Diferencias de Género En Pacientes Con Síndrome de Fatiga Crónica. *Reumatol. Clin.* **2016**, *12*, 72–77. [CrossRef]
8. Janse, A.; Nikolaus, S.; Wiborg, J.F.; Heins, M.; van der Meer, J.W.M.; Bleijenberg, G.; Tummers, M.; Twisk, J.; Knoop, H. Long-Term Follow-up after Cognitive Behaviour Therapy for Chronic Fatigue Syndrome. *J. Psychosom. Res.* **2017**, *97*, 45–51. [CrossRef]
9. Price, J.R.; Mitchell, E.; Tidy, E.; Hunot, V. Cognitive Behaviour Therapy for Chronic Fatigue Syndrome in Adults. *Cochrane Database Syst. Rev.* **2008**, *2021*, CD001027. [CrossRef]
10. Crawford, J. Internet-Based CBT for Adolescents with Chronic Fatigue Syndrome. *Lancet* **2012**, *380*, 561–562. [CrossRef]
11. Sharpe, M. Cognitive Behavior Therapy for Chronic Fatigue Syndrome: Efficacy and Implications. *Am. J. Med.* **1998**, *105*, 104S–109S. [CrossRef]
12. Larun, L.; Brurberg, K.G.; Odgaard-Jensen, J.; Price, J.R. Exercise Therapy for Chronic Fatigue Syndrome. *Cochrane Database Syst. Rev.* **2017**, *4*, CD003200. [CrossRef]
13. Chalder, T.; Goldsmith, K.A.; White, P.D.; Sharpe, M.; Pickles, A.R. Rehabilitative Therapies for Chronic Fatigue Syndrome: A Secondary Mediation Analysis of the PACE Trial. *Lancet Psychiatry* **2015**, *2*, 141–152. [CrossRef]
14. Schreurs, K.M.G.; Veehof, M.M.; Passade, L.; Vollenbroek-Hutten, M.M.R. Cognitive Behavioural Treatment for Chronic Fatigue Syndrome in a Rehabilitation Setting: Effectiveness and Predictors of Outcome. *Behav. Res. Ther.* **2011**, *49*, 908–913. [CrossRef] [PubMed]
15. Fernie, B.A.; Murphy, G.; Wells, A.; Nikčević, A.V.; Spada, M.M. Treatment Outcome and Metacognitive Change in CBT and GET for Chronic Fatigue Syndrome. *Behav. Cogn. Psychother.* **2016**, *44*, 397–409. [CrossRef]
16. White, P.; Goldsmith, K.; Johnson, A.; Potts, L.; Walwyn, R.; DeCesare, J.; Baber, H.; Burgess, M.; Clark, L.; Cox, D.; et al. Comparison of Adaptive Pacing Therapy, Cognitive Behaviour Therapy, Graded Exercise Therapy, and Specialist Medical Care for Chronic Fatigue Syndrome (PACE): A Randomised Trial. *Lancet* **2011**, *377*, 823–836. [CrossRef]
17. Galeoto, G.; Sansoni, J.; Valenti, D.; Mollica, R.; Valente, D.; Parente, M.; Servadio, A. The Effect of Physiotherapy on Fatigue and Physical Functioning in Chronic Fatigue Syndrome Patients: A Systematic Review. *La Clin. Ter.* **2018**, *169*, e184–e188. [CrossRef]
18. Smith, M.E.B.; Haney, E.; McDonagh, M.; Pappas, M.; Daeges, M.; Wasson, N.; Fu, R.; Nelson, H.D. Treatment of Myalgic Encephalomyelitis/Chronic Fatigue Syndrome: A Systematic Review for a National Institutes of Health Pathways to Prevention Workshop. *Ann. Intern. Med.* **2015**, *162*, 841–850. [CrossRef]
19. Mandarano, A.H.; Maya, J.; Giloteaux, L.; Peterson, D.L.; Maynard, M.; Gottschalk, C.G.; Hanson, M.R. Myalgic Encephalomyelitis/Chronic Fatigue Syndrome Patients Exhibit Altered T Cell Metabolism and Cytokine Associations. *J. Clin. Investig.* **2020**, *130*, 1491–1505. [CrossRef]
20. Maes, M.; Mihaylova, I.; Leunis, J. Chronic Fatigue Syndrome Is Accompanied by an IgM-Related Immune Response Directed against Neopitopes Formed by Oxidative or Nitrosative Damage to Lipids and Proteins. *Neuro. Endocrinol. Lett.* **2006**, *27*, 615–621.
21. Lorusso, L.; Mikhaylova, S.V.; Capelli, E.; Ferrari, D.; Ngonga, G.K.; Ricevuti, G. Immunological Aspects of Chronic Fatigue Syndrome. *Autoimmun. Rev.* **2009**, *8*, 287–291. [CrossRef]
22. Brenu, E.W.; van Driel, M.L.; Staines, D.R.; Ashton, K.J.; Hardcastle, S.L.; Keane, J.; Tajouri, L.; Peterson, D.; Ramos, S.B.; Marshall-Gradisnik, S.M. Longitudinal Investigation of Natural Killer Cells and Cytokines in Chronic Fatigue Syndrome/Myalgic Encephalomyelitis. *J. Transl. Med.* **2012**, *10*, 88. [CrossRef]
23. Wirth, K.; Scheibenbogen, C. A Unifying Hypothesis of the Pathophysiology of Myalgic Encephalomyelitis/Chronic Fatigue Syndrome (ME/CFS): Recognitions from the Finding of Autoantibodies against ß2-Adrenergic Receptors. *Autoimmun. Rev.* **2020**, *19*, 102527. [CrossRef]
24. Loebel, M.; Grabowski, P.; Heidecke, H.; Bauer, S.; Hanitsch, L.G.; Wittke, K.; Meisel, C.; Reinke, P.; Volk, H.-D.; Fluge, Ø.; et al. Antibodies to β Adrenergic and Muscarinic Cholinergic Receptors in Patients with Chronic Fatigue Syndrome. *Brain Behav. Immun.* **2016**, *52*, 32–39. [CrossRef]
25. Scheibenbogen, C.; Loebel, M.; Freitag, H.; Krueger, A.; Bauer, S.; Antelmann, M.; Doehner, W.; Scherbakov, N.; Heidecke, H.; Reinke, P.; et al. Immunoadsorption to Remove ß2 Adrenergic Receptor Antibodies in Chronic Fatigue Syndrome CFS/ME. *PLoS ONE* **2018**, *13*, e0193672. [CrossRef]
26. Maes, M.; Twisk, F.N.M.; Kubera, M.; Ringel, K. Evidence for Inflammation and Activation of Cell-Mediated Immunity in Myalgic Encephalomyelitis/Chronic Fatigue Syndrome (ME/CFS): Increased Interleukin-1, Tumor Necrosis Factor-α, PMN-Elastase, Lysozyme and Neopterin. *J. Affect. Disord.* **2012**, *136*, 933–939. [CrossRef]
27. Kerr, J.R.; Barah, F.; Mattey, D.L.; Laing, I.; Hopkins, S.J.; Hutchinson, I.V.; Tyrrell, D.A.J. Circulating Tumour Necrosis Factor-α and Interferon-γ Are Detectable during Acute and Convalescent Parvovirus B19 Infection and Are Associated with Prolonged and Chronic Fatigue. *J. Gen. Virol.* **2001**, *82*, 3011–3019. [CrossRef] [PubMed]

28. Skowera, A.; Cleare, A.; Blair, D.; Bevis, L.; Wessely, S.C.; Peakman, M. High Levels of Type 2 Cytokine-Producing Cells in Chronic Fatigue Syndrome. *Clin. Exp. Immunol.* **2004**, *135*, 294–302. [CrossRef] [PubMed]
29. Klimas, N.G.; Salvato, F.R.; Morgan, R.; Fletcher, M.A. Immunologic Abnormalities in Chronic Fatigue Syndrome. *J. Clin. Microbiol.* **1990**, *28*, 1403–1410. [CrossRef] [PubMed]
30. Torres-Harding, S.; Sorenson, M.; Jason, L.A.; Maher, K.; Fletcher, M.A. Evidence for T-Helper 2 Shift and Association with Illness Parameters in Chronic Fatigue Syndrome (CFS). *Bull. IACFS/ME* **2008**, *16*, 19–33.
31. Nguyen, T.; Johnston, S.; Clarke, L.; Smith, P.; Staines, D.; Marshall-Gradisnik, S. Impaired Calcium Mobilization in Natural Killer Cells from Chronic Fatigue Syndrome/Myalgic Encephalomyelitis Patients Is Associated with Transient Receptor Potential Melastatin 3 Ion Channels. *Clin. Exp. Immunol.* **2017**, *187*, 284–293. [CrossRef] [PubMed]
32. Rivas, J.L.; Palencia, T.; Fernández, G.; García, M. Association of T and NK Cell Phenotype With the Diagnosis of Myalgic Encephalomyelitis/Chronic Fatigue Syndrome (ME/CFS). *Front. Immunol.* **2018**, *9*, 1028. [CrossRef] [PubMed]
33. Brenu, E.W.; van Driel, M.L.; Staines, D.R.; Ashton, K.J.; Ramos, S.B.; Keane, J.; Klimas, N.G.; Marshall-Gradisnik, S.M. Immunological Abnormalities as Potential Biomarkers in Chronic Fatigue Syndrome/Myalgic Encephalomyelitis. *J. Transl. Med.* **2011**, *9*, 81. [CrossRef] [PubMed]
34. Kennedy, G.; Khan, F.; Hill, A.; Underwood, C.; Belch, J.J.F. Biochemical and Vascular Aspects of Pediatric Chronic Fatigue Syndrome. *Arch. Pediatrics Adolesc. Med.* **2010**, *164*, 817–823. [CrossRef]
35. Yang, T.; Yang, Y.; Wang, D.; Li, C.; Qu, Y.; Guo, J.; Shi, T.; Bo, W.; Sun, Z.; Asakawa, T. The Clinical Value of Cytokines in Chronic Fatigue Syndrome. *J. Transl. Med.* **2019**, *17*, 1–12. [CrossRef] [PubMed]
36. Prins, J.B.; van der Meer, J.W.; Bleijenberg, G. Chronic Fatigue Syndrome. *Lancet* **2006**, *367*, 346–355. [CrossRef]
37. Maes, M.; Mihaylova, I.; Kubera, M.; Leunis, J.-C.; Geffard, M. IgM-Mediated Autoimmune Responses Directed against Multiple Neoepitopes in Depression: New Pathways That Underpin the Inflammatory and Neuroprogressive Pathophysiology. *J. Affect. Disord.* **2011**, *135*, 414–418. [CrossRef]
38. Broderick, G.; Katz, B.Z.; Fernandes, H.; Fletcher, M.A.; Klimas, N.; Smith, F.A.; O'Gorman, M.R.; Vernon, S.D.; Taylor, R. Cytokine Expression Profiles of Immune Imbalance in Post-Mononucleosis Chronic Fatigue. *J. Transl. Med.* **2012**, *10*, 191. [CrossRef]
39. Broderick, G.; Fuite, J.; Kreitz, A.; Vernon, S.D.; Klimas, N.; Fletcher, M.A. A Formal Analysis of Cytokine Networks in Chronic Fatigue Syndrome. *Brain Behav. Immun.* **2010**, *24*, 1209–1217. [CrossRef]
40. Rasmussen, A.K.; Nielsen, H.; Andersen, V.; Barington, T.; Bendtzen, K.; Hansen, M.B.; Nielsen, L.; Pedersen, B.K.; Wiik, A. Chronic Fatigue Syndrome—A Controlled Cross Sectional Study. *J. Rheumatol.* **1994**, *21*, 1527–1531.
41. Patarca, R.; Klimas, N.G.; Lugtendorf, S.; Antoni, M.; Fletcher, M.A. Dysregulated Expression of Tumor Necrosis Factor in Chronic Fatigue Syndrome: Interrelations with Cellular Sources and Patterns of Soluble Immune Mediator Expression. *Clin. Infect. Dis.* **1994**, *18*, S147–S153. [CrossRef] [PubMed]
42. Moss, R.B.; Mercandetti, A.; Vojdani, A. TNF-Alpha and Chronic Fatigue Syndrome. *J. Clin. Immunol.* **1999**, *19*, 314–316. [CrossRef] [PubMed]
43. Hornig, M.; Montoya, J.G.; Klimas, N.G.; Levine, S.; Felsenstein, D.; Bateman, L.; Peterson, D.L.; Gottschalk, C.G.; Schultz, A.F.; Che, X.; et al. Distinct Plasma Immune Signatures in ME/CFS Are Present Early in the Course of Illness. *Sci. Adv.* **2015**, *1*, e1400121. [CrossRef] [PubMed]
44. Sullivan, P.F.; Evengard, B.; Jacks, A.; Pedersen, N.L. Twin Analyses of Chronic Fatigue in a Swedish National Sample. *Psychol. Med.* **2005**, *35*, 1327–1336. [CrossRef] [PubMed]
45. Glassford, J.A.G. The Neuroinflammatory Etiopathology of Myalgic Encephalomyelitis/Chronic Fatigue Syndrome (ME/CFS). *Front. Physiol.* **2017**, *8*, 88. [CrossRef]
46. Blomberg, J.; Gottfries, C.-G.; Elfaitouri, A.; Rizwan, M.; Rosén, A. Infection Elicited Autoimmunity and Myalgic Encephalomyelitis/Chronic Fatigue Syndrome: An Explanatory Model. *Front. Immunol.* **2018**, *9*, 229. [CrossRef] [PubMed]
47. Dubois, R.E.; Seeley, J.K.; Brus, I.; Sakamoto, K.; Ballow, M.; Harada, S.; Bechtold, T.A.; Pearson, G.; Purtilo, D.T. Chronic Mononucleosis Syndrome. *South. Med. J.* **1984**, *77*, 1376–1382. [CrossRef]
48. Manian, F.A. Simultaneous Measurement of Antibodies to Epstein-Barr Virus, Human Herpesvirus 6, Herpes Simplex Virus Types 1 and 2, and 14 Enteroviruses in Chronic Fatigue Syndrome: Is There Evidence of Activation of a Nonspecific Polyclonal Immune Response? *Clin. Infect. Dis.* **1994**, *19*, 448–453. [CrossRef]
49. Loebel, M.; Strohschein, K.; Giannini, C.; Koelsch, U.; Bauer, S.; Doebis, C.; Thomas, S.; Unterwalder, N.; von Baehr, V.; Reinke, P.; et al. Deficient EBV-Specific B- and T-Cell Response in Patients with Chronic Fatigue Syndrome. *PLoS ONE* **2014**, *9*, e85387. [CrossRef]
50. Niller, H.H.; Wolf, H.; Ay, E.; Minarovits, J. Epigenetic Dysregulation of Epstein-Barr Virus Latency and Development of Autoimmune Disease. In *Epigenetic Contributions in Autoimmune Disease*; Springer: Boston, MA, USA, 2011.
51. Kerr, J.R. The Role of Parvovirus B19 in the Pathogenesis of Autoimmunity and Autoimmune Disease. *J. Clin. Pathol.* **2016**, *69*, 279–291. [CrossRef]
52. Kerr, J.R.; Bracewell, J.; Laing, I.; Mattey, D.L.; Bernstein, R.M.; Bruce, I.N.; Tyrrell, D.A.J. Chronic Fatigue Syndrome and Arthralgia Following Parvovirus B19 Infection. *J. Rheumatol.* **2002**, *29*, 595–602.
53. Seishima, M.; Mizutani, Y.; Shibuya, Y.; Arakawa, C. Chronic Fatigue Syndrome after Human Parvovirus B19 Infection without Persistent Viremia. *Dermatology* **2008**, *216*, 341–346. [CrossRef]

54. Cameron, B.; Flamand, L.; Juwana, H.; Middeldorp, J.; Naing, Z.; Rawlinson, W.; Ablashi, D.; Lloyd, A. Serological and Virological Investigation of the Role of the Herpesviruses EBV, CMV and HHV-6 in Post-Infective Fatigue Syndrome. *J. Med. Virol.* **2010**, *82*, 1684–1688. [CrossRef]
55. Clauw, D.J. Perspectives on Fatigue from the Study of Chronic Fatigue Syndrome and Related Conditions. *PMR* **2010**, *2*, 414–430. [CrossRef] [PubMed]
56. de Meirleir, K.; Bisbal, C.; Campine, I.; de Becker, P.; Salehzada, T.; Demettre, E.; Lebleu, B. A 37 KDa 2-5A Binding Protein as a Potential Biochemical Marker for Chronic Fatigue Syndrome. *Am. J. Med.* **2000**, *108*, 99–105. [CrossRef]
57. Suhadolnik, R.J.; Peterson, D.L.; O'Brien, K.; Cheney, P.R.; Herst, C.V.T.; Reichenbach, N.L.; Kon, N.; Horvath, S.E.; Iacono, K.T.; Adelson, M.E.; et al. Biochemical Evidence for a Novel Low Molecular Weight 2-5A-Dependent RNase L in Chronic Fatigue Syndrome. *J. Interferon Cytokine Res.* **1997**, *17*, 377–385. [CrossRef] [PubMed]
58. Nijhof, S.L.; Rutten, J.M.T.M.; Uiterwaal, C.S.P.M.; Bleijenberg, G.; Kimpen, J.L.L.; Putte, E.M. van de The Role of Hypocortisolism in Chronic Fatigue Syndrome. *Psychoneuroendocrinology* **2014**, *42*, 199–206. [CrossRef] [PubMed]
59. Kennedy, G.; Spence, V.A.; McLaren, M.; Hill, A.; Underwood, C.; Belch, J.J.F. Oxidative Stress Levels Are Raised in Chronic Fatigue Syndrome and Are Associated with Clinical Symptoms. *Free Radic. Biol. Med.* **2005**, *39*, 584–589. [CrossRef]
60. Marshall-Gradisnik, S.; Huth, T.; Chacko, A.; Smith, P.; Staines, D.; Johnston, S. Natural Killer Cells and Single Nucleotide Polymorphisms of Specific Ion Channels and Receptor Genes in Myalgic Encephalomyelitis/Chronic Fatigue Syndrome. *Appl. Clin. Genet.* **2016**, *9*, 39–47. [CrossRef]
61. Maes, M. Inflammatory and Oxidative and Nitrosative Stress Pathways Underpinning Chronic Fatigue, Somatization and Psychosomatic Symptoms. *Curr. Opin. Psychiatry* **2009**, *22*, 75–83. [CrossRef]
62. Maes, M.; Leunis, J.; Geffard, M.; Berk, M. Evidence for the Existence of Myalgic Encephalomyelitis/Chronic Fatigue Syndrome (ME/CFS) with and without Abdominal Discomfort (Irritable Bowel) Syndrome. *Neuro Endocrinol. Lett.* **2014**, *35*, 445–453.
63. Cairns, R.; Hotopf, M. A Systematic Review Describing the Prognosis of Chronic Fatigue Syndrome. *Occup. Med.* **2005**, *55*, 20–31. [CrossRef]
64. Sotzny, F.; Blanco, J.; Capelli, E.; Castro-Marrero, J.; Steiner, S.; Murovska, M.; Scheibenbogen, C. Myalgic Encephalomyelitis/Chronic Fatigue Syndrome—Evidence for an Autoimmune Disease. *Autoimmun. Rev.* **2018**, *17*, 601–609. [CrossRef]
65. Loebel, M.; Eckey, M.; Sotzny, F.; Hahn, E.; Bauer, S.; Grabowski, P.; Zerweck, J.; Holenya, P.; Hanitsch, L.G.; Wittke, K.; et al. Serological Profiling of the EBV Immune Response in Chronic Fatigue Syndrome Using a Peptide Microarray. *PLoS ONE* **2017**, *12*, e0179124. [CrossRef] [PubMed]
66. Ascherio, A.; Munger, K.L. EBV and Autoimmunity. In *Epstein Barr Virus*; Springer: Cham, Switzerland, 2015.
67. Wallis, A.; Ball, M.; McKechnie, S.; Butt, H.; Lewis, D.P.; Bruck, D. Examining Clinical Similarities between Myalgic Encephalomyelitis/Chronic Fatigue Syndrome and d-Lactic Acidosis: A Systematic Review. *J. Transl. Med.* **2017**, *15*, 1–22. [CrossRef] [PubMed]
68. Stussman, B.; Williams, A.; Snow, J.; Gavin, A.; Scott, R.; Nath, A.; Walitt, B. Characterization of Post–Exertional Malaise in Patients With Myalgic Encephalomyelitis/Chronic Fatigue Syndrome. *Front. Neurol.* **2020**, *11*, 1025. [CrossRef] [PubMed]
69. Nijs, J.; Nees, A.; Paul, L.; de Kooning, M.; Ickmans, K.; Meeus, M.; van Oosterwijck, J. Altered Immune Response to Exercise in Patients with Chronic Fatigue Syndrome/Myalgic Encephalomyelitis: A Systematic Literature Review. *Exerc. Immunol. Rev.* **2014**, *20*, 94–116.
70. White, A.T.; Light, A.R.; Hughen, R.W.; Bateman, L.; Martins, T.B.; Hill, H.R.; Light, K.C. Severity of Symptom Flare after Moderate Exercise Is Linked to Cytokine Activity in Chronic Fatigue Syndrome. *Psychophysiology* **2010**, *47*, 615–624. [CrossRef]
71. van de Putte, E.; van Doornen, L.; Engelbert, R.; Kuis, W.; Kimpen, J.; Uiterwaal, C. Mirrored Symptoms in Mother and Child with Chronic Fatigue Syndrome. *Pediatrics* **2006**, *117*, 2074–2079. [CrossRef]
72. Albright, F.; Light, K.; Light, A.; Bateman, L.; Cannon-Albright, L.A. Evidence for a Heritable Predisposition to Chronic Fatigue Syndrome. *BMC Neurol.* **2011**, *11*, 62. [CrossRef]
73. Wang, T.; Yin, J.; Miller, A.H.; Xiao, C. A Systematic Review of the Association between Fatigue and Genetic Polymorphisms. *Brain Behav. Immun.* **2017**, *62*, 230–244. [CrossRef]
74. Dibble, J.J.; McGrath, S.J.; Ponting, C.P. Genetic Risk Factors of ME/CFS: A Critical Review. *Hum. Mol. Genet.* **2020**, *29*, R118–R125. [CrossRef]
75. Hall, K.T.; Kossowsky, J.; Oberlander, T.F.; Kaptchuk, T.J.; Saul, J.P.; Wyller, V.B.; Fagermoen, E.; Sulheim, D.; Gjerstad, J.; Winger, A.; et al. Genetic Variation in Catechol-O-Methyltransferase Modifies Effects of Clonidine Treatment in Chronic Fatigue Syndrome. *Pharm. J.* **2016**, *16*, 454–460. [CrossRef]
76. Falkenberg, V.R.; Whistler, T.; Murray, J.R.; Unger, E.R.; Rajeevan, M.S. Acute Psychosocial Stress-Mediated Changes in the Expression and Methylation of Perforin in Chronic Fatigue Syndrome. *Genet. Epigenet.* **2013**, *1*, 1–9. [CrossRef]
77. Herrera, S.; de Vega, W.; Ashbrook, D.; Vernon, S.; McGowan, P. Genome-Epigenome Interactions Associated with Myalgic Encephalomyelitis/Chronic Fatigue Syndrome. *Epigenetics* **2018**, *13*, 1174–1190. [CrossRef] [PubMed]
78. Smith, A.K.; Fang, H.; Whistler, T.; Unger, E.R.; Rajeevan, M.S. Convergent Genomic Studies Identify Association of GRIK2 and NPAS2 with Chronic Fatigue Syndrome. *Neuropsychobiology* **2011**, *64*, 183–194. [CrossRef] [PubMed]
79. Schlauch, K.A.; Khaiboullina, S.F.; de Meirleir, K.L.; Rawat, S.; Petereit, J.; Rizvanov, A.A.; Blatt, N.; Mijatovic, T.; Kulick, D.; Palotás, A.; et al. Genome-Wide Association Analysis Identifies Genetic Variations in Subjects with Myalgic Encephalomyelitis/Chronic Fatigue Syndrome. *Transl. Psychiatry* **2016**, *6*, e730. [CrossRef] [PubMed]

80. Meyer, B.; Nguyen, C.; Moen, A.; Fagermoen, E.; Sulheim, D.; Nilsen, H.; Wyller, V.; Gjerstad, J. Maintenance of Chronic Fatigue Syndrome (CFS) in Young CFS Patients Is Associated with the 5-HTTLPR and SNP Rs25531 A > G Genotype. *PLoS ONE* **2015**, *10*, e0140883. [CrossRef] [PubMed]
81. Löbel, M.; Mooslechner, A.A.; Bauer, S.; Günther, S.; Letsch, A.; Hanitsch, L.G.; Grabowski, P.; Meisel, C.; Volk, H.D.; Scheibenbogen, C. Polymorphism in COMT Is Associated with IgG3 Subclass Level and Susceptibility to Infection in Patients with Chronic Fatigue Syndrome. *J. Transl. Med.* **2015**, *13*, 264. [CrossRef] [PubMed]
82. De Luca, C.; Gugliandolo, A.; Calabrò, C.; Currò, M.; Ientile, R.; Raskovic, D.; Korkina, L.; Caccamo, D. Role of Polymorphisms of Inducible Nitric Oxide Synthase and Endothelial Nitric Oxide Synthase in Idiopathic Environmental Intolerances. *Mediat. Inflamm.* **2015**, *2015*, 245308. [CrossRef] [PubMed]
83. Fukuda, S.; Horiguchi, M.; Yamaguti, K.; Nakatomi, Y.; Kuratsune, H.; Ichinose, H.; Watanabe, Y. Association of Monoamine-Synthesizing Genes with the Depression Tendency and Personality in Chronic Fatigue Syndrome Patients. *Life Sci.* **2013**, *92*, 183–186. [CrossRef]
84. Smith, A.; Dimulescu, I.; Falkenberg, V.; Narasimhan, S.; Heim, C.; Vernon, S.; Rajeevan, M. Genetic Evaluation of the Serotonergic System in Chronic Fatigue Syndrome. *Psychoneuroendocrinology* **2008**, *33*, 188–197. [CrossRef]
85. Carlo-Stella, N.; Badulli, C.; de Silvestri, A.; Bazzichi, L.; Martinetti, M.; Lorusso, L.; Bombardieri, S.; Salvaneschi, L.; Cuccia, M. A First Study of Cytokine Genomic Polymorphisms in CFS: Positive Association of TNF-857 and IFNgamma 874 Rare Alleles. *Clin. Exp. Rheumatol.* **2006**, *24*, 179–182. [PubMed]
86. Perez, M.; Jaundoo, R.; Hilton, K.; Del Alamo, A.; Gemayel, K.; Klimas, N.G.; Craddock, T.J.A.; Nathanson, L. Genetic Predisposition for Immune System, Hormone, and Metabolic Dysfunction in Myalgic Encephalomyelitis/Chronic Fatigue Syndrome: A Pilot Study. *Front. Pediatrics* **2019**, *7*, 206. [CrossRef] [PubMed]
87. Carlo-Stella, N.; Bozzini, S.; de Silvestri, A.; Sbarsi, I.; Pizzochero, C.; Lorusso, L.; Martinetti, M.; Cuccia, M. Molecular Study of Receptor for Advanced Glycation Endproduct Gene Promoter and Identification of Specific HLA Haplotypes Possibly Involved in Chronic Fatigue Syndrome. *Int. J. Immunopathol. Pharmacol.* **2009**, *22*, 745–754. [CrossRef] [PubMed]
88. Sommerfeldt, L.; Portilla, H.; Jacobsen, L.; Gjerstad, J.; Wyller, V. Polymorphisms of Adrenergic Cardiovascular Control Genes Are Associated with Adolescent Chronic Fatigue Syndrome. *Acta Paediatr.* **2011**, *100*, 293–298. [CrossRef] [PubMed]
89. Caswell, A.; Daniels, J. Anxiety and Depression in Chronic Fatigue Syndrome: Prevalence and Effect on Treatment. A Systematic Review, Meta-Analysis and Meta-Regression. In Proceedings of the British Association of Behavioural and Cognitive Psychotherapy, Glasgow, UK, 18–20 July 2018.
90. Griffith, J.; Zarrouf, F. A Systematic Review of Chronic Fatigue Syndrome: Don't Assume It's Depression. *Prim. Care Companion J. Clin. Psychiatry* **2008**, *10*, 120–128. [CrossRef] [PubMed]
91. Bair, M.; Robinson, R.; Katon, W.; Kroenke, K. Depression and Pain Comorbidity: A Literature Review. *Arch. Intern. Med.* **2003**, *163*, 2433–2445. [CrossRef]
92. Brites, D.; Fernandes, A. Neuroinflammation and Depression: Microglia Activation, Extracellular Microvesicles and MicroRNA Dysregulation. *Front. Cell. Neurosci.* **2015**, *9*, 1–20. [CrossRef] [PubMed]
93. Chaves-Filho, A.; Macedo, D.; de Lucena, D.; Maes, M. Shared Microglial Mechanisms Underpinning Depression and Chronic Fatigue Syndrome and Their Comorbidities. *Behav. Brain Res.* **2019**, *372*, 111975. [CrossRef]
94. Maes, M.; Kubera, M.; Leunis, J.C.; Berk, M. Increased IgA and IgM Responses against Gut Commensals in Chronic Depression: Further Evidence for Increased Bacterial Translocation or Leaky Gut. *J. Affect. Disord.* **2012**, *141*, 55–62. [CrossRef] [PubMed]
95. Landrø, N.; Stiles, T.; Sletvold, H. Memory Functioning in Patients with Primary Fibromyalgia and Major Depression and Healthy Controls. *J. Psychosom. Res.* **1997**, *42*, 297–306. [CrossRef]
96. Morris, G.; Maes, M. A Neuro-Immune Model of Myalgic Encephalomyelitis/Chronic Fatigue Syndrome. *Metab. Brain Dis.* **2013**, *28*, 523–540. [CrossRef]
97. Nakatomi, Y.; Mizuno, K.; Ishii, A.; Wada, Y.; Tanaka, M.; Tazawa, S.; Onoe, K.; Fukuda, S.; Kawabe, J.; Takahashi, K.; et al. Neuroinflammation in Patients with Chronic Fatigue Syndrome/Myalgic Encephalomyelitis: An 11 C-(R)-PK11195 PET Study. *J. Nucl. Med.* **2014**, *55*, 945–950. [CrossRef]
98. Chaudhuri, A.; Behan, P.O. Fatigue in Neurological Disorders. *Lancet* **2004**, *363*, 978–988. [CrossRef]
99. Maes, M.; Twisk, F.; Ringel, K. Inflammatory and Cell-Mediated Immune Biomarkers in Myalgic Encephalomyelitis/Chronic Fatigue Syndrome and Depression: Inflammatory Markers Are Higher in Myalgic Encephalomyelitis/Chronic Fatigue Syndrome than in Depression. *Psychother. Psychosom.* **2012**, *81*, 286–295. [CrossRef]
100. Robertson, M.; Schacterle, R.; Mackin, G.; Wilson, S.; Bloomingdale, K.; Ritz, J.; Komaroff, A. Lymphocyte Subset Differences in Patients with Chronic Fatigue Syndrome, Multiple Sclerosis and Major Depression. *Clin. Exp. Immunol.* **2005**, *141*, 326–332. [CrossRef]
101. Scott, L.; Salahuddin, F.; Cooney, J.; Svec, F.; Dinan, T. Differences in Adrenal Steroid Profile in Chronic Fatigue Syndrome, in Depression and in Health. *J. Affect. Disord.* **1999**, *54*, 129–137. [CrossRef]
102. Iacob, E.; Light, A.; Donaldson, G.; Okifuji, A.; Hughen, R.; White, A.; Light, K. Gene Expression Factor Analysis to Differentiate Pathways Linked to Fibromyalgia, Chronic Fatigue Syndrome, and Depression in a Diverse Patient Sample. *Arthritis Care Res.* **2016**, *68*, 132–140. [CrossRef] [PubMed]

103. Morris, G.; Berk, M.; Puri, B. A Comparison of Neuroimaging Abnormalities in Multiple Sclerosis, Major Depression and Chronic Fatigue Syndrome (Myalgic Encephalomyelitis): Is There a Common Cause? *Mol. Neurobiol.* **2018**, *55*, 3592–3609. [CrossRef] [PubMed]
104. Costa, D.; Tannock, C.; Brostoff, J. Brainstem Perfusion Is Impaired in Chronic Fatigue Syndrome. *QJM Mon. J. Assoc. Physicians* **1995**, *88*, 767–773.
105. Goldstein, J.A.; Mena, I.; Jouanne, E.; Lesser, I. The Assessment of Vascular Abnormalities in Late Life Chronic Fatigue Syndrome by Brain SPECT: Comparison with late life major depressive disorder. *J. Chronic Fatigue Syndr.* **2011**, *1*, 55–79. [CrossRef]
106. MacHale, S.; Lawrie, S.; Cavanagh, J.; Glabus, M.; Murray, C.; Goodwin, G.; Ebmeier, K. Cerebral Perfusion in Chronic Fatigue Syndrome and Depression. *Br. J. Psychiatry* **2000**, *176*, 550–556. [CrossRef] [PubMed]
107. Castro-Marrero, J.; Sáez-Francàs, N.; Santillo, D.; Alegre, J. Treatment and Management of Chronic Fatigue Syndrome/Myalgic Encephalomyelitis: All Roads Lead to Rome. *Br. J. Pharmacol.* **2017**, *174*, 345–369. [CrossRef]
108. Theoharides, T.C.; Asadi, S.; Weng, Z.; Zhang, B. Serotonin-Selective Reuptake Inhibitors and Nonsteroidal Anti-Inflammatory Drugs-Important Considerations of Adverse Interactions Especially for the Treatment of Myalgic Encephalomyelitis/Chronic Fatigue Syndrome. *J. Clin. Psychopharmacol.* **2011**, *31*, 403–405. [CrossRef] [PubMed]
109. Boneva, R.; Lin, J.; Maloney, E.; Jones, J.; Reeves, W. Use of Medications by People with Chronic Fatigue Syndrome and Healthy Persons: A Population-Based Study of Fatiguing Illness in Georgia. *Health Qual. Life Outcomes* **2009**, *7*, 67. [CrossRef]
110. Nijs, J.; Crombez, G.; Meeus, M.; Knoop, H.; Van Damme, S.; Cauwenbergh, V.; Bleijenberg, G. Pain in Patients with Chronic Fatigue Syndrome: Time for Specific Pain Treatment? *Pain Physician* **2012**, *15*, E677–E686. [CrossRef]
111. Rao, S.G.; Clauw, D.J. The Management of Fibromyalgia. *Drugs Today* **2004**, *40*, 539–554. [CrossRef]
112. Nijs, J.; George, S.Z.; Clauw, D.J.; Fernández-de-las-Peñas, C.; Kosek, E.; Ickmans, K.; Fernández-Carnero, J.; Polli, A.; Kapreli, E.; Huysmans, E.; et al. Central Sensitisation in Chronic Pain Conditions: Latest Discoveries and Their Potential for Precision Medicine. *Lancet Rheumatol.* **2021**, *3*, e383–e392. [CrossRef]
113. Schwartzman, R.J.; Grothusen, J.; Kiefer, T.R.; Rohr, P. Neuropathic Central Pain. *Arch. Neurol.* **2001**, *58*, 1547–1550. [CrossRef]
114. Ranjbar, E.; Memari, A.; Hafizi, S.; Shayestehfar, M.; Mirfazeli, F.; Eshghi, M. Depression and Exercise: A Clinical Review and Management Guideline. *Asian J. Sports Med.* **2015**, *6*, 1–6. [CrossRef]
115. Vink, M.; Vink-Niese, F. Graded Exercise Therapy Does Not Restore the Ability to Work in ME/CFS—Rethinking of a Cochrane Review. *Work* **2020**, *66*, 283–308. [CrossRef]
116. Deale, A.; Husain, K.; Chalder, T.; Wessely, S. Long-Term Outcome of Cognitive Behavior Therapy versus Relaxation Therapy for Chronic Fatigue Syndrome: A 5-Year Follow-up Study. *Am. J. Psychiatry* **2001**, *158*, 2038–2042. [CrossRef]
117. Nijhof, S.L.; Priesterbach, L.P.; Uiterwaal, C.S.P.M.; Bleijenberg, G.; Kimpen, J.L.L.; van de Putte, E.M. Internet-Based Therapy for Adolescents With Chronic Fatigue Syndrome: Long-Term Follow-Up. *Pediatrics* **2013**, *131*, e1788–e1795. [CrossRef]
118. Stoll, S.V.E.; Crawley, E.; Richards, V.; Lal, N.; Brigden, A.; Loades, M.E. What Treatments Work for Anxiety in Children with Chronic Fatigue Syndrome/Myalgic Encephalomyelitis (CFS/ME)? Systematic Review. *BMJ Open* **2017**, *7*, e015481. [CrossRef] [PubMed]
119. Knoop, H.; Stulemeijer, M.; Prins, J.B.; van der Meer, J.W.M.; Bleijenberg, G. Is Cognitive Behaviour Therapy for Chronic Fatigue Syndrome Also Effective for Pain Symptoms? *Behav. Res. Ther.* **2007**, *45*, 2034–2043. [CrossRef] [PubMed]
120. O'Dowd, H.; Gladwell, P.; Rogers, C.; Hollinghurst, S.; Gregory, A. Cognitive Behavioural Therapy in Chronic Fatigue Syndrome: A Randomised Controlled Trial of an Outpatient Group Programme. *Health Technol. Assess.* **2006**, *10*, 1–121. [CrossRef] [PubMed]
121. Loades, M.; Sheils, E.; Crawley, E. Treatment for Paediatric Chronic Fatigue Syndrome or Myalgic Encephalomyelitis (CFS/ME) and Comorbid Depression: A Systematic Review. *BMJ Open* **2016**, *6*, e012271. [CrossRef] [PubMed]
122. Knight, S.; Scheinberg, A.; Harvey, A. Interventions in Pediatric Chronic Fatigue Syndrome/Myalgic Encephalomyelitis: A Systematic Review. *J. Adolesc. Health Off. Publ. Soc. Adolesc. Med.* **2013**, *53*, 154–165. [CrossRef]
123. Chalder, T.; Tong, J.; Deary, V. Family Cognitive Behaviour Therapy for Chronic Fatigue Syndrome: An Uncontrolled Study. *Arch. Dis. Child.* **2002**, *86*, 95–97. [CrossRef] [PubMed]
124. Rollnik, J. [Chronic Fatigue Syndrome: A Critical Review]. *Fortschr. Neurol. Psychiatr.* **2017**, *85*, 79–85. [CrossRef]
125. Pae, C.; Marks, D.; Patkar, A.; Masand, P.; Luyten, P.; Serretti, A. Pharmacological Treatment of Chronic Fatigue Syndrome: Focusing on the Role of Antidepressants. *Expert Opin. Pharmacother.* **2009**, *10*, 1561–1570. [CrossRef]
126. Klimas, N.; Morgan, R.; van Riel, F.; Fletcher, M. Observations regarding use of an antidepressant, fluoxetine, in chronic fatigue syndrome. In *Chronic Fatigue and Related Immune Deficiency Syndromes*; Goodnick, P.J., Klimas, N.G., Eds.; American Psychiatric Association: Washington, DC, USA, 1993; pp. 95–108.
127. Goodnick, P.; Sandoval, R.; Brickman, A.; Klimas, N. Bupropion Treatment of Fluoxetine-Resistant Chronic Fatigue Syndrome. *Biol. Psychiatry* **1992**, *32*, 834–838. [CrossRef]
128. Richman, S.; Morris, M.; Broderick, G.; Craddock, T.; Klimas, N.; Fletcher, M. Pharmaceutical Interventions in Chronic Fatigue Syndrome: A Literature-Based Commentary. *Clin. Ther.* **2019**, *41*, 798–805. [CrossRef]
129. Chrousos, G.P. Stress and Disorders of the Stress System. *Nat. Rev. Endocrinol.* **2009**, *5*, 374–381. [CrossRef]
130. Tomas, C.; Newton, J.; Watson, S. A Review of Hypothalamic-Pituitary-Adrenal Axis Function in Chronic Fatigue Syndrome. *ISRN Neurosci.* **2013**, *2013*, 784520. [CrossRef] [PubMed]
131. Ruiz-Núñez, B.; Tarasse, R.; Vogelaar, E.F.; Janneke Dijck-Brouwer, D.A.; Muskiet, F.A.J. Higher Prevalence of "Low T3 Syndrome" in Patients With Chronic Fatigue Syndrome: A Case–Control Study. *Front. Endocrinol.* **2018**, *9*, 97. [CrossRef] [PubMed]

132. Boneva, R.S.; Maloney, E.M.; Lin, J.-M.; Jones, J.F.; Wieser, F.; Nater, U.M.; Heim, C.M.; Reeves, W.C. Gynecological History in Chronic Fatigue Syndrome: A Population-Based Case-Control Study. *J. Women's Health* **2011**, *20*, 21–28. [CrossRef] [PubMed]
133. Cleare, A.J. The HPA Axis and the Genesis of Chronic Fatigue Syndrome. *Trends Endocrinol. Metab.* **2004**, *15*, 55–59. [CrossRef] [PubMed]
134. Samaras, A.; Espírito Santo, C.; Papandroulakis, N.; Mitrizakis, N.; Pavlidis, M.; Höglund, E.; Pelgrim, T.N.M.; Zethof, J.; Spanings, F.A.T.; Vindas, M.A.; et al. Allostatic Load and Stress Physiology in European Seabass (*Dicentrarchus Labrax* L.) and Gilthead Seabream (*Sparus Aurata* L.). *Front. Endocrinol.* **2018**, *9*, 451. [CrossRef] [PubMed]
135. Arroll, M.A. Allostatic Overload in Myalgic Encephalomyelitis/Chronic Fatigue Syndrome (ME/CFS). *Med. Hypotheses* **2013**, *81*, 506–508. [CrossRef] [PubMed]
136. Navaneetharaja, N.; Griffiths, V.; Wileman, T.; Carding, S. A Role for the Intestinal Microbiota and Virome in Myalgic Encephalomyelitis/Chronic Fatigue Syndrome (ME/CFS)? *J. Clin. Med.* **2016**, *5*, 55. [CrossRef] [PubMed]
137. Giloteaux, L.; Goodrich, J.K.; Walters, W.A.; Levine, S.M.; Ley, R.E.; Hanson, M.R. Reduced Diversity and Altered Composition of the Gut Microbiome in Individuals with Myalgic Encephalomyelitis/Chronic Fatigue Syndrome. *Microbiome* **2016**, *4*, 1–12. [CrossRef]
138. Nagy-Szakal, D.; Williams, B.L.; Mishra, N.; Che, X.; Lee, B.; Bateman, L.; Klimas, N.G.; Komaroff, A.L.; Levine, S.; Montoya, J.G.; et al. Fecal Metagenomic Profiles in Subgroups of Patients with Myalgic Encephalomyelitis/Chronic Fatigue Syndrome. *Microbiome* **2017**, *5*, 1–17. [CrossRef]
139. Lupo, G.F.D.; Rocchetti, G.; Lucini, L.; Lorusso, L.; Manara, E.; Bertelli, M.; Puglisi, E.; Capelli, E. Potential Role of Microbiome in Chronic Fatigue Syndrome/Myalgic Encephalomyelits (CFS/ME). *Sci. Rep.* **2021**, *11*, 7043. [CrossRef]
140. Frémont, M.; Coomans, D.; Massart, S.; de Meirleir, K. High-Throughput 16S RRNA Gene Sequencing Reveals Alterations of Intestinal Microbiota in Myalgic Encephalomyelitis/Chronic Fatigue Syndrome Patients. *Anaerobe* **2013**, *22*, 50–56. [CrossRef]
141. du Preez, S.; Corbitt, M.; Cabanas, H.; Eaton, N.; Staines, D.; Marshall-Gradisnik, S. A Systematic Review of Enteric Dysbiosis in Chronic Fatigue Syndrome/Myalgic Encephalomyelitis. *Syst. Rev.* **2018**, *7*, 241. [CrossRef]
142. Mandarano, A.H.; Giloteaux, L.; Keller, B.A.; Levine, S.M.; Hanson, M.R. Eukaryotes in the Gut Microbiota in Myalgic Encephalomyelitis/Chronic Fatigue Syndrome. *PeerJ* **2018**, *6*, e4282. [CrossRef]
143. Lucas, K.; Maes, M. Role of the Toll like Receptor (TLR) Radical Cycle in Chronic Inflammation: Possible Treatments Targeting the TLR4 Pathway. *Mol. Neurobiol.* **2013**, *48*, 190–204. [CrossRef]
144. Maes, M.; Mihaylova, I.; Leunis, J.C. Increased Serum IgA and IgM against LPS of Enterobacteria in Chronic Fatigue Syndrome (CFS): Indication for the Involvement of Gram-Negative Enterobacteria in the Etiology of CFS and for the Presence of an Increased Gut-Intestinal Permeability. *J. Affect. Disord.* **2007**, *99*, 237–240. [CrossRef] [PubMed]
145. Mohammad, S.; Thiemermann, C. Role of Metabolic Endotoxemia in Systemic Inflammation and Potential Interventions. *Front. Immunol.* **2021**, *11*, 594150. [CrossRef] [PubMed]
146. Munford, R. Endotoxemia-Menace, Marker, or Mistake? *J. Leukoc. Biol.* **2016**, *100*, 687–698. [CrossRef] [PubMed]
147. Lakhan, S.E.; Kirchgessner, A. Gut Inflammation in Chronic Fatigue Syndrome. *Nutr. Metab.* **2010**, *7*, 1–10. [CrossRef] [PubMed]
148. Morris, G.; Maes, M. Oxidative and Nitrosative Stress and Immune-Inflammatory Pathways in Patients with Myalgic Encephalomyelitis (ME)/Chronic Fatigue Syndrome (CFS). *Curr. Neuropharmacol.* **2014**, *12*, 168–185. [CrossRef]
149. Maes, M.; Leunis, J.-C. Normalization of Leaky Gut in Chronic Fatigue Syndrome (CFS) Is Accompanied by a Clinical Improvement: Effects of Age, Duration of Illness and the Translocation of LPS from Gram-Negative Bacteria. *Neuro Endocrinol. Lett.* **2008**, *29*, 902.
150. Boudry, G.; Hamilton, M.K.; Chichlowski, M.; Wickramasinghe, S.; Barile, D.; Kalanetra, K.M.; Mills, D.A.; Raybould, H.E. Bovine Milk Oligosaccharides Decrease Gut Permeability and Improve Inflammation and Microbial Dysbiosis in Diet-Induced Obese Mice. *J. Dairy Sci.* **2017**, *100*, 2471–2481. [CrossRef]
151. Cani, P.; Possemiers, S.; van de Wiele, T.; Guiot, Y.; Everard, A.; Rottier, O.; Geurts, L.; Naslain, D.; Neyrinck, A.; Lambert, L.; et al. Changes in Gut Microbiota Control Inflammation in Obese Mice through a Mechanism Involving GLP-2-Driven Improvement of Gut Permeability. *Gut* **2009**, *58*, 1091–1103. [CrossRef]
152. Yu, T.; Wang, Y.; Chen, X.; Xiong, W.; Tang, Y.; Lin, L. Spirulina Platensis Alleviates Chronic Inflammation with Modulation of Gut Microbiota and Intestinal Permeability in Rats Fed a High-Fat Diet. *J. Cell. Mol. Med.* **2020**, *24*, 8603–8613. [CrossRef]
153. Zhang, Z.; Lin, T.; Meng, Y.; Hu, M.; Shu, L.; Jiang, H.; Gao, R.; Ma, J.; Wang, C.; Zhou, X. FOS/GOS Attenuates High-Fat Diet Induced Bone Loss via Reversing Microbiota Dysbiosis, High Intestinal Permeability and Systemic Inflammation in Mice. *Metab. Clin. Exp.* **2021**, *119*, 154767. [CrossRef]
154. Borody, T.J.; Nowak, A.; Finlayson, S. The GI Microbiome and Its Role in Chronic Fatigue Syndrome: A Summary of BacteriotherapyThe GI Microbiome and Its Role in Chronic Fatigue Syndrome: A Summary of Bacteriotherapy. *ACNEM J.* **2012**, *31*, 3–8.
155. Imdad, A.; Nicholson, M.; Tanner-Smith, E.; Zackular, Z.; Gomez-Duarte, O.; Beaulieu, S.; Acra, S. Fecal Transplantation for Treatment of Inflammatory Bowel Disease. *Cochrane Database Syst. Rev.* **2018**, *11*, CD012774. [CrossRef] [PubMed]
156. Shen, Z.-H.; Zhu, C.-X.; Quan, Y.-S.; Yang, Z.-Y.; Wu, S.; Luo, W.-W.; Tan, B.; Wang, X.-Y. Relationship between Intestinal Microbiota and Ulcerative Colitis: Mechanisms and Clinical Application of Probiotics and Fecal Microbiota Transplantation. *World J. Gastroenterol.* **2018**, *24*, 14. [CrossRef] [PubMed]

157. Tan, P.; Li, X.; Shen, J.; Feng, Q. Fecal Microbiota Transplantation for the Treatment of Inflammatory Bowel Disease: An Update. *Front. Pharmacol.* **2020**, *11*, 1409. [CrossRef] [PubMed]
158. Evrensel, A.; Ceylan, M.E. Fecal Microbiota Transplantation and Its Usage in Neuropsychiatric Disorders. *Clin. Psychopharmacol. Neurosci.* **2016**, *14*, 231–237. [CrossRef]
159. Aroniadis, O.C.; Brandt, L.J. Fecal Microbiota Transplantation: Past, Present and Future. *Curr. Opin. Gastroenterol.* **2013**, *29*, 79–84. [CrossRef]
160. Mattick, J.S.; Makunin, I.V. Non-Coding RNA. *Hum. Mol. Genet.* **2006**, *15* (Suppl. 1), R17–R29. [CrossRef] [PubMed]
161. Al-Rawaf, H.A.; Alghadir, A.H.; Gabr, S.A. MicroRNAs as Biomarkers of Pain Intensity in Patients with Chronic Fatigue Syndrome. *Pain Pract.* **2019**, *19*, 848–860. [CrossRef]
162. Paulmurugan, R. MicroRNAs—A New Generation Molecular Targets for Treating Cellular Diseases. *Theranostics* **2013**, *3*, 927–929. [CrossRef]
163. Ji, R.R.; Kohno, T.; Moore, K.A.; Woolf, C.J. Central Sensitization and LTP: Do Pain and Memory Share Similar Mechanisms? *Trends Neurosci.* **2003**, *26*, 696–705. [CrossRef]
164. Gravelsina, S.; Nora-Krukle, Z.; Vilmane, A.; Svirskis, S.; Vecvagare, K.; Krumina, A.; Murovska, M. Potential of Activin B as a Clinical Biomarker in Myalgic Encephalomyelitis/Chronic Fatigue Syndrome (ME/CFS). *Biomolecules* **2021**, *11*, 1189. [CrossRef]
165. Lidbury, B.A.; Kita, B.; Lewis, D.P.; Hayward, S.; Ludlow, H.; Hedger, M.P.; de Kretser, D.M. Activin B Is a Novel Biomarker for Chronic Fatigue Syndrome/Myalgic Encephalomyelitis (CFS/ME) Diagnosis: A Cross Sectional Study. *J. Transl. Med.* **2017**, *15*, 1–10. [CrossRef] [PubMed]
166. Brenu, E.W.; Ashton, K.J.; Batovska, J.; Staines, D.R.; Marshall-Gradisnik, S.M. High-Throughput Sequencing of Plasma MicroRNA in Chronic Fatigue Syndrome/Myalgic Encephalomyelitis. *PLoS ONE* **2014**, *9*, e102783. [CrossRef] [PubMed]
167. Cheema, A.K.; Sarria, L.; Bekheit, M.; Collado, F.; Almenar-Pérez, E.; Martín-Martínez, E.; Alegre, J.; Castro-Marrero, J.; Fletcher, M.A.; Klimas, N.G.; et al. Unravelling Myalgic Encephalomyelitis/Chronic Fatigue Syndrome (ME/CFS): Gender-specific Changes in the MicroRNA Expression Profiling in ME/CFS. *J. Cell. Mol. Med.* **2020**, *24*, 5865–5877. [CrossRef] [PubMed]
168. Petty, R.D.; McCarthy, N.E.; le Dieu, R.; Kerr, J.R. MicroRNAs Hsa-MiR-99b, Hsa-MiR-330, Hsa-MiR-126 and Hsa-MiR-30c: Potential Diagnostic Biomarkers in Natural Killer (NK) Cells of Patients with Chronic Fatigue Syndrome (CFS)/Myalgic Encephalomyelitis (ME). *PLoS ONE* **2016**, *11*, e0150904. [CrossRef]
169. Blauensteiner, J.; Bertinat, R.; León, L.E.; Riederer, M.; Sepúlveda, N.; Westermeier, F. Altered Endothelial Dysfunction-Related MiRs in Plasma from ME/CFS Patients. *Sci. Rep.* **2021**, *11*, 10604. [CrossRef]
170. Nepotchatykh, E.; Elremaly, W.; Caraus, I.; Godbout, C.; Leveau, C.; Chalder, L.; Beaudin, C.; Kanamaru, E.; Kosovskaia, R.; Lauzon, S.; et al. Profile of Circulating MicroRNAs in Myalgic Encephalomyelitis and Their Relation to Symptom Severity, and Disease Pathophysiology. *Sci. Rep.* **2020**, *10*, 19620. [CrossRef]
171. Yang, C.-A.; Bauer, S.; Ho, Y.-C.; Sotzny, F.; Chang, J.-G.; Scheibenbogen, C. The Expression Signature of Very Long Non-Coding RNA in Myalgic Encephalomyelitis/Chronic Fatigue Syndrome. *J. Transl. Med.* **2018**, *16*, 1–8. [CrossRef]
172. Del Rio, C.; Collins, L.F.; Malani, P. Long-Term Health Consequences of COVID-19. *JAMA* **2020**, *324*, 1723–1724. [CrossRef]
173. Marshall, M. The Lasting Misery of Coronavirus Long-Haulers. *Nature* **2020**, *585*, 339–341. [CrossRef] [PubMed]
174. Rubin, R. As Their Numbers Grow, COVID-19 "Long Haulers" Stump Experts. *JAMA* **2020**, *324*, 1381–1383. [CrossRef] [PubMed]
175. Townsend, L.; Dyer, A.H.; Jones, K.; Dunne, J.; Mooney, A.; Gaffney, F.; O'Connor, L.; Leavy, D.; O'Brien, K.; Dowds, J.; et al. Persistent Fatigue Following SARS-CoV-2 Infection Is Common and Independent of Severity of Initial Infection. *PLoS ONE* **2020**, *15*, e0240784. [CrossRef] [PubMed]
176. Carfì, A.; Bernabei, R.; Landi, F. Persistent Symptoms in Patients After Acute COVID-19. *JAMA* **2020**, *324*, 603–605. [CrossRef] [PubMed]
177. Logue, J.K.; Franko, N.M.; McCulloch, D.J.; McDonald, D.; Magedson, A.; Wolf, C.R.; Chu, H.Y. Sequelae in Adults at 6 Months After COVID-19 Infection. *JAMA Netw. Open* **2021**, *4*, e210830. [CrossRef] [PubMed]
178. Hickie, I.; Davenport, T.; Wakefield, D.; Vollmer-Conna, U.; Cameron, B.; Vernon, S.D.; Reeves, W.C.; Lloyd, A. Post-Infective and Chronic Fatigue Syndromes Precipitated by Viral and Non-Viral Pathogens: Prospective Cohort Study. *BMJ* **2006**, *333*, 575. [CrossRef]
179. Katz, B.Z.; Collin, S.M.; Murphy, G.; Moss-Morris, R.; Wyller, V.B.; Wensaas, K.-A.; Hautvast, J.L.A.; Bleeker-Rovers, C.P.; Vollmer-Conna, U.; Buchwald, D.; et al. The International Collaborative on Fatigue Following Infection (COFFI). *Fatigue Biomed. Health Behav.* **2018**, *6*, 106–121. [CrossRef]
180. O'Sullivan, O. Long-Term Sequelae Following Previous Coronavirus Epidemics. *Clin. Med.* **2021**, *21*, e68–e70. [CrossRef]
181. Ahmed, H.; Patel, K.; Greenwood, D.; Halpin, S.; Lewthwaite, P.; Salawu, A.; Eyre, L.; Breen, A.; O'Connor, R.; Jones, A.; et al. Long-Term Clinical Outcomes in Survivors of Severe Acute Respiratory Syndrome and Middle East Respiratory Syndrome Coronavirus Outbreaks after Hospitalisation or ICU Admission: A Systematic Review and Meta-Analysis. *J. Rehabil. Med.* **2020**, *52*, jrm00063. [CrossRef]
182. Lam, M.H.-B. Mental Morbidities and Chronic Fatigue in Severe Acute Respiratory Syndrome Survivors. *Arch. Intern. Med.* **2009**, *169*, 2142–2147. [CrossRef]
183. Rogers, J.P.; Chesney, E.; Oliver, D.; Pollak, T.A.; McGuire, P.; Fusar-Poli, P.; Zandi, M.S.; Lewis, G.; David, A.S. Psychiatric and Neuropsychiatric Presentations Associated with Severe Coronavirus Infections: A Systematic Review and Meta-Analysis with Comparison to the COVID-19 Pandemic. *Lancet Psychiatry* **2020**, *7*, 611–627. [CrossRef]

184. Poenaru, S.; Abdallah, S.J.; Corrales-Medina, V.; Cowan, J. COVID-19 and Post-Infectious Myalgic Encephalomyelitis/Chronic Fatigue Syndrome: A Narrative Review. *Ther. Adv. Infect. Dis.* **2021**, *8*, 20499361211009385. [CrossRef]
185. Araja, D.; Berkis, U.; Lunga, A.; Murovska, M. Shadow Burden of Undiagnosed Myalgic Encephalomyelitis/Chronic Fatigue Syndrome (ME/CFS) on Society: Retrospective and Prospective—In Light of COVID-19. *J. Clin. Med.* **2021**, *10*, 3017. [CrossRef]
186. González-Hermosillo, J.A.; Martínez-López, J.P.; Carrillo-Lampón, S.A.; Ruiz-Ojeda, D.; Herrera-Ramírez, S.; Amezcua-Guerra, L.M.; Martínez-Alvarado, M. del R. Post-Acute COVID-19 Symptoms, a Potential Link with Myalgic Encephalomyelitis/Chronic Fatigue Syndrome: A 6-Month Survey in a Mexican Cohort. *Brain Sci.* **2021**, *11*, 760. [CrossRef] [PubMed]
187. Mantovani, E.; Mariotto, S.; Gabbiani, D.; Dorelli, G.; Bozzetti, S.; Federico, A.; Zanzoni, S.; Girelli, D.; Crisafulli, E.; Ferrari, S.; et al. Chronic Fatigue Syndrome: An Emerging Sequela in COVID-19 Survivors? *J. Neuro Virol.* **2021**, *27*, 631–637. [CrossRef]
188. Simani, L.; Ramezani, M.; Darazam, I.A.; Sagharichi, M.; Aalipour, M.A.; Ghorbani, F.; Pakdaman, H. Prevalence and Correlates of Chronic Fatigue Syndrome and Post-Traumatic Stress Disorder after the Outbreak of the COVID-19. *J. Neuro Virol.* **2021**, *27*, 154–159. [CrossRef]
189. Petracek, L.S.; Suskauer, S.J.; Vickers, R.F.; Patel, N.R.; Violand, R.L.; Swope, R.L.; Rowe, P.C. Adolescent and Young Adult ME/CFS After Confirmed or Probable COVID-19. *Front. Med.* **2021**, *8*, 525. [CrossRef] [PubMed]

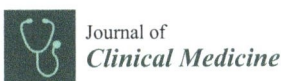

Review

Prevalence of Chronic Fatigue Syndrome (CFS) in Korea and Japan: A Meta-Analysis

Eun-Jin Lim [1] and Chang-Gue Son [2],*

[1] Department of Integrative Medicine, Graduate School of Integrative Medicine, CHA University, 120 Haeryong-ro, Kyeong-gi, Pocheon 11160, Korea; eunjinlimsydney@gmail.com
[2] Department of Korean Medicine, Institute of Bioscience and Integrative Medicine, Daejeon University, 62 Daehak-ro, Dong-gu, Daejeon 300-716, Korea
* Correspondence: ckson@dju.kr; Tel.: +82-42-229-6484; Fax: +82-42-257-6398

Abstract: Background: Myalgic encephalomyelitis/chronic fatigue syndrome (ME/CFS) is a long-term disabling illness accompanied by fatigue unsolved by rest. However, ME/CFS is a poorly understood illness that lacks a universally accepted pathophysiology and treatment. A lack of CFS-related studies have been conducted in Asian countries. This study aimed to estimate and compare the prevalence of ME/CFS in Korea and Japan and conducted a meta-analysis. Methods: We searched PubMed, EMBASE, Cochrane, and KMBASE for population-based prevalence studies of the two countries and synthesized the data according to the Fukuda case definition. Results: Of the eight studies (five in Korea, three in Japan) included, the total prevalence rate of Korean studies was 0.77% (95% CI 0.34–1.76), and 0.76% (95% CI 0.46–1.25) for the Japanese studies. The prevalence rate in females was approximately two-fold higher than males in Korean studies (1.31% female vs. 0.60% male), while the gender difference was less obvious in Japanese studies (0.76% female vs. 0.65% male). Conclusions: Further epidemiology studies on the female ME/CFS prevalence rate between countries may be required.

Keywords: chronic fatigue syndrome; CFS; ME/CFS; prevalence; Korea and Japan; meta-analysis

Citation: Lim, E.-J.; Son, C.-G. Prevalence of Chronic Fatigue Syndrome (CFS) in Korea and Japan: A Meta-Analysis. *J. Clin. Med.* **2021**, *10*, 3204. https://doi.org/10.3390/jcm10153204

Academic Editors: Giovanni Ricevuti and Lorenzo Lorusso

Received: 25 June 2021
Accepted: 19 July 2021
Published: 21 July 2021

Publisher's Note: MDPI stays neutral with regard to jurisdictional claims in published maps and institutional affiliations.

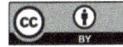

Copyright: © 2021 by the authors. Licensee MDPI, Basel, Switzerland. This article is an open access article distributed under the terms and conditions of the Creative Commons Attribution (CC BY) license (https://creativecommons.org/licenses/by/4.0/).

1. Introduction

Fatigue is a common complaint in both the general population and people with disorders [1]. Fatigue generally disappears after rest or treatment; however, uncontrolled chronic fatigue, particularly when lacking a medical explanation, substantially impairs health-related quality of life [2]. Among fatigue-related disorders, chronic fatigue syndrome (CFS) is the most debilitating, resulting in unemployment in half of the affected patients and a seven-fold higher risk of suicide compared to healthy subjects [3]. Until recently, there has been trivialization of CFS, with a debate on the origin of the illness (psychological vs. neurological) [4]. Currently, the Institute of Medicine (IOM) in the U.S. defines CFS as a complex multisystem neurological disorder [5].

The CFS prevalence may vary depending on country, ethnicity, sex, age, and especially diagnostic criteria [6]. To date, the prevalence of CFS has been found to be approximately 0.9%, and there are 1.5 to 2 times more women than men affected by CFS worldwide [7]. Most CFS-related studies have been conducted in the United States and United Kingdom, and the prevalence in Asian populations is uncertain due to the lack of studies. Korea and Japan are located near each other, but their ethnicities differ, and some epidemiologic differences in diseases have been reported between the two countries [8].

In order to expand the demographic knowledge of CFS, we sought to estimate and compare the prevalence of CFS in the Korean and Japanese populations.

2. Methods

2.1. Data Sources and Keywords

Using a domestic database (KMBASE, https://kmbase.medric.or.kr/ (accessed on 4 January 2021)) and three international databases (PubMed, EMBASE, Cochrane), we searched for publications reporting the prevalence of CFS in Japan and Korea and then performed a meta-analysis. The search term was "[[Chronic fatigue syndrome [MeSH term] AND Prevalence] AND [Japan OR Korea]]" and included studies published between January 1994 and January 2021 due to the Fukuda case definition, which was developed in 1994. All references listed in any included study were also then searched to identify titles matching our study question.

2.2. Eligibility and Exclusion Criteria

Papers were initially assessed according to the inclusion criteria. After reading the title and abstract, full articles that met the criteria were thoroughly read and screened by the exclusion criteria. The inclusion criteria were a population-based clinical study, and a prevalence study of ME/CFS in Japan and Korea. For consistency of the data, we included studies used only the Fukuda criteria (also known as CDC-1994 criteria). The exclusion criteria were nonclinical-based studies, randomized controlled studies, and studies focusing on clinical features or biological aspects of ME/CFS (Figure 1).

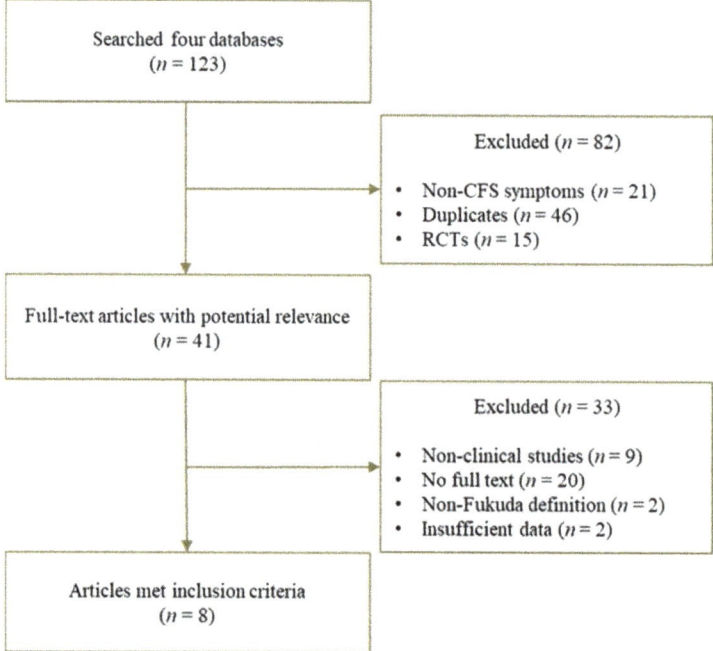

Figure 1. Flow chart for selection of articles.

2.3. Review Process

Two authors searched databases and selected the eligible articles according to the above criteria. The prevalence rate by country, the number of participants and patients, and their gender were collected from the selected articles. The final decision in extracting the data was made based upon the consensus of the two authors.

2.4. Statistical Analysis

The number of participants and ME/CFS patients from the included articles were organized to compare Korea vs. Japan and male vs. female to estimate the number of populations and the prevalence. A meta-analysis using the random effects model by the Comprehensive Meta Analysis (CMA) program was conducted to estimate heterogeneity of the data.

3. Results

3.1. Study Characteristics

In total, eight studies, five in Korea [9–13] and three in Japan [14–16] were included, which involved a total of 72,669 participants (6319 Korean and 66,350 Japanese). The sex ratios (male vs. female) of participants were very similar in both Korean studies (52% vs. 48%) and Japanese studies (50% vs. 50%), but the average number of participants was much higher in studies of Japanese (22,365 ± 37,369) than Korean (1264 ± 496). The mean age of participants was younger in Korean studies (30.3 ± 11.9 years) than Japanese (46.7 ± 10.4 years) (Table 1).

Table 1. Characteristics of the studies reporting the prevalence of ME/CFS in Korea and Japan.

Group	Korea	Japan	Total
Number of studies included (%)	5 (63)	3 (37)	8 (100)
Community	2 (25)	2 (25)	4 (50)
Primary care	3 (38)	1 (12)	4 (50)
Total number of participants	6319	66,350	72,669
(Average ± SD)	(1264 ± 496)	(22,365 ± 37,369)	(9173 ± 22,766)
Number of participants Male/Female	3276/3043	33,177/33,173	36,453/36,216
(male: female Ratio %)	(52:48)	(50:50)	(50:50)
Mean age of participants ±	30.3 ± 11.9	46.7 ± 10.4	38.5 ± 14.9
Year of publication (N. of participants)			
1994–2000	2 (2056)	2 (64,920)	4 (66,976)
2001–2010	3 (4263)		3 (4263)
2011–2018		1 (1430)	1 (1430)
Diagnostic method			
Interview (medical test −)	2 (2615)	2 (64,920)	4 (67,535)
Interview (medical test +)	3 (3704)	1 (1430)	4 (5134)

± Estimated from either the reported mean age for each gender or the mean age of both sexes. The age of children and adolescents was excluded.

3.2. CFS Prevalence

From the results of the meta-analysis, the overall prevalence rate of CFS in the Korean studies was 0.77% (95% CI 0.34–1.76), being slightly higher than the 0.76% reported in the Japanese studies (95% CI 0.46–1.25) (Figure 2). As expected, there was an approximately two-fold female predominance (1.31% female vs. 0.60% male) in Korean studies, while this sex difference was less obvious in Japanese studies, with 0.76% female and 0.65% male (Figures 3 and 4).

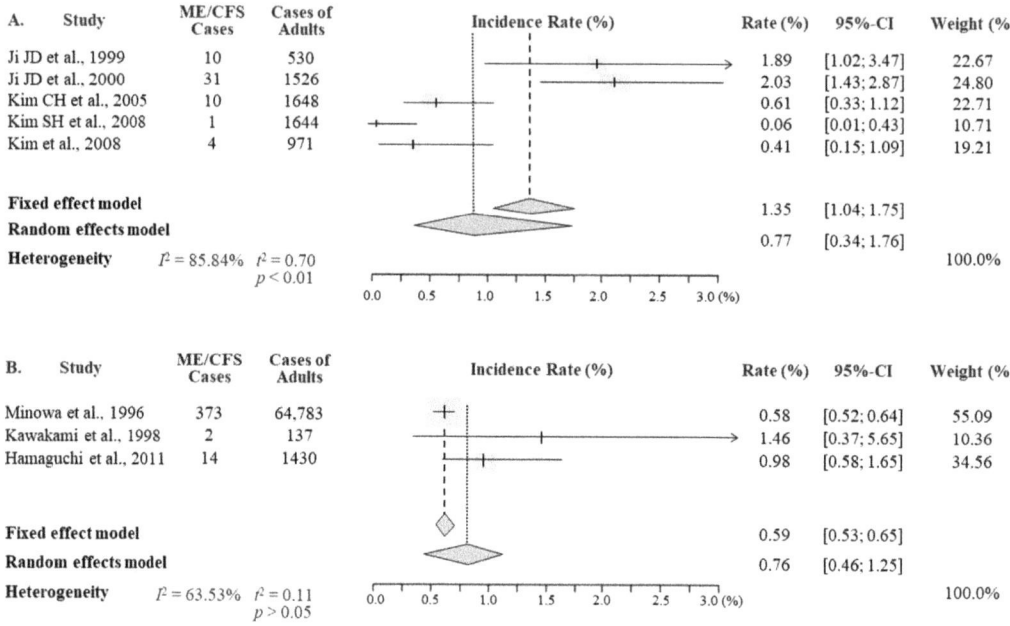

Figure 2. Meta-analysis of the ME/CFS total prevalence in Korea (**A**) and Japan (**B**).

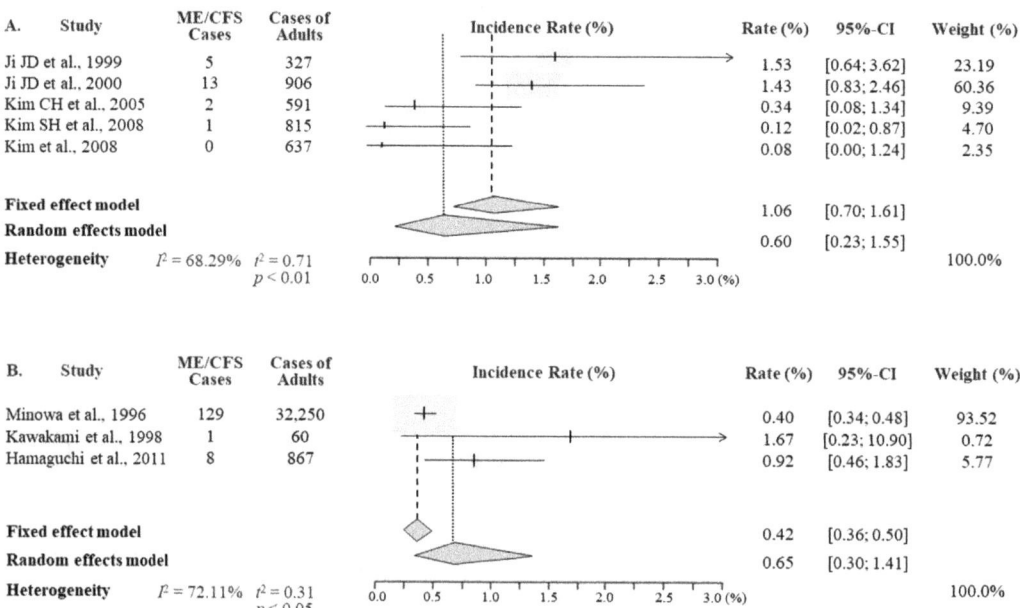

Figure 3. Meta-analysis of the ME/CFS prevalence in males in Korea (**A**) and Japan (**B**).

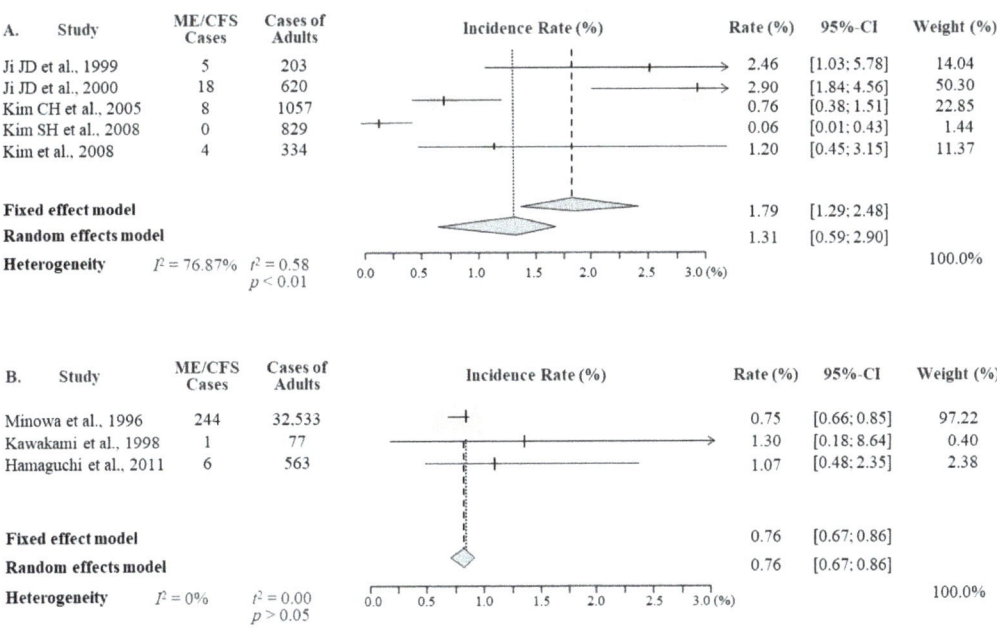

Figure 4. Meta-analysis of the ME/CFS prevalence in females in Korea (**A**) and Japan (**B**).

4. Discussion

As we expected, the prevalence rate in Korea (0.77%) and Japan (0.76%) of CFS was similar to those already reported worldwide (approximately 1%) [17]. We previously reported that CFS prevalence could be strongly affected by the diagnostic method or case definition used; the difference between using the Fukuda (CDC-1994) and Holmes (CDC-1988) criteria yielded rates of 0.89% vs. 0.17%, respectively [6]. In the present analysis, all the included eight studies used the Fukuda criteria. The Fukuda criteria relies on the presence of four or more of the eight main symptoms [18], which are the most commonly used criteria for the diagnosis of CFS in clinics including clinical trials [19].

All eight studies used interviews as the diagnostic method, and four studies additionally conducted or included the results of medical tests according to CDC-1994 guideline [18], three of the five Korean studies [9–11] and one of the three Japanese studies [16]. This means that Korean studies applied stricter criteria for the diagnosis of CFS than Japanese studies, which can be considered as leading to a reduction in the CFS prevalence rate of Korean data. However, in this study, we found the prevalence rates in Korea (0.77%, 95% CI 0.34–1.76) and Japan (0.76%, 95% CI 0.46–1.25) were very similar. This result is somewhat different from our previous meta-analysis for global CFS prevalence; we found the slight difference in the prevalence rate depends on the diagnostic methods, for example: diagnosed by primarily interview (1.14%) vs. interview conducted with medical tests (0.95%) [6]. This might tell the fact that inclusion of medical tests for CFS diagnosis may not have much of an impact on the overall prevalence rate. Lim et al.'s study included a total of 28 studies (interviews, 19 studies, vs. interviews with medical tests, nine studies) [6], whereas only eight (four vs. four, respectively) were included in this study (Table 1). Additionally, the prevalence rate among the studies using the same diagnostic method, that is with medical tests of the primary care participants, showed widely varied prevalence rates (ex, 0.61% Kim CH 2005 vs. 2.03% Ji JD 2000) between the studies [10,11]. In addition to the diagnostic method, race as a factor is another important aspect of CFS prevalence. This study shows that the meta-analysis results of each study in Korea and

Japan were widely varied, ranging from 0.06% to 1.46% for the subjects diagnosed by interview (four studies), and 0.61% to 1.89% (four studies) for interviews with medical tests. We compared these results to the studies of Western countries (mainly the UK and USA), using CDC-1994 and an adult general population recruited from both primary care and community settings. Those results ranged from 0.23% to 2.74% (five studies) and 0.42% to 2.62% (six studies), which indicates a somewhat higher prevalence than in Korea and Japan [6]. Being the female gender is a well-known predisposing factor of CFS [20], and an approximate two-fold female predominance of CFS was observed in Korean studies, while this female predominance was very low in Japanese studies (0.76% female and 0.65% male). We could anticipate that the large difference in CFS prevalence in females between Korea and Japan (1.31% vs. 0.76%) might be due to genetic and/or social factors. Comparative studies have reported slightly higher prevalence rates of four noncommunicable diseases in Korea than Japan, including hypertension (17.6% in Korea vs. 15.2% in Japan), diabetes (5.7% vs. 4.8%), hyperlipidemia (9.2% vs. 6.9%), and angina pectoris, and their general risk factors (1.7% vs. 1.5%). However, the sex-related risk was different according to the disease; for example, the male-to-female odds ratio was 0.88 in Korea vs. 0.64 in Japan for hypertension but 1.05 vs. 1.39 for diabetes [21].

The present study has some limitations: the original epidemiologic studies included were outdated (conducted 10 to 25 years ago) using the CDC-1994 case definition, and the average sample size, especially in Korean studies, was relatively small (1264 ± 496). One Japanese study was performed on a large scale (65,500 participants) [14], but the other two studies (1430 and 147 participants) were small. The results of a large gender difference are limited to Korea and Japan in this study, which should not be generalized to world data.

Despite those limitations, we systematically estimated the overall prevalence rate of CFS in Korea and Japan and identified differences. This information would be helpful for epidemiological research on CFS in the future. Further studies may be required on the rationales for the genetic and social factors that cause the gender difference in prevalence rate of CFS between Korea and Japan. Moreover, investigation of the prevalence rate using updated case definitions may also be needed.

Author Contributions: E.-J.L. searched the literature, collected data, conducted meta-analysis, and wrote the manuscript. C.-G.S. supervised the study and contributed to writing the manuscript. Both authors have read and agreed to the published version of the manuscript.

Funding: The authors would like to thank the Ministry of Education, Science and Technology the National Research Foundation of Korea (2018R1A6A1A03025221) for supporting this research.

Conflicts of Interest: There are no potential conflicts of interest to disclose.

References

1. Van't Leven, M.; Zielhuis, G.A.; van der Meer, J.W.; Verbeek, A.L.; Bleijenberg, G. Fatigue and chronic fatigue syndrome-like complaints in the general population. *Eur. J. Public Health* **2010**, *20*, 251–257. [CrossRef] [PubMed]
2. Jorgensen, R. Chronic fatigue: An evolutionary concept analysis. *J. Adv. Nurs.* **2008**, *63*, 199–207. [CrossRef] [PubMed]
3. Kapur, N.; Webb, R. Suicide risk in people with chronic fatigue syndrome. *Lancet* **2016**, *387*, 1596–1597. [CrossRef]
4. Speight, N. Myalgic encephalomyelitis/chronic fatigue syndrome: Review of history, clinical features, and controversies. *Saudi J. Med. Med. Sci.* **2013**, *1*, 11–13. [CrossRef]
5. Institute of Medicine. Beyond Myalgic Encephalomyelitis/Chronic Fatigue Syndrome; Redefining an Illness. Institute of Medicine of the National Academies, 2015. Available online: www.nap.edu (accessed on 4 January 2021).
6. Lim, E.J.; Ahn, Y.C.; Jang, E.S.; Lee, S.W.; Lee, S.H.; Son, C.G. Systematic review and meta-analysis of the prevalence of chronic fatigue syndrome/myalgic encephalomyelitis (CFS/ME). *J. Transl. Med.* **2020**, *18*, 100. [CrossRef] [PubMed]
7. Jason, L.A.; Porter, N.; Brown, M.; Anderson, V.; Brown, A.; Hunnell, J.; Lerch, A. CFS: A review of epidemiology and natural history studies. *Bull. IACFS/ME* **2009**, *17*, 88–106.
8. Kim, H.; Ryu, D.R. Difference in stroke incidence between Korean and Japanese patients initiating dialysis—Era or ethnic effect? *Int. J. Cardiol.* **2016**, *202*, 942. [CrossRef] [PubMed]
9. Ji, J.D.; Choi, S.J.; Lee, Y.H.; Song, G.G. Incidence and clinical manifestations of chronic fatigue in Korea. *Korean J. Med.* **1999**, *56*, 738–744.

10. Ji, J.D.; Choi, Y.S.; Chun, B.C.; Choi, S.J.; Lee, Y.H.; Song, G.G. The prevalence and clinical manifestations of chronic fatigue syndrome in persons who visited health management center. *Korean J. Med.* **2000**, *59*, 529–534.
11. Kim, C.H.; Shin, H.C.; Won, C.W. Prevalence of chronic fatigue and chronic fatigue syndrome in Korea: Community-based primary care study. *J. Korean Med. Sci.* **2005**, *20*, 529–534. [CrossRef]
12. Kim, S.H. Prevalence of chronic widespread pain and chronic fatigue syndrome in young Korean adults. *J. Musculoskelet. Pain* **2008**, *16*, 149–153. [CrossRef]
13. Kim, S.H.; Lee, K.; Lim, H.S. Prevalence of chronic widespread pain and chronic fatigue syndrome in Korean livestock raisers. *J. Occup. Health* **2008**, *50*, 525–528. [CrossRef]
14. Minowa, M.; Jiamo, M. Descriptive epidemiology of chronic fatigue syndrome based on a nationwide survey in Japan. *J. Epidemiol.* **1996**, *6*, 75–80. [CrossRef] [PubMed]
15. Kawakami, N.; Iwata, N.; Fujihara, S.; Kitamura, T. Prevalence of chronic fatigue syndrome in a community population in Japan. *Tohoku J. Exp. Med.* **1998**, *186*, 33–42. [CrossRef] [PubMed]
16. Hamaguchi, M.; Kawahito, Y.; Takeda, N.; Kato, T.; Kojima, T. Characteristics of chronic fatigue syndrome in a Japanese community population. *Clin. Rheumatol.* **2011**, *30*, 895–906. [CrossRef] [PubMed]
17. GBD 2016 Multiple Sclerosis Collaborators. Global, regional, and national burden of multiple sclerosis 1990–2016: A systematic analysis for the Global Burden of Disease Study 2016. *Lancet Neurol.* **2019**, *18*, 269–285. [CrossRef]
18. Fukuda, K.; Straus, S.E.; Hickie, I.; Sharpe, M.C.; Dobbins, J.G.; Komarof, A. The chronic fatigue syndrome: A comprehensive approach to its definition and study. *Ann. Intern. Med.* **1994**, *121*, 953–959. [CrossRef] [PubMed]
19. Kim, D.Y.; Lee, J.S.; Park, S.Y.; Kim, S.J.; Son, C.G. Systematic review of randomized controlled trials for chronic fatigue syndrome/myalgic encephalomyelitis (CFS/ME). *J. Transl. Med.* **2020**, *18*, 7. [CrossRef]
20. Bested, A.C.; Marshall, L.M. Review of myalgic encephalomyelitis/chronic fatigue syndrome: An evidence-based approach to diagnosis and management by clinicians. *Rev. Environ. Health* **2015**, *30*, 223–249. [CrossRef] [PubMed]
21. Ma, D.; Sakai, H.; Wakabayashi, C.; Kwon, J.S.; Lee, Y.; Liu, S.; Wan, Q.; Sasao, K.; Ito, K.; Nishihara, K.; et al. The prevalence and risk factor control associated with noncommunicable diseases in China, Japan, and Korea. *J. Epidemiol.* **2017**, *27*, 568–573. [CrossRef] [PubMed]

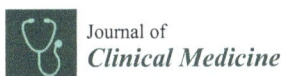

Review

The Prospects of the Two-Day Cardiopulmonary Exercise Test (CPET) in ME/CFS Patients: A Meta-Analysis

Eun-Jin Lim [1], Eun-Bum Kang [2], Eun-Su Jang [1] and Chang-Gue Son [1,*]

1. Department of Korean Medicine, Institute of Bioscience and Integrative Medicine, Daejeon University, 62 Daehak-ro, Dong-gu, Daejeon 34520, Korea; eunjinlimsydney@gmail.com (E.-J.L.); jang.ensu2@gmail.com (E.-S.J.)
2. Department of Health and Exercise Management, Daejeon University, 62 Daehak-ro, Dong-gu, Daejeon 34520, Korea; kbume23@naver.com
* Correspondence: ckson@dju.ac.kr; Tel.: +82-42-229-6484; Fax: +82-42-257-6398

Received: 10 November 2020; Accepted: 11 December 2020; Published: 14 December 2020

Abstract: Background: The diagnosis of myalgic encephalomyelitis/chronic fatigue syndrome (ME/CFS) is problematic due to the lack of established objective measurements. Postexertional malaise (PEM) is a hallmark of ME/CFS, and the two-day cardiopulmonary exercise test (CPET) has been tested as a tool to assess functional impairment in ME/CFS patients. This study aimed to estimate the potential of the CPET. Methods: We reviewed studies of the two-day CPET and meta-analyzed the differences between ME/CFS patients and controls regarding four parameters: volume of oxygen consumption and level of workload at peak (VO_{2peak}, $Workload_{peak}$) and at ventilatory threshold ($VO_2@VT$, $Workload@VT$). Results: The overall mean values of all parameters were lower on the 2nd day of the CPET than the 1st in ME/CFS patients, while it increased in the controls. From the meta-analysis, the difference between patients and controls was highly significant at $Workload@VT$ (overall mean: −10.8 at Test 1 vs. −33.0 at Test 2, $p < 0.05$), which may reflect present the functional impairment associated with PEM. Conclusions: Our results show the potential of the two-day CPET to serve as an objective assessment of PEM in ME/CFS patients. Further clinical trials are required to validate this tool compared to other fatigue-inducing disorders, including depression, using well-designed large-scale studies.

Keywords: cardiopulmonary exercise test; chronic fatigue syndrome; myalgic encephalomyelitis; postexertional malaise

1. Introduction

Myalgic encephalomyelitis/chronic fatigue syndrome (ME/CFS) is a debilitating multisystem disease that affects more than 20 million people of all ages and races worldwide [1,2]. The core symptoms are severe fatigue, unrefreshing sleep, postexertional malaise (PEM), and cognitive dysfunction for more than 6 months [3]. Approximately 30% of the patients are housebound, and 50% are unable to work full time [4]. Despite the seriousness of the illness, ME/CFS has no established pathophysiology or diagnostic tests yet [4]. Moreover, the diagnosis of ME/CFS is often confused with other fatigue-related or comorbid illnesses (e.g., depression) due to the overlapping symptoms [5].

Although the clinical presentation of ME/CFS can be ambiguous, a 2015 report by the Institute of Medicine (IOM) states that PEM is a hallmark of this disease and helps distinguish it from other conditions [3]. PEM consists of exertional intolerance and worsening of symptoms following minor physical or cognitive exertion, which can be severe enough to leave the patients bedridden [6,7]. Studies on the prevalence of PEM in ME/CFS reported that more than 80% of all ME/CFS patients had experienced this symptom at some point in their illness [8,9]. The underlying pathophysiology of PEM is not clearly understood, but researchers have adapted the two-day cardiopulmonary exercise test (CPET) as a strategy for objectively measuring PEM [3,10–12].

The CPET was developed as a tool to measure the functional capacity of the body through analysis of gas exchange (e.g., oxygen, and carbon dioxide) during exercise for athletes and people with cardiac, pulmonary, vascular, and metabolic disorders [13]. In general, the CPET is performed on a single day for the above purposes; however, the two-day CPET has received attention particularly for ME/CFS since 2007 [10]. It can assess recovery capacity using two exercise tests administered 24 h apart [14]. A number of one-day CPET studies reported a lack of significant differences between ME/CFS patients and controls [15–18]; however, significantly different responses were observed in the 2nd test of the two-day CPET [10,19,20]. This may indicate impaired recovery, reduced energy production, and likely PEM in ME/CFS patients [14]. Multiple studies have reported an association with mitochondrial dysfunction as a potential pathophysiology in ME/CFS patients [21,22].

A previous review study assessed one parameter (the volume of oxygen consumption at peak, VO_{2peak}) between ME/CFS patients and controls by combining the two different tests (one-day and two-day CPET studies) [23]. However, considering the possible differences in the results of one-day and two-day CPET, two-day CPET data may need to be analyzed separately in various parameters.

Therefore, we meta-analyzed the parameters of VO_2 and workload both at peak (VO_{2peak}, Workload$_{peak}$) and at ventilatory threshold (VO_2@VT, Workload@VT) in two-day CPET studies to assess the potential use of this test as a diagnostic tool for ME/CFS.

2. Methods

2.1. Search Strategy, Inclusion and Exclusion Criteria

We conducted a systematic search in five public databases and two search sources: PubMed, the Cochrane Library, the Cumulative Index to Nursing and Allied Health Literature (CINAHL), Medline, Google Scholar, a hand search, and the reference lists of the included studies. The search was conducted from February to June 2020. The search keywords were 'Chronic fatigue syndrome' [MeSH terms] AND 'cardiopulmonary exercise test' or 'CEPT' [MeSH terms]. For the Google Scholar search in particular, we restricted the search criteria to reduce the initial abundant numbers and selected the studies not searched by PubMed. Papers were screened using the following inclusion criteria: (a) studies of cross-sectional, case–control, prospective studies that conducted the CPET to measure diagnostic parameters for ME/CFS, (b) two-day CPET with the two sessions conducted 24 h apart, (c) studies that measured the four parameters (VO_{2peak}, Workload$_{peak}$, VO_2@VT, and Workload@VT) for the test. The exclusion criteria were as follows: (a) non clinical-based studies, (b) studies for other than ME/CFS, and studies with (c) single CPET, (d) no controls and that failed to state the four parameter values, (e) less than 5 participants, (f) studies that measured other than the four parameters. The search and data extraction were performed by E-J. L. and C-G. S., and any disagreements were resolved by discussions.

2.2. Data Extraction and Outcome Measures

The main features of the studies were extracted and compiled including; authors, year of publication, and the number of participants, the age and body mass index (BMI) of the participants, and the methodology of selecting the participants (Table 1). The primary outcome measures were the four parameters: VO_{2peak}, Workload$_{peak}$, VO_2@VT, and Workload@VT. These parameters are involved in measuring activity limitations of ME/CFS patients [24]. These are defined as follows: (1) VO_{2peak} is the highest value of oxygen uptake obtained during the exercise. (2) VO_2 at ventilatory threshold (VT) is the volume of oxygen at VT, which is the point which ventilation starts to increase at a faster rate than oxygen consumption. (3) Workload$_{peak}$ is the power output produced by the participant at peak. (4) Workload@VT is the level of power output produced at VT [11,14].

2.3. Statistical Analysis

We calculated the mean difference and meta-analyzed the four parameters of ME/CFS patients and controls as of Testes 1 and 2 (Tables 2–4). The four parameters was estimated with a random-effects model to account for the heterogeneity of the data, and we compared the I^2 and significance (p values) of those groups. I^2 higher than 50% is considered substantially heterogeneous [25]. A forest plot was used to show the estimated overall mean number of the parameters, and p value < 0.05 is considered significant. The data were analyzed using the meta-analysis program version 5.3 Review Manager (The Cochrane Collaboration, Oxford, UK) [26].

2.4. Assessment of Quality of Studies

The quality of studies included was assessed according to the Newcastle Ottawa Scale (NOS) guideline for case-control studies, which judges studies on the following perspectives: selection of the groups, the comparability of the groups, and the ascertainment of exposure [27] (Table 1).

3. Results

3.1. Characteristics of Included Studies

In total, 218 studies were initially selected as candidates for this meta-analysis; ultimately, 5 studies were included (Figure 1). All studies used the same study protocol (an incremental cycling protocol with an interval of 24 h) and case definition (Fukuda) for inclusion of participants. Two studies additionally used the International Consensus Criteria (ICC) [28] and/or the Canadian Consensus Criteria (CCC) [6]. The total number of participants across the five studies was 98 ME/CFS patients (90 female and 8 male) and 51 controls (45 female and 6 male). The total mean age and BMI of the participants were comparable between the patient and control groups (Table 1).

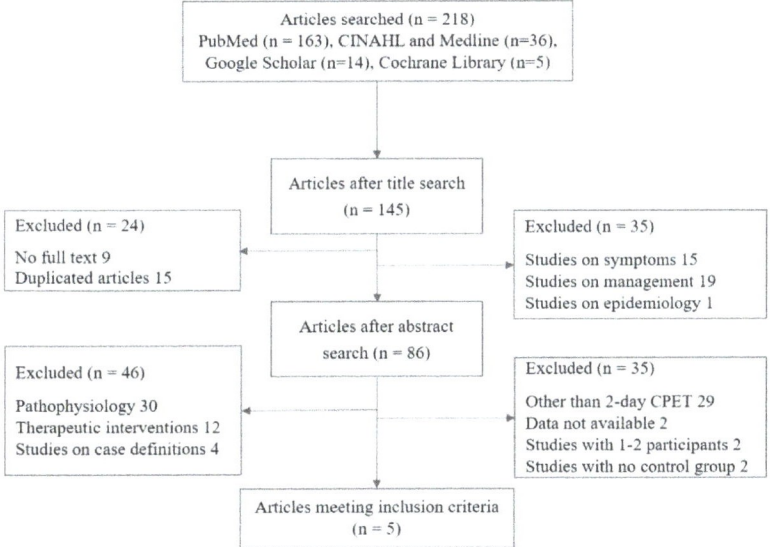

Figure 1. Flow chart of the study selection process.

Table 1. Characteristics and assessment of quality of studies.

	ME/CFS +	Control	Newcastle Ottawa Scale [§]							
			S				C		E	
			1	2	3	4	5	6	7	8
No. of studies	5	5								
No. of participants (Female/Male)	98 (90/8)	51 (45/6)								
Age (y) [#]	42.3 ± 11.6	41.3 ± 12.4								
BMI (kg/m^2) [#]	25.3 ± 4.8	25.6 ± 4.2								
	Selection of participants									
	ME/CFS	Control								
Van Ness (2007) [10]	Physician diagnosis and Fukuda	Healthy sedentary	*	*	*	*	*	*	*	*
Vermeulen (2010) [19]	CDC-SI 59.5 ± 13.1 [‡] Fukuda, infectious disease onset	CDC-SI 5.0 ± 4.5	*	*	*	*	*	*	*	*
Snell (2013) [29]	Sedentary [※] Fukuda, Presence of PEM	Sedentary [※]	*	*	*	*	*	*	*	*
Hodges (2017) [30]	Fukuda, (CCC and ICC) [α] De Paul Questionnaire, SF-36	Healthy	*	*	-	-	*	*	*	*
Nelson (2019) [20]	Sedentary [†] Physician diagnosis Fukuda/(CCC/ICC) [α]	Sedentary [†]	*	*	*	*	*	*	*	*

+ ME/CFS, Myalgic encephalomyelitis/chronic fatigue syndrome. [§] A star system at the included studies are judged on 3 perspectives: S, selection of groups. C, comparability of groups. * checked and confirmed. E, exposure. CDC-SI, Centers for Disease Control and Prevention-Symptom Inventory questionnaire. [#] Estimated from the mean ages of the individual studies. [†] Four ME/CFS fatigue symptoms ≥7.5. [※] <30 min exercise/per week. [‡] <150 min of moderate exercise/per week. [α] CCC, Canadian consensus criteria. ICC, International consensus criteria.

Table 2. Studies that performed the two-day cardiopulmonary exercise test (CPET) in ME/CFS patients and controls.

#	Study	Participants (Patients/Controls)	VO$_{2peak}$ Test 1/Test 2 (T2-T1) (mL kg^{-1} min^{-1})	VO$_2$@VT Test 1/Test 2 (T2-T1) (mL kg^{-1} min^{-1})	Workload$_{peak}$ Test 1/Test 2 (T2-T1) (Watt)	Workload@VT Test 1/Test 2 (T2-T1) (Watt)
1	Van Ness (2007) [10]	6(F) 6(F)	26.2 ± 4.9/20.5 ± 1.8 (−5.8) 28.4 ± 7.2/28.9 ± 8.0 (+0.5)	15.0 ± 4.9/11.0 ± 3.4 (−4.0) 17.6 ± 4.9/18.0 ± 5.3 (+0.4)	-	-
2	Vermeulen (2010) [19]	15(F) 15(F)	22.3 ± 5.7/20.9 ± 5.5 (−1.3) 31.2 ± 7.0/31.9 ± 7.4 (+0.7)	12.8 ± 3.0/11.9 ± 2.9 (−0.9) 16.7 ± 4.0/18.0 ± 4.6 (+1.3)	132.0 ± 30.0/125.0 ± 35.0 (−7.0) 188.0 ± 46.0/196.0 ± 51.0 (+8.0)	58.6 ± 24.2/54.5 ± 20.9 (−4.1) 82.9 ± 29.1/92.9 ± 31.4 (+10.0)
3	Snell (2013) [29]	51(F) 10(F)	21.5 ± 4.1/20.4 ± 4.5 (−1.1) 25.0 ± 4.4/24.0 ± 4.3 (−1.0)	12.7 ± 2.9/11.4 ± 2.9 (−1.3) 13.8 ± 2.8/14.1 ± 3.3 (+0.3)	109.6 ± 28.9/101.6 ± 30.7 (−8.0) 137.2 ± 23.2/140.0 ± 25.0 (+2.8)	49.5 ± 20.4/22.2 ± 18.1 (−27.3) 58.0 ± 16.7/63.5 ± 19.5 (+5.5)
4	Hodges (2017) [30]	9(F)/1(M) 9(F)/1(M)	25.0 ± 8.9/26.3 ± 7.8 (+1.3) 32.0 ± 10.9/33.1 ± 12.5 (+1.1)	21.0 ± 4.3/22.2 ± 6.2 (+1.2) 23.6 ± 9.0/28.5 ± 12.5 (+4.9)	135.0 ± 43.0/126.0 ± 45.0 (−9.0) 164.0 ± 40.0/167.0 ± 41.0 (+3.0)	105.0 ± 30.0/93.0 ± 37.0 (−12.0) 119.0 ± 28.0/132.0 ± 42.0 (+13.0)
5	Nelson (2019) [20]	9(F)/7(M) 5(F)/5(M)	27.3 ± 9.2/27.4 ± 8.8 (+0.1) 29.9 ± 6.1/30.3 ± 6.2 (+0.4)	15.9 ± 4.1/15.4 ± 3.4 (−0.5) 16.5 ± 2.0/15.9 ± 1.5 (−0.6)	154.4 ± 56.0/152.5 ± 51.7 (−1.9) 172.0 ± 35.5/174.0 ± 36.6 (+2.0)	87.8 ± 29.6/72.5 ± 27.7 (−15.3) 90.5 ± 17.1/88.0 ± 16.7 (−2.5)
	Total	90(F)/8(M) 45(F)/6(M)	24.5 ± 6.6/23.1 ± 5.7 (−1.4) 29.3 ± 7.1/29.6 ± 7.7 (+0.3)	15.5 ± 3.8/14.4 ± 3.8 (−1.1) 17.6 ± 4.5/18.9 ± 5.4 (+1.3)	132.8 ± 39.5/126.3 ± 40.6 (−6.5) 165.3 ± 36.2/169.3 ± 38.4 (+4.0)	75.2 ± 26.1/60.6 ± 25.9 (−14.6) 87.6 ± 22.7/94.1 ± 27.4 (+6.5)

ME/CFS, Myalgic encephalomyelitis/chronic fatigue syndrome. VO$_{2peak}$, volume of oxygen uptake at peak. @VT, at ventilatory threshold. The units of parameter for VO$_2$ is mL kg^{-1} min^{-1}, and for Workload is Watt. F, female. M, male. All results are rounded to one decimal place. Exercise mode: cycle ergometer.

Table 3. Meta-analysis of two-day CPET (test 2−test 1) for the comparisons between the ME/CFS patients and controls.

#	Study		Weight (%)				Mean Difference			
			VO$_{2peak}$	@VT	WL$_{peak}$	@VT	VO$_{2peak}$	@VT	WL$_{peak}$	@VT
1	Van Ness (2007) [10]	P	16	3.5	-	-	−5.7 (−1.5, −9.9)	−4.0 (0.8, −8.8)	-	-
		C	8.2	4.3	-	-	0.5 (9.1, −8.1)	0.4 (6.2, −5.4)	-	-
2	Vermeulen (2010) [19]	P	17.1	17.9	17.2	26.2	−0.9 (1.2, −3.0)	−1.4 (2.6, −5.4)	−7.0 (16.3, −30.3)	−4.1 (12.1, −20.3)
		C	23.0	15.0	17.0	18.4	0.7 (5.9, −4.5)	1.3 (4.4, −1.8)	8.0 (42.8, −26.8)	10.0 (31.6, −11.6)
3	Snell (2013) [29]	P	53.1	63.1	69.8	38.6	−1.1 (0.6, −2.8)	−1.3 (−0.2, −2.4)	−8.0 (3.6, −19.6)	−27.3 (−19.8, −34.8)
		C	42.0	19.8	46.0	33.8	−1.0 (2.8, −4.8)	0.3 (3.0, −2.4)	2.8 (23.9, −18.3)	5.5 (21.4, −10.4)
4	Hodges (2017) [30]	P	5.9	3.7	6.3	13.4	1.3 (8.6, −6.0)	1.2 (5.9, −3.5)	−9.0 (29.6, −47.6)	−12.0 (17.5, −41.5)
		C	5.8	1.6	16.3	8.7	1.1 (11.4, −9.2)	4.9 (14.5, −4.7)	3.0 (38.5, −32.5)	13.0 (44.3, −18.3)
5	Nelson (2019) [20]	P	7.9	11.7	6.7	21.7	0.1 (6.3, −6.1)	−0.5 (2.1, −3.1)	−1.9 (35.5, −39.3)	−15.3 (4.6, −35.2)
		C	21.0	59.4	20.6	39.0	0.4 (5.8, −5.0)	−0.6 (1.0, −2.2)	2.0 (33.6, −29.6)	−2.5 (12.3, −17.3)
	Overall values for P Heterogeneity (I^2) p value		19% 0.30	0 0.61	0% 0.99	60% 0.06	−1.7 (0.2, −3.5)	−1.1 (−0.2, −2.0)	−7.5 (2.2, −17.2)	−16.6 (−3.6, −29.5)
	Overall values for C Heterogeneity (I^2) p value		0% 0.98	0% 0.67	0% 0.99	0% 0.71	−0.1 (2.4, −2.5)	−0.01 (1.2, −1.2)	3.6 (17.9, −10.8)	3.9 (13.1, −5.4)
	P vs. C p value		0.23	0.10	0.83	0.01 **				

ME/CFS, Myalgic encephalomyelitis/chronic fatigue syndrome. CPET, Cardiopulmonary exercise testing. #, Number of studies. VO$_{2peak}$, volume of oxygen uptake at peak. @VT, at ventilatory threshold. WL$_{peak}$, workload at peak. The units of parameter for VO$_2$ is mL × kg^{-1} × min^{-1}, and for Workload or WL is Watt. P, patient. C, control. All results are rounded to one decimal place. **, p value < 0.01.

Table 4. Meta-analysis (of ME/CFS patient control) for the comparisons between the two-day CPET 1 and 2.

#	Study		Weight (%)				Mean Difference			
			VO_{2peak}	@VT	WL_{peak}	@VT	VO_{2peak}	@VT	WL_{peak}	@VT
1	VanNess (2007) [19]	T1	11.9	5.4	-	-	−2.2 (−9.2, 4.8)	−2.6 (−8.1, 2.9)	-	-
		T2	16.4	15	-	-	−8.4 (−14.7, −1.8)	−7.0 (−12.0, −2.0)	-	-
2	Vermeulen (2010) [19]	T1	23.4	23.9	22.8	18.7	−8.9 (−13.37, −4.3)	−3.9 (−6.4, −1.4)	−56.0 (−83.79, −28.2)	−24.3 (−43.5, −5.2)
		T2	23.1	23.9	22.3	25.5	−11.0 (−15.7, −6.3)	−6.1 (−8.9, −3.4)	−71.0 (−102.3, 39.7)	−38.4 (−57.4, −19.4)
3	Snell (2013) [29]	T1	41.0	39.3	47.2	49.5	−3.5 (−6.5, −0.6)	−1.1 (−3.0, 0.8)	−27.6 (−44.0, −11.2)	−8.5 (−20.3, 3.3)
		T2	31.0	26.3	40.5	34.8	−3.6 (−6.5, −0.7)	−2.7 (−4.9, −0.5)	−38.4 (−56.0, −20.8)	−41.3 (−54.4, −28.2)
4	Hodges (2017) [30]	T1	8.0	4.3	14.6	10.6	−7.0 (−15.7, 1.7)	−2.6 (−8.8, 3.6)	−29.0 (−65.4, 7.4)	−14.0 (−39.4, 11.4)
		T2	10.5	7.4	17.2	11.6	−6.8 (−15.9, 2.3)	−6.3 (−15.0, 2.4)	−41.0 (−78.7, −3.3)	−39.0 (−73.7, −4.3)
5	Nelson (2019) [20]	T1	15.8	27.1	15.4	21.2	−2.6 (−8.5, 3.3)	−0.6 (−3.0, 1.8)	−17.6 (−52.8, 17.6)	−2.7 (−20.7, 15.3)
		T2	18.9	27.4	20.0	28.2	−2.9 (−8.7, 2.9)	−0.5 (−2.4, 1.4)	−21.5 (−55.5, 12.5)	−15.5 (−32.6, 1.6)
	Overall values for T1 Heterogeneity (I^2) T1 p value		22% 0.27	7% 0.37	21% 0.28	0% 0.41	−4.8 (−7.3, −2.2)	−1.8 (−3.1, −0.5)	−3−32.7 (−47.6, −17.8)	−10.8 (−19.1, −2.5)
	Overall values for T2 Heterogeneity (I^2) T2 p value		53% 0.07	72% 0.01**	38% 0.18	50% 0.11	−6.3 (−9.8, −2.9)	−3.8 (−6.5, −1.1)	−42.8 (−61.0, −24.5)	−33.0 (−46.4, −19.6)
	T1 vs. T2 p value		0.42	0.14	0.46	0.03 *				

ME/CFS, Myalgic encephalomyelitis/chronic fatigue syndrome. CPET, Cardiopulmonary exercise testing. VO_{2peak}, volume of oxygen uptake at peak. @VT, at ventilatory threshold. WL_{peak}, workload at peak. The units of parameter for VO_2 is mL·kg^{-1}·min^{-1}, and for Workload or WL is Watt. T1, Test 1. T2, Test 2. All results are rounded to one decimal place. *, p value < 0.05. **, p value < 0.01.

3.2. Comparisons of the Four Parameters

The four parameters as of Test 1 and Test 2, as well as their differences between sessions, are summarized in Table 2. From Test 1 to Test 2, all four measures (VO_{2peak}, $VO_2@VT$, $Workload_{peak}$, and Workload@VT) increased in the control group but decreased in the patient group. Among the four parameters, the Workload@VT of the patient group showed an especially marked decrease on Test 2 compared to Test 1, with a difference (Test 2–Test 1) of −14.6 in patients and +6.5 in controls (Table 2).

3.3. Outcomes of Meta-Analysis

From the meta-analysis, we evaluated the differences in parameters from Test 2 to Test 1 in ME/CFS patients compared to the control group (Figure 2). The values of all four parameters increased as of the 2nd test (Test 2) in the control group, while ME/CFS patients showed notable decreases in all parameters at Test 2 (Figure 2, Tables 2 and 3).

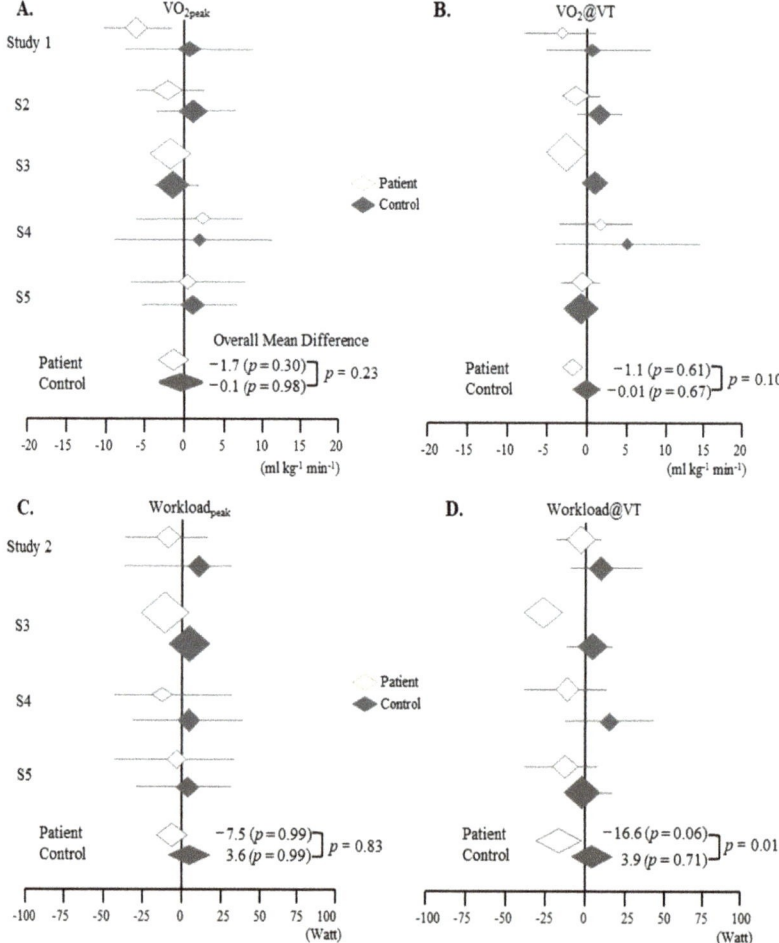

Figure 2. Meta analyzed overall mean differences of the four parameters (A-D) from the scores of the two-day CPET (test 2–test 1) for the ME/CFS (Myalgic encephalomyelitis/chronic fatigue syndrome) patients and controls: (**A**). VO_2peak, (**B**). $VO_2@VT$, (**C**). Workloadpeak, (**D**). Workload@VT. *p*, *p* value. Refer to Table 3 for details.

In general, the differences between patients and controls were greater at VT than at peak and greater for workload than for VO$_2$ (Figures 2 and 3). From the meta-analysis focused on the difference between Test 2–Test 1 (using the data from patients and controls), Workload@VT showed the most notable significant difference ($p < 0.05$) (Figures 2 and 3).

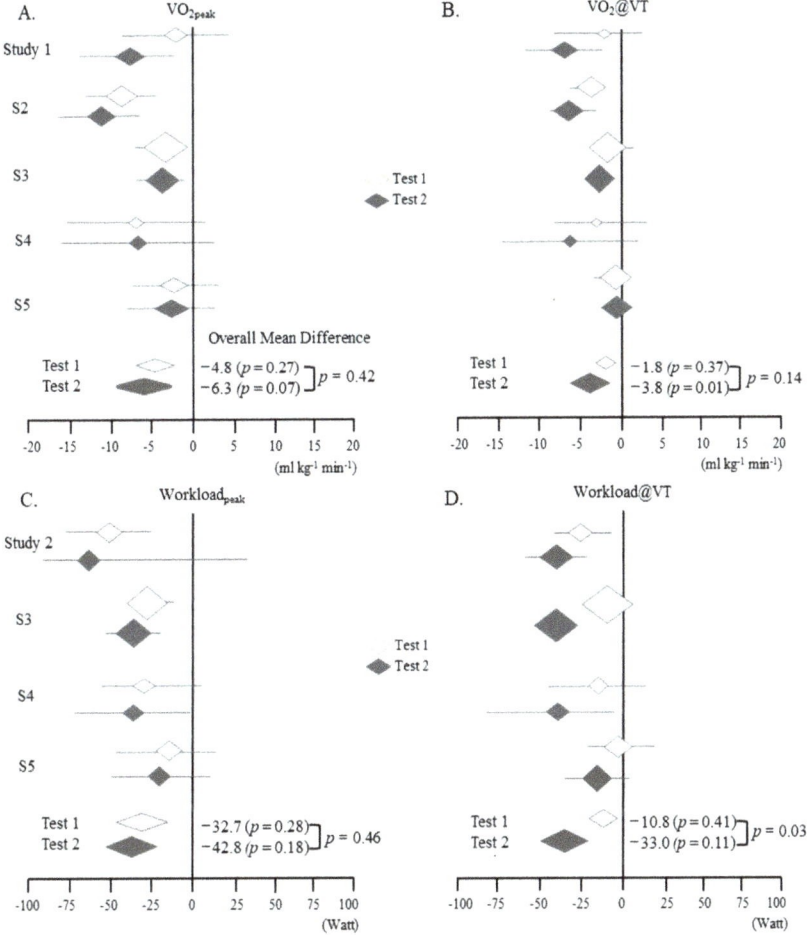

Figure 3. Meta analyzed overall mean differences of the four parameters (A-D) from the scores of the ME/CFS patients—controls for the two-day CPET 1 and 2: (**A**). VO$_2$peak, (**B**). VO$_2$@VT, (**C**). Workloadpeak, (**D**). Workload@VT. p, p value. Refer to Table 4 for details.

4. Discussion

From our meta-analysis of five studies of two-day CPET, we identified the following three key features. First, ME/CFS patients appeared to have lower levels of all parameters than controls, especially on Test 2. Second, on Test 2, the difference between the patients and controls was observed to be larger at VT than at peak. Third, on a more specific level, Workload@VT was notably different between the two tests and between the two groups (Figures 2 and 3, Tables 2–4). These data may indicate the potential of Workload@VT value as an objective measurement in ME/CFS.

The reduced levels of parameters in the ME/CFS patient group on Test 2 shows that they failed to reproduce their work capacity from Test 1 [19]. Such reduced work capacity in general is likely linked to a lack of cellular adenosine triphosphate (ATP) production, which normally occurs through aerobic and anaerobic metabolism [31]. Imbalanced ATP production can be caused by functional impairment of mitochondria in patients with ME/CFS [32]. Studies have reported conflicted results regarding mitochondrial impairment; some have provided evidence of actual mitochondrial dysfunction affecting oxidative phosphorylation [21,33], while other studies found no abnormal indicators of altered mitochondrial function or mitochondrial DNA mutation [19,34,35]. In fact, a number of researchers suggested a possible problem in the pathway of oxygen or glucose transportation into the cells, which may inhibit the function of mitochondria in ME/CFS patients [10,19,29,30,35,36]. The hypothesized factors inhibiting mitochondria ATP production include viral/bacterial infection [37], high levels of proinflammatory cytokines [38], reactive oxygen species (ROS) [39], and decreased levels of enzymes (such as pyruvate dehydrogenase, PDH) needed in the process of aerobic cellular respiration [40].

Lower work capacity on Test 2 than on Test 1 seems to be a unique feature of ME/CFS and is indicated as a cardinal feature for the diagnosis of PEM [3]. Patients with lung, heart, or kidney diseases presented no significant differences between Tests 1 and 2 in repeated CPETs [41–43]. Moreover, patients with other fatigue-inducing conditions such as multiple sclerosis (MS) and positive human immunodeficiency virus (HIV) status showed improved Workload@VT values on Test 2, in contrast to ME/CFS patients [30,44]. The present meta-analysis consists exclusively of data from studies containing control groups. Several other studies, despite having no control groups with larger patient group [45,46], and male ME/CFS patient group [46], produced similar outcomes, with ME/CFS patients' lower values of Workload@VT on Test 2 than on Test 1.

Although mitochondria-associated alterations have been observed, the underlying pathophysiology of PEM has not been explored in detail. Most recently, several groups have investigated metabolic changes in ME/CFS patients with PEM [12,47]. Naviaux et al. found reduced concentrations of specific metabolites in the plasma of 45 ME/CFS patients [47]. McGregor et al. also found altered glycolysis, a low level of acetate, and a positive correlation between urine metabolites and the severity of PEM [12]. These metabolite-based findings have been applied to the development of diagnostic tools. The metabolic response showed high validity in a diagnostic test for ME/CFS, achieving accuracy of over 95% [47]. Esfandyarpour et al. demonstrated the use of a nanoneedle to measure a metabolite-based biomarker from a small volume of blood in ME/CFS patients [48]. The present data might support a link between PEM symptom and alterations in metabolism and mitochondrial ATP production in ME/CFS.

5. Conclusions

The meta-analysis indicates a significant alteration of workload at VT especially on the 2nd day of CPET in ME/CFS patients. Accordingly, the two-day CPET could be considered as one of the potential objective assessment tools for PEM in ME/CFS patients. The present study may be of value in suggesting a direction for the development of ME/CFS diagnostic tools. However, we should consider the limitations of this study, the relatively small number of participants and the studies included. Additionally, the absence of percent predicted values for different genders should also be noted as another weak point of this study. For further studies, the following should be cautiously considered: the selection of the participants using appropriate diagnostic criteria, the severity of symptoms, the comparison of males and females, and the comparison with other fatigue-inducing disorders. Studies at larger scales with more rigorous methodology are needed.

Author Contributions: E.-J.L. searched the literature, analyzed the extracted data, and wrote manuscript. E.-B.K. and E.-S.J. participated in discussion. C.-G.S. supported writing manuscript. All authors agreed to publish the manuscript. All authors have read and agreed to the published version of the manuscript.

Funding: This study was supported by the National Research Foundation of Korea (NRF) funded by the Oriental Medicine R&D Project (NRF-2018R1A6A1A03025221).

Conflicts of Interest: There are no potential conflict of interest to disclose.

References

1. Osoba, T.; Pheby, D.; Gray, S.; Nacul, L. The Development of an Epidemiological Definition for Myalgic Encephalomyelitis/Chronic Fatigue Syndrome. *J. Chronic Fatigue Syndr.* **2007**, *14*, 61–84.
2. American ME and CFS Society. How Many People Have ME/CFS? American ME and CFS Society U.S. (U.S.): 2019. Available online: https://ammes.org/how-many-people-have-mecfs/ (accessed on 30 June 2019).
3. Institute of Medicine of the National Academes. *Beyond Myalgic Encephalomyelitis/Chronic Fatigue Syndrome; Redefining an Illness*; Committee on the Diagnostic Criteria for ME/CFS; Institute of Medicine: Washington, DC, USA; The National Academies Press: Washington, DC, USA, 2015.
4. Bethesda, M. Myalgic Encephalomyelitis/Chronic Fatigue Syndrome (ME/CFS) Research. Workshop Report. In *State of the Knowledge Workshop*; National Institutes of Health (Maryland, U.S.): Bethesda, MD, USA, 2011.
5. Devasahayam, A.; Lawn, T.; Murphy, M.; White, P.D. Alternative diagnoses to chronic fatigue syndrome in referrals to a specialist service: Service evaluation survey. *JRSM Short Rep.* **2012**, *3*, 4. [PubMed]
6. Carruthers, B.M.; Jain, A.K.; De Meirleir, K.L.; Peterson, D.L.; Klimas, N.G.; Lerner, A.M.; Bested, A.C.; Flor-Henry, P.; Joshi, P.; Powles, A.P.; et al. Myalgic Encephalomyelitis/Chronic Fatigue Syndrome. *J. Chronic Fatigue Syndr.* **2003**, *11*, 7–115.
7. Food and Drug Administration (FDA). *The Voice of the Patient: Chronic Fatigue Syndrome and Myalgic Encephalomyelitis*; Center for Drug Evaluation and Research (CDER): Bethesda, MD, USA, 2013.
8. Jason, L.A.; Porter, N.; Hunnell, J.; Brown, A.; Rademaker, A.; Richman, J.A. A natural history study of chronic fatigue syndrome. *Rehabil. Psychol.* **2011**, *56*, 32–42.
9. Jason, L.A.; Sunnquist, M.; Brown, A.; Evans, M.; Vernon, S.D.; Furst, J.D.; Simonis, V. Examining case definition criteria for chronic fatigue syndrome and myalgic encephalomyelitis. *Fatigue* **2014**, *2*, 40–56.
10. Van Ness, J.M.; Snell, C.R.; Stevens, S.R. Diminished Cardiopulmonary Capacity during Post-Exertional Malaise. *J. Chronic Fatigue Syndr.* **2007**, *14*, 77–85.
11. Ella, A. Decoding the 2-Day Cardiopulmonary Exercise Test (CPET) in Chronic Fatigue Syndrome (ME/CFS). Health Rising Finding Answers for ME/CFS and FM. 2019. Available online: https://www.healthrising.org/blog/2019/01/17/decoding-2-day-cpet-chronic-fatigue-syndrome/ (accessed on 15 February 2020).
12. McGregor, N.R.; Armstrong, C.W.; Lewis, D.P.; Gooley, P.R. Post-Exertional Malaise Is Associated with Hypermetabolism, Hypoacetylation and Purine Metabolism Deregulation in ME/CFS Cases. *Diagn. (BaselSwitz.)* **2019**, *9*, 70.
13. Albouaini, K.; Egred, M.; Alahmar, A.; Wright, D.J. Cardiopulmonary exercise testing and its application. *Postgrad. Med. J.* **2007**, *83*, 675–682.
14. Stevens, S.; Snell, C.; Stevens, J.; Keller, B.; VanNess, J.M. Cardiopulmonary Exercise Test Methodology for Assessing Exertion Intolerance in Myalgic Encephalomyelitis/Chronic Fatigue Syndrome. *Front. Pediatr.* **2018**, *6*, 242.
15. Bazelmans, E.; Bleijenberg, G.; Van Der Meer, J.W.; Folgering, H. Is physical deconditioning a perpetuating factor in chronic fatigue syndrome? A controlled study on maximal exercise performance and relations with fatigue, impairment and physical activity. *Psychol. Med.* **2001**, *31*, 107–114.
16. Cook, D.B.; Nagelkirk, P.R.; Peckerman, A.; Poluri, A.; Lamanca, J.J.; Natelson, B.H. Perceived exertion in fatiguing illness: Civilians with chronic fatigue syndrome. *Med. Sci. Sports Exerc.* **2003**, *35*, 563–568. [PubMed]
17. Cook, D.B.; Nagelkirk, P.R.; Peckerman, A.; Poluri, A.; Lamanca, J.J.; Natelson, B.H. Perceived exertion in fatiguing illness: Gulf War veterans with chronic fatigue syndrome. *Med. Sci. Sports Exerc.* **2003**, *35*, 569–574. [PubMed]
18. Moneghetti, K.J.; Skhiri, M.; Contrepois, K.; Kobayashi, Y.; Maecker, H.; Davis, M.; Snyder, M.; Haddad, F.; Montoya, J.G. Value of Circulating Cytokine Profiling During Submaximal Exercise Testing in Myalgic Encephalomyelitis/Chronic Fatigue Syndrome. *Sci. Rep.* **2018**, *8*, 2779. [PubMed]
19. Vermeulen, R.C.W.; Kurk, R.M.; Visser, F.C.; Sluiter, W.; Scholte, H.R. Patients with chronic fatigue syndrome performed worse than controls in a controlled repeated exercise study despite a normal oxidative phosphorylation capacity. *J. Transl. Med.* **2010**, *8*, 93.
20. Nelson, M.J.; Buckley, J.D.; Thomson, R.L.; Clark, D.; Kwiatek, R.; Davison, K. Diagnostic sensitivity of 2-day cardiopulmonary exercise testing in Myalgic Encephalomyelitis/Chronic Fatigue Syndrome. *J. Transl. Med.* **2019**, *17*, 80.

21. Myhill, S.; Booth, N.E.; McLaren-Howard, J. Chronic fatigue syndrome and mitochondrial dysfunction. *Int. J. Clin. Exp. Med.* **2009**, *2*, 1–16.
22. Booth, N.E.; Myhill, S.; McLaren-Howard, J. Mitochondrial dysfunction and the pathophysiology of Myalgic Encephalomyelitis/Chronic Fatigue Syndrome (ME/CFS). *Int. J. Clin. Exp. Med.* **2012**, *5*, 208–220.
23. Franklin, J.D.; Atkinson, G.; Atkinson, J.M.; Batterham, A.M. Peak oxygen uptake in chronic fatigue syndrome/myalgic encephalomyelitis: A meta-analysis. *Int. J. Clin. Exp. Med.* **2019**, *40*, 77–87.
24. Jones, D.E.; Hollingsworth, K.G.; Jakovljevic, D.G.; Fattakhova, G.; Pairman, J.; Blamire, A.M.; Trenell, M.I.; Newton, J.L. Loss of capacity to recover from acidosis on repeat exercise in chronic fatigue syndrome: A case-control study. *Eur. J. Clin. Investig.* **2012**, *42*, 186–194.
25. Higgins, J.P.T.; Thompson, S.G. Quantifying heterogeneity in a meta-analysis. *Stat. Med.* **2002**, *21*, 1539–1558.
26. The Cochrane Collaboration. *Review Manager (RevMan)*; Computer program, Version 5.3; The Cochrane Collaboration: London, UK, 2020.
27. Wells, G.A.; Shea, B.; O'Connell, D.; Peterson, J.; Welch, V.; Losos, M.; Tugwell, P. The Newcastle-Ottawa Scale (NOS) for Assessing the Quality of Nonrandomized Studies in Meta-Analyses. Available online: http://www.ohri.ca/programs/clinical_epidemiology/oxford.asp (accessed on 20 June 2020).
28. Carruthers, B.M.; van de Sande, M.I.; De Meirleir, K.L.; Klimas, N.G.; Broderick, G.; Mitchell, T.; Staines, D.; Powles, A.P.; Speight, N.; Vallings, R.; et al. Myalgic encephalomyelitis: International Consensus Criteria. *J. Intern. Med.* **2011**, *270*, 327–338. [CrossRef] [PubMed]
29. Snell, C.R.; Stevens, S.R.; Davenport, T.E.; Van Ness, J.M. Discriminative Validity of Metabolic and Workload Measurements for Identifying People with Chronic Fatigue Syndrome. *Phys. Ther.* **2013**, *93*, 1484–1492. [CrossRef] [PubMed]
30. Hodges, L.D.; Nielsen, T.; Baken, D. Physiological measures in participants with chronic fatigue syndrome, multiple sclerosis and healthy controls following repeated exercise: A pilot study. *Clin. Physiol. Funct. Imaging* **2018**, *38*, 639–644. [CrossRef] [PubMed]
31. Spriet, L.L. Anaerobic metabolism during exercise. In *Exercise Metabolism*, 2nd ed.; Hargreaves, M., Spriet, L.L., Eds.; Human Kinetics: Champaign, IL, USA, 2006; pp. 7–27.
32. Stephens, C. *MEA Summary Review: The role of Mitochondria in ME/CFS*; The ME Association: Buckinghamshire, UK, 12 July 2019; Available online: https://meassociation.org.uk/2019/07/mea-summary-review-the-role-of-mitochondria-in-me-cfs-13-july-2019/ (accessed on 10 July 2020).
33. Tomas, C.; Brown, A.; Strassheim, V.; Elson, J.L.; Newton, J.; Manning, P. Cellular bioenergetics is impaired in patients with chronic fatigue syndrome. *PLoS ONE* **2017**, *12*, e0186802. [CrossRef] [PubMed]
34. Billing-Ross, P.; Germain, A.; Ye, K.; Keinan, A.; Gu, Z.; Hanson, M.R. Mitochondrial DNA variants correlate with symptoms in myalgic encephalomyelitis/chronic fatigue syndrome. *J. Transl. Med.* **2016**, *14*, 19. [CrossRef]
35. Tomas, C.; Elson, J.L. The role of mitochondria in ME/CFS: A perspective. *Fatigue Biomed. Health Behav.* **2019**, *7*, 52–58. [CrossRef]
36. Lawson, N.; Hsieh, C.-H.; March, D.; Wang, X. Elevated Energy Production in Chronic Fatigue Syndrome Patients. *J. Nat. Sci.* **2016**, *2*, e221.
37. Rasa, S.; Nora-Krukle, Z.; Henning, N.; Eliassen, E.; Shikova, E.; Harrer, T.; Scheibenbogen, C.; Murovska, M.; Prusty, B.K. Chronic viral infections in myalgic encephalomyelitis/chronic fatigue syndrome (ME/CFS). *J. Transl. Med.* **2018**, *16*, 268. [CrossRef]
38. Morris, G.; Maes, M. Mitochondrial dysfunctions in myalgic encephalomyelitis/chronic fatigue syndrome explained by activated immuno-inflammatory, oxidative and nitrosative stress pathways. *Metab. Brain Dis.* **2014**, *29*, 19–36. [CrossRef]
39. Morris, G.; Stubbs, B.; Köhler, C.A.; Walder, K.; Slyepchenko, A.; Berk, M.; Carvalho, A.F. The putative role of oxidative stress and inflammation in the pathophysiology of sleep dysfunction across neuropsychiatric disorders: Focus on chronic fatigue syndrome, bipolar disorder and multiple sclerosis. *Sleep Med. Rev.* **2018**, *41*, 255–265. [CrossRef]
40. Fluge, Ø.; Mella, O.; Bruland, O.; Risa, K.; Dyrstad, S.E.; Alme, K.; Rekeland, I.G.; Sapkota, D.; Røsland, G.V.; Fosså, A.; et al. Metabolic profiling indicates impaired pyruvate dehydrogenase function in myalgic encephalopathy/chronic fatigue syndrome. *JCI Insight* **2016**, *1*, e89376. [CrossRef] [PubMed]
41. Koufaki, P.; Naish, P.F.; Mercer, T.H. Reproducibility of exercise tolerance in patients with end-stage renal disease. *Arch. Phys. Med. Rehabil.* **2001**, *82*, 1421–1424. [CrossRef] [PubMed]

42. Selig, S.E.; Carey, M.F.; Menzies, D.G.; Patterson, J.; Geerling, R.H.; Williams, A.D.; Bamroongsuk, V.; Toia, D.; Krum, H.; Hare, D.L. Reliability of isokinetic strength and aerobic power testing for patients with chronic heart failure. *J. Cardiopulm. Rehabil.* **2002**, *22*, 282–289. [CrossRef] [PubMed]
43. Hansen, J.E.; Sun, X.G.; Yasunobu, Y.; Garafano, R.P.; Gates, G.; Barst, R.J.; Wasserman, K. Reproducibility of cardiopulmonary exercise measurements in patients with pulmonary arterial hypertension. *Chest* **2004**, *126*, 816–824. [CrossRef] [PubMed]
44. Larson, B.; Davenport, T.E.; Stevens, S.R.; Van Ness, J.M.; Snell, C.R. Reproducibility of measurements obtained during cardiopulmonary exercise testing in individuals with and without fatiguing health conditions: A case series. *Cardiopulm. Phys. Ther. J.* **2019**, *30*, 145–152. [CrossRef]
45. Keller, B.A.; Pryor, J.L.; Giloteaux, L. Inability of myalgic encephalomyelitis/chronic fatigue syndrome patients to reproduce VO$_2$peak indicates functional impairment. *J. Transl. Med.* **2014**, *12*, 104. [CrossRef] [PubMed]
46. van Campen, C.; Rowe, P.; Visser, F. Validity of 2-Day Cardiopulmonary Exercise Testing in Male Patients with Myalgic Encephalomyelitis/Chronic Fatigue Syndrome. *Adv. Phys. Educ.* **2020**, *10*, 68–80. [CrossRef]
47. Naviaux, R.K.; Naviaux, J.C.; Li, K.; Bright, A.T.; Alaynick, W.A.; Wang, L.; Baxter, A.; Nathan, N.; Anderson, W.; Gordon, E. Metabolic features of chronic fatigue syndrome. *Proc. Natl. Acad. Sci. USA* **2016**, *113*, E5472–E5480. [CrossRef]
48. Esfandyarpour, R.; Kashi, A.; Nemat-Gorgani, M.; Wilhelmy, J.; Davis, R.W. A nanoelectronics-blood-based diagnostic biomarker for myalgic encephalomyelitis/chronic fatigue syndrome (ME/CFS). *Proc. Natl. Acad. Sci. USA* **2019**, *116*, 10250–10257. [CrossRef]

Publisher's Note: MDPI stays neutral with regard to jurisdictional claims in published maps and institutional affiliations.

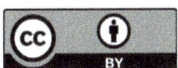

© 2020 by the authors. Licensee MDPI, Basel, Switzerland. This article is an open access article distributed under the terms and conditions of the Creative Commons Attribution (CC BY) license (http://creativecommons.org/licenses/by/4.0/).

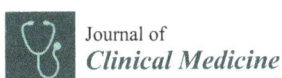

Review

Systematic Review of Primary Outcome Measurements for Chronic Fatigue Syndrome/Myalgic Encephalomyelitis (CFS/ME) in Randomized Controlled Trials

Do-Young Kim [1], Jin-Seok Lee [2] and Chang-Gue Son [2,*]

[1] Department of Korean Medicine, Korean Medical College of Daejeon University, 62, Daehak-ro, Dong-gu, Daejeon 34520, Korea; 95kent@naver.com
[2] Institute of Bioscience & Integrative Medicine, Dunsan Oriental Hospital of Daejeon University, 75, Daedeok-daero 176, Seo-gu, Daejeon 35235, Korea; neptune@dju.kr
* Correspondence: ckson@dju.ac.kr

Received: 9 October 2020; Accepted: 26 October 2020; Published: 28 October 2020

Abstract: Background: Due to its unknown etiology, the objective diagnosis and therapeutics of chronic fatigue syndrome/myalgic encephalomyelitis (CFS/ME) are still challenging. Generally, the patient-reported outcome (PRO) is the major strategy driving treatment response because the patient is the most important judge of whether changes are meaningful. Methods: In order to determine the overall characteristics of the main outcome measurement applied in clinical trials for CFS/ME, we systematically surveyed the literature using two electronic databases, PubMed and the Cochrane Library, throughout June 2020. We analyzed randomized controlled trials (RCTs) for CFS/ME focusing especially on main measurements. Results: Fifty-two RCTs out of a total 540 searched were selected according to eligibility criteria. Thirty-one RCTs (59.6%) used single primary outcome and others adapted ≥2 kinds of measurements. In total, 15 PRO-derived tools were adapted (50 RCTs; 96.2%) along with two behavioral measurements for adolescents (4 RCTs; 7.7%). The 36-item Short Form Health Survey (SF-36; 16 RCTs), Checklist Individual Strength (CIS; 14 RCTs), and Chalder Fatigue Questionnaire (CFQ; 11 RCTs) were most frequently used as the main outcomes. Since the first RCT in 1996, Clinical Global Impression (CGI) and SF-36 have been dominantly used each in the first and following decade (26.1% and 28.6%, respectively), while both CIS and Multidimensional Fatigue Inventory (MFI) have been the preferred instruments (21.4% each) in recent years (2016 to 2020). Conclusions: This review comprehensively provides the choice pattern of the assessment tools for interventions in RCTs for CFS/ME. Our data would be helpful practically in the design of clinical studies for CFS/ME-related therapeutic development.

Keywords: chronic fatigue syndrome; myalgic encephalomyelitis; RCT; measurement

1. Introduction

Chronic fatigue syndrome/myalgic encephalomyelitis (CFS/ME) is a debilitating disease characterized by medically unexplained chronic severe fatigue for at least 6 months along with key symptoms such as unrefreshing sleep, postexertion malaise (PEM), impairments in memory or concentration, and/or orthostatic intolerance [1]. The daily lives of patients are heavily impeded, which leads to unemployment for approximately half of patients and being home- or bed-bound for one quarter [2]. The prevalence of CFS/ME is suggested to be approximately 1–2% worldwide [3], and the annual economic cost for medical care is estimated to be up to USD 10,000 per patient in the US [4].

Although various etiologies of CFS/ME, such as autonomic and neurological dysfunction, abnormalities in mitochondrial function, and aberrant gut microbiota, have been hypothesized, they have not yet been clearly revealed [5]. Recently, this disease has become considered a multisystem neuroimmune disease [1]. To date, various randomized controlled trials (RCTs) for therapeutics have been conducted; however, no effective therapy for CFS/ME exists [6]. Recently, the PACE trial, a large-scale clinical study of cognitive behavior therapy (CBT) and graded-exercise therapy (GET), was reported to be effective for CFS/ME [7]. There is however a fair amount of controversy surrounding this PACE trial, likely due to the debates regarding its efficacy and criticisms by researchers and patients due to judgments of restoration as well as side effects [8].

On the other hand, the absence of objective biomarkers of CFS/ME raises a problem for the actual diagnosis of this illness. In addition, clinical evaluations of treatment responses are also dependent on self-reported assessments of symptom severity, leading to potential trouble during the investigation of new therapeutics [9]. Accordingly, methodologically well-designed tools to assess the valuable responses of treatments for CFS/ME are very important. To date, diverse patient-reported outcome (PRO) measurements have been developed and used to assess fatigue status in clinics, such as the Checklist Individual Strength (CIS) scale, Chalder Fatigue Questionnaire (CFQ), and Multidimensional Fatigue Inventory (MFI) [10–12]. Many clinical studies, however, have adopted various fatigue-nonspecific instruments, including the 36-item Short Form Health Survey (SF-36), Clinical Global Impression (CGI), and Sickness Impact Profile-8 (SIP-8) [13–15]. In fact, researchers need to carefully review the available measurements and choose the most optimized one for the purpose of their own clinical studies. However, it is not easy for researchers to choose the appropriate measurement instruments for CFS/ME-related studies due to the absence of well-established international guidelines.

To identify the assessment tools that help in the clinical study process for CFS/ME, we comprehensively reviewed the primary measurements used in RCTs and determined changes in the use of these measurements.

2. Methods

2.1. Data Sources and Search Terms

In accordance with the Preferred Reporting Items for Systematic Reviews and Meta-Analysis (PRISMA) guidelines [16], a systematic literature survey was performed using two electronic literature databases, PubMed and the Cochrane Library, throughout June 2020. The search terms were encephalomyelitis/chronic fatigue syndrome, ME/CFS, encephalomyelitis, ME, chronic fatigue syndrome, CFS, randomized controlled trial, RCT, and clinical trial. The trial type was limited to RCTs, and all languages were included.

2.2. Eligibility Criteria

Selected articles for this study were determined by the following inclusion criteria: (1) RCTs or randomized controlled crossover trials, (2) patients with CFS/ME as participants, (3) an evaluation of the efficacy of the intervention for CFS/ME treatment, and (4) fatigue-related measurement or outcome. The exclusion criteria were as follows: (1) articles with no full text and (2) studies without mention of the primary or main outcome. We did not have a criterion based on the number of participants in RCTs.

2.3. Data Extraction and Analysis

We extracted data on general features of RCTs, such as the number of participants, age, intervention, and treatment period, along with the primary outcome measurement instrument (subscales, items, range of scores, versions, and application of cutoff scores for recruitment).

As a descriptive analysis, this study did not need to apply statistical analyses. Regarding the treatment period, the mean and standard deviation (SD) are presented.

3. Results

3.1. General Characteristics of RCTs

A total of 540 articles were initially identified from the PubMed and Cochran databases, and 52 articles met the inclusion criteria for this study (Figure 1). Forty-eight RCTs (92.3%) were performed with adult patients ($n = 5872$), while 4 RCTs (7.7%) were performed with adolescent subjects ($n = 387$). Twenty-six RCTs evaluated the efficacy of pharmacologic interventions, and 27 RCTs were conducted to evaluate nonpharmacologic interventions. The mean treatment period was 15.0 ± 9.3 weeks (Table 1).

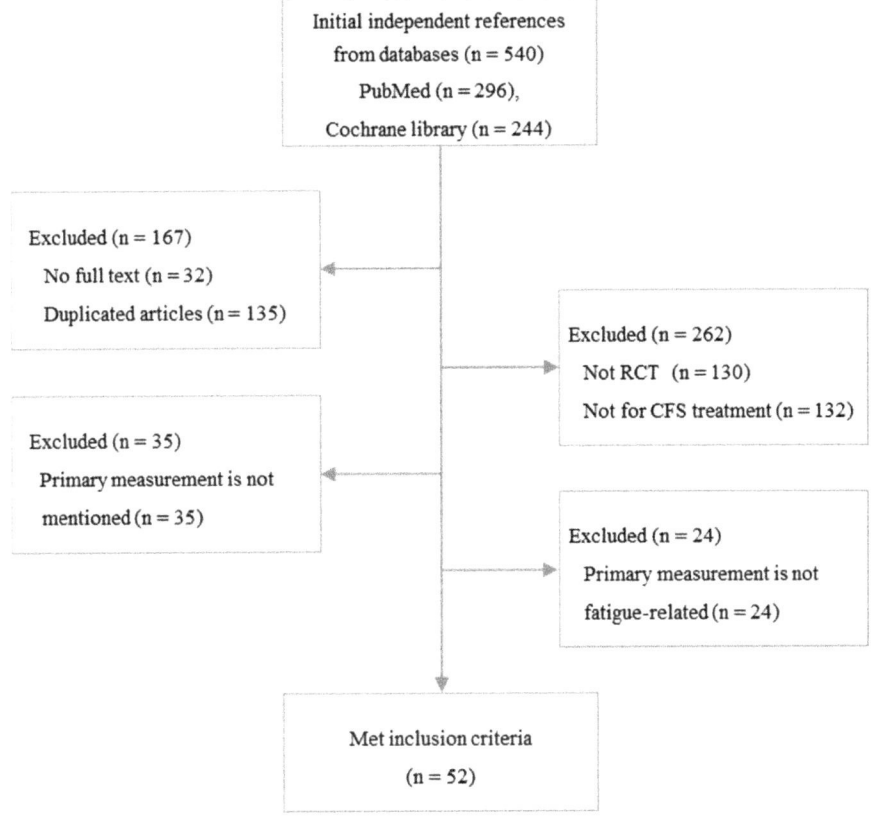

Figure 1. Flow chart of the study.

In terms of the number of primary outcomes in RCTs, 31 RCTs (59.6%) used a single primary outcome (29 RCTs with adults and 2 RCTs with adolescents). Fifteen RCTs (28.8%) adopted two kinds of main measurements (with adult patients), while six RCTs (11.5%) used three kinds of measurements (four RCTs with adults and two with adolescents) as a primary outcome (Table 1).

Table 1. Study characteristics.

Items	Adults	Adolescents	Total
[A] Total RCT (%)	48 (92.3)	4 (7.7)	52 (100.0)
N. of participants (female)	5872 (4437)	387 (302)	6259 (4739)
Treatment period (mean weeks)	14.1 ± 8.2	25.3 ± 16.4	15.0 ± 9.3
RCT for pharmaceutical intervention (%)	25 (96.2)	1 (3.8)	[B] 26 (100.0)
RCT for nonpharmaceutical intervention (%)	24 (88.9)	3 (11.1)	[B] 27 (100.0)
N. of primary outcomes in RCT (%)			
One primary measurement	29 (93.5)	2 (6.5)	31 (100.0)
Two primary measurements	15 (100.0)	0 (0.0)	15 (100.0)
Three primary measurements	4 (66.7)	2 (33.3)	6 (100.0)
Methodological classification of measurement instrument (%)			
RCT with behavioral measurement	0 (0.0)	4 (100.0)	4 (100.0)
Kinds of measurement	0 (0.0)	2 (100.0)	2 (100.0)
RCT with survey-based measurement	48 (96.0)	2 (4.0)	50 (100.0)
[C] Kinds of measurement	14 (93.3)	3 (20.0)	15 (100.0)
Criteria for participant recruitment (%)			
[D] RCT used measurement-based cutoff score	17 (94.4)	1 (5.6)	18 (100.0)
Behavioral score	0 (0.0)	1 (100.0)	1 (100.0)
[C] Survey-based score	6 (85.7)	2 (28.6)	7 (100.0)

[A] The detailed information for the whole RCT list is summarized in Supplementary Table S1. [B] One RCT used both pharmacologic and nonpharmacologic interventions (fluoxetine + graded exercise therapy). [C] Some items were applied multiple times; thus, the total percentage was larger than 100%. [D] Eighteen RCTs applied a cutoff score for inclusion criteria.

3.2. Characteristics of Primary Measurements in RCTs

As shown in Figure 2, the 52 RCTs used 17 kinds of methodological instruments, which were classified into survey-based measurements (15 instruments in 50 RCTs) and behavioral measurements (two instruments in four RCTs). All RCTs with adults adopted survey-based measurements, while four RCTs with adolescent patients adopted behavioral (two RCTs) and/or survey-based (two RCTs) measurements (Table 1).

Among the 17 kinds of instruments, the SF-36 was most frequently used (30.8%), followed by the CIS (26.9%), CFQ (21.2%), CGI (13.5%), MFI (11.5%), and SIP-8 (11.5%) (Table 2). Twenty-four RCTs adopted at least one subscale score from these measurement instruments, most commonly the fatigue severity score of CIS (12 RCTs) or physical function score of SF-36 (10 RCTs) (Table 2). Alternatively, these instrument-derived scores were applied as cutoff scores for participant inclusion, such as the fatigue severity score of the CIS (11 RCTs), total score of the SIP-8 (six RCTs), physical function score of the SF-36 (four RCTs), and total score of the CFQ (four RCTs) (Supplementary Table S1).

Table 2. Measurement instruments in RCTs.

Scale	N. of RCTs (%)	Measurement and Structure of Items	Subscale for Primary Outcome (N. of RCTs) (Reference)
SF-36	16 (30.8)	Assess functional impairment in eight areas summarized as physical and mental function.	Total score (4) [17–20] Physical function (10) [7,21–29] Physical + social function (1) [30] [A] Mental health summary (1) [31]
CIS	14 (26.9)	Covers several aspects of fatigue, such as severity, concentration, motivation, and physical activity.	Total score (2) [32,33] Fatigue severity (12) [17,23,25,28,30,34–40]
CFQ	11 (21.2)	Measures fatigue severity with items categorized into physical and mental fatigue.	Total score (10) [7,21,24,26,27,41–45] Physical score (1) [46]
CGI	7 (13.5)	Provides a global rating of illness severity and improvement through single Likert scale.	Single item score (7) [44,47–52]
MFI	6 (11.5)	Evaluates five dimensions of fatigue: general, physical, mental fatigue, reduced motivation, and reduced activity.	Total score (4) [53–56] General fatigue (2) [57,58]
SIP-8	6 (11.5)	Measures dysfunction through everyday behavior. Items are summarized into psychosocial, physical, and independent dimensions.	Total score (6) [23,25,37–40]
FSS	4 (7.7)	Measures the severity of fatigue and its effect on a person's activities and lifestyle, with no particular subscales.	Total score (4) [53,59–61]
VAS	4 (7.7)	Through Likert scale items, assesses subjective characteristics that cannot be directly measured.	Single item score (2) [33,53] Fatigue symptom (2) [20,62]
SAR	3 (5.8)	Measures overall health status of adolescents with school attendance rate.	Attendance rate (3) [28,36,63]
[B] APS	2 (3.8)	Measures fatigue status through survey designed by authors of RCT according to 1994 CDC criteria.	Fatigue severity (1) [64] Symptom checklist (1) [39]
BRIEF-A	1 (2.0)	Evaluates an adult's executive functions of self-regulation in everyday environment of patient. Subscales are summarized in behavioral regulation and metacognition.	Total score (1) [65]
CHQ-CF	1 (2.0)	Measures health-related quality of life for adolescents. Items are within 9 subscales that focus on neurologic and psychologic domains.	Physical function (1) [36]
CPRS-15	1 (2.0)	Assesses severity of psychiatric symptoms and observed behavior. Items focus on symptoms of mental disorder.	Total score (1) [50]
FIS	1 (2.0)	Measures the symptom of fatigue as part of an underlying chronic disease or condition. Items are divided into cognitive, physical, and psychosocial functioning.	Total score (1) [66]
MFS	1 (2.0)	Has strength in evaluating psychiatric symptoms with no subcategorization of 15 items.	Total score (1) [47]
N. of steps	1 (2.0)	Evaluates general health status by measuring the number of steps per day.	Number of steps per day (1) [67]

[A] Mental health summary includes vitality, social function, role function/emotional, and mental health subscales.
[B] There were 2 kinds of nonestablished measurements which authors of RCTs produced. APS: author-produced scale, BRIEF-A: Behavior Rating Inventory of Executive Function—Adult version, CFQ: Chalder Fatigue Questionnaire, CGI: Clinical Global Impression, CHQ-CF: Child Health Questionnaire—Child Form, CIS: Checklist Individual Strength, CPRS-15: Comprehensive Psychopathological Rating Scale-15, FIS: Fatigue Impact Scale, FSS: Fatigue Severity Scale, MFI: Multidimensional Fatigue Inventory, MFS: Mental Fatigue Scale, SAR: school attendance rate, SF-36: 36-item Short Form Health Survey, SIP-8: Sickness Impact Profile-8, VAS: visual analog scale.

3.3. Quinquennial Distribution of Primary Measurements for RCTs

Since the first report of an RCT for CFS/ME using GET in 1997, the number of RCTs has increased, reaching a maximum from 2011 to 2015 (17 RCTs) (Figure 2). In the earliest decade (1996–2005), the CGI was dominantly used as a measurement instrument as the primary outcome in RCTs (6 out of 15 RCTs). During the following decade (2006–2015), the SF-36, CIS, and CFQ were preferred (19 out of 27 RCTs). In the last 5 years (2016–2020), the CIS and MFI have been frequently employed as primary outcome measurements (6 out of 10 RCTs) (Figure 2).

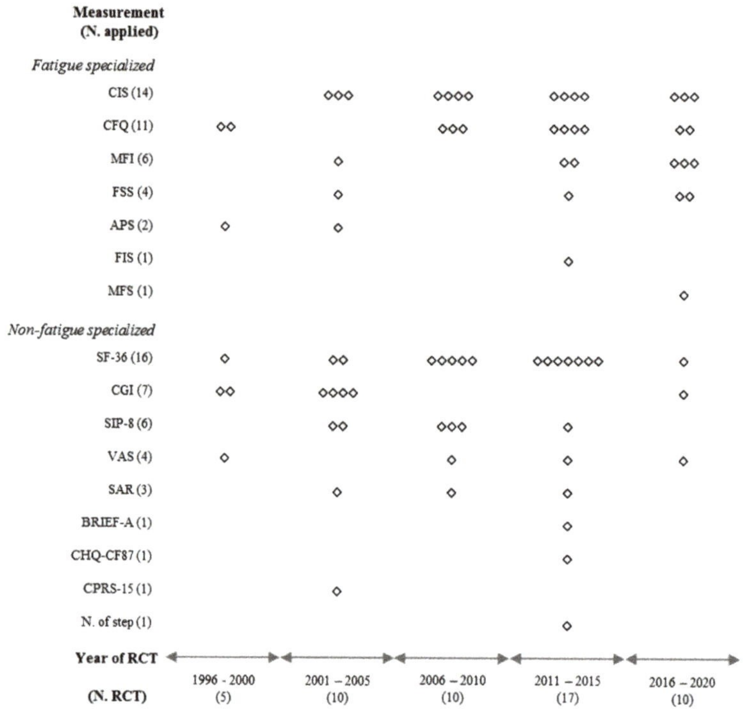

Measurement (N. applied)	1996 – 2000	2001 – 2005	2006 – 2010	2011 – 2015	2016 – 2020
Fatigue specialized					
CIS (14)		◇◇◇	◇◇◇◇	◇◇◇◇	◇◇◇
CFQ (11)	◇◇		◇◇◇	◇◇◇◇	◇◇
MFI (6)		◇		◇◇	◇◇◇
FSS (4)		◇		◇	◇◇
APS (2)	◇	◇			
FIS (1)				◇	
MFS (1)					◇
Non-fatigue specialized					
SF-36 (16)	◇	◇◇	◇◇◇◇◇	◇◇◇◇◇◇◇	◇
CGI (7)	◇◇	◇◇◇◇			◇
SIP-8 (6)		◇◇	◇◇◇	◇	
VAS (4)	◇		◇	◇	◇
SAR (3)		◇	◇	◇	
BRIEF-A (1)				◇	
CHQ-CF87 (1)				◇	
CPRS-15 (1)		◇			
N. of step (1)			◇		
Year of RCT (N. RCT)	1996 – 2000 (5)	2001 – 2005 (10)	2006 – 2010 (10)	2011 – 2015 (17)	2016 – 2020 (10)

Figure 2. Graphical display for quinquennial distribution of primary measurements.

4. Discussion

In terms of CFS/ME, a symptom-based approach is a key strategy for not only therapy but also diagnosis because of its unknown etiology [1]. The Centers for Disease Control and Prevention (CDC) recommended symptomatic treatment based on the case definition of the Institute of Medicine (IOM) for providing alternative care for patients [68]. The subjective complaints and comprehension of the PROs are crucial in the diagnostic process as well as in evaluating therapeutic responses in clinical practice for CFS/ME. To provide practical guidance in choosing a suitable measurement in clinical studies for CFS/ME, we analyzed the primary outcome measurements in RCTs conducted to date.

Unlike common guidelines recommending single primary outcome measurement in RCTs [69], 21 (40.4%) of the 52 RCTs employed multiple primary measurements (Table 1). This might be due to the absence of a well-established measurement tool specialized for CFS/ME. Among the 17 tools used in the 52 RCTs, only two behavioral measurements (school attendance rate and the number of steps per day) were adopted in four RCTs that enrolled only adolescent participants (Table 1). It is generally well known that adolescent patients show a poorer school attendance rate than healthy controls [70]. The remaining RCTs (50 RCTs with 15 different tools) employed survey-based PRO measurements, likely for many subjective symptoms or disorders, including migraine, major depressive disorder, or anxiety [71–73]. We classified the measurements into two groups: nine nonfatigue specialized tools employed mainly in an earlier decade (1996 to 2005) and eight fatigue-specialized measurements which have been dominant since 2016 (Figure 2).

The SF-36, not specialized for fatigue, is the most frequently used measurement based on our data (16 RCTs) (Table 2). It has been broadly applied for measuring patients' general health status in reference to health-related quality of life (HRQOL). It is well recognized that the HRQOL of CFS/ME sufferers is notoriously poor and has been linked to a 7-fold higher risk of suicide than healthy controls [74,75]. Therefore, the SF-36, especially the physical functioning subscale, was steadily employed as a primary measurement until 2015, often supportively combined with other fatigue-specialized measurements (10 RCTs), such as the CIS or CFQ. Likewise, the SIP-8 score assessing dysfunction of daily behaviors has been used as part of the primary outcome coupled with fatigue-specialized tools (Supplementary Table S1).

In regard to fatigue-specialized instruments, the fatigue severity subscale of the CIS and the total score of the CFQ (11-item version) were dominantly employed (Table 2). Both have been commonly endorsed for the evaluation of psychometric fatigue status in RCTs for CFS/ME and other disorders, including rheumatoid arthritis and fibromyalgia [76]. Both instruments assess not only physical but also mental fatigue status, such as concentration and motivation, and they are known to show a very high correlation in assessing fatigue severity [77]. In particular, the CFQ was employed mostly in trials conducted in the UK (9/11 adoptions), while the CIS was preferred in the Netherlands (12/14 adoptions). On the other hand, the MFI, markedly preferred in recent studies along with the CIS, was originally developed for assessing multifarious fatigue status in patients with cancer [12]. The MFI was one of the measures in the Wichita clinical study assessing over 30 kinds of measurements or parameters for CFS/ME in 2005, and the MFI was proven as a valid measurement [78]. Recently, the MFI was applied in a large-scale study to explore the cytokine signature that showed a positive correlation between serum levels of TGF-β and the severity of CFS/ME [79]. Both the MFI and CIS were created by Dutch researchers and contain 20 nearly identical questionnaire items. However, they have some differences in measurement method strategies: a maximum of 140 points with 7-point scales on the CIS versus a maximum of 100 points with 5-point scales on the MFI (Supplementary Table S2). Unlike the CFQ-11, the MFI and CIS adopt both positive and negative questions and measure PEM-related symptoms such as "I am tired very quickly or easily", which is focused on as one of the recently established hallmark symptoms of CFS/ME [1].

In fact, numerous studies certified the validity and reliability of these commonly used instruments for CFS/ME, such as the CFQ-11, CIS, and MFI [10,78,80], while some researchers have pointed out the ceiling effects of these measurements, especially in clinical trials for treatments [81,82]. They are concerned with the possibility that sufferers of CFS/ME tend to report scores close to maximum, thereby hindering the accurate reflection of treatment response and the baseline condition. Most measurement tools (including CFS/ME-specific instruments) have non-CFS/ME-specific questionnaires, such as "I feel tired" or "I feel weak", which are frequently complained of among general populations. Accordingly, many trials (most RCTs adopted CIS-based primary outcome) used cutoff scores in the process of participant inclusion (Supplementary Table S1). On the other hand, responders to the CFQ-11 will obtain high scores due to comparisons with "usual" or "last well-state". Because most CFS patients have experienced many years of the disease with fluctuating symptoms, assessment methods involving comparisons to "usual" can hardly reflect not only deterioration in status but also treatment response [2]. Thus, some studies have adopted a modified CFQ-11 as a 10-point Likert scale (from 0 points for healthy conditions to 9 points for the worst status) in RCTs for drug development related to CFS/ME [41].

Although no confirmative pathophysiology of CFS/ME has been identified, some new findings have been highlighted, such as aberrant composition of the gut microbiome and altered serotonergic metabolism within the brain [83,84]. In addition, several studies investigating objective parameters for diagnostic and severity assessments, including elevated levels of TGF-β and nanoelectronic assays, have been conducted [79,85]. One group also found a reduction of red blood cell deformability in patients with CFS/ME [86]. Along with these advances in knowledge, it is necessary that a CFS/ME-specialized measurement instrument be developed to reflect the clinical severity and treatment response and objective biomarkers be discovered to ensure CFS/ME.

5. Conclusions

This systematic review provides a comprehensive overview of the choice of primary measurements in RCTs for CFS/ME to date. Approximately 40% of RCTs applied multiple primary measurements.

Of the 17 kinds of measurement tools, the SF-36 (nonfatigue specific measurement) had been most frequently applied through 2015, while two fatigue-specific measurements, the CIS and MFI, have been frequently employed in recent trials. Our data will be helpful in the practical design of clinical studies for CFS/ME-related therapeutic development.

Supplementary Materials: The following are available online at http://www.mdpi.com/2077-0383/9/11/3463/s1, Table S1: Summary of RCTs included in this review, Table S2: General characteristics of self-reported survey measurements used in RCTs.

Author Contributions: D.-Y.K. searched the literature, then extracted and analyzed the data. J.-S.L. participated in discussion. D.-Y.K. and C.-G.S. wrote the manuscript. C.-G.S. supervised the whole process of this study with initial design. All authors have read and agreed to the published version of the manuscript.

Funding: This research was supported by the National Research Foundation of Korea (NRF) grant funded by the Ministry of Science, ICT & Future Planning (NRF-2018R1A6A1A03025221).

Conflicts of Interest: The authors have no conflicts of interest to declare.

References

1. Institute of Medicine of the National Academes. *Beyond Myalgic Encephalomyelitis/Chronic Fatigue Syndrome: Redefining an Illness*; Committee on the diagnostic criteria for ME/CFS; Institute of Medicine: Washington, DC, USA, 2015.
2. Castro-Marrero, J.; Faro, M.; Zaragozá, M.C.; Aliste, L.; De Sevilla, T.F.; Alegre, J. Unemployment and work disability in individuals with chronic fatigue syndrome/myalgic encephalomyelitis: A community-based cross-sectional study from Spain. *BMC Public Health* **2019**, *19*, 1–13. [CrossRef] [PubMed]
3. Lim, E.-J.; Ahn, Y.-C.; Jang, E.-S.; Lee, S.-W.; Lee, S.-H.; Son, C.-G. Systematic review and meta-analysis of the prevalence of chronic fatigue syndrome/myalgic encephalomyelitis (CFS/ME). *J. Transl. Med.* **2020**, *18*, 1–15. [CrossRef] [PubMed]
4. Jason, L.A.; Benton, M.C.; Valentine, L.M.; Johnson, A.; Torres-Harding, S.R. The Economic impact of ME/CFS: Individual and societal costs. *Dyn. Med.* **2008**, *7*, 6. [CrossRef] [PubMed]
5. Missailidis, D.; Annesley, S.J.; Fisher, P.R. Pathological Mechanisms Underlying Myalgic Encephalomyelitis/Chronic Fatigue Syndrome. *Diagnostics* **2019**, *9*, 80. [CrossRef] [PubMed]
6. Kim, D.-Y.; Lee, J.-S.; Park, S.-Y.; Kim, S.-J.; Son, C.-G. Systematic review of randomized controlled trials for chronic fatigue syndrome/myalgic encephalomyelitis (CFS/ME). *J. Transl. Med.* **2020**, *18*, 7–12. [CrossRef]
7. White, P.D.; Goldsmith, K.A.; Johnson, A.L.; Potts, L.; Walwyn, R.; De Cesare, J.C.; Baber, H.L.; Burgess, M.; Clark, L.V.; Cox, D.L.; et al. Comparison of adaptive pacing therapy, cognitive behavior therapy, graded exercise therapy, and specialist medical care for chronic fatigue syndrome (PACE): A randomised trial. *Lancet* **2011**, *377*, 823–836. [CrossRef]
8. Shepherd, C.B. PACE trial claims for recovery in myalgic encephalomyelitis/chronic fatigue syndrome—true or false? It's time for an independent review of the methodology and results. *J. Health Psychol.* **2017**, *22*, 1187–1191. [CrossRef]
9. Cleare, A.J.; Reid, S.; Chalder, T.; Hotopf, M.; Wessely, S. Chronic fatigue syndrome. *BMJ Clin. Evid.* **2015**, *2015*, 1101.
10. Vercoulen, J.H.; Swanink, C.M.; Fennis, J.F.; Galama, J.M.; Van Der Meer, J.W.; Bleijenberg, G. Dimensional assessment of chronic fatigue syndrome. *J. Psychosom. Res.* **1994**, *38*, 383–392. [CrossRef]
11. Chalder, T.; Berelowitz, G.; Pawlikowska, T.; Watts, L.; Wessely, S.; Wright, D.; Wallace, E. Development of a fatigue scale. *J. Psychosom. Res.* **1993**, *37*, 147–153. [CrossRef]
12. Smets, E.; Garssen, B.; Bonke, B.; De Haes, J. The multidimensional Fatigue Inventory (MFI) psychometric qualities of an instrument to assess fatigue. *J. Psychosom. Res.* **1995**, *39*, 315–325. [CrossRef]
13. Stewart, A.L.; Hays, R.D.; Ware, J.E. The MOS Short-form General Health Survey. *Med. Care* **1988**, *26*, 724–735. [CrossRef]
14. Guy, W. *ECDEU Assessment Manual for Psychopharmacology*; U.S. Department of Health, Education, and Welfare: Washington, DC, USA, 1976.
15. Bergner, M.; Bobbitt, R.A.; Carter, W.B.; Gilson, B.S. The Sickness Impact Profile: Development and Final Revision of a Health Status Measure. *Med. Care* **1981**, *19*, 787–805. [CrossRef]

16. Moher, D.; Liberati, A.; Tetzlaff, J.; Altman, D.G.; Prisma Group. Preferred reporting items for systematic reviews and meta-analyses: The PRISMA statement. *BMJ* **2009**, *339*, b2535. [CrossRef]
17. Vos-Vromans, D.C.W.M.; Smeets, R.J.E.M.; Huijnen, I.P.J.; Köke, A.J.; Hitters, W.M.G.C.; Rijnders, L.J.M.; Pont, M.; Winkens, B.; Knottnerus, J.A. Multidisciplinary rehabilitation treatment versus cognitive behavioural therapy for patients with chronic fatigue syndrome: A randomized controlled trial. *J. Intern. Med.* **2015**, *279*, 268–282. [CrossRef]
18. Núñez, M.; Fernández-Solà, J.; Nuñez, E.; Fernández-Huerta, J.-M.; Godás-Sieso, T.; Gómez-Gil, E. Health-related quality of life in patients with chronic fatigue syndrome: Group cognitive behavioural therapy and graded exercise versus usual treatment. A randomised controlled trial with 1 year of follow-up. *Clin. Rheumatol.* **2011**, *30*, 381–389. [CrossRef]
19. O'Dowd, H.; Gladwell, P.; Rogers, C.A.; Hollinghurst, S.; Gregory, A. Cognitive behavioural therapy in chronic fatigue syndrome: A randomised controlled trial of an outpatient group programme. *Health Technol. Assess.* **2006**, *10*, 1–121. [CrossRef]
20. Peterson, P.K.; Pheley, A.; Schroeppel, J.; Schenck, C.; Marshall, P.; Kind, A.; Haugland, J.M.; Lambrecht, L.J.; Swan, S.; Goldsmith, S. A preliminary placebo-controlled crossover trial of fludrocortisone for chronic fatigue syndrome. *Arch. Intern. Med.* **1998**, *158*, 908–914. [CrossRef]
21. Clark, L.V.; Pesola, F.; Thomas, J.M.; Vergara-Williamson, M.; Beynon, M.; White, P.D. Guided graded exercise self-help plus specialist medical care versus specialist medical care alone for chronic fatigue syndrome (GETSET): A pragmatic randomised controlled trial. *Lancet* **2017**, *390*, 363–373. [CrossRef]
22. Pinxsterhuis, I.; Sandvik, L.; Strand, E.B.; Bautz-Holter, E.; Sveen, U. Effectiveness of a group-based self-management program for people with chronic fatigue syndrome: A randomised controlled trial. *Clin. Rehabil.* **2016**, *31*, 93–103. [CrossRef]
23. Wiborg, J.F.; Van Bussel, J.; Van Dijk, A.; Bleijenberg, G.; Knoop, H. Randomised Controlled Trial of Cognitive Behaviour Therapy Delivered in Groups of Patients with Chronic Fatigue Syndrome. *Psychother. Psychosom.* **2015**, *84*, 368–376. [CrossRef]
24. Burgess, M.; Andiappan, M.; Chalder, T. Cognitive Behaviour Therapy for Chronic Fatigue Syndrome in Adults: Face to Face versus Telephone Treatment—A Randomized Controlled Trial. *Behav. Cogn. Psychother.* **2011**, *40*, 175–191. [CrossRef]
25. Tummers, M.; Knoop, H.; Bleijenberg, G. Effectiveness of stepped care for chronic fatigue syndrome: A randomized noninferiority trial. *J. Consult. Clin. Psychol.* **2010**, *78*, 724–731. [CrossRef]
26. Wearden, A.; Dowrick, C.; Chew-Graham, C.; Bentall, R.P.; Morriss, R.K.; Peters, S.; Riste, L.; Richardson, G.; Lovell, K.; Dunn, G.; et al. Nurse led, home based self help treatment for patients in primary care with chronic fatigue syndrome: Randomised controlled trial. *BMJ* **2010**, *340*, c1777. [CrossRef]
27. Hobday, R.A.; Thomas, S.; O'Donovan, A.; Murphy, M.; Pinching, A.J. Dietary intervention in chronic fatigue syndrome. *J. Hum. Nutr. Diet.* **2008**, *21*, 141–149. [CrossRef]
28. Stulemeijer, M.; Jong, L.W.A.M.D.; Fiselier, T.J.W.; Hoogveld, S.W.B.; Bleijenberg, G. Cognitive behaviour therapy for adolescents with chronic fatigue syndrome: Randomised controlled trial. *BMJ* **2004**, *330*, 14. [CrossRef]
29. Powell, P.; Bentall, R.P.; Nye, F.J.; Edwards, R.H.T. Randomised controlled trial of patient education to encourage graded exercise in chronic fatigue syndrome. *BMJ* **2001**, *322*, 387. [CrossRef]
30. Tummers, M.; Knoop, H.; Van Dam, A.; Bleijenberg, G. Implementing a minimal intervention for chronic fatigue syndrome in a mental health centre: A randomized controlled trial. *Psychol. Med.* **2012**, *42*, 2205–2215. [CrossRef]
31. Walach, H.; Bösch, H.; Lewith, G.; Naumann, J.; Schwarzer, B.; Falk, S.; Kohls, N.; Haraldsson, E.; Wiesendanger, H.; Nordmann, A.; et al. Effectiveness of Distant Healing for Patients with Chronic Fatigue Syndrome: A Randomised Controlled Partially Blinded Trial (EUHEALS). *Psychother. Psychosom.* **2008**, *77*, 158–166. [CrossRef]
32. Montoya, J.G.; Anderson, J.N.; Adolphs, D.L.; Bateman, L.; Klimas, N.; Levine, S.M.; Garvert, D.W.; Kaiser, J.D. KPAX002 as a treatment for Myalgic Encephalomyelitis/Chronic Fatigue Syndrome (ME/CFS): A prospective, randomized trial. *Int. J. Clin. Exp. Med.* **2018**, *11*, 2890–2900.
33. Blockmans, D.; Persoons, P.; Van Houdenhove, B.; Bobbaers, H. Does Methylphenidate Reduce the Symptoms of Chronic Fatigue Syndrome? *Am. J. Med.* **2006**, *119*, 167.e23–167.e30. [CrossRef] [PubMed]

34. Janse, A.; Worm-Smeitink, M.; Bleijenberg, G.; Donders, R.; Knoop, H. Efficacy of web-based cognitive–behavioural therapy for chronic fatigue syndrome: Randomised controlled trial. *Br. J. Psychiatry* **2018**, *212*, 112–118. [CrossRef]
35. Roerink, M.E.; Bredie, S.J.; Heijnen, M.; Dinarello, C.A.; Knoop, H.; Van Der Meer, J.W. Cytokine Inhibition in Patients With Chronic Fatigue Syndrome. *Ann. Intern. Med.* **2017**, *166*, 557. [CrossRef] [PubMed]
36. Nijhof, S.L.; Bleijenberg, G.; Uiterwaal, C.S.P.M.; Kimpen, J.L.L.; Van De Putte, E.M. Effectiveness of internet-based cognitive behavioural treatment for adolescents with chronic fatigue syndrome (FITNET): A randomised controlled trial. *Lancet* **2012**, *379*, 1412–1418. [CrossRef]
37. The, G.K.H.; Bleijenberg, G.; Buitelaar, J.K.; Van Der Meer, J.W.M. The Effect of Ondansetron, a 5-HT 3 Receptor Antagonist, in Chronic Fatigue Syndrome. *J. Clin. Psychiatry* **2010**, *71*, 528–533. [CrossRef] [PubMed]
38. The, G.K.H.; Bleijenberg, G.; Van Der Meer, J.W.M. The Effect of Acclydine in Chronic Fatigue Syndrome: A Randomized Controlled Trial. *PLoS Clin. Trials* **2007**, *2*, e19. [CrossRef]
39. Brouwers, F.; Van Der Werf, S.; Bleijenberg, G.; Van Der Zee, L.; Van Der Meer, J. The effect of a polynutrient supplement on fatigue and physical activity of patients with chronic fatigue syndrome: A double-blind randomized controlled trial. *QJM Int. J. Med.* **2002**, *95*, 677–683. [CrossRef]
40. Prins, J.B.; Bleijenberg, G.; Bazelmans, E.; Elving, L.D.; De Boo, T.M.; Severens, J.L.; Krabbenborg, L.; Spinhoven, P.; Van Der Meer, J.W. Cognitive behaviour therapy for chronic fatigue syndrome: A multicentre randomised controlled trial. *Lancet* **2001**, *357*, 841–847. [CrossRef]
41. Joung, J.-Y.; Lee, J.-S.; Cho, J.-H.; Lee, D.-S.; Ahn, Y.-C.; Son, C.-G. The Efficacy and Safety of Myelophil, an Ethanol Extract Mixture of Astragali Radix and Salviae Radix, for Chronic Fatigue Syndrome: A Randomized Clinical Trial. *Front. Pharmacol.* **2019**, *10*. [CrossRef]
42. Ng, S.-M.; Yiu, Y.-M. Acupuncture for chronic fatigue syndrome: A randomized, sham-controlled trial with single-blinded design. *Altern. Ther. Health Med.* **2013**, *19*, 21–26.
43. Rimes, K.A.; Wingrove, J. Mindfulness-Based Cognitive Therapy for People with Chronic Fatigue Syndrome Still Experiencing Excessive Fatigue after Cognitive Behaviour Therapy: A Pilot Randomized Study. *Clin. Psychol. Psychother.* **2011**, *20*, 107–117. [CrossRef] [PubMed]
44. Cleare, A.J.; Heap, E.; Malhi, G.S.; Wessely, S.; O'Keane, V.; Miell, J. Low-dose hydrocortisone in chronic fatigue syndrome: A randomised crossover trial. *Lancet* **1999**, *353*, 455–458. [CrossRef]
45. Wearden, A.J.; Morriss, R.K.; Mullis, R.; Strickland, P.L.; Pearson, D.J.; Appleby, L.; Campbell, I.T.; Morris, J.A. Randomised, double-blind, placebo-controlled treatment trial of fluoxetine and graded exercise for chronic fatigue syndrome. *Br. J. Psychiatry* **1998**, *172*, 485–490. [CrossRef] [PubMed]
46. McDermott, C.; Richards, S.; Thomas, P.W.; Montgomery, J.; Lewith, G. A placebo-controlled, double-blind, randomized controlled trial of a natural killer cell stimulant (BioBran MGN-3) in chronic fatigue syndrome. *QJM Int. J. Med.* **2006**, *99*, 461–468. [CrossRef] [PubMed]
47. Nilsson, M.K.L.; Zachrisson, O.; Gottfries, C.-G.; Matousek, M.; Peilot, B.; Forsmark, S.; Schuit, R.C.; Carlsson, M.L.; Kloberg, A.; Carlsson, A. A randomised controlled trial of the monoaminergic stabiliser (−)-OSU6162 in treatment of myalgic encephalomyelitis/chronic fatigue syndrome. *Acta Neuropsychiatr.* **2017**, *30*, 148–157. [CrossRef] [PubMed]
48. Moss-Morris, R.; Sharon, C.; Tobin, R.; Baldi, J.C. A Randomized Controlled Graded Exercise Trial for Chronic Fatigue Syndrome: Outcomes and Mechanisms of Change. *J. Health Psychol.* **2005**, *10*, 245–259. [CrossRef]
49. Blacker, C.V.R.; Greenwood, D.T.; Wesnes, K.A.; Wilson, R.; Woodward, C.; Howe, I.; Ali, T. Effect of Galantamine Hydrobromide in Chronic Fatigue Syndrome. *JAMA* **2004**, *292*, 1195–1204. [CrossRef]
50. Zachrisson, O.C.; Regland, B.; Jahreskog, M.; Jonsson, M.; Kron, M.; Gottfries, C.-G. Treatment with staphylococcus toxoid in fibromyalgia/chronic fatigue syndrome–a randomised controlled trial. *Eur. J. Pain* **2002**, *6*, 455–466. [CrossRef]
51. Rowe, P.C.; Calkins, H.; DeBusk, K.; McKenzie, R.; Anand, R.; Sharma, G.; Cuccherini, B.A.; Soto, N.; Hohman, P.; Snader, S.; et al. Fludrocortisone Acetate to Treat Neurally Mediated Hypotension in Chronic Fatigue Syndrome. *JAMA* **2001**, *285*, 52–59. [CrossRef]
52. Fulcher, K.Y.; White, P.D. Randomised controlled trial of graded exercise in patients with the chronic fatigue syndrome. *BMJ* **1997**, *314*, 1647. [CrossRef]

53. Park, S.B.; Kim, K.-N.; Sung, E.; Lee, S.Y.; Shin, H.C. Human Placental Extract as a Subcutaneous Injection Is Effective in Chronic Fatigue Syndrome: A Multi-Center, Double-Blind, Randomized, Placebo-Controlled Study. *Biol. Pharm. Bull.* **2016**, *39*, 674–679. [CrossRef] [PubMed]
54. Windthorst, P.; Mazurak, N.; Kuske, M.; Hipp, A.; Giel, K.E.; Enck, P.; Nieß, A.; Zipfel, S.; Teufel, M. Heart rate variability biofeedback therapy and graded exercise training in management of chronic fatigue syndrome: An exploratory pilot study. *J. Psychosom. Res.* **2017**, *93*, 6–13. [CrossRef] [PubMed]
55. Montoya, J.G.; Kogelnik, A.M.; Bhangoo, M.; Lunn, M.R.; Flamand, L.; Merrihew, L.E.; Watt, T.; Kubo, J.; Paik, J.; Desai, M. Randomized clinical trial to evaluate the efficacy and safety of valganciclovir in a subset of patients with chronic fatigue syndrome. *J. Med. Virol.* **2013**, *85*, 2101–2109. [CrossRef] [PubMed]
56. Weatherley-Jones, E.; Nicholl, J.P.; Thomas, K.J.; Parry, G.J.; McKendrick, M.W.; Green, S.T.; Stanley, P.J.; Lynch, S.P. A randomised, controlled, triple-blind trial of the efficacy of homeopathic treatment for chronic fatigue syndrome. *J. Psychosom. Res.* **2004**, *56*, 189–197. [CrossRef]
57. Ostojic, S.M.; Stojanovic, M.; Drid, P.; Hoffman, J.R.; Sekulic, D.; Zenic, N. Supplementation with Guanidinoacetic Acid in Women with Chronic Fatigue Syndrome. *Nutrients* **2016**, *8*, 72. [CrossRef]
58. Arnold, L.M.; Blom, T.J.; Welge, J.A.; Mariutto, E.; Heller, A. A Randomized, Placebo-Controlled, Double-Blinded Trial of Duloxetine in the Treatment of General Fatigue in Patients with Chronic Fatigue Syndrome. *Psychosomatics* **2015**, *56*, 242–253. [CrossRef]
59. Friedberg, F.; Adamowicz, J.L.; Caikauskaite, I.; Seva, V.; Napoli, A. Efficacy of two delivery modes of behavioral self-management in severe chronic fatigue syndrome. *Fatigue Biomed. Health Behav.* **2016**, *4*, 158–174. [CrossRef]
60. Kim, J.-E.; Seo, B.-K.; Choi, J.-B.; Kim, H.-J.; Kim, T.H.; Lee, M.-H.; Kang, K.-W.; Kim, J.-H.; Shin, K.-M.; Lee, S.H.; et al. Acupuncture for chronic fatigue syndrome and idiopathic chronic fatigue: A multicenter, nonblinded, randomized controlled trial. *Trials* **2015**, *16*, 314. [CrossRef]
61. Olson, L.G.; Ambrogetti, A.; Sutherland, D. A Pilot Randomized Controlled Trial of Dexamphetamine in Patients With Chronic Fatigue Syndrome. *J. Psychosom. Res.* **2003**, *44*, 38–43. [CrossRef]
62. Fluge, Ø.; Bruland, O.; Risa, K.; Storstein, A.; Kristoffersen, E.K.; Sapkota, D.; Næss, H.; Dahl, O.; Nyland, H.; Mella, O. Benefit from B-Lymphocyte Depletion Using the Anti-CD20 Antibody Rituximab in Chronic Fatigue Syndrome. A Double-Blind and Placebo-Controlled Study. *PLoS ONE* **2011**, *6*, e26358. [CrossRef]
63. Chalder, T.; Deary, V.; Husain, K.; Walwyn, R. Family-focused cognitive behaviour therapy versus psycho-education for chronic fatigue syndrome in 11- to 18-year-olds: A randomized controlled treatment trial. *Psychol. Med.* **2009**, *40*, 1269–1279. [CrossRef] [PubMed]
64. Forsyth, L.M.; Preuss, H.G.; MacDowell, A.L.; Chiazze, L.; Birkmayer, G.D.; Bellanti, J.A. Therapeutic effects of oral NADH on the symptoms of patients with chronic fatigue syndrome. *Ann. Allergy Asthma Immunol.* **1999**, *82*, 185–191. [CrossRef]
65. Young, J.L. Use of lisdexamfetamine dimesylate in treatment of executive functioning deficits and chronic fatigue syndrome: A double blind, placebo-controlled study. *Psychiatry Res.* **2013**, *207*, 127–133.
66. Castro-Marrero, J.; Cordero, M.D.; Segundo, M.J.; Sáez-Francàs, N.; Calvo, N.; Román-Malo, L.; Aliste, L.; De Sevilla, T.F.; Alegre, J. Does Oral Coenzyme Q10 Plus NADH Supplementation Improve Fatigue and Biochemical Parameters in Chronic Fatigue Syndrome? *Antioxid. Redox Signal.* **2015**, *22*, 679–685. [CrossRef] [PubMed]
67. Sulheim, D.; Fagermoen, E.; Winger, A.; Andersen, A.M.; Godang, K.; Müller, F.; Rowe, P.C.; Saul, J.P.; Skovlund, E.; Øie, M.G.; et al. Disease Mechanisms and Clonidine Treatment in Adolescent Chronic Fatigue Syndrome. *JAMA Pediatr.* **2014**, *168*, 351–360. [CrossRef] [PubMed]
68. Centers for Disease Control and Prevention. Treatment of ME/CFS. Available online: https://www.cdc.gov/me-cfs/treatment/index.html (accessed on 20 July 2020).
69. Schulz, K.F.; Altman, D.G.; Moher, D.; CONSORT Group. CONSORT 2010 Statement: Updated guidelines for reporting parallel group randomised trials. *BMJ* **2010**, *340*, c332. [CrossRef] [PubMed]
70. Knight, S.; Politis, J.; Garnham, C.; Scheinberg, A.; Tollit, M.A. School Functioning in Adolescents with Chronic Fatigue Syndrome. *Front. Pediatr.* **2018**, *6*, 302. [CrossRef]
71. Peng, K.-P.; Wang, S.-J. Migraine diagnosis: Screening items, instruments, and scales. *Acta Anaesthesiol. Taiwanica* **2012**, *50*, 69–73. [CrossRef]

72. Lee, Y.; Rosenblat, J.D.; Lee, J.; Carmona, N.E.; Subramaniapillai, M.; Shekotikhina, M.; Mansur, R.B.; Brietzke, E.; Lee, J.-H.; Ho, R.C.; et al. Efficacy of antidepressants on measures of workplace functioning in major depressive disorder: A systematic review. *J. Affect. Disord.* **2018**, *227*, 406–415. [CrossRef]
73. Lazor, T.; Tigelaar, L.; Pole, J.D.; De Souza, C.; Tomlinson, D.; Sung, L. Instruments to measure anxiety in children, adolescents, and young adults with cancer: A systematic review. *Support. Care Cancer* **2017**, *25*, 2921–2931. [CrossRef]
74. Hvidberg, M.F.; Brinth, L.S.; Olesen, A.V.; Petersen, K.; Ehlers, L. The Health-Related Quality of Life for Patients with Myalgic Encephalomyelitis/Chronic Fatigue Syndrome (ME/CFS). *PLoS ONE* **2015**, *10*, e0132421. [CrossRef] [PubMed]
75. Kapur, N.; Webb, R. Suicide risk in people with chronic fatigue syndrome. *Lancet* **2016**, *387*, 1596–1597. [CrossRef]
76. Hewlett, S.; Dures, E.; Almeida, C. Measures of fatigue: Bristol Rheumatoid Arthritis Fatigue Multi-Dimensional Questionnaire (BRAF MDQ), Bristol Rheumatoid Arthritis Fatigue Numerical Rating Scales (BRAF NRS) for severity, effect, and coping, Chalder Fatigue Questionnaire (CFQ), Checklist Individual Strength (CIS20R and CIS8R), Fatigue Severity Scale (FSS), Functional Assessment Chronic Illness Therapy (Fatigue) (FACIT-F), Multi-Dimensional Assessment of Fatigue (MAF), Multi-Dimensional Fatigue Inventory (MFI), Pediatric Quality Of Life (PedsQL) Multi-Dimensional Fatigue Scale, Profile of Fatigue (ProF), Short form 36 Vitality Subscale (SF-36 VT), and Visual Analog Scales (VAS). *Arthritis Care Res. (Hoboken)* **2011**, *63*, S263–S286. [CrossRef]
77. De Vries, J.; Michielsen, H.J.; Van Heck, G.L. Assessment of fatigue among working people: A comparison of six questionnaires. *Occup. Environ. Med.* **2003**, *60*, 10–15. [CrossRef]
78. Reeves, W.C.; Wagner, D.; Nisenbaum, R.; Jones, J.F.; Gurbaxani, B.M.; Solomon, L.; Papanicolaou, D.A.; Unger, E.R.; Vernon, S.D.; Heim, C. Chronic Fatigue Syndrome—A clinically empirical approach to its definition and study. *BMC Med.* **2005**, *3*, 19. [CrossRef]
79. Montoya, J.G.; Holmes, T.H.; Anderson, J.N.; Maecker, H.T.; Rosenberg-Hasson, Y.; Valencia, I.J.; Chu, L.; Younger, J.W.; Tato, C.M.; Davis, M.M. Cytokine signature associated with disease severity in chronic fatigue syndrome patients. *Proc. Natl. Acad. Sci. USA* **2017**, *114*, E7150–E7158. [CrossRef] [PubMed]
80. Cella, M.; Chalder, T. Measuring fatigue in clinical and community settings. *J. Psychosom. Res.* **2010**, *69*, 17–22. [CrossRef]
81. Murdock, K.W.; Wang, X.S.; Shi, Q.; Cleeland, C.S.; Fagundes, C.P.; Vernon, S.D. The utility of patient-reported outcome measures among patients with myalgic encephalomyelitis/chronic fatigue syndrome. *Qual. Life Res.* **2016**, *26*, 913–921. [CrossRef] [PubMed]
82. Sasusa. *PACE: The Research That Sparked a Patient Rebellion and Challenged Medicine*; Sense about Science USA: New York, NY, USA, 2016.
83. Giloteaux, L.; Goodrich, J.K.; Walters, W.A.; Levine, S.M.; Ley, R.E.; Hanson, M.R. Reduced diversity and altered composition of the gut microbiome in individuals with myalgic encephalomyelitis/chronic fatigue syndrome. *Microbiome* **2016**, *4*, 1–12. [CrossRef] [PubMed]
84. Kashi, A.A.; Davis, R.W.; Phair, R. The IDO Metabolic Trap Hypothesis for the Etiology of ME/CFS. *Diagnostics* **2019**, *9*, 82. [CrossRef] [PubMed]
85. Esfandyarpour, R.; Kashi, A.; Nemat-Gorgani, M.; Wilhelmy, J.; Davis, R.W. A nanoelectronics-blood-based diagnostic biomarker for myalgic encephalomyelitis/chronic fatigue syndrome (ME/CFS). *Proc. Natl. Acad. Sci. USA* **2019**, *116*, 10250–10257. [CrossRef] [PubMed]
86. Saha, A.K.; Schmidt, B.R.; Wilhelmy, J.; Nguyen, V.; Abugherir, A.; Do, J.K.; Nemat-Gorgani, M.; Davis, R.W.; Ramasubramanian, A.K. Red blood cell deformability is diminished in patients with Chronic Fatigue Syndrome. *Clin. Hemorheol. Microcirc.* **2019**, *71*, 113–116. [CrossRef] [PubMed]

Publisher's Note: MDPI stays neutral with regard to jurisdictional claims in published maps and institutional affiliations.

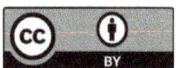

© 2020 by the authors. Licensee MDPI, Basel, Switzerland. This article is an open access article distributed under the terms and conditions of the Creative Commons Attribution (CC BY) license (http://creativecommons.org/licenses/by/4.0/).

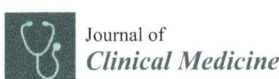

Brief Report

Male vs. Female Differences in Responding to Oxygen–Ozone Autohemotherapy (O$_2$-O$_3$-AHT) in Patients with Myalgic Encephalomyelitis/Chronic Fatigue Syndrome (ME/CFS)

Salvatore Chirumbolo [1,*], Luigi Valdenassi [2], Marianno Franzini [2], Sergio Pandolfi [2,3], Giovanni Ricevuti [2,4] and Umberto Tirelli [5]

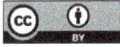

Citation: Chirumbolo, S.; Valdenassi, L.; Franzini, M.; Pandolfi, S.; Ricevuti, G.; Tirelli, U. Male vs. Female Differences in Responding to Oxygen–Ozone Autohemotherapy (O$_2$-O$_3$-AHT) in Patients with Myalgic Encephalomyelitis/Chronic Fatigue Syndrome (ME/CFS). *J. Clin. Med.* 2022, 11, 173. https://doi.org/10.3390/jcm11010173

Academic Editor: Simona Bonavita

Received: 23 November 2021
Accepted: 27 December 2021
Published: 29 December 2021

Publisher's Note: MDPI stays neutral with regard to jurisdictional claims in published maps and institutional affiliations.

Copyright: © 2021 by the authors. Licensee MDPI, Basel, Switzerland. This article is an open access article distributed under the terms and conditions of the Creative Commons Attribution (CC BY) license (https://creativecommons.org/licenses/by/4.0/).

[1] Department of Neurosciences, Biomedicine and Movement Sciences, University of Verona, 37134 Verona, Italy
[2] Italian Society of Oxygen Ozone Therapy (SIOOT), University of Pavia, 27100 Pavia, Italy; luigi.valdenassi@unipv.it (L.V.); marianno.franzini@gmail.com (M.F.); sergiopandolfis2@gmail.com (S.P.); giovanni.ricevuti@unipv.it (G.R.)
[3] Villa Mafalda Clinics, Via Monte delle Gioie 5 Rome, 00199 Roma, Italy
[4] School of Pharmacy, Department of Drug Sciences, University of Pavia, 27100 Pavia, Italy
[5] Tirelli Medical Group, 33170 Pordenone, Italy; utirelli@cro.it
* Correspondence: salvatore.chirumbolo@univr.it

Abstract: (1) Background: Myalgic Encephalomyelitis/Chronic Fatigue Syndrome (ME/CFS) is a syndrome that has fatigue as its major symptom. Evidence suggests that ozone is able to relieve ME/CFS-related fatigue in affected patients. (2) Objective: To evaluate whether differences exist between males and females in ozone therapy outputs in ME/CFS. (3) Methods: In total, 200 patients previously diagnosed with ME/CFS (mean age 33 ± 13 SD years) underwent treatment with oxygen–ozone autohemotherapy (O$_2$-O$_3$-AHT). Fatigue was investigated via an FSS 7-scoring questionnaire before and following 1 month after treatment. (4) Results: The Mann-Whitney test (MW test) assessed the significance of this difference (H = 13.8041, p = 0.0002), and female patients showed better outcomes than males. This difference was particularly striking in the youngest age cohort (14–29 years), and a KW test resulted in H = 7.1609, p = 0.007 for the Δ = 28.3% (males = 3.8, females = 5.3). (5) Conclusions: When treated with O$_2$-O$_3$-AHT, females respond better than males.

Keywords: ME/CFS; ozone; oxygen–ozone therapy; fatigue; clinical trial

1. The Myalgic Encephalomyelitis/Chronic Fatigue Syndrome (ME/CFS) Challenge

Myalgic encephalomyelitis/chronic fatigue syndrome (ME/CFS) is a complex pathology, and was recently reviewed in [1]. ME/CFS must be considered a serious and long-term syndrome, which is characterized by fatigue and debilitating muscular–skeletal pain, conditions that affect many fundamental aspects of people's social habits [2–4]. Fatigue is a major symptom in ME/CFS and its treatment is accounted for in many forerunners in Italy [5–16]. Tirelli et al. performed a study with 82 CFS patients living in northern Italy, showing that early symptoms occur between 24 and 40 years and that ME/CFS is primarily (3:1) observed in female subjects [15]. However, ME/CFS diagnosis is particularly burdensome, as patients with fatigue and other clinical signs are more often misdiagnosed with other chronic illnesses [17,18]; this is despite official diagnostic criteria for ME/CFS from the Centers for Disease Control and Prevention, the so-called IOM 2015 Diagnostic Criteria, having been updated in the CDC's 1994 guidelines, which can be consulted elsewhere [19]. Fatigue is the leading symptom of ME/CFS, alongside other physical symptoms, such as headaches, tender lymph nodes, sore throat, poor sleep, poor concentration, reduced attention or memory, post-exertional malaise, muscular–skeletal pain and polyarthralgia, [20–23]. The diagnosis of ME/CFS therefore almost entirely based on fatigue-related symptoms [24,25].

The burdensome task to achieve a proper and sound diagnosis affects the therapeutic approach [26], despite some commendable attempts [5,7,11]; however, ME/CFS remains a considerable concern for clinics. Promising attempts in treating ME/CFS fatigue with oxygen–ozone autohemotherapy (O_2-O_3-AHT) were successfully performed by our group and others [27–29]. O_2-O_3-AHT may affect many complex issues in terms of immunity, most of which characterize the pathogenetic mechanisms causing ME/CFS [30,31]. Interestingly, ME/CFS might also have an oxidative stress causative pathogenesis [32,33]. This evidence, linked to the increasing awareness that ozone is able to regulate inflammation by targeting the oxidative stress signaling [32], thus suggesting several encouraging pieces of evidence for ME/CFS diagnoses [27], compelled us to treat fatigue in patients with O_2-O_3-AHT and investigate whether therapy outputs showed differences between male and female patients.

2. Materials and Methods

2.1. Patient Recruitment

In total, 224 outpatients (mean age from the clinical centers of Pordenone and Gorle (Bergamo) were enrolled, having met the eligibility criteria agreed for the present study. Male mean age was 32.04 ± 18.45 SD and female mean age was 29.65 ± 11.54 SD ($p = 0.354$, in a Wilcoxon test). Of these patients, 200 entered the study; 19 escaped the study design because they referred to other therapy centers and were excluded. Five were formally accepted but never started for family and private reasons. Mean age was 33.08 ± 13.50 SD years [CI_{95} = 31.20–34.97], and median age was 33.14 years, comprising 69 men (34.5%) and 131 women. All patients were made aware of the therapy protocol and the use of the data for research purposes, according the recommendations of the Declaration of Helsinki.

2.2. Inclusion and Exclusion Criteria

Inclusion criteria were represented by outpatients referred to our clinical healthcare who were previously diagnosed with ME/CFS [23,34] and suffering from fatigue. These patients accepted and signed the informed consent for therapy and allowed for their data to be shared for research purposes. Exclusion criteria were represented by patients without ME/CFS, with other chronic and inflammation diseases, such as tumors or other immunological disorders and those who had taken pharmaceutical drugs in the previous 72 h; other exclusion criteria were those with chronic inflammatory and immune ailments such as autoimmunity, cancer or chronic inflammatory illness and pregnancy.

2.3. Sample Size

Sample size was calculated to achieve an error range of about 10%. Referring to a population proportion of 51%, forecast data resulted in a 13.86% error with 50 patients, whereas there was an error of 9.80% (<10%) with 103 patients; therefore, 200 patients were within the minimal sample size with $p < 0.001$. The Cohen d statistics for the two independent groups, i.e., before O_2-O_3-AHT and following O_2-O_3-AHT, were successfully implemented ($p = 0.004323$ or Hedges' g value). Moreover, Glass' delta was $p = 0.012444$ ($p < 0.02$).

2.4. Patient Evaluation of Fatigue Symptomatology

An anamnestic interview and complete visitation of about 20–30 min were performed. Fatigue was the major symptom evaluated in the study as it was able to highlight patients' overall clinical status in the most sound and reliable manner; this is due to its optimal performance features, stability over time and scant possibility of being overshadowed by other minor symptoms. Each patient was asked to respond to a 7-point scoring system, the Fatigue Severity Scale (FSS), before undergoing therapy and one month following therapy [35,36]. Results were collected as scores and statistically evaluated.

2.5. Patients' Treatment with Oxygen–Ozone Autohemotherapy (O_2-O_3-AHT)

Patients underwent no fewer than two weekly sessions of major oxygen–ozone autohemotherapy, according to the protocol previously assessed by the Italian Society of Oxygen–Ozone Therapy (SIOOT) [27]. Briefly speaking, each patient underwent a treatment option requiring an ozone generator, compressed oxygen as a medical grade, a venipuncture syringe and a certified bag with an intravenous cannula for ozone therapy via autohemotherapy. A maximal volume of 200 mL of blood was usually withdrawn from each patient and collected in a CE-certified SANO3 bag, with automatic gentle mixing then immediately treated with 45 µg/mL of an O_3 mixture in O_2 (Multioxygen Medical 95 CPS, Gorle, Italy). This was finally reintroduced into the circulatory blood directly and within a few minutes [27,37]. Patients were followed up after 30 days following the second O_2-O_3-AHT session, and were asked to complete the FSS questionnaire, as previously agreed.

2.6. Statistics

Data were collected and expressed as mean ± standard deviation, for quantitative values. Sample size was evaluated by assessing data and forecasting evaluations with Cohen d statistics and a Glass' delta. Statistical inference, if any, was evaluated following non-parametric tests. Scores were evaluated by a Mann–Whitney test for two independent groups, with $p < 0.05$. Data were elaborated with SPSS v 24 software and Stata software for graphs.

3. Results

Figure 1 shows the difference (DELTA) in FSS score between female patients and male patients undergoing O_2-O_3-AHT. The average score was 5.14 ± 1.18 SD for females (CI_{95} = 4.865–5.4209) and 4.03 ± 1.80 SD for males (CI_{95} = 3.606–4.450) (mode: 6 and 5, respectively, median 5.5 and 5.0, respectively). The Mann–Whitney (MW) test assessed the significance at $p < 0.05$ of this difference ($p = 0.0001$), and female patients showed a better outcome than males. This difference was particularly striking in the youngest age cohort (14–29 years), as the MW test resulted in a $p = 0.006$ for the Δ = 28.3% (males = 3.8, females = 5.3). By arranging age groups into three clusters, i.e., 14–29 years, 30–49 years and $\geq$50, no difference in FSS score was reported for either females or males. Due to it having the highest heterogeneity in FSS response, the male group (see Figure 1), i.e., the MW test in the male age clusters, lacked statistical significance ($p = 0.76$). The O_2-O_3-AHT works optimally in an independent way with respect to elderly subjects of those of different ages.

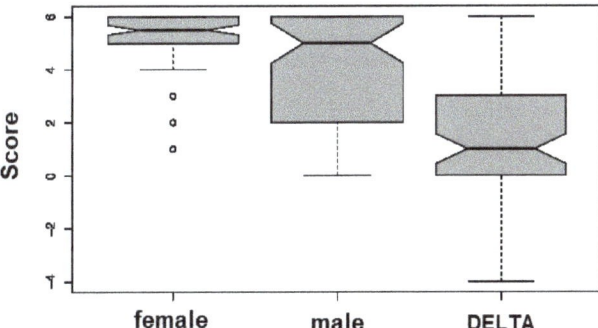

Figure 1. Box plot representation of the FSS differential response between male and female patients with ME/CFS treated with O_2-O_3-AHT.

4. Discussion

Our results suggest that O_2-O_3-AHT is able to relieve fatigue in almost half of the whole cohort of ME/CFS patients. Female patients showed a higher ability, particularly during youth (14–29 years), to respond to O_2-O_3-AHT than males. Age clusters did not significantly affect the influence of O_2-O_3-AHT on both sexes. Thus far, no sound explanation can be attained to explain why female patients show better outcomes with O_2-O_3-AHT. This fact might be explained by the different endocrine endowment in males compared to females, at least in terms of ER receptors and their effect on T cell activation and NK cell functional activity [11]. The modulation of immunity may be a sound solution to counter ME/CFS fatigue, and ozone may be a possible approach [5,6,27]. We are therefore unable to fully elucidate how ozone can restore wellness in patients suffering from ME/CFS-related fatigue [27]. Cell biology should suggest that, in ME/CFS mitochondria, activity is greatly disturbed, generating an impairment in fundamental mitochondria-related activities, such as ROS signaling [38], leading to inflammation disorders [39,40]. During ME/CFS, an increase in $CD4^+CD25^+Foxp3^+$ T regulatory (Treg) cells occurs [41], a circumstance that may be modulated by ozone [42]. ME/CFS pathogenesis involves the impairment of Th17 cells. The $CCR6^+$ Th17 cells in ME/CFS secrete less IL-17 with respect to healthy subjects; moreover, their cell frequency in blood is lower and ozone can restore their numbers [43,44]. The immune micro-environment in ME/CFS is therefore fundamental for proper therapy [9–11]. Furthermore, 4-hydroxynonenal (4-HNE) induces the thioredoxin reductase 1 via Nrf2 signaling, and then increases the level of Tregs [45,46]. The ability of ozone to modulate immunity and inflammation via the Nrf2 system is particularly well noted [32]. Ozone may regulate nitric oxide (NO) and eNOS [32]. That said, ME/CFS patients should have normal NO alongside normal IL-6 levels, both before and after physical exercise upon fatigue symptoms, but should also show high levels of F2-isoprostanes, i.e., oxidative stress biomarkers, which are probably quenched by the activity of ozone on the Nrf2/Keap1/ARE system [47–49].

The ability of O_2-O_3-AHT to elicit a greater response in females than males may involve ER-beta signaling on T reg biology [50], and may signal the possible involvement of Nrf2 signaling, as elicited by O_2-O_3-AHT. This represents another issue that should be investigated in future studies [51,52].

5. Conclusions

Patients suffering from ME/CFS fatigue and being treated with O_2-O_3-AHT experience rapid relief of their symptoms. Female subjects are able to respond to O_2-O_3-AHT and reduce fatigue symptoms better than males. Further insights are needed to elucidate the mechanism by which these differences occur.

Author Contributions: Conceptualization, U.T. and S.C.; methodology, U.T., M.F., L.V. and S.C.; software, S.C.; validation, U.T., G.R. and S.C.; formal analysis, S.C. and S.P.; investigation, U.T. and M.F.; resources, U.T., M.F. and L.V.; data curation, S.C. and S.P.; writing—original draft preparation, S.C.; writing—review and editing, U.T., S.C. and S.P.; visualization, U.T.; supervision, U.T., M.F., L.V., S.P., G.R. and S.C.; project administration, U.T.; funding acquisition, M.F. and L.V. All authors have read and agreed to the published version of the manuscript.

Funding: This research was funded by SIOOT, Gorle (BG).

Institutional Review Board Statement: The study was conducted according to the guidelines of the Declaration of Helsinki and approved by the Institutional Review Board of the Tirelli Clinical Group (code TIR18APR).

Informed Consent Statement: Informed consent was obtained from all subjects involved in the study. All subjects were outpatients of our healthcare institution, and made their own decisions and were aware of the purpose of undergoing treatment with oxygen–ozone, which is not an experimental therapy. Therefore, patients were simply asked to agree and sign a consent form to use their data for research purposes. All subjects gave their informed consent for optional inclusion in the research before they participated in the study, which was conducted in accordance with the Declaration of Helsinki.

Data Availability Statement: Data repository can be requested to the Prof Umberto Tirelli, at your disposal and to Prof M Franzini at SIOOT (Bergamo).

Acknowledgments: A special thank to all the caregivers and health personnel involved in the management of the study.

Conflicts of Interest: The authors declare no conflict of interest.

References

1. Deumer, U.S.; Varesi, A.; Floris, V.; Savioli, G.; Mantovani, E.; López-Carrasco, P.; Rosati, G.M.; Prasad, S.; Ricevuti, G. Myalgic Encephalomyelitis/Chronic Fatigue Syndrome (ME/CFS): An Overview. *J. Clin. Med.* **2021**, *10*, 4786. [CrossRef]
2. Barhorst, E.E.; Boruch, A.E.; Cook, D.B.; Lindheimer, J.B. Pain-related post-exertional malaise in Myalgic Encephalomyelitis/Chronic Fatigue Syndrome (ME/CFS) and Fibromyalgia: A systematic review and three-level meta-analysis. *Pain Med.* **2021**, pnab308. [CrossRef]
3. Noor, N.; Urits, I.; Degueure, A.; Rando, L.; Kata, V.; Cornett, E.M.; Kaye, A.D.; Imani, F.; Narimani-Zamanabadi, M.; Varrassi, G.; et al. A Comprehensive Update of the Current Understanding of Chronic Fatigue Syndrome. *Anesth. Pain Med.* **2021**, *11*, e113629. [CrossRef] [PubMed]
4. Lim, E.J.; Son, C.G. Prevalence of Chronic Fatigue Syndrome (CFS) in Korea and Japan: A Meta-Analysis. *J. Clin. Med.* **2021**, *10*, 3204. [CrossRef] [PubMed]
5. Tirelli, U.; Lleshi, A.; Berretta, M.; Spina, M.; Talamini, R.; Giacalone, A. Treatment of 741 Italian patients with chronic fatigue syndrome. *Eur. Rev. Med. Pharmacol. Sci.* **2013**, *17*, 2847–2852. [PubMed]
6. Tirelli, U.; Cirrito, C.; Pavanello, M.; Del Pup, L.; Lleshi, A.; Berretta, M. Oxygen-ozone therapy as support and palliative therapy in 50 cancer patients with fatigue—A short report. *Eur. Rev. Med. Pharmacol. Sci.* **2018**, *22*, 8030–8033.
7. Arpino, C.; Carrieri, M.P.; Valesini, G.; Pizzigallo, E.; Rovere, P.; Tirelli, U.; Conti, F.; Dialmi, P.; Barberio, A.; Rusconi, N.; et al. Idiopathic chronic fatigue and chronic fatigue syndrome: A comparison of two case-definitions. *Ann. Ist. Super. Sanita* **1999**, *35*, 435–441. [PubMed]
8. Tirelli, U.; Chierichetti, F.; Tavio, M.; Simonelli, C.; Bianchin, G.; Zanco, P.; Ferlin, G. Brain positron emission tomography (PET) in chronic fatigue syndrome: Preliminary data. *Am. J. Med.* **1998**, *105*, 54S–58S. [CrossRef]
9. Montoya, J.G.; Holmes, T.H.; Anderson, J.N.; Maecker, H.T.; Rosenberg-Hasson, Y.; Valencia, I.J.; Chu, L.; Younger, J.W.; Tato, C.M.; Davis, M.M. Cytokine signature associated with disease severity in chronic fatigue syndrome patients. *Proc. Natl. Acad. Sci. USA* **2017**, *114*, E7150–E7158. [CrossRef]
10. Tirelli, U.; Marotta, G.; Improta, S.; Pinto, A. Immunological abnormalities in patients with chronic fatigue syndrome. *Scand. J. Immunol.* **1994**, *40*, 601–608. [CrossRef]
11. Tirelli, V.; Pinto, A.; Marotta, G.; Crovato, M.; Quaia, M.; De Paoli, P.; Galligioni, E.; Santini, G. Clinical and immunologic study of 205 patients with chronic fatigue syndrome: A case series from Italy. *Arch. Intern. Med.* **1993**, *153*, 116–120. [CrossRef]
12. Estévez-López, F.; Mudie, K.; Wang-Steverding, X.; Bakken, I.J.; Ivanovs, A.; Castro-Marrero, J.; Nacul, L.; Alegre, J.; Zalewski, P.; Słomko, J.; et al. Systematic Review of the Epidemiological Burden of Myalgic Encephalomyelitis/Chronic Fatigue Syndrome Across Europe: Current Evidence and EUROMENE Research Recommendations for Epidemiology. *J. Clin. Med.* **2020**, *9*, 1557. [CrossRef]
13. Vincent, A.; Brimmer, D.J.; Whipple, M.O.; Jones, J.F.; Boneva, R.; Lahr, B.D.; Maloney, E.; St Sauver, J.L.; Reeves, W.C. Prevalence, incidence, and classification of chronic fatigue syndrome in Olmsted County, Minnesota, as estimated using the Rochester Epidemiology Project. *Mayo Clin. Proc.* **2012**, *87*, 1145–1152. [CrossRef]
14. Lim, E.J.; Ahn, Y.C.; Jang, E.S.; Lee, S.W.; Lee, S.H.; Son, C.G. Systematic review and meta-analysis of the prevalence of chronic fatigue syndrome/myalgic encephalomyelitis (CFS/ME). *J. Transl. Med.* **2020**, *18*, 100. [CrossRef] [PubMed]
15. Capelli, E.; Lorusso, L.; Ghitti, M.; Venturini, L.; Cusa, C.; Ricevuti, G. Chronic fatigue syndrome: Features of a population of patients from northern Italy. *Int. J. Immunopathol. Pharmacol.* **2015**, *28*, 53–59. [CrossRef]
16. Spazzapan, S.; Bearz, A.; Tirelli, U. Fatigue in cancer patients receiving chemotherapy. An analysis of published studies. *Ann. Oncol.* **2004**, *15*, 1576. [PubMed]
17. Solomon, L.; Reeves, W.C. Factors influencing the diagnosis of chronic fatigue syndrome. *Arch. Intern. Med.* **2004**, *164*, 2241–2245. [CrossRef] [PubMed]
18. Brenna, E.; Araja, D.; Pheby, D.F.H. Comparative Survey of People with ME/CFS in Italy, Latvia, and the UK: A Report on Behalf of the Socioeconomics Working Group of the European ME/CFS Research Network (EUROMENE). *Medicina* **2021**, *57*, 300. [CrossRef]
19. Kennedy, G.; Abbot, N.C.; Spence, V.; Underwood, C.; Belch, J.J. The specificity of the CDC-1994 criteria for chronic fatigue syndrome: Comparison of health status in three groups of patients who fulfill the criteria. *Ann. Epidemiol.* **2004**, *14*, 95–100. [CrossRef]
20. Kuratsune, H. Diagnosis and Treatment of Myalgic Encephalomyelitis/Chronic Fatigue Syndrome. *Brain Nerve* **2018**, *70*, 11–18.
21. Carruthers, B.M.; van de Sande, M.I.; De Meirleir, K.L.; Klimas, N.G.; Broderick, G.; Mitchell, T.; Staines, D.; Powles, A.C.; Speight, N.; Vallings, R.; et al. Myalgic encephalomyelitis: International Consensus Criteria. *J. Intern. Med.* **2011**, *270*, 327–338. [CrossRef]

22. Bruun Wyller, V.; Bjørneklett, A.; Brubakk, O.; Festvåg, L.; Follestad, I.; Malt, U.; Malterud, K.; Nyland, H.; Rambøl, H.; Stubhaug, B.; et al. *Diagnosis and Treatment of Chronic Fatigue Syndrome/Myalgic Encephalopathy (CFS/ME)*; Report from Norwegian Knowledge Centre for the Health Services (NOKC) No. 09-2006; Knowledge Centre for the Health Services at The Norwegian Institute of Public Health (NIPH): Oslo, Norway, 2006.
23. Chew-Graham, C.; Dowrick, C.; Wearden, A.; Richardson, V.; Peters, S. Making the diagnosis of Chronic Fatigue Syndrome/Myalgic Encephalitis in primary care: A qualitative study. *BMC Fam. Pract.* **2010**, *11*, 16. [CrossRef]
24. Son, C.G. Differential diagnosis between "chronic fatigue" and "chronic fatigue syndrome". *Integr. Med. Res.* **2019**, *8*, 89–91. [CrossRef] [PubMed]
25. Nelsen, D.A., Jr. Differential diagnosis for chronic fatigue syndrome. *Am. Fam. Physician* **2003**, *67*, 252, author reply 252.
26. Craig, T.; Kakumanu, S. Chronic fatigue syndrome: Evaluation and treatment. *Am. Fam. Physician* **2002**, *65*, 1083–1089. [PubMed]
27. Tirelli, U.; Cirrito, C.; Pavanello, M. Ozone therapy is an effective therapy in chronic fatigue syndrome: Result of an Italian study in 65 patients. *Ozon Ther.* **2018**, *3*, 27–30. [CrossRef]
28. Morelli, L.; Bramani, S.C.; Morelli, F.C. Oxygen-ozone therapy in meningoencephalitis and chronic fatigue syndrome. Treatment in the field of competitive sports: Case report. *Ozone Ther.* **2019**, *4*, 20–23. [CrossRef]
29. Borrelli, E.; Bocci, V. A novel therapeutic option for Chronic Fatigue Syndrome and Fibromyalgia. *Rivista Ital. Ossig-Ozonoterap.* **2002**, *1*, 149–153.
30. Viebahn-Haensler, R.; León Fernández, O.S. Ozone in Medicine. The Low-Dose Ozone Concept and Its Basic Biochemical Mechanisms of Action in Chronic Inflammatory Diseases. *Int. J. Mol. Sci.* **2021**, *22*, 7890. [CrossRef]
31. Bjørklund, G.; Dadar, M.; Pivina, L.; Doşa, M.D.; Semenova, Y.; Maes, M. Environmental, Neuro-immune, and Neuro-oxidative Stress Interactions in Chronic Fatigue Syndrome. *Mol. Neurobiol.* **2020**, *57*, 4598–4607. [CrossRef]
32. Chirumbolo, S.; Valdenassi, L.; Simonetti, V.; Bertossi, D.; Ricevuti, G.; Franzini, M.; Pandolfi, S. Insights on the mechanisms of action of ozone in the medical therapy against COVID-19. *Int. Immunopharmacol.* **2021**, *96*, 107777. [CrossRef]
33. Paul, B.D.; Lemle, M.D.; Komaroff, A.L.; Snyder, S.H. Redox imbalance links COVID-19 and myalgic encephalomyelitis/chronic fatigue syndrome. *Proc. Natl. Acad. Sci. USA* **2021**, *118*, e2024358118. [CrossRef] [PubMed]
34. Baker, R.; Shaw, E.J. Diagnosis and management of chronic fatigue syndrome or myalgic encephalomyelitis (or encephalopathy): Summary of NICE guidance. *BMJ* **2007**, *335*, 446–448. [CrossRef]
35. Neuberger, G.B. Measures of fatigue in Arthritis and Rheumatisms. *Arthr. Care Res.* **2003**, *48*, S175–S183. [CrossRef]
36. Tirelli, U.; Franzini, M.; Valdenassi, L.; Pisconti, S.; Taibi, R.; Torrisi, C.; Pandolfi, S.; Chirumbolo, S. Fatigue in post-acute sequelae of SARS-CoV2 (PASC) treated with oxygen-ozone autohemotherapy-Preliminary results on 100 patients. *Eur. Rev. Med. Pharmacol. Sci.* **2021**, *25*, 5871–5875. [PubMed]
37. Lvis, A.M.; Ekta, J.S. Ozone therapy: A clinical review. *J. Nat. Sci. Biol. Med.* **2011**, *2*, 66–70.
38. Anderson, G.; Maes, M. Mitochondria and immunity in chronic fatigue syndrome. *Prog. Neuro-Psychopharmacol. Biol. Psychiatry* **2020**, *103*, 109976. [CrossRef]
39. Maes, M.; Twisk, F.N.; Kubera, M.; Ringel, K. Evidence for inflammation and activation of cell-mediated immunity in Myalgic Encephalomyelitis/Chronic Fatigue Syndrome (ME/CFS): Increased interleukin-1, tumor necrosis factor-α, PMN-elastase, lysozyme and neopterin. *J. Affect. Disord.* **2012**, *136*, 933–939. [CrossRef] [PubMed]
40. Maes, M.; Twisk, F.N.; Ringel, K. Inflammatory and cell-mediated immune biomarkers in myalgic encephalomyelitis/chronic fatigue syndrome and depression: Inflammatory markers are higher in myalgic encephalomyelitis/chronic fatigue syndrome than in depression. *Psychother. Psychosom.* **2012**, *81*, 286–295. [CrossRef]
41. Brenu, E.W.; Huth, T.K.; Hardcastle, S.L.; Fuller, K.; Kaur, M.; Johnston, S.; Ramos, S.B.; Staines, D.R.; Marshall-Gradisnik, S.M. Role of adaptive and innate immune cells in chronic fatigue syndrome/myalgic encephalomyelitis. *Int. Immunol.* **2014**, *26*, 233–242. [CrossRef] [PubMed]
42. Wei, M.; Tu, L.; Liang, Y.H.; Liu, J.; Gong, Y.J.; Zhang, J.H.; Zhang, Y.H. Effects of ozone exposure on percentage of CD4(+)CD25(high)Foxp3(+) regulatory T cells and mRNA expression of Foxp3 in asthmatic rats. *Zhonghua Lao Dong Wei Sheng Zhi Ye Bing Za Zhi* **2013**, *31*, 693–696.
43. Broderick, G.; Fuite, J.; Kreitz, A.; Vernon, S.D.; Klimas, N.; Fletcher, M.A. A formal analysis of cytokine networks in chronic fatigue syndrome. *Brain Behav. Immun.* **2010**, *24*, 1209–1217. [CrossRef]
44. Izadi, M.; Tahmasebi, S.; Pustokhina, I.; Yumashev, A.V.; Lakzaei, T.; Alvanegh, A.G.; Roshangar, L.; Dadashpour, M.; Yousefi, M.; Ahmadi, M. Changes in Th17 cells frequency and function after ozone therapy used to treat multiple sclerosis patients. *Mult. Scler. Relat. Disord.* **2020**, *46*, 102466. [CrossRef] [PubMed]
45. Chen, Z.H.; Saito, Y.; Yoshida, Y.; Sekine, A.; Noguchi, N.; Niki, E. 4-Hydroxynonenal induces adaptive response and enhances PC12 cell tolerance primarily through induction of thioredoxin reductase 1 via activation of Nrf2. *J. Biol. Chem.* **2005**, *280*, 41921–41927. [CrossRef]
46. Wang, X.; Dong, H.; Li, Q.; Li, Y.; Hong, A. Thioredoxin induces Tregs to generate an immunotolerant tumor microenvironment in metastatic melanoma. *Oncoimmunology* **2015**, *4*, e1027471. [CrossRef]
47. Meeus, M.; Van Eupen, I.; Hondequin, J.; De Hauwere, L.; Kos, D.; Nijs, J. Nitric oxide concentrations are normal and unrelated to activity level in chronic fatigue syndrome: A case-control study. *In Vivo* **2010**, *24*, 865–869.

48. Robinson, M.; Gray, S.R.; Watson, M.S.; Kennedy, G.; Hill, A.; Belch, J.J.; Nimmo, M.A. Plasma IL-6, its soluble receptors and F2-isoprostanes at rest and during exercise in chronic fatigue syndrome. *Scand. J. Med. Sci. Sports* **2010**, *20*, 282–290. [CrossRef] [PubMed]
49. Milne, G.L.; Musiek, E.S.; Morrow, J.D. F2-isoprostanes as markers of oxidative stress in vivo: An overview. *Biomarkers* **2005**, *10* (Suppl. S1), S10–S23. [CrossRef] [PubMed]
50. Goodman, W.A.; Bedoyan, S.M.; Havran, H.L.; Richardson, B.; Cameron, M.J.; Pizarro, T.T. Impaired estrogen signaling underlies regulatory T cell loss-of-function in the chronically inflamed intestine. *Proc. Natl. Acad. Sci. USA* **2020**, *117*, 17166–17176. [CrossRef]
51. Gräns, H.; Nilsson, M.; Dahlman-Wright, K.; Evengård, B. Reduced levels of oestrogen receptor beta mRNA in Swedish patients with chronic fatigue syndrome. *J. Clin. Pathol.* **2007**, *60*, 195–198. [CrossRef]
52. Ishii, T.; Warabi, E. Mechanism of Rapid Nuclear Factor-E2-Related Factor 2 (Nrf2) Activation via Membrane-Associated Estrogen Receptors: Roles of NADPH Oxidase 1, Neutral Sphingomyelinase 2 and Epidermal Growth Factor Receptor (EGFR). *Antioxidants* **2019**, *8*, 69. [CrossRef] [PubMed]

MDPI
St. Alban-Anlage 66
4052 Basel
Switzerland
Tel. +41 61 683 77 34
Fax +41 61 302 89 18
www.mdpi.com

Journal of Clinical Medicine Editorial Office
E-mail: jcm@mdpi.com
www.mdpi.com/journal/jcm

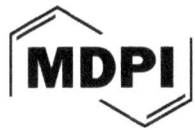